Atlas of PET-CT Imaging in Oncology

Tamer Özülker • Filiz Özülker

Atlas of PET-CT Imaging in Oncology

A Case-Based Guide to Image Interpretation

Springer

Tamer Özülker
Nuclear Medicine
Okmeydani Training and Research Hospital
Istanbul
Turkey

Filiz Özülker
Nuclear Medicine
Okmeydani Training and Research Hospital
Istanbul
Turkey

ISBN 978-3-319-36093-5   ISBN 978-3-319-18994-9 (eBook)
DOI 10.1007/978-3-319-18994-9

Springer Cham Heidelberg New York Dordrecht London

Softcover reprint of the hardcover 1st edition 2015

Printed on acid-free paper

Springer International Publishing AG Switzerland is part of Springer Science+Business Media (www.springer.com)

To our son C. Güney

Foreword

Introduction of combined PET/CT scanner at the beginning of the millennium, which means combination of functional metabolic information and anatomical data, ushered in a new epoch in the field of medicine, particularly oncology. Shortly after its emerging from academic research centers, it became an indispensable tool in oncologic imaging. As practicing nuclear medicine physicians, we realized that both radiology and nuclear medicine students and physicians facing the practice of PET/CT require a book that can help them to overcome the diagnostic dilemmas. Our book, *Atlas of PET-Imaging in Oncology-A Case-Based Guide to Image Interpretation*, presents a variety of clinical examples of studies done with ^{18}F-FDG PET/CT for the diagnosis and management of patients with malignancies. This book does not cover the whole range of positron emitters available but focuses only on the role of ^{18}F-FDG. Today, 95 % of FDG PET applications are in the field of oncology. This technology is also increasingly being utilized for clinical applications in the cardiovascular system, the central nervous system, and infection imaging, but these are outside the scope of our book. All of the cases included in this atlas have been collected from studies performed since year 2007. Part I covers the fundamentals of PET-CT imaging with FDG including physiologic distribution of ^{18}F-FDG, normal variants, benign findings, and technical artifacts. Since the main problematic of oncologic ^{18}F-FDG PET/CT studies is to distinguish benign and malignant lesions, it is of particular importance to be familiar with the normal signs and variants. For this purpose, a wide variety of normal and benign findings that an interpreter would confront while reporting PET studies, is presented in this part. Part II covers a variety of clinical applications in oncology including common indications and rare findings. Each case presentation has an identical organization including a brief history, description of findings at images, interpretation of these findings, and finally a teaching point which is often supported by relevant literature. All of the diagnosis are histopathologically verified and some of them are notified under the heading of "result."

Residents and practitioners in nuclear medicine, radiology, oncology, radiation oncology, and nuclear medicine technology will benefit a lot from this book.

Filiz Özülker
Tamer Özülker

İstanbul, Turkey

List of Editors and Contributors

Tamer Özülker, M.D.
Assoc. Prof. of Nuclear Medicine
Department of Nuclear Medicine
Okmeydani Training & Research Hospital, Darülaceze Street 25,
34384 Istanbul, Turkey
E-Mail: tozulker@gmail.com

Filiz Özülker, M.D.
Nuclear Medicine Specialist
Department of Nuclear Medicine
Okmeydani Training & Research Hospital, Darülaceze Street 25,
34384 Istanbul, Turkey
E-Mail: fozulker@gmail.com

Mehmet Tarık Tatoğlu, M.D.,
Nuclear Medicine Specialist
Department of Nuclear Medicine
Istanbul Medeniyet University, Goztepe Training and Research Hospital
Merdivenkoy Polyclinics, Ressam Salih Ermez Street,
34722 Kadikoy, İstanbul, Turkey
E-Mail: tariktatoglu@gmail.com

Introduction

Background

Molecular imaging emerged by the beginning of 1990s and ^{18}fluorine-fluorodeoxyglucose (^{18}F-FDG) positron emission tomography (PET) scan has become unquestionably one of the most amazing methods in this field, with its great impact on clinical management of the diseases.

Following the discovery of positron emission from radioactive nuclei in 1933, coincidence detection techniques with positron emitters were first used for localization of brain tumors in 1951.

In 1924, Otto Warburg, a German biochemist, observed that cancer cells use glucose as their primary energy substrate and produce lactic acid as its by-product. The increased glycolysis in cancer cells even in the presence of oxygen was named as Warburg effect. Energy requirements of dividing tumor cell increases and this gives rise to an increase in the number of transmembrane GLUT transporters that facilitate glucose transport into the cell. Hexokinase activity in the tumor cell is also elevated which in turn results in increased rate of phosphorylation. All of these facts result in a net effect of significant increase in glucose metabolism in tumor cells, and this has been exploited clinically by ^{18}F-FDG PET scanning. FDG is a glucose analog labeled to the fluorine-18 which is a radioactive positron emitter. The first radiosynthesis of ^{18}F-FDG was achieved in 1976 and afterwards it became the key radiopharmaceutical of PET studies. At the present time, more than 95 % of PET procedures all around the world are performed with ^{18}F-FDG.

FDG, similarly to glucose, is transported into the normal or malignant cells via facilitated transport by using GLUT transport proteins. Once FDG is internalized into the cell, it is converted to FDG-6-phosphate intracellularly by hexokinase, but unlike glucose it does not undergo significant enzymatic reactions and remains trapped in tissue because of the negative charge from the phosphate group on FDG-6-phosphate. Glucose-6-phosphatase levels are low in cancer cells but dephosphorylation of FDG is also slow in normal myocardium and brain tissue.

The primary route of excretion of ^{18}F-FDG occurs by urinary system, although excretion through the bowel also takes place to some extent. When the renal functions are normal, 50 % of the radioactivity reaches the bladder by 2 h after administration of radiotracer. In a normal individual glucose is not excreted by kidneys since it is freely filtered by glomeruli and absorbed by nephron, but FDG is not reabsorbed after filtration, resulting in detection of significant activity in urinary system.

Patient Preparation

The main logic of patient preparation is keeping FDG uptake at normal tissues at minimum level while providing an optimum tracer uptake at tumor tissues. For this purpose the patient should fast 4–6 h prior to injection of FDG. Blood glucose levels should be less than 200 mg/dl before examination, otherwise circulating blood glucose may compete with FDG and cause a decrease in overall FDG uptake, so measurement of blood glucose levels should be performed prior to injection of FDG to be sure that the patient is in fasting state and to detect elevated blood glucose levels. Hyperinsulinemia should also be avoided because it results in increased FDG uptake into skeletal muscle. The tracer should be administered at least 4 h after the last insulin administration in order not to observe any altered biokinetics of FDG in terms of muscle, liver, or tumor uptake. Although there are no restrictions for intake of prescribed daily medications, stopping the oral antidiabetic drug metformin at least 3 days before the examination will prevent unwanted increased physiological bowel uptake.

The patient should be hydrated adequately to decrease the concentration of FDG in urine for having less artifacts and lowering radiation exposure.

Strenuous exercise must be avoided for 24 h before the FDG PET/CT study. During the administration of tracer and the subsequent 45 min period, the patient should remain seated or lie still. During the uptake phase talking or chewing may cause increased accumulation of tracer at laryngeal and neck muscles which may confound the interpretation of the lesions at head and neck area. If the patient is tense during this time physiological uptake within the muscles of the neck can be seen, and to reduce this uptake it is suggested that patients be given 5–10 mg diazepam orally 1 h before FDG injection. The patient should be kept warm starting 30–60 min before the injection of FDG and continuing throughout the uptake period and examination to avoid unwanted FDG accumulation in brown fat due to sympathetic activation.

The dose of FDG is calculated according to the system, time per bed position, and body weight of the patient. In most of the centers patients are administered 140 μCi/kg of FDG with a minimum of 10 mCi and a maximum of 20 mCi. For oncologic imaging, FDG-PET scans are performed approximately 60 min following the intravenous administration of FDG. Acquisition time may vary depending on the FDG dose administered to the patient but usually in a PET/CT scanner, a 2–3 min/bed position is used for patients up to 90 kg, and emission acquisition time per bed is increased to 4 min/bed position for those greater than 90 kg.

A traditional whole body scan is carried out from the skull base to the mid-thighs. This is because the brain metastases are difficult to distinguish from surrounding brain tissue which has already intense uptake, and metastatic lesions at lower limbs are infrequently seen. The limitation of acquisition area in the body also provides less radiation exposure to the patient and saving of time. Malignant melanoma and multiple myeloma require whole body scanning as head-to-toe imaging. For malignancies that have high chance of involvement of structures at abdomen or pelvis, intraluminal gastrointestinal contrast agent may be given to improve visualization of the gastrointestinal tract on CT and discriminate bowel from mass lesions and other intraabdominal structures. In some centers iv contrast is used and injection of the contrast agent is performed either during the acquisition of CT data used for attenuation correction or after the CT and PET acquisition is completed.

Pregnancy is an absolute contraindication for ^{18}F-FDG PET/CT studies. Breastfeeding of the baby should be discontinued for 24 h following the injection.

Normal Distribution

Normal brain, particularly gray matter, shows intense FDG uptake because it uses glucose as the sole energy source. Metastatic lesions at CNS can be detected in less than 1 % of patients on FDG PET studies performed for evaluation of malignant diseases. Mild FDG uptake is usually detected at lingual and palatine tonsils and base of the tongue which represents the lymphatic tissue in Waldeyer's ring. Mild to moderate tracer uptake also occurs at salivary glands, mylohyoid muscle, and soft palate. The symmetrical appearance of the activities in the head and neck region and evaluation of images together with the corresponding CT slices help to distinguish them from malignant lesions. Mild diffuse FDG uptake can be observed at thyroid gland in normal individuals. Intensely diffuse uptake generally indicates thyroiditis. Focal

FDG uptake at thyroid gland must be cautiously evaluated since one in every third focal hypermetabolic lesion at thyroid gland turns out to be malignant.

Moderately increased diffuse FDG uptake at breast is seen in young premenopausal women. The breast uptake can be intense in lactating patients.

In the fasting state, myocardium preferentially uses fatty acids as energy source, so cardiac uptake is expected to be minimal theoretically, but most of the time significant myocardial FDG uptake is encountered. Excretion of FDG through kidneys without any reabsorption unlike glucose causes accumulation of activity at kidneys, ureters, and bladder. Intravenous hydration and furosemide injection may help to decrease this unwanted uptake. While evaluating the patients with bladder cancer catheterization may improve diagnostic accuracy.

Liver and spleen display mild FDG uptake in normal patient. Spleen may show increased uptake when there is hematopoietic activation. Spleen/liver SUVmax ratio is 0.85 in normal individuals.

FDG uptake at skeletal muscle increases after insulin administration, eating, and exercise. Diaphragmatic crus uptake may be increased as a result of hyperventilation. Extraocular muscle uptake is usually seen because of intense eye movement. Cervical muscle uptake can be confounding especially when it is unilateral due to torticollis. Symmetrical FDG uptake is noted at vocal cords due to talking during uptake phase, meanwhile unilateral uptake can be seen due to contralateral recurrent laryngeal nerve palsy.

Brown fat has the capacity to generate heat upon activation of the sympathetic nervous system by cold or secretion of excess catecholamines due to any other reason. This may cause increased FDG uptake at deep cervical, supraclavicular, interscapular, paravertebral regions, and interatrial septum.

Physiological uptake at gastrointestinal tract can be seen in varying intensity and patterns. Moderate diffuse uptake at gastric walls is frequently seen in normal patients but if the uptake is intense or focal, inflammatory or malignant conditions should be considered. Diffuse bowel uptake is usually observed. Although exact mechanisms of uptake are not very well understood, the activity in the bowel is probably related to lymphoid tissue and smooth muscle uptake as well as activity in the intraluminal contents. Focal accumulations of FDG at bowel is suspicious for malignant lesions, whereas segmental uptake is indicative of inflammatory disease.

Mild symmetric testicular uptake in young men is usually seen. In women, FDG uptake at ovaries during ovulation and uterus uptake during menstruation are usual findings.

^{18}F-FDG accumulates in activated lymphocytes, neutrophils, and macrophages infiltrating various inflammatory and infectious lesions and this may result in misinterpretation of the benign lesions as malignant. Surgical interventions may cause increased FDG uptake due to inflammation, so FDG PET studies should be performed at least 6 weeks after an operation. Fractures of bone, benign tumors like pleomorphic adenoma, Warthin tumor, diverticulitis of bowel, and surrenal adenomas are some of the benign conditions that may cause false-positive results by resembling metastasis when exploring the metastatic sites in cancer patients.

Standardized Uptake Value (SUV)

The SUV is a semiquantitative measurement which is calculated by normalizing the amount of FDG accumulation in a certain region of interest to the total injected dose and the patient body weight/surface area. SUV reflects the relative amount of activity in a lesion and it is one of the criteria that is used to identify the malignant nature of the lesion.

The formula of SUV is:

$$\frac{\text{Region of interest}\left(\text{ROI}\right)\text{activity}\left(\text{mCi / ml}\right)\text{x}}{\text{Injected dose}\left(\text{mCi}\right)/\text{body weight}\left(\text{g}\right)}$$

SUVmax reflects part of the tumor with the highest intensity of activity and it gives less variable results than SUVmean. There are several factors affecting SUV measurement:

- As the body weight of the patient increases, SUV measurements give erroneously high results since body of a heavy patient contains higher proportion of fat tissue which is less metabolically active than muscle tissue.
- Plasma glucose levels has an inverse correlation with SUV, as the nonlabeled glucose cause a decrease in FDG uptake by competitive inhibition.
- Extravasation of dose causes calculation of SUV falsely lower than it should be.
- After the injection of FDG, SUV values increases with time, especially for the first 120 min and then plateaus, so earlier measurements give falsely low SUV results.
- If the lesion is less than 2–3 cm in size, SUV might be calculated erroneously low due to partial volume effect.
- SUV measurements from images reconstructed with filtered back projection (FBP) are lower than the real values.

Indications for ^{18}F-FDG PET CT in Oncological Applications

- Identification of the malignant nature of a lesion
- Pretreatment staging of a patient with a known malignancy
- Restaging of a malignancy when there is a suspicion for recurrence either detected by anatomical imaging or elevated tumor markers
- Posttreatment evaluation of therapy response in a known malignancy
- Early prediction of therapy response
- Searching for carcinoma of unknown primary when a metastatic lesion is detected and primary lesion is not found with conventional investigations
- Finding primary malignancy when a patient presents with a paraneoplastic syndrome
- Differentiating recurrent or residual tumor from posttreatment fibrosis or necrosis
- Guiding radiation therapy planning
- Guiding biopsy by showing the most metabolically active part of the tumor

Acknowledgement

We thank Assoc. Prof. Dr. Tevfik Özpaçacı, MD for his contributions to our medical education and we appreciate the opportunities he afforded us.

We thank Prof. Dr. İbrahim Gözükara, MD for his contributions to our medical education.

We wish to thank Prof. Dr. Metin Halaç for his contributions to our training in PET and for encouraging us in the field of academic research.

We thank Dr. Mehmet Tarık Tatoğlu for his technical support which made this book possible.

We would like to express appreciation and gratitude to all our colleagues and residents in the field of Nuclear Medicine, particularly Dr. Özgür Eker.

We wish to express our gratitude to all clinicians and oncologists who referred their patients to us.

We sincerely send our gratitudes to Assoc. Prof. Dr. Mine Adaş, MD, Assoc. Prof. Dr. Meral Mert, MD, Asst. Prof. Dr. Ebru Özgönenel, MD, Dr. Hülya Yıldız, Dr. Yasemin Gökden, Dr. Ferhan Mantar, Dr. Filiz Cebeci and Dr. Aysun Küçüköz Uzun for their contributions and friendship.

We would like to thank all of the PET staff including nurses, secretaries, and technologists, especially Emrah Karapınar, Leyla Yıldız and Ebru Çelik for their technical assistance in acquiring the images shown in this book.

We send our gratitudes to our beloved teacher Prof. Dr. Ali Tan Işıtman, MD who inspired and encouraged us in our academic studies and passed away before the edition of this book.

Finally, we would like to cordially thank Sylvana Freyberg from Springer for her input in the preparation of this book.

Contents

Part I

Fundamentals

1 Physiologic Distribution of ^{18}F-FDG

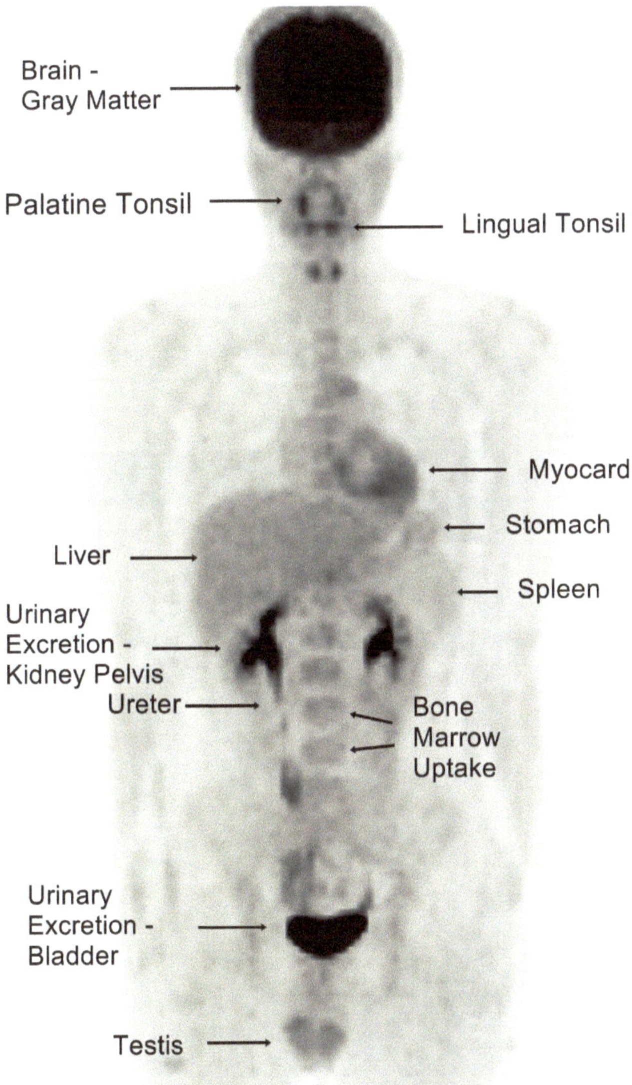

Fig. 1.1 MIP image of normal distribution of ^{18}F-FDG for man

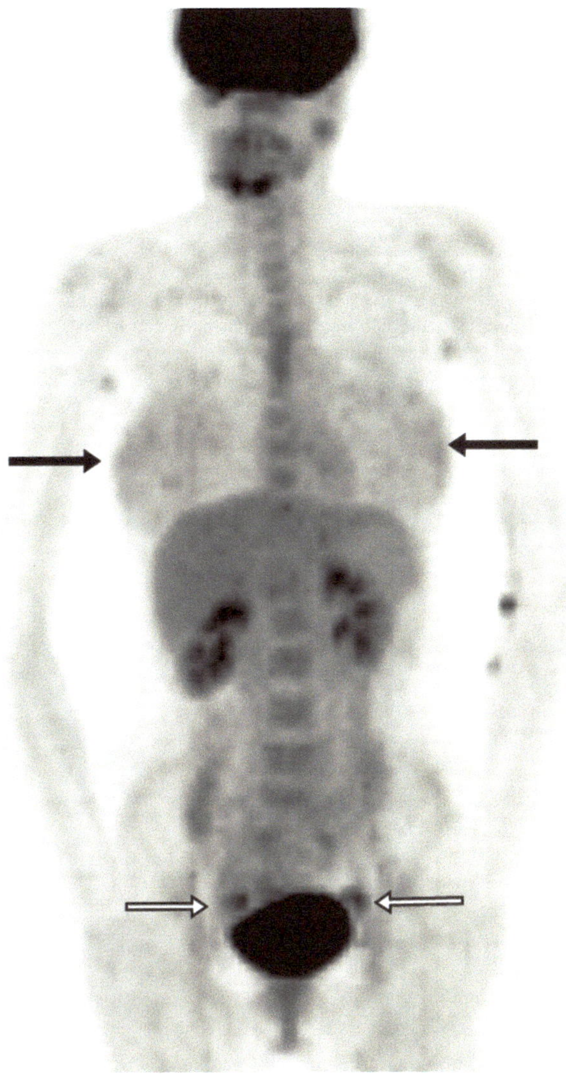

Fig. 1.2 MIP image of normal distribution of ^{18}F-FDG for woman. Physiologic FDG uptake at breasts is seen (*arrows*), being more prominent in young or lactating patients. During ovulation, ovaries display increased FDG uptake (*empty arrows*)

T. Özülker, F. Özülker, *Atlas of PET-CT Imaging in Oncology: A Case-Based Guide to Image Interpretation*,
DOI 10.1007/978-3-319-18994-9_1

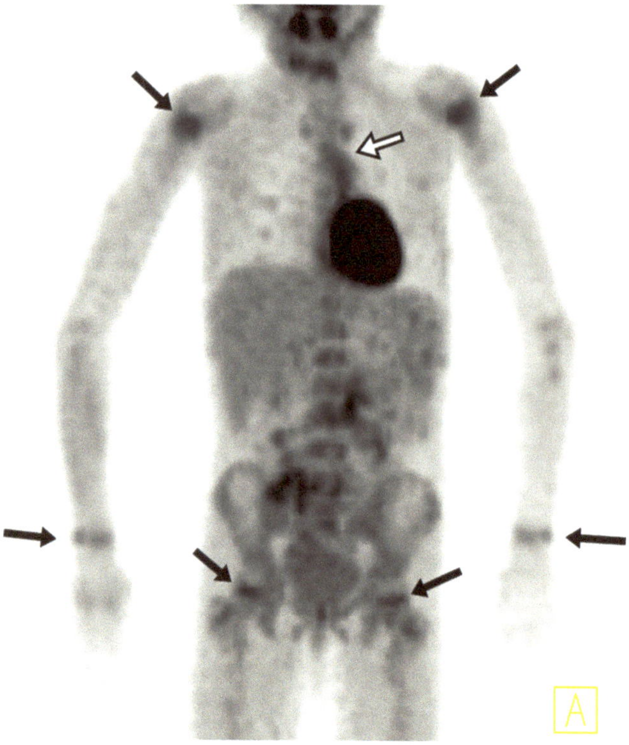

Fig. 1.3 MIP image of normal distribution of ^{18}F-FDG for a 7-year-old girl. Mild uptake at epiphyseal plates normally can be seen (*arrows*). There is physiologic thymus uptake which is also normal for this age (*empty arrow*)

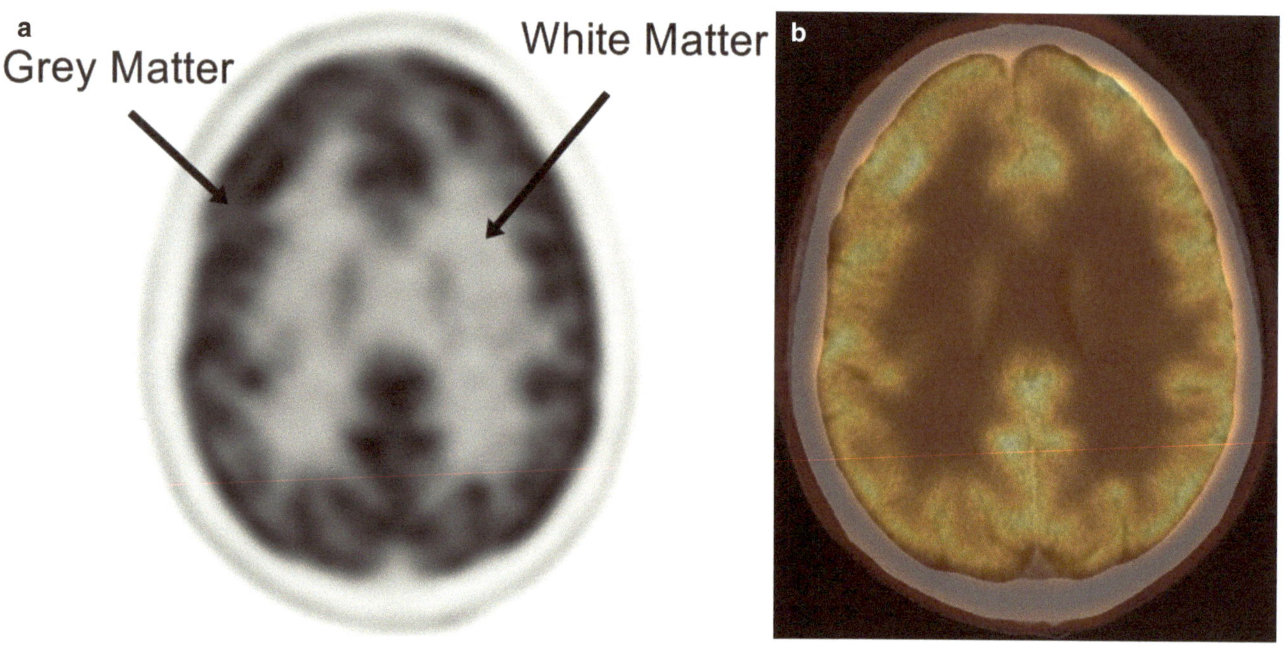

Fig. 1.4 Axial PET and fusion images (**a**, **b**). Since the main energy source of brain is glucose, very intense FDG uptake in gray matter, basal ganglia and thalami is seen

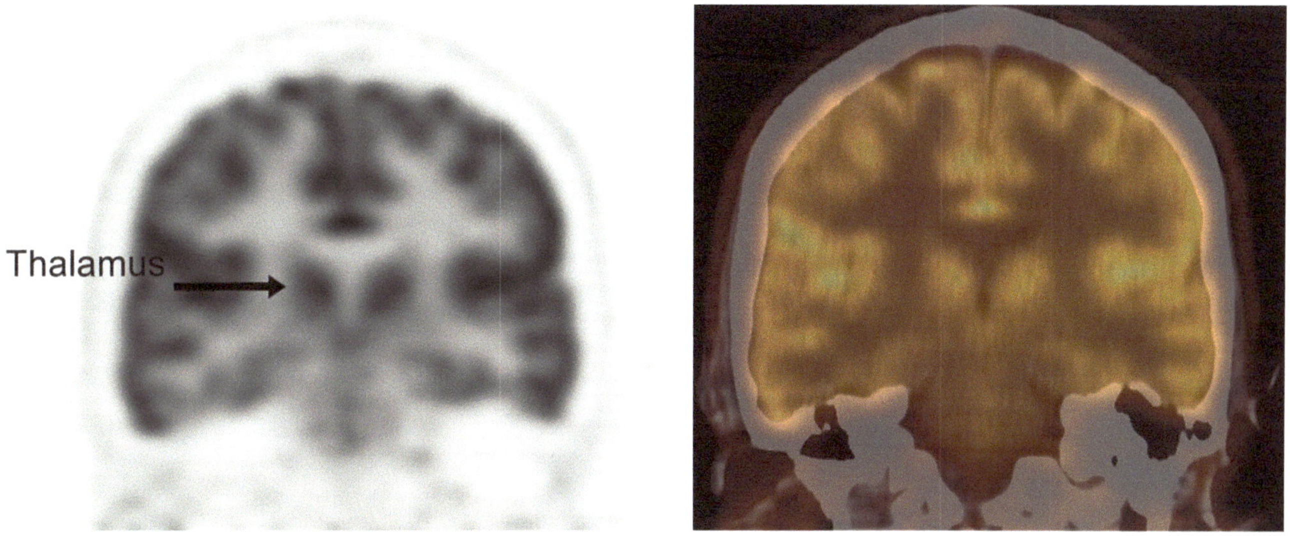

Fig. 1.5 Coronal PET and fusion images

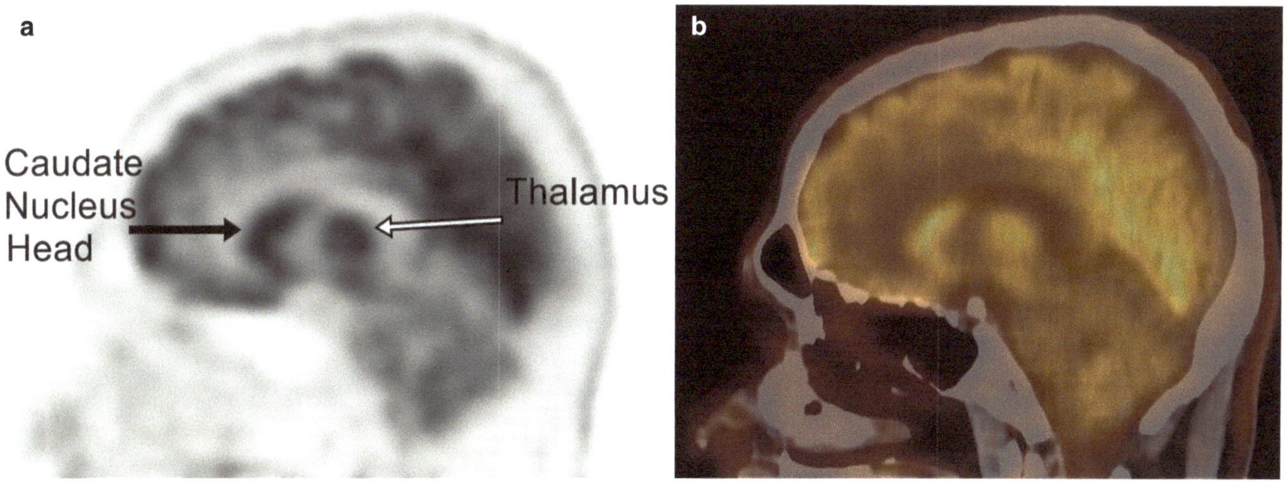

Fig. 1.6 Sagittal PET and fusion images (**a**, **b**)

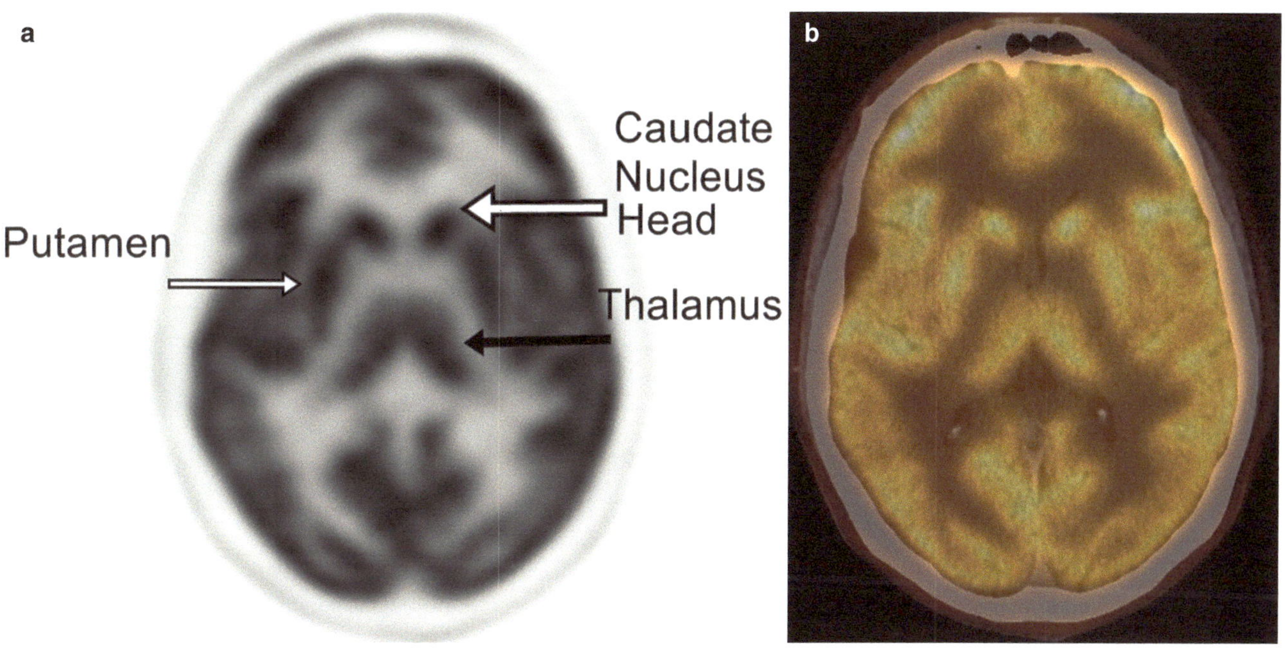

Fig. 1.7 Axial PET and fusion images (**a**, **b**)

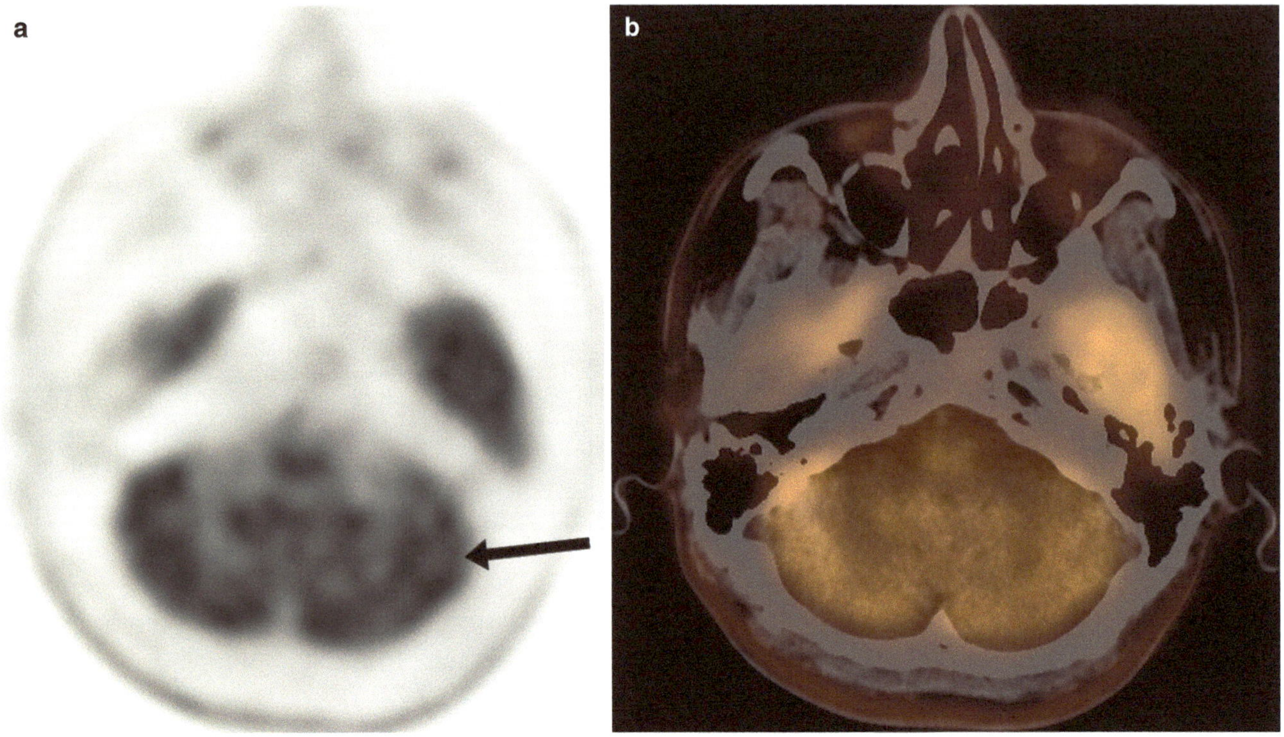

Fig. 1.8 Axial PET and fusion images show normal FDG uptake at cerebellum (*arrow*) (**a**, **b**)

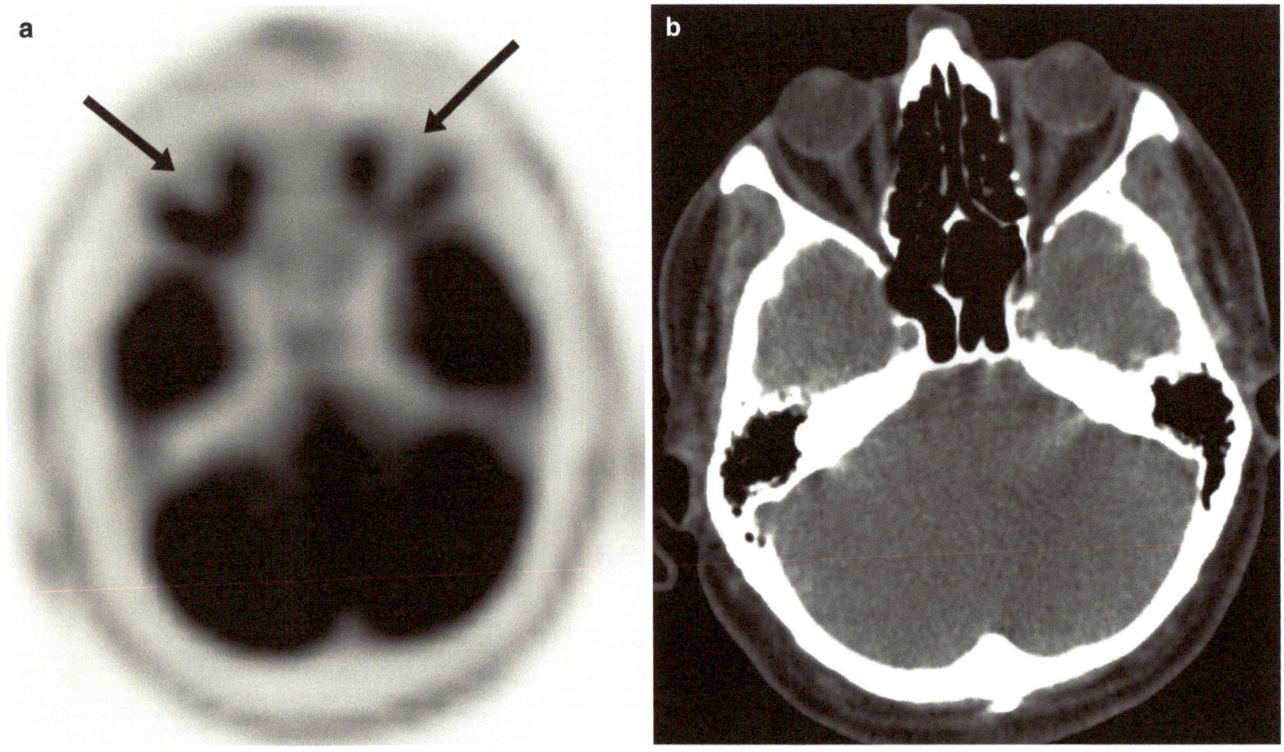

Fig. 1.9 Physiologic uptake at extraocular muscles (**a**, **b**). The 20 min period after administration of FDG is uptake phase. In this period waiting with eyes closed is very important to minimalize FDG uptake of extraocular muscles

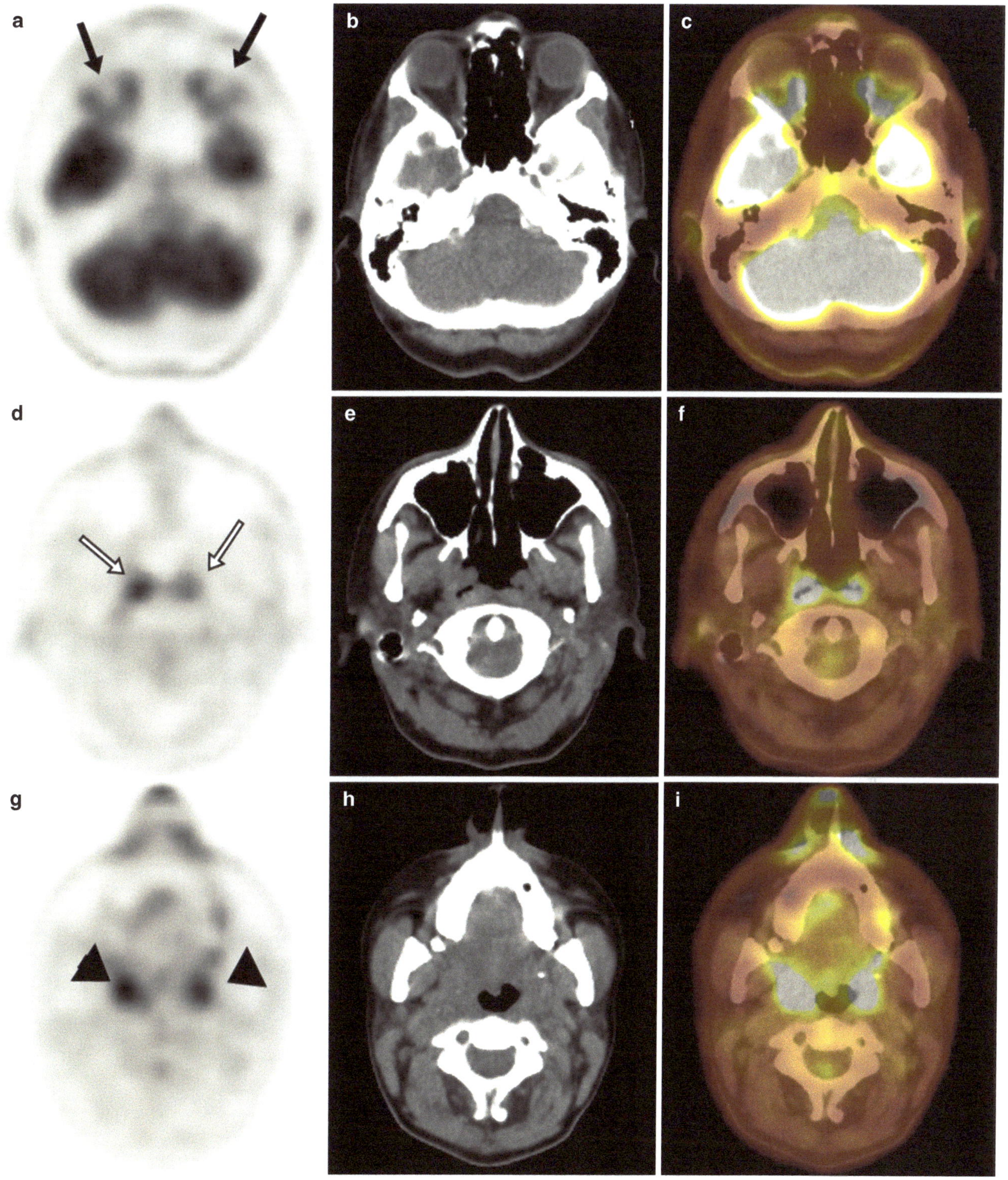

Fig. 1.10 Axial slices of PET, CT, and fusion images show extraocular muscle uptake (*arrow*) (**a–c**), bilateral uptake at nasopharynx (*empty arrows*) (**d–f**), and bilateral uptake at palatin tonsils (*arrow heads*) (**g–i**). Generally bilateral intense uptake can be seen in lingual and palatin tonsils. If significant asymmetric uptake is seen in these areas, clinical correlation should be done to differentiate pathological condition

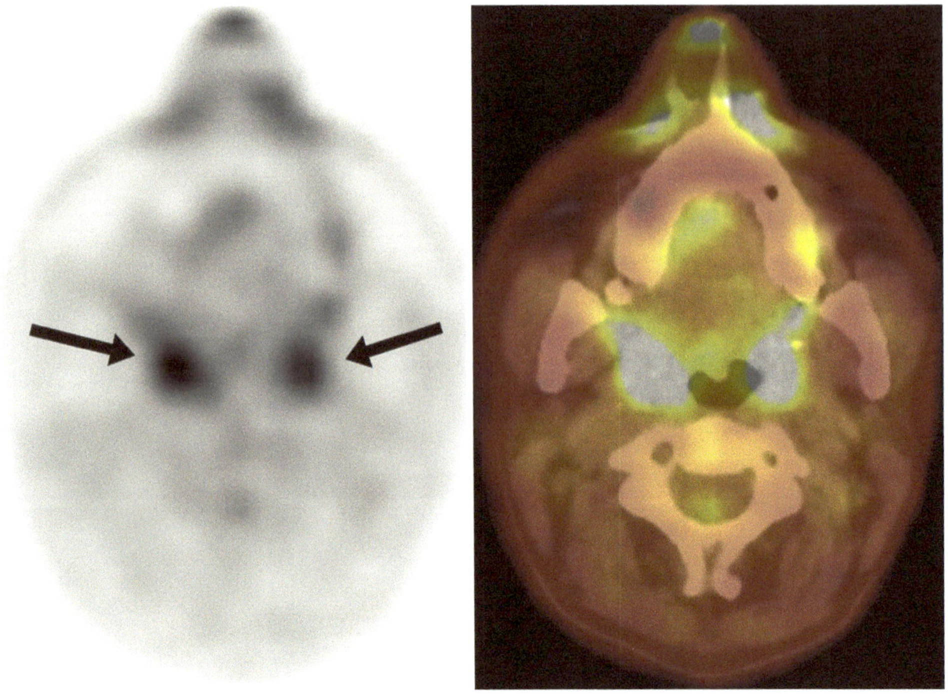

Fig. 1.11 Physiologic bilateral palatin tonsil uptake (*arrows*)

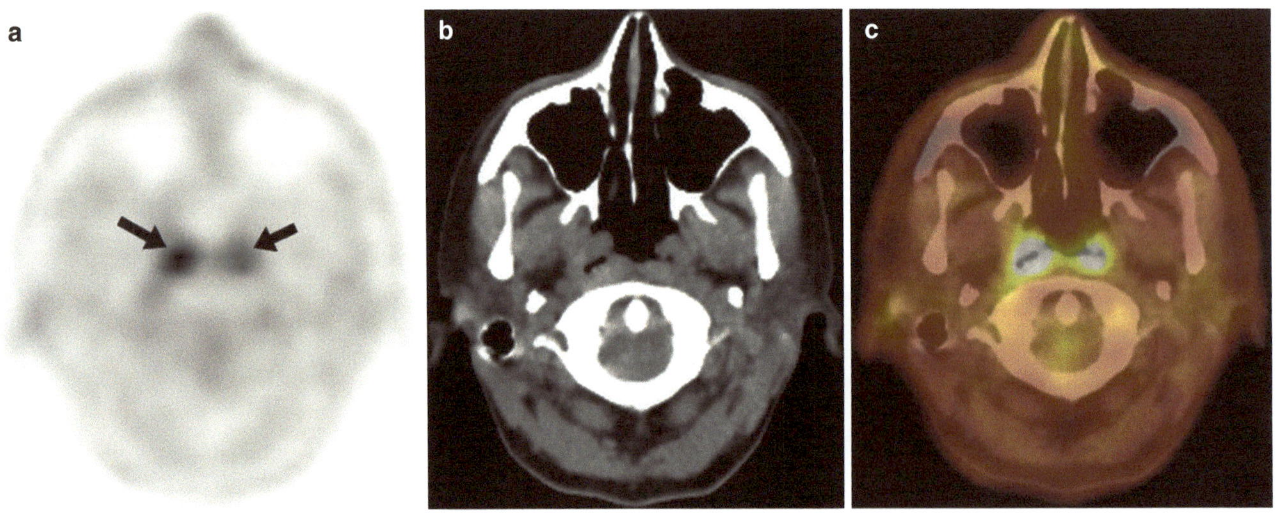

Fig. 1.12 Bilateral uptake at nasopharynx (*arrows*) (**a**–**c**)

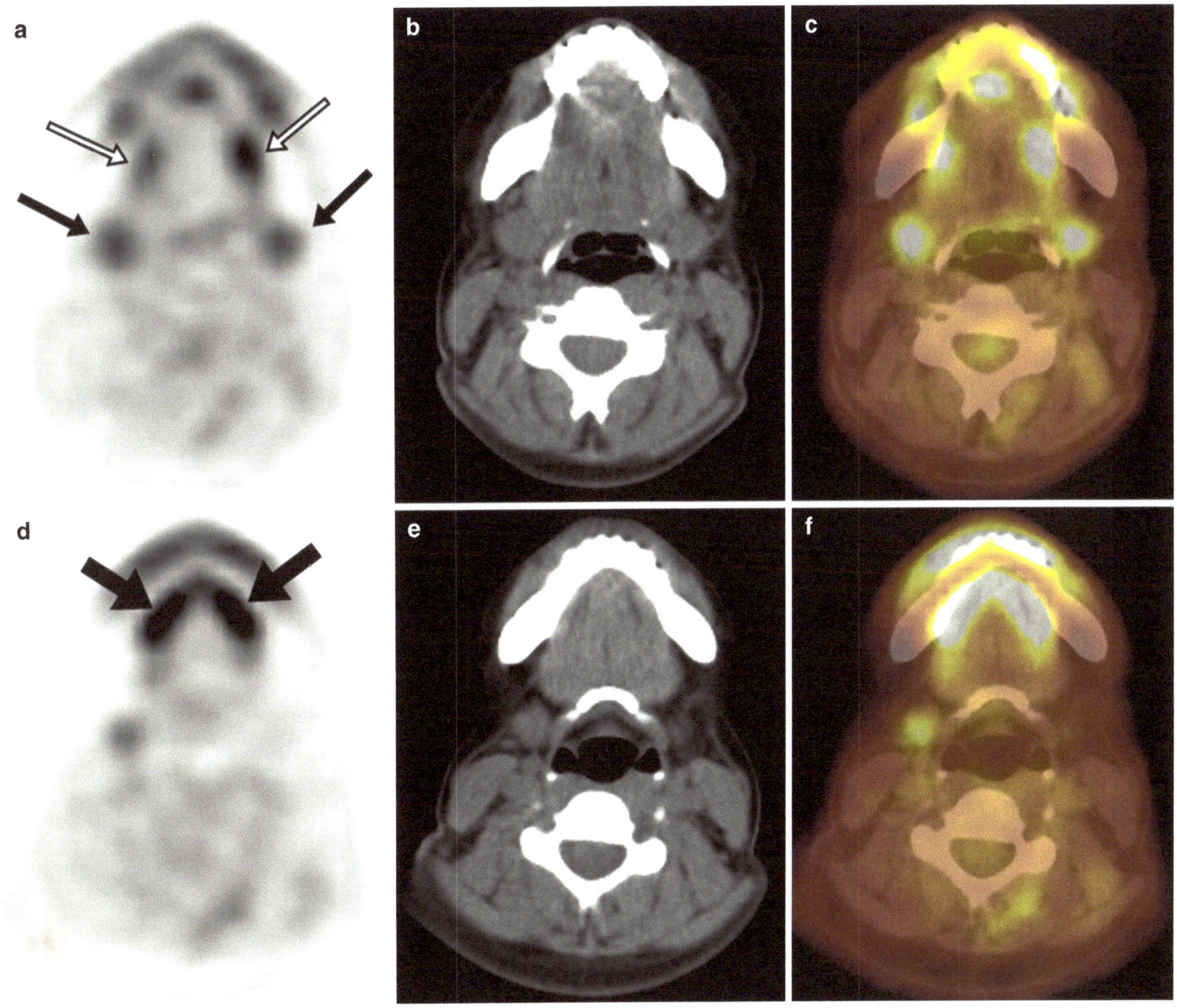

Fig. 1.13 Inverted V shape uptake medial to mandibula reflects mylohyoid muscle (*empty arrows* and *thick arrows*). There is bilateral mild uptake at submandibular glands (*arrows*) (**a–f**)

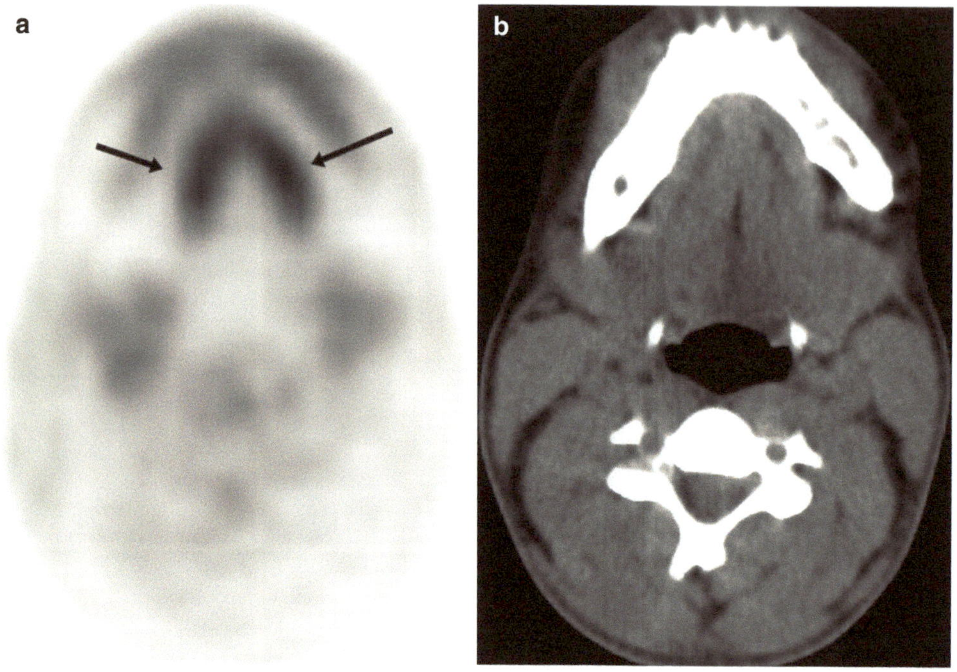

Fig. 1.14 Mylohyoid muscle uptake (*arrows*) (**a**, **b**)

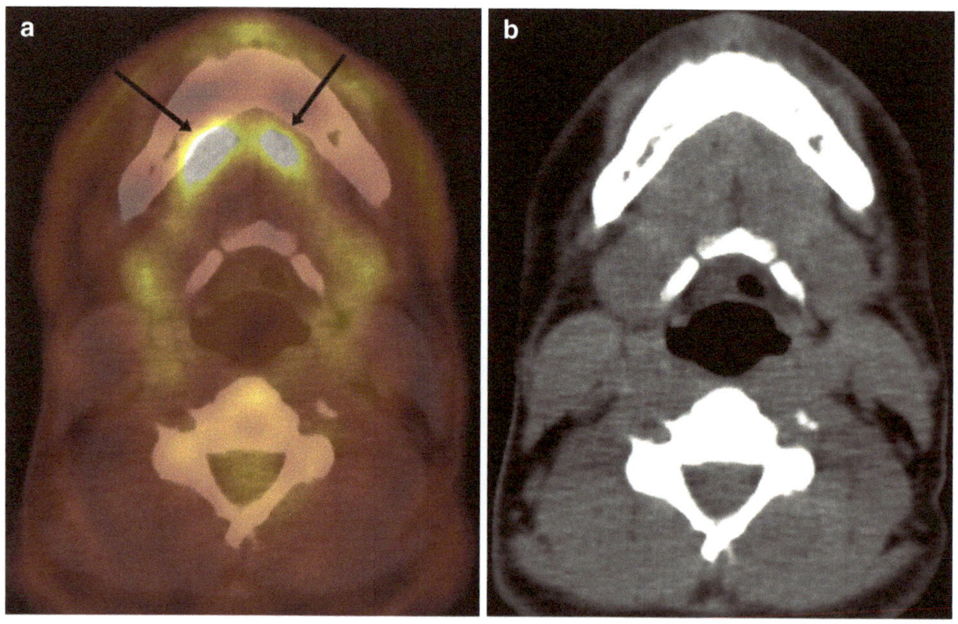

Fig. 1.15 Bilateral focal uptake medial to mandibula represents sublingual glands (*arrows*) (**a**, **b**). Sublingual glands resembles mylohyoid muscle but mylohyoid muscle is usually linear, and located inferior to sublingual glands

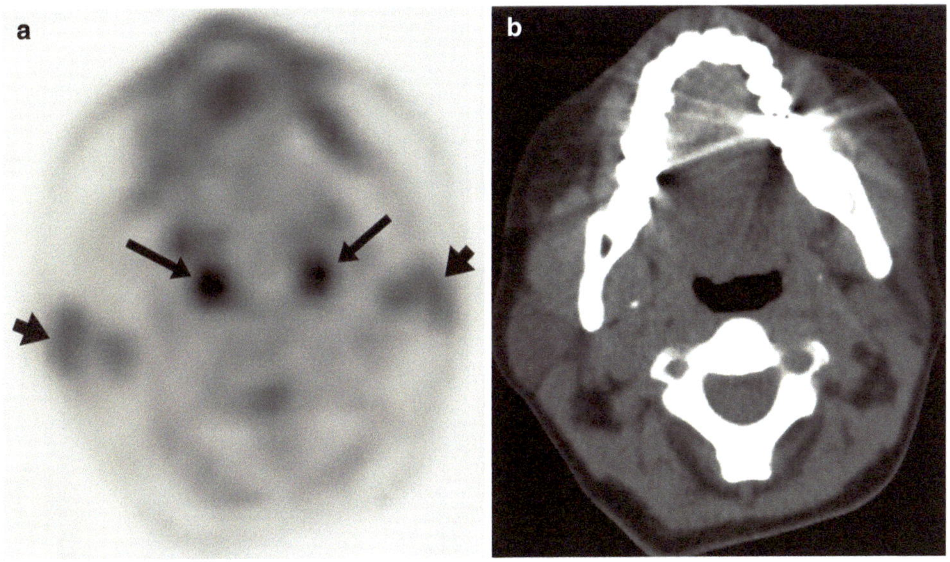

Fig. 1.16 Uptake at bilateral palatin tonsils (*arrows*) and parotid glands (*short arrows*) (**a**, **b**)

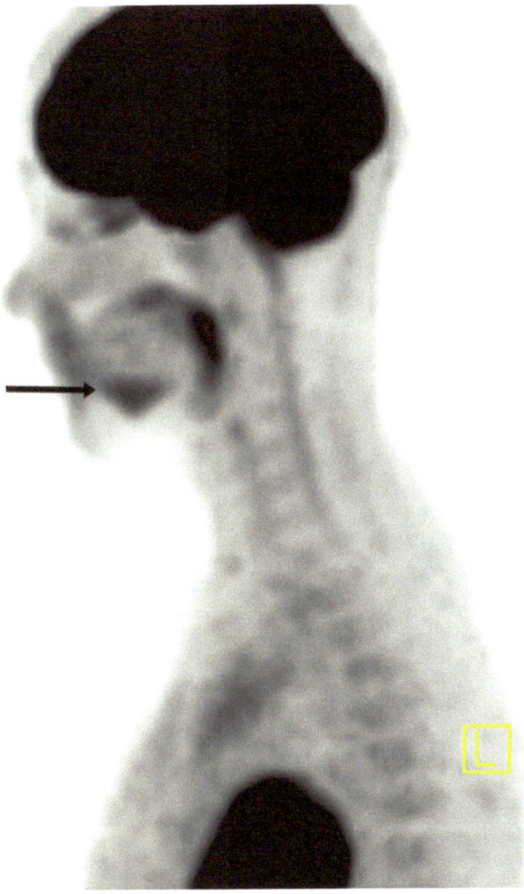

Fig. 1.17 Mild uptake at tongue muscle (*arrow*)

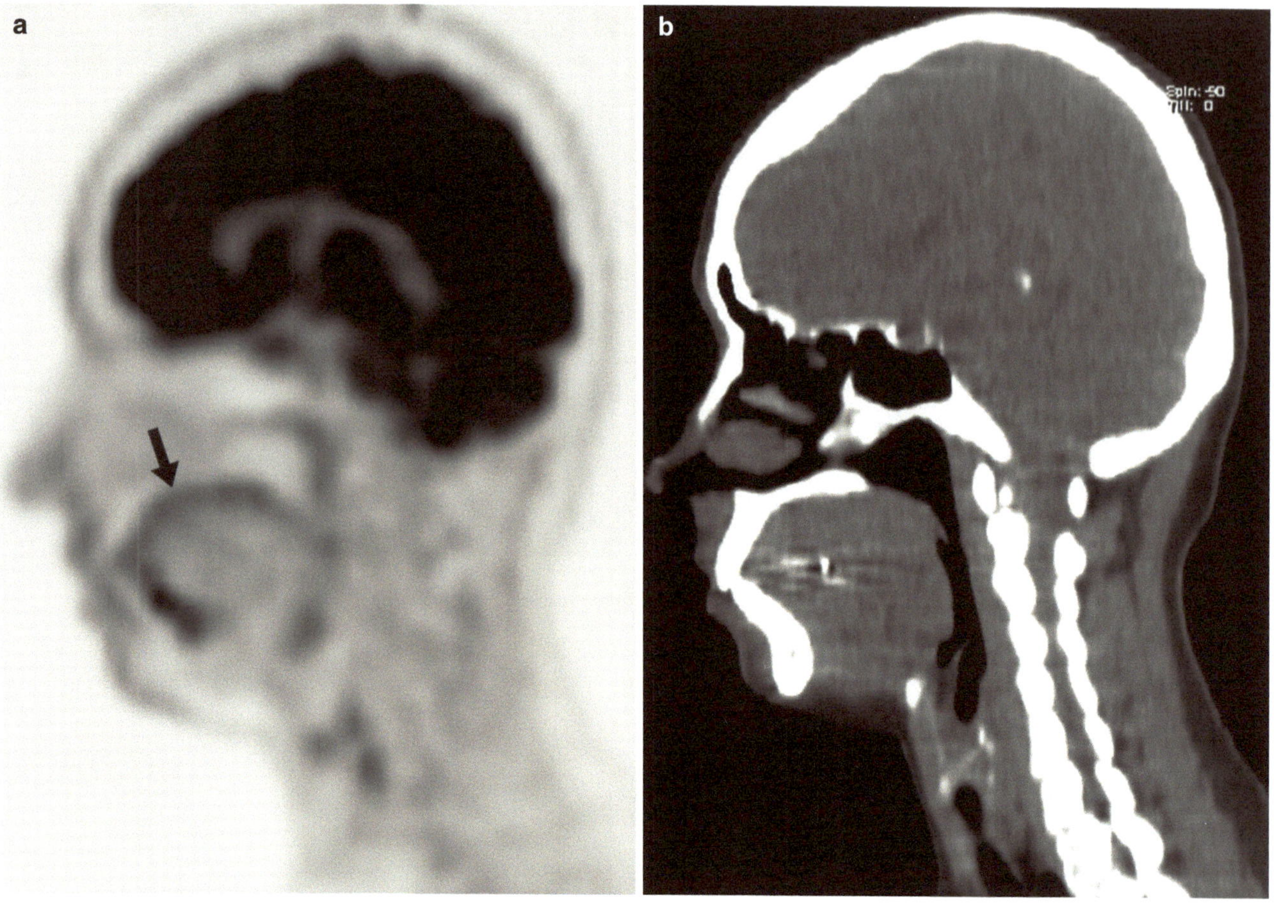

Fig. 1.18 Physiologic uptake at hard palate (*arrow*) (**a**, **b**)

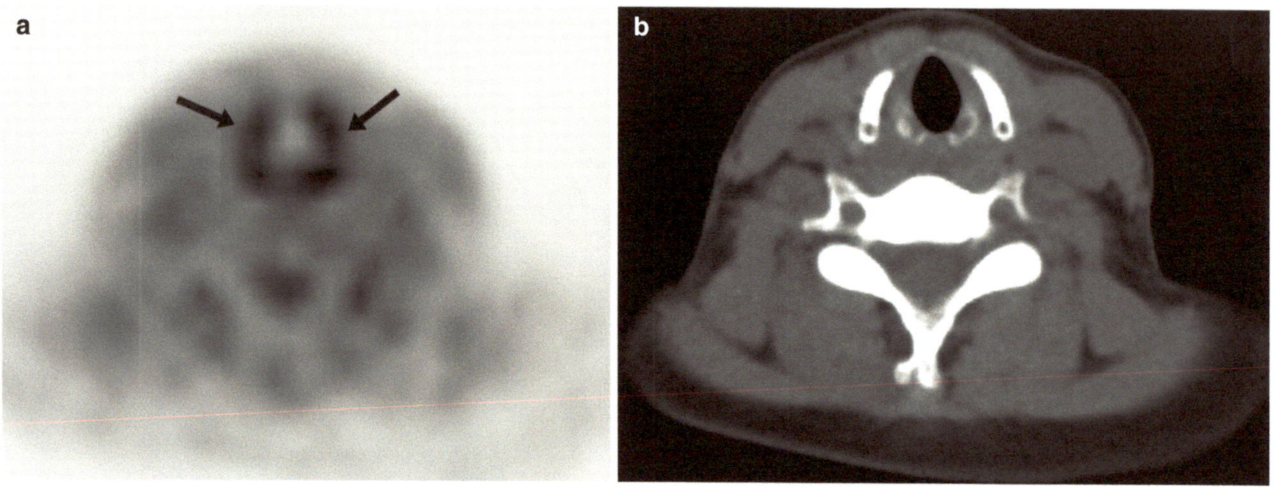

Fig. 1.19 Bilateral uptake at vocal cords (*arrows*) (**a**, **b**)

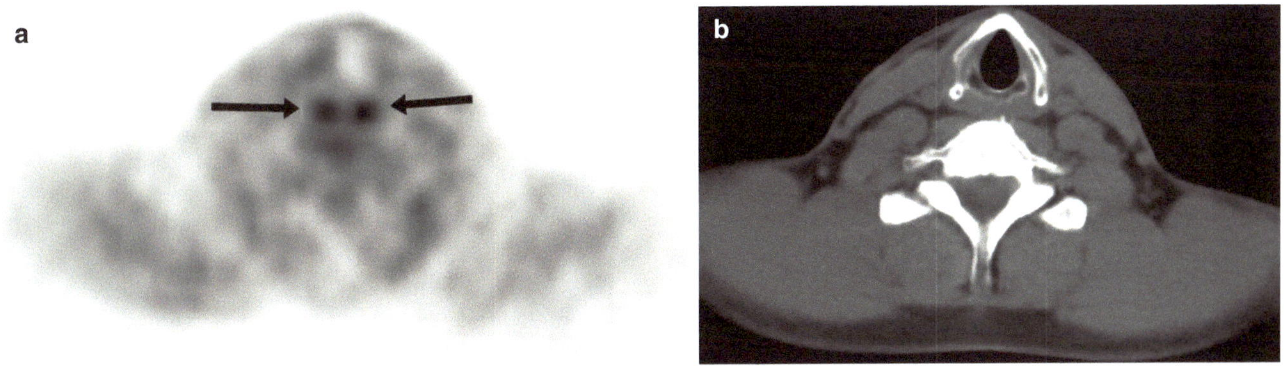

Fig. 1.20 Bilateral uptake at posterior cricoarytenoid muscles (*arrows*) (**a**, **b**). If the patient talks before imaging, intense uptake can be seen at posterior cricoarytenoid muscles and vocal cords. Patients should avoid talking during this period

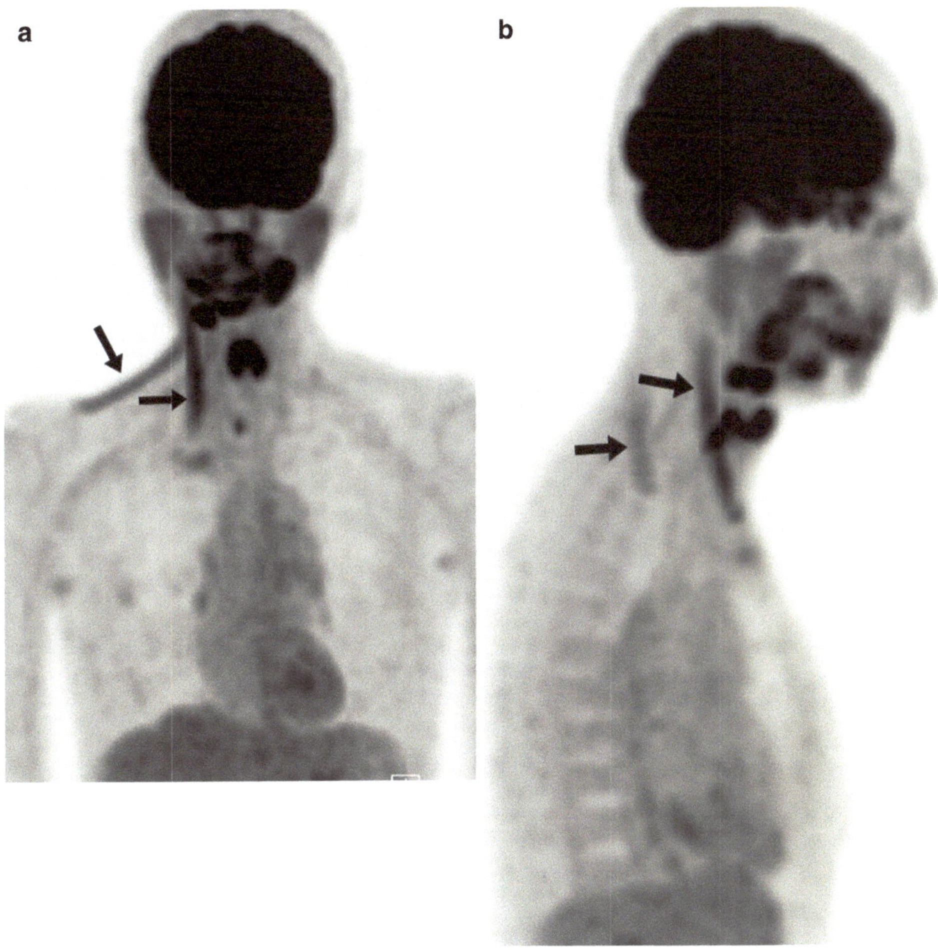

Fig. 1.21 Unilateral uptake at cervical neck muscles due to tension (*arrows*). Normally low FDG uptake is seen at rest (**a**, **b**). Hiccuping, exercise, hyperventilation, torticollis, and involuntary movement can cause increased FDG uptake at muscles

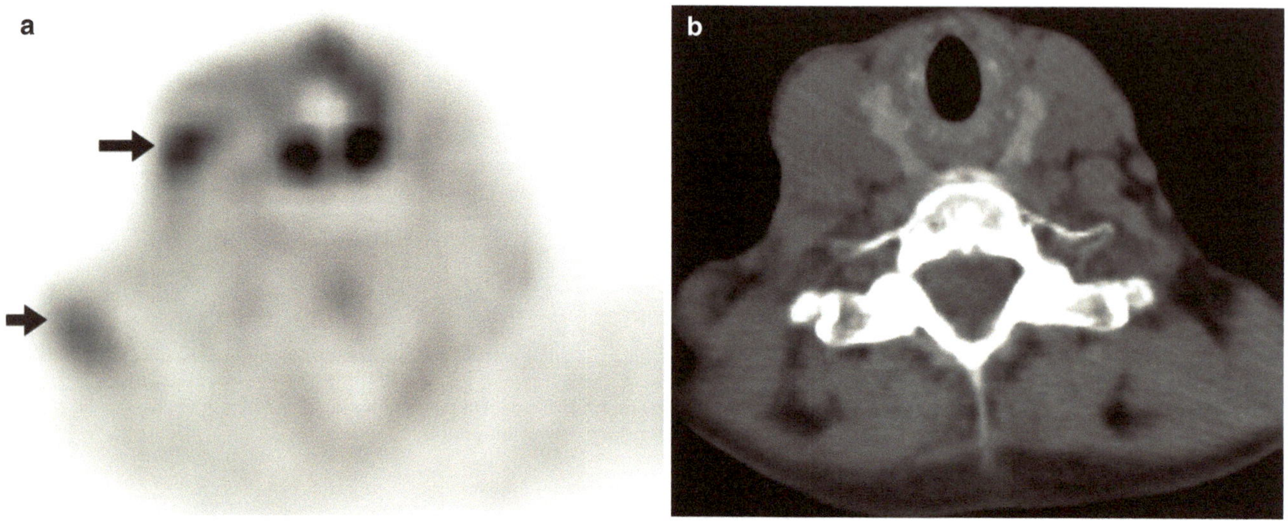

Fig. 1.22 Axial slices of PET and CT images show hypermetabolic foci at right side of the neck which represents physiologic muscle uptake (**a**, **b**). The focal uptake at neck should be further evaluated by reviewing the MIP images, otherwise physiologic muscle uptake can be misinterpreted as pathological

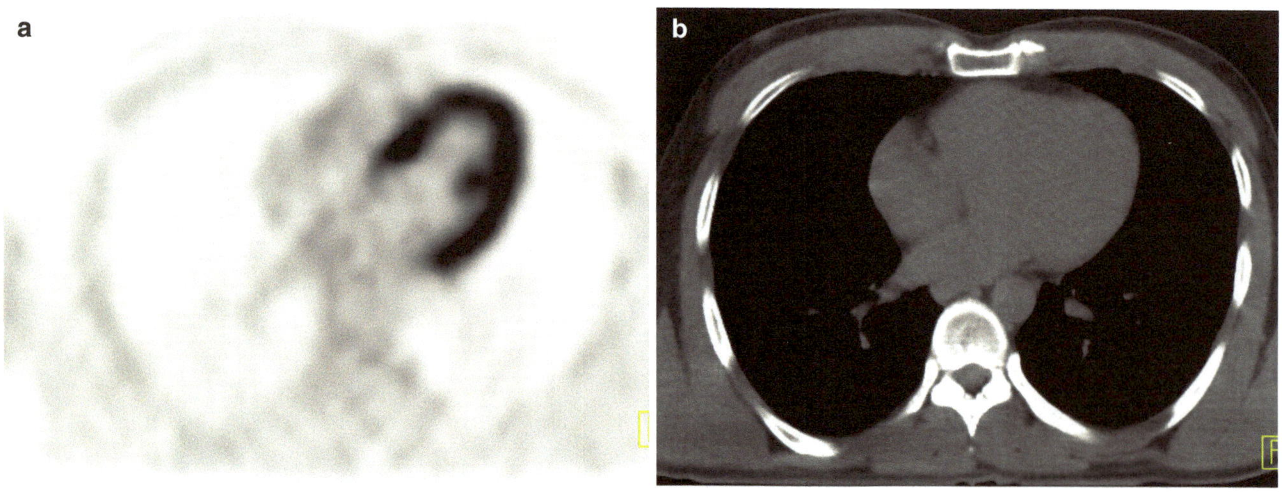

Fig. 1.23 Usually homogenous activity is seen in the left ventricle (**a**, **b**). In fed state, myocardium use glucose as energy source so increased FDG uptake is seen, whereas less FDG uptake is seen in long fasting state since myocardium uses fatty acid as energy source instead of glucose. Hypermetabolic focus noted in left ventricle belongs to papillary muscle uptake

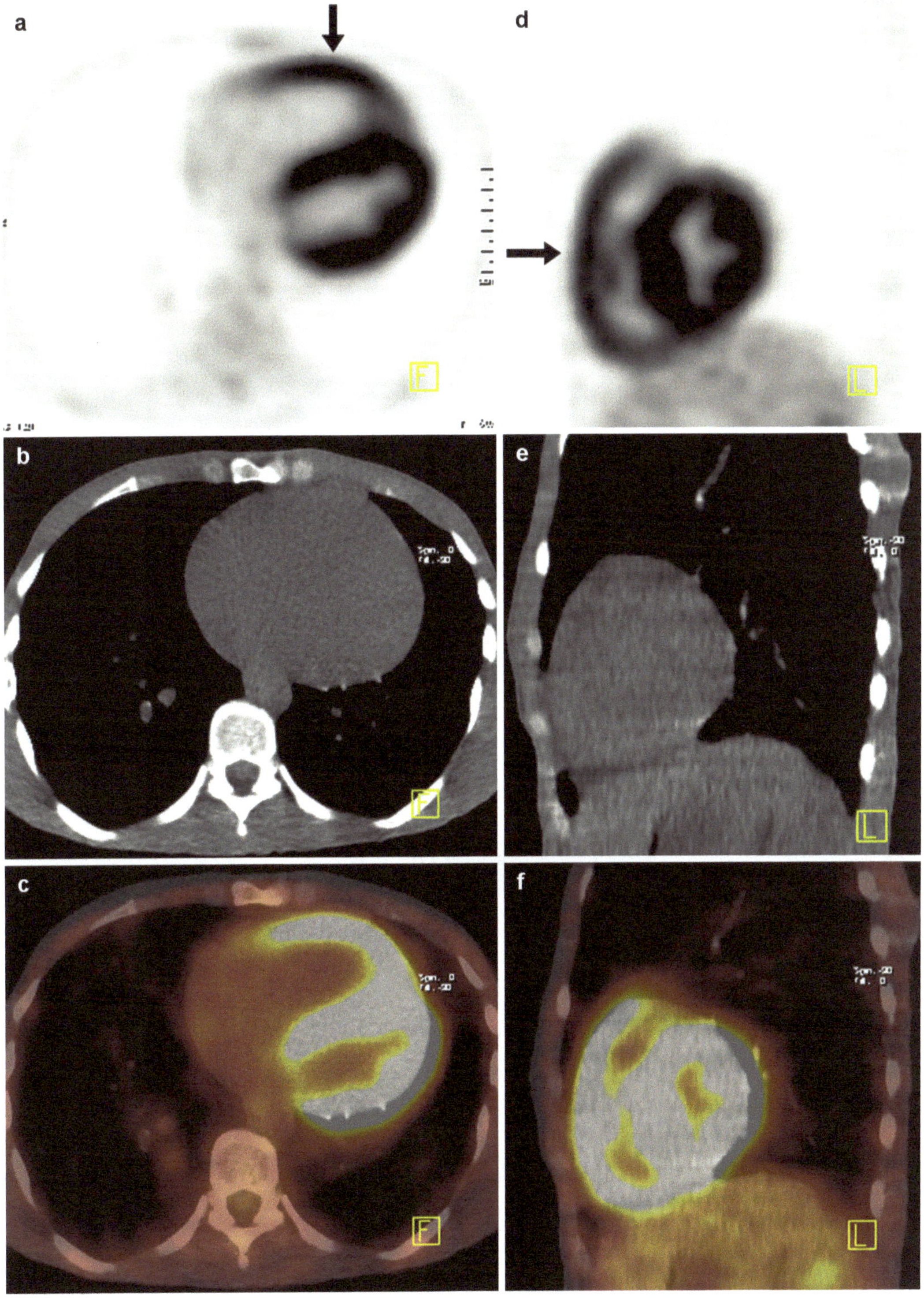

Fig. 1.24 Physiologic uptake at left ventricle. Less frequently right ventricle uptake also can be seen (*arrow*) (**a–f**)

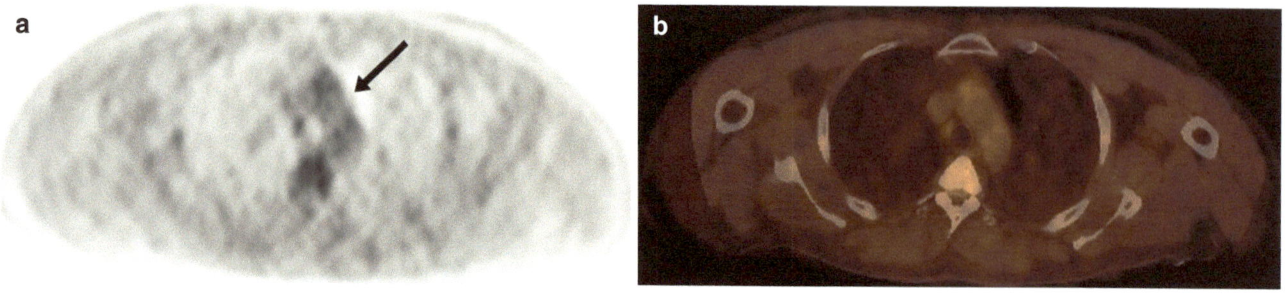

Fig. 1.25 Mild blood pool activity can be seen in the great vessels (**a**, **b**). Sometimes this activity may be intense (*arrows*)

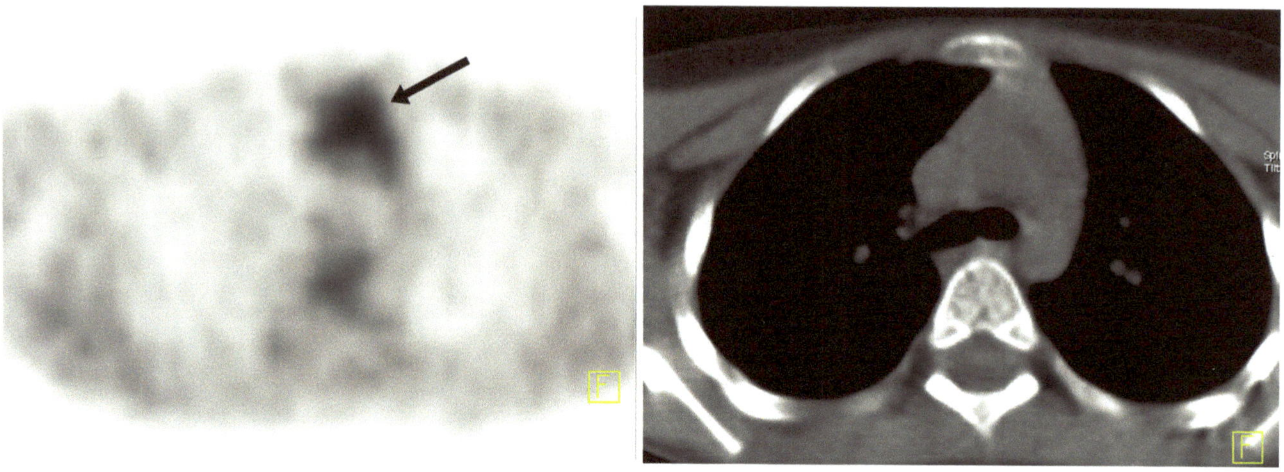

Fig. 1.26 Physiologic thymus uptake is frequently seen in young patients (*arrow*) (**a**, **b**)

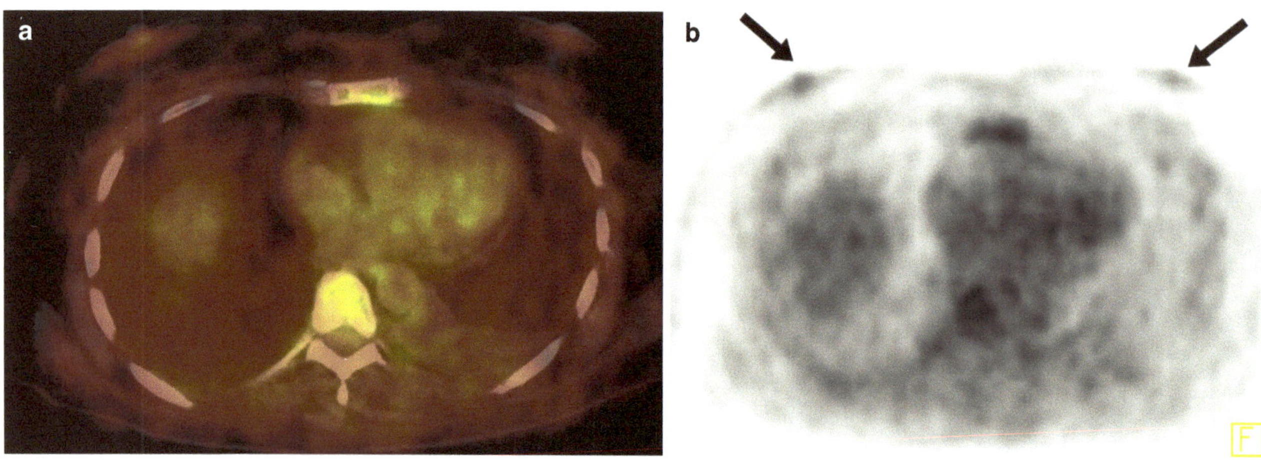

Fig. 1.27 Nipple uptake at both breasts (*arrows*) (**a**, **b**)

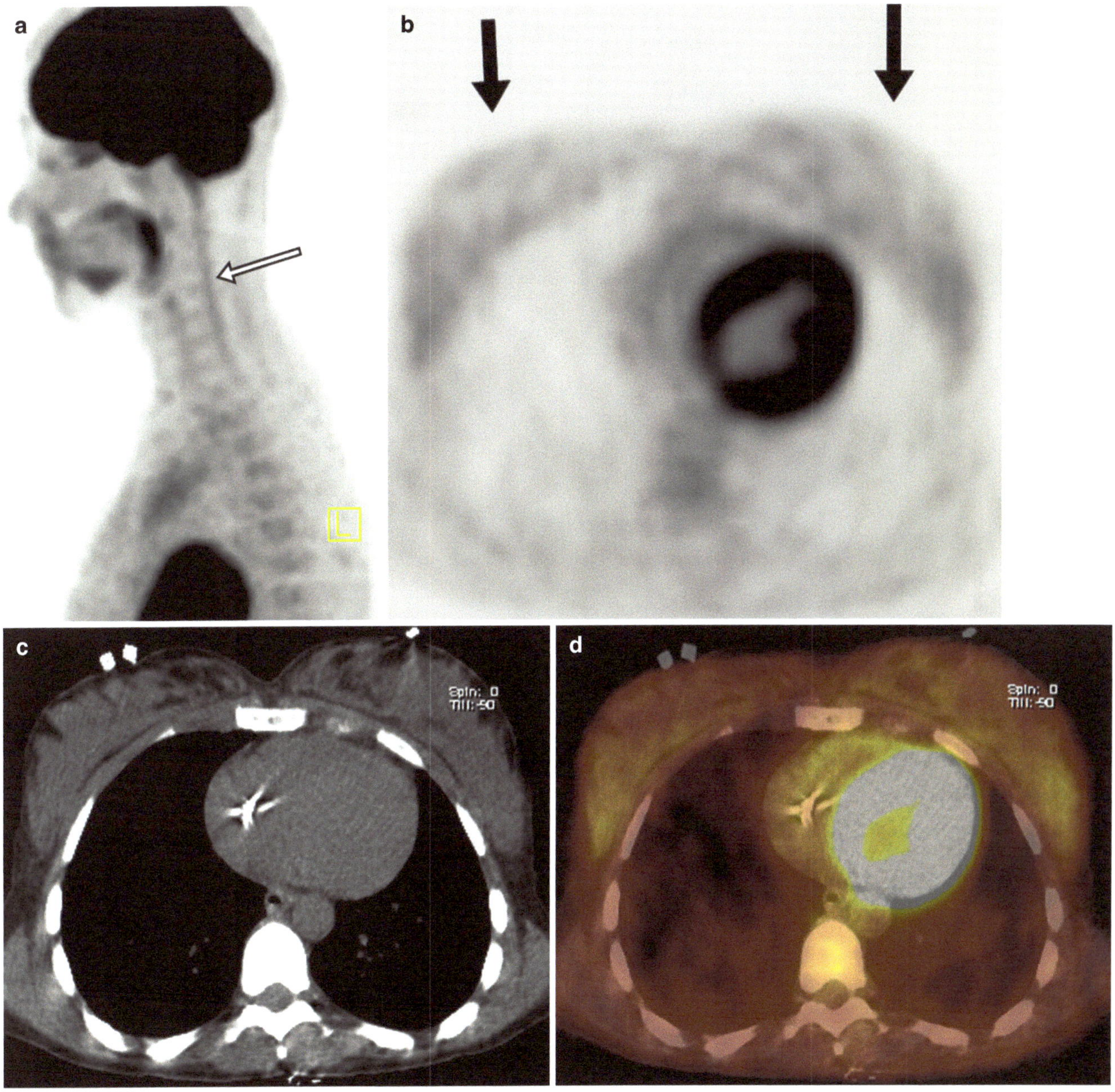

Fig. 1.28 Sometimes mild FDG uptake can be seen at spinal cord (*empty arrow*) (**a**). In young females diffuse uptake at breasts are seen (*arrows*) (**b–d**)

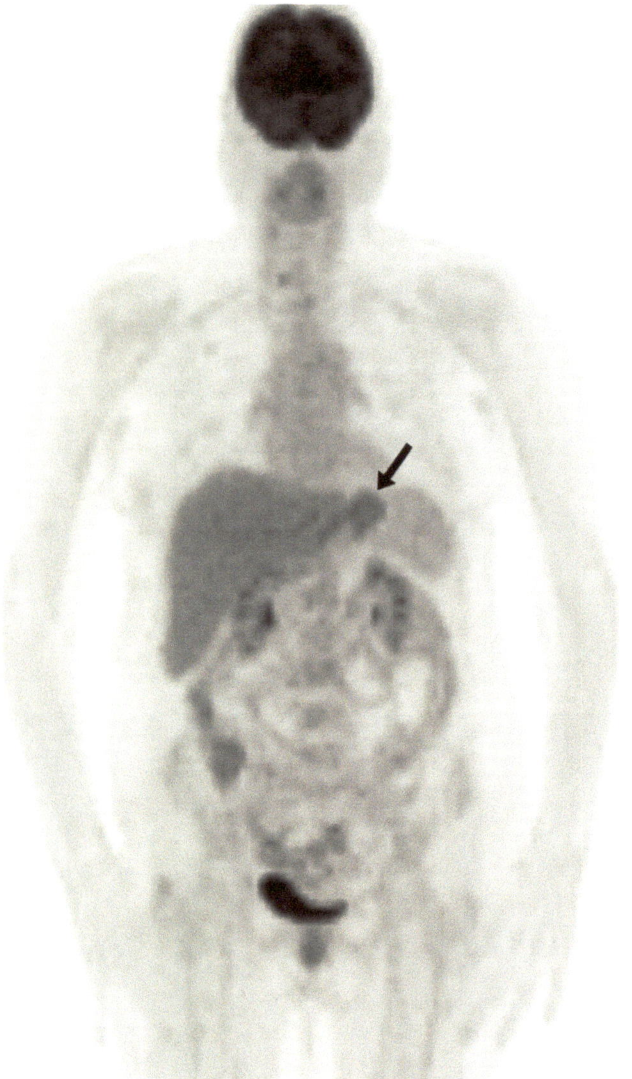

Fig. 1.29 Variable FDG uptake can be seen in stomach (*arrow*). If stomach is empty and contracted uptake may be more intense

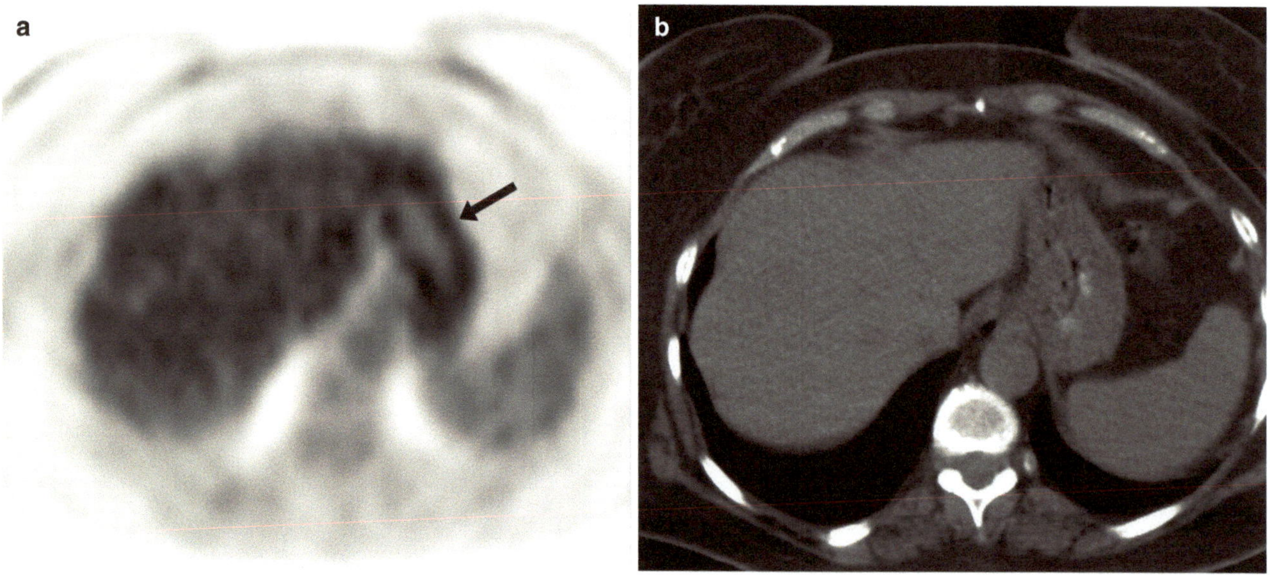

Fig. 1.30 Faint uptake at gastric wall (*arrow*). Mild FDG uptake is seen in liver (**a, b**). Uptake in spleen is normally less than that of liver

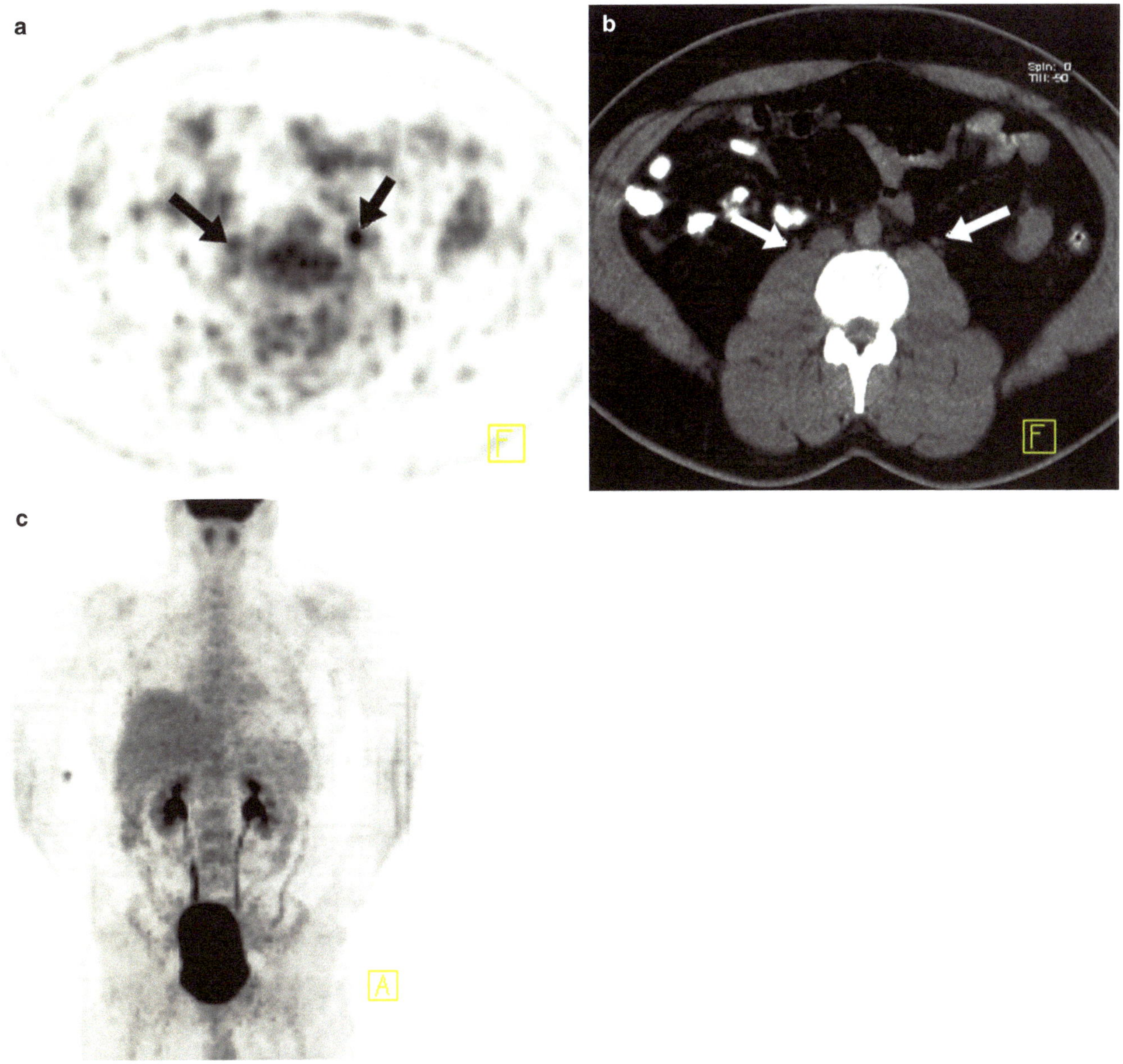

Fig. 1.31 FDG is filtered by the glomerulus but not reabsorbed by the tubules of the kidney, therefore intense FDG activity seen in collecting system, ureters (*arrows*), and bladder (**a**–**c**)

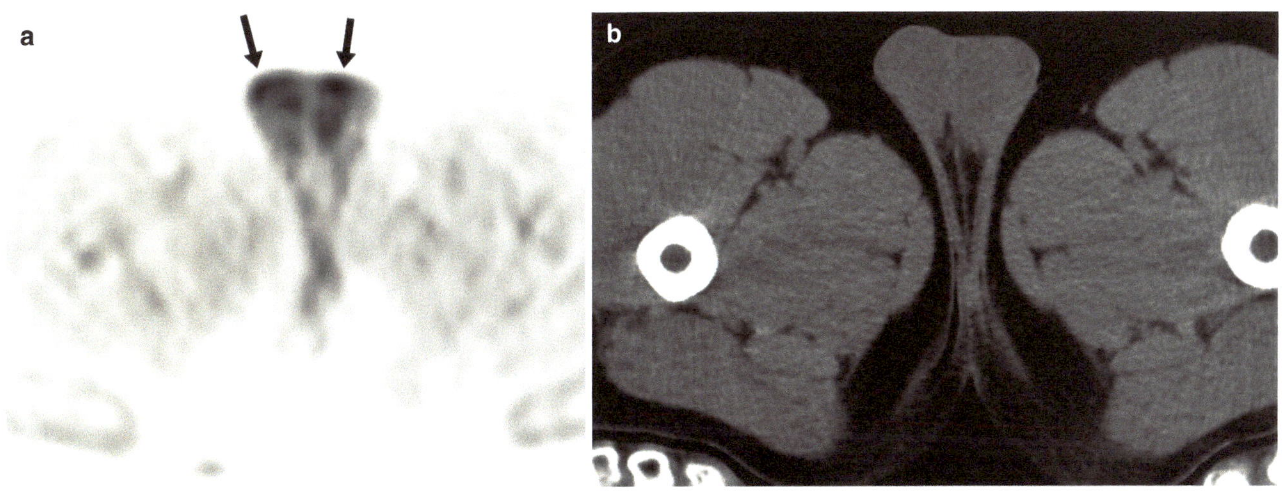

Fig. 1.32 Mild uptake can occur in testes (*arrows*) (**a**, **b**); in young patients FDG uptake can be higher

2 Normal Variants and Benign Findings

2.1 Head and Neck

Cerebrovascular Infarct

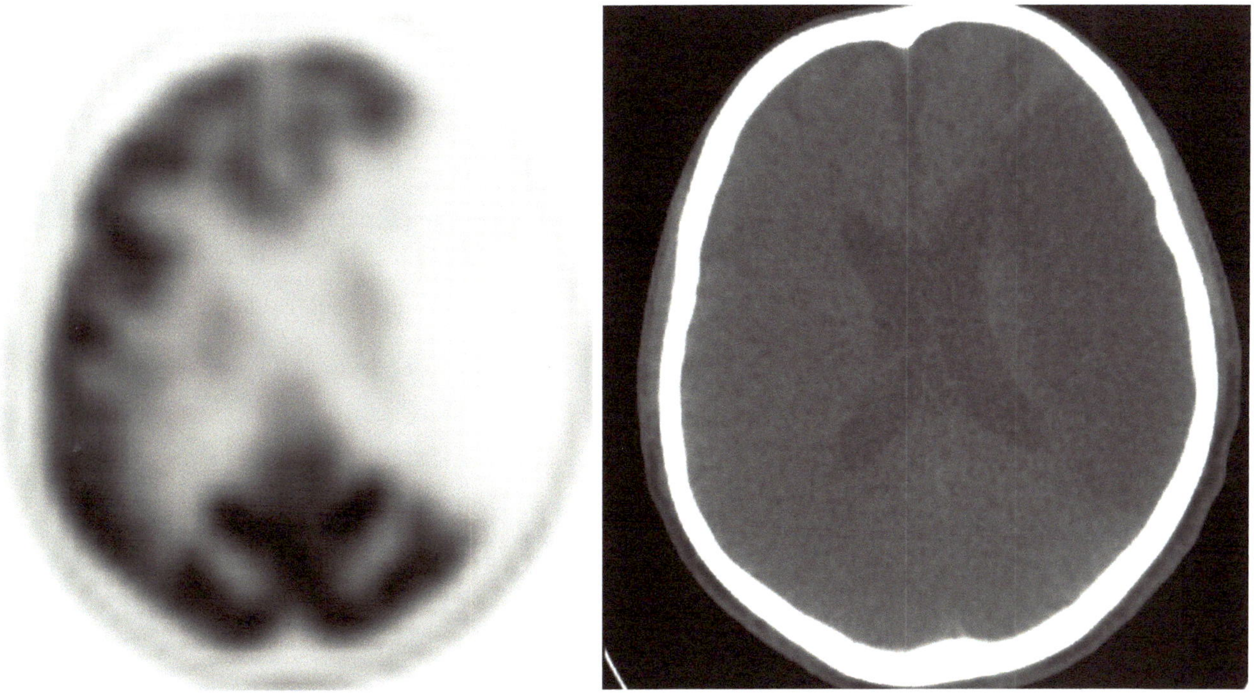

Fig. 2.1 Previously diagnosed remote cerebrovascular infarction presenting with diminished FDG uptake corresponding to the hypodense area on CT at left parietal and frontal lobes

T. Özülker, F. Özülker, *Atlas of PET-CT Imaging in Oncology: A Case-Based Guide to Image Interpretation*,
DOI 10.1007/978-3-319-18994-9_2

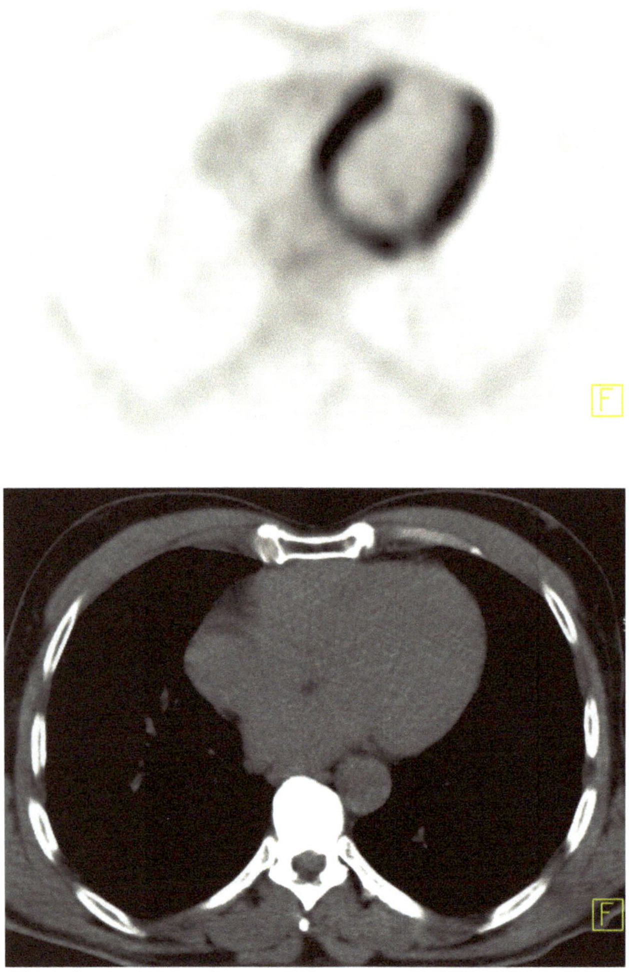

Fig. 2.2 Axial ^{18}F-FDG PET/CT image of the same patient at Fig. 2.1 showing hypometabolism at apicoseptal wall of left ventricle representing an infarct

Arachnoid Cyst

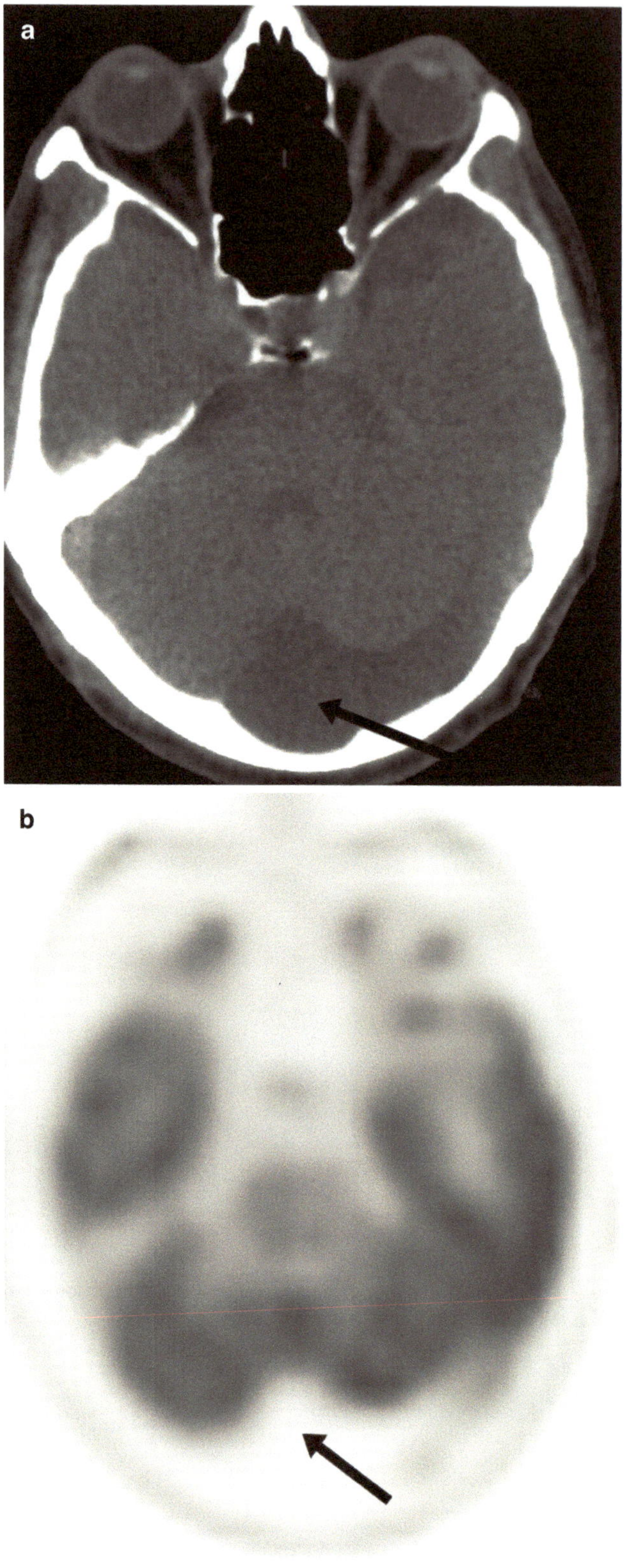

Fig. 2.3 Axial CT image (**a**) shows collection of CSF-attenuation fluid in posterior fossa (*arrow*) without any FDG uptake at the corresponding PET image (**b**), which is consistent with left retrocerebellar arachnoid cyst. Arachnoid cysts are congenital abnormalities that constitutes 1 % of all intracranial lesions. FDG PET can show hypometabolism corresponding to an arachnoid cyst, with the adjacent compressed brain parenchyma showing relatively normal FDG activity

Microadenoma

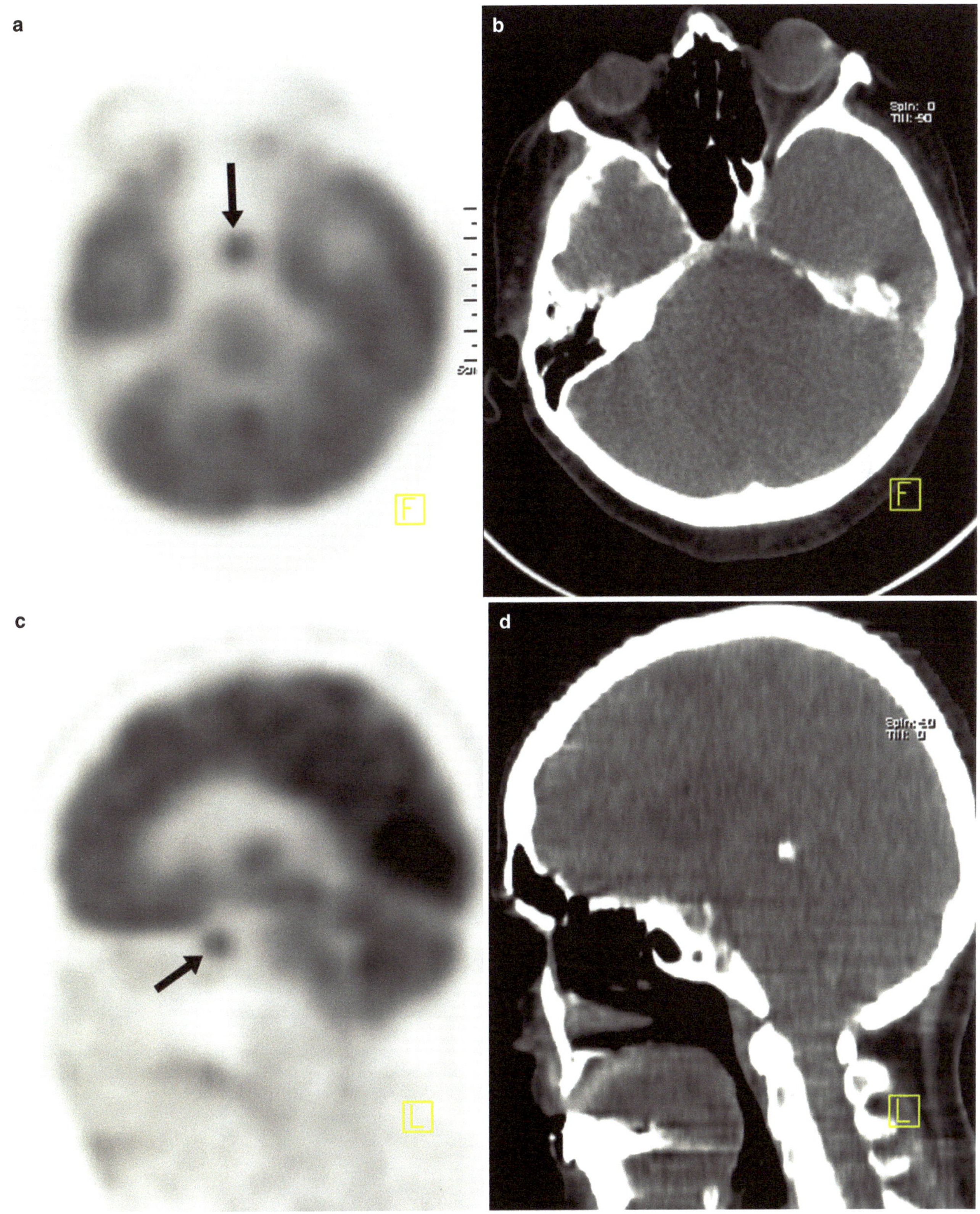

Fig. 2.4 Axial (**a**, **b**) and sagittal (**c**, **d**) PET and CT images of a patient showing a focus of mild hypermetabolism in the sellar region representing a microadenoma of pituitary gland (*arrow*)

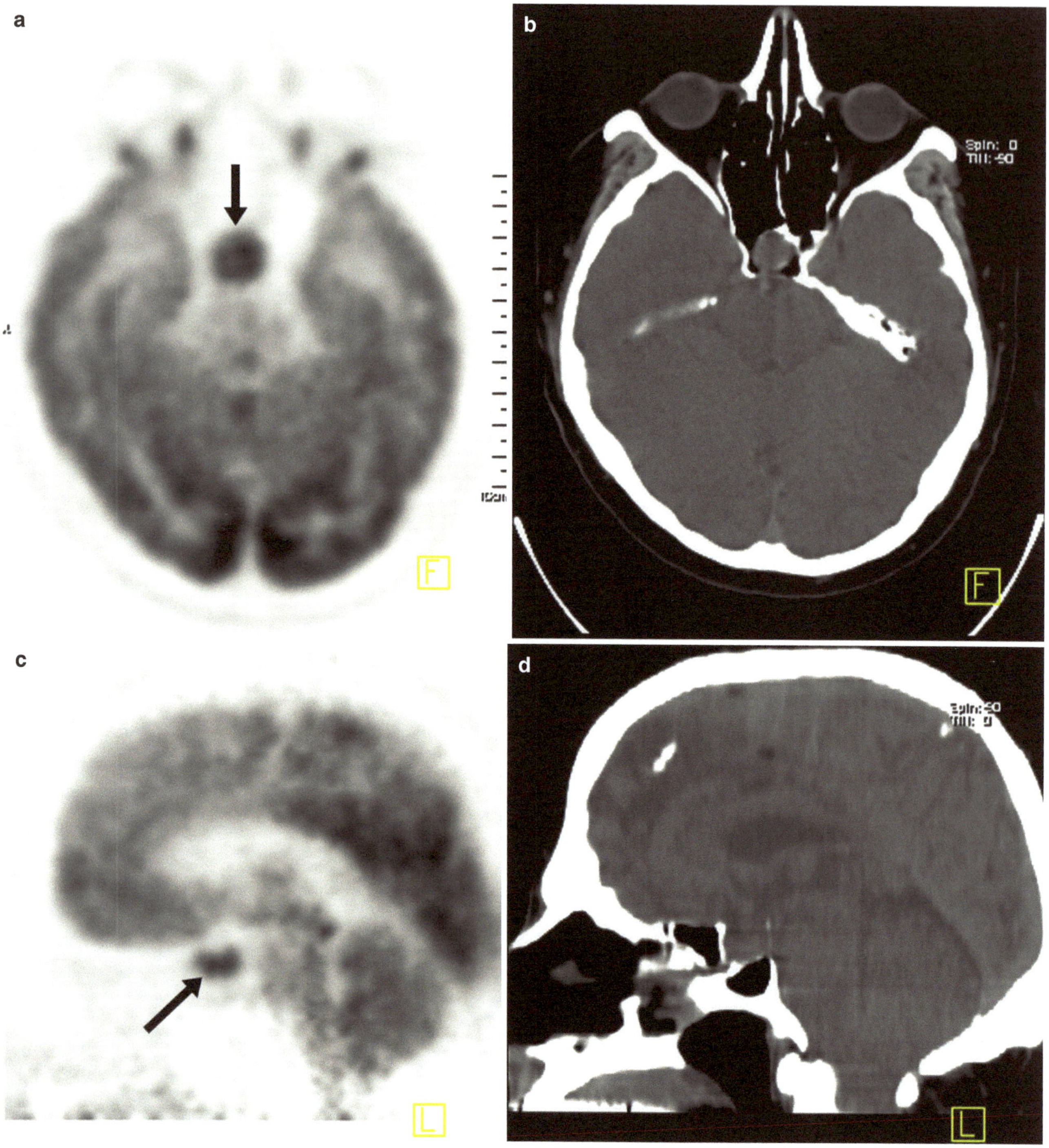

Fig. 2.5 Axial (**a**, **b**) and sagittal (**c**, **d**) PET and CT images of a patient showing a focus of intense hypermetabolism in the sellar region representing a macroadenoma of pituitary gland (*arrow*). Pituitary incidentalomas <10 mm are classified as microadenomas, and those >10 mm are macroadenomas. They are also classified according to their hormone secretion status as functioning or nonfunctioning adenomas. Macroadenomas show higher FDG uptake than microadenomas

Mastoiditis

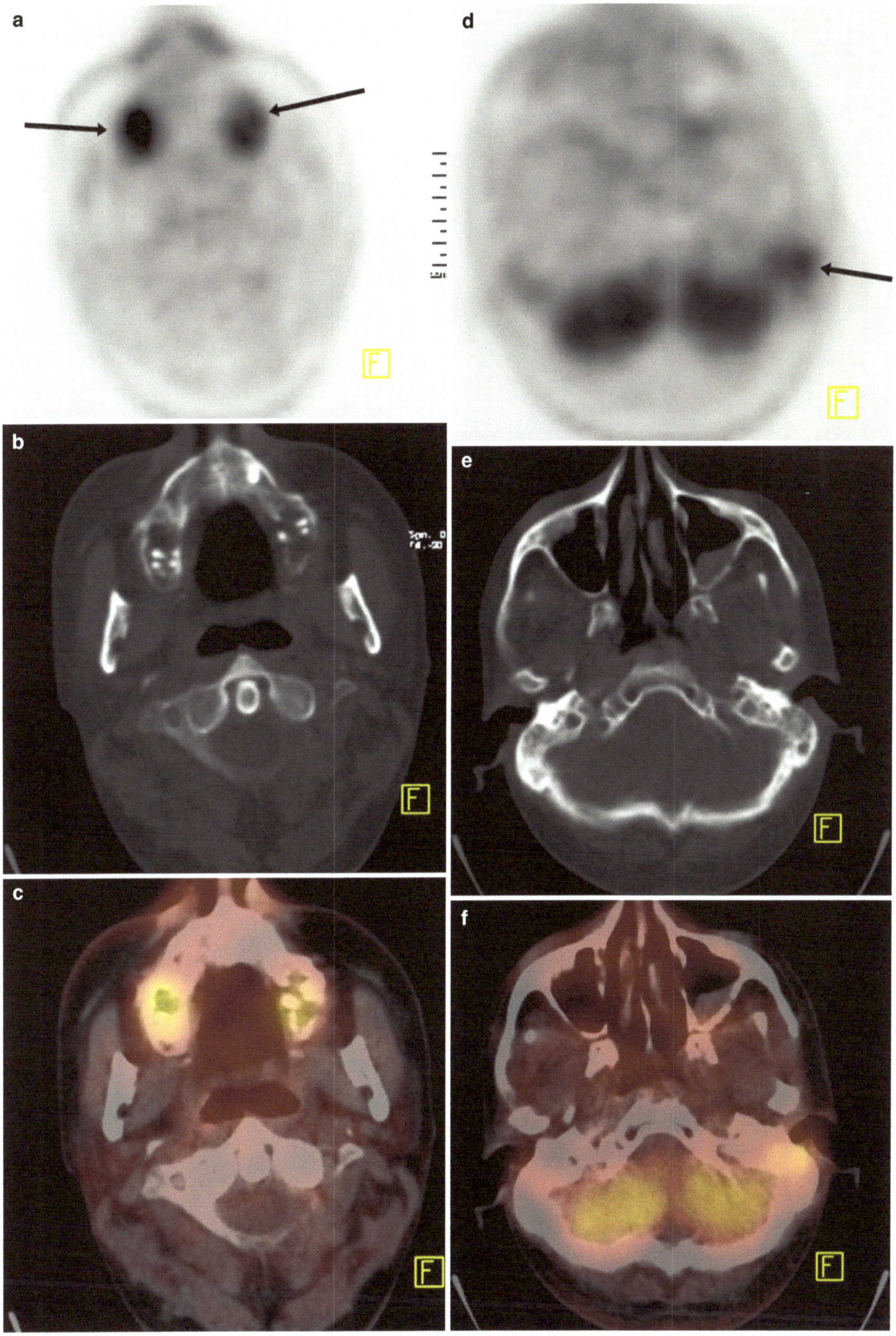

Fig. 2.6 Axial PET, CT, and fusion images showing increased FDG uptake at bilateral alveoli at maxilla due to tooth extraction (*arrows*) (**a–c**), axial PET, CT, and fusion images showing increased FDG uptake at left mastoid bone representing mastoiditis (*arrow*) (**d–f**)

Increased Activity at Masticatory Muscles

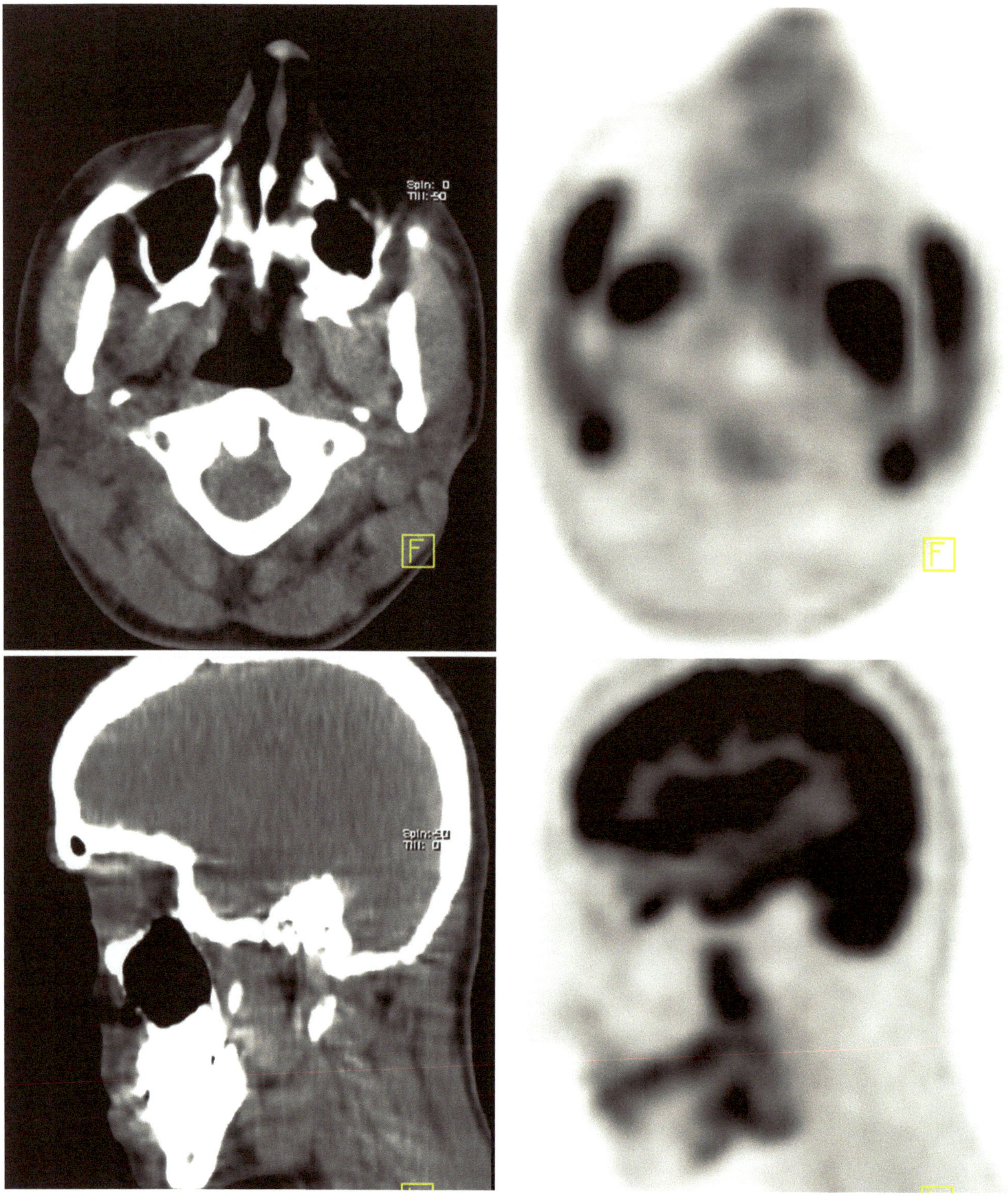

Fig. 2.7 The patient was chewing gum prior to imaging which caused increased masseter and pterygoid muscle activity

Maxillary Retention Cyst

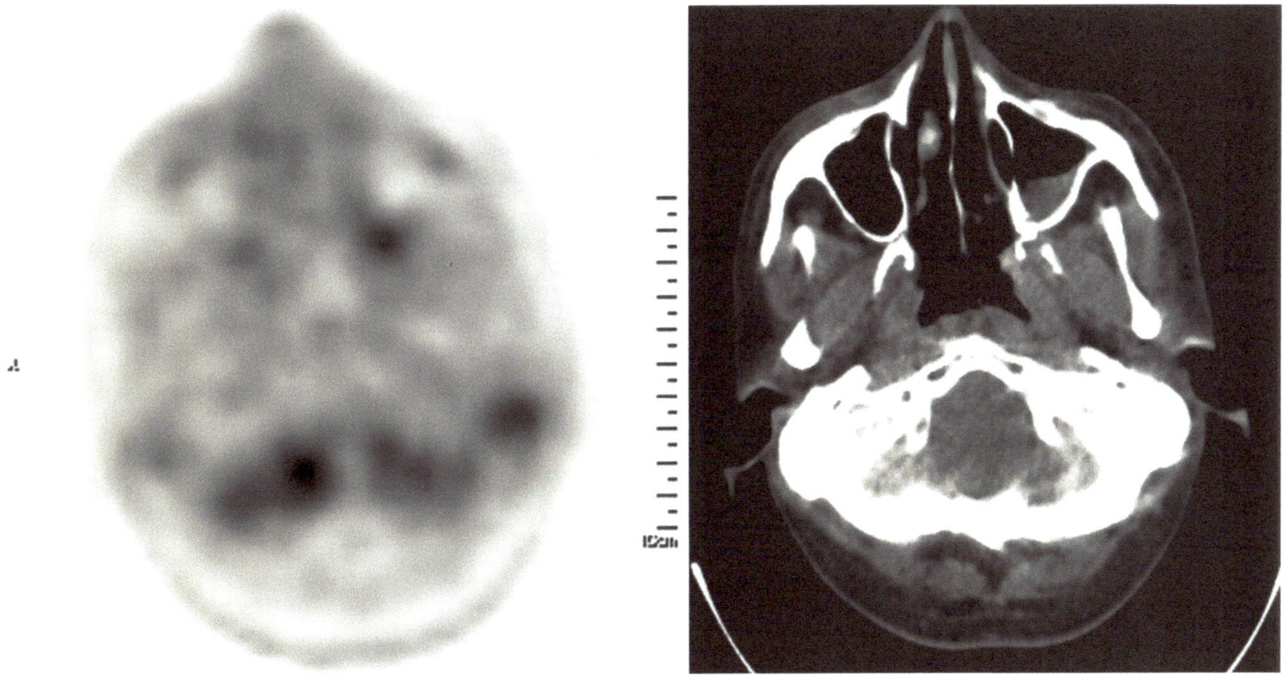

Fig. 2.8 Maxillary retention cyst at left maxillary sinus showing mild FDG uptake

Pleomorphic Adenoma

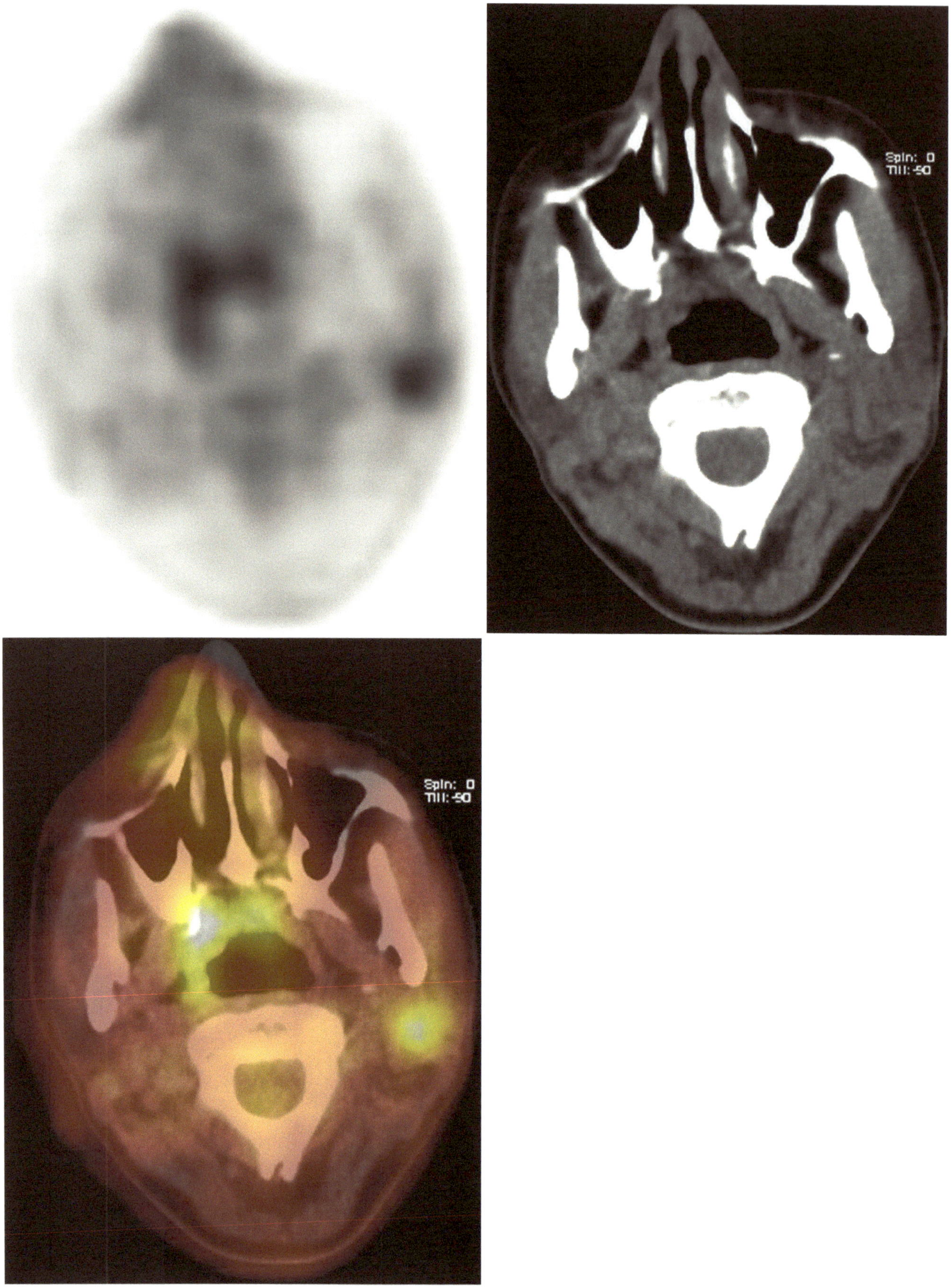

Fig. 2.9 Pleomorphic adenoma at left parotid gland showing mildly increased FDG uptake (SUVmax 2.9)

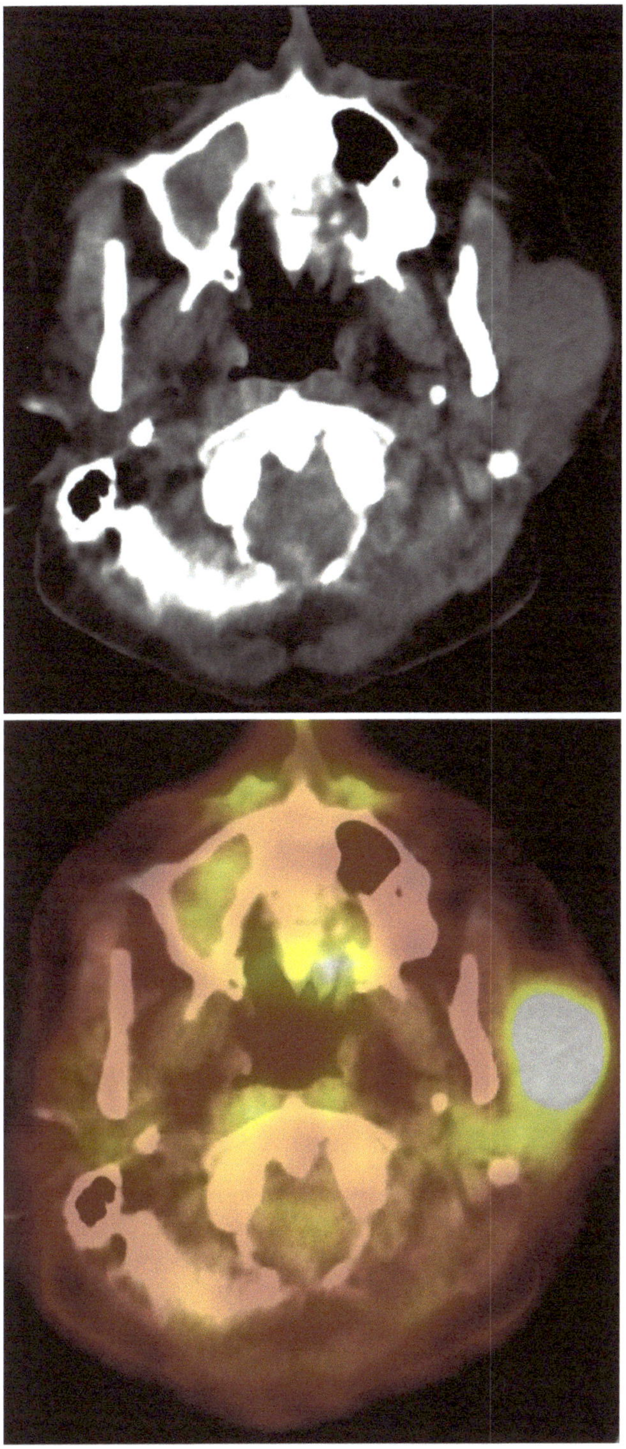

Fig. 2.10 Pleomorphic adenoma at left parotid gland showing significantly increased FDG uptake (SUVmax 5.5). Pleomorphic adenomas are FDG avid benign lesions causing false positive appearance at FDG PET and their metabolic activity increases as the size of the lesion increases

Warthin Tumor

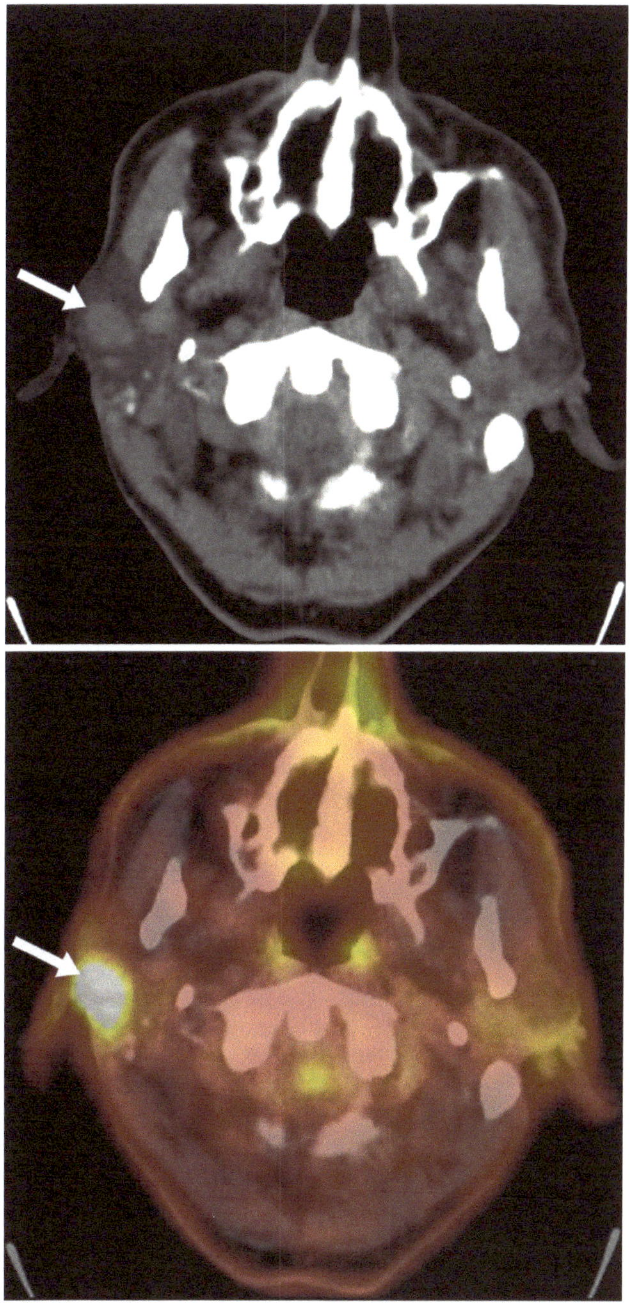

Fig. 2.11 Axial CT and fusion images of a 75-year-old male with Warthin tumor of the right parotid gland (*arrow*) (SUV max 6.5)

Sjögren's Syndrome

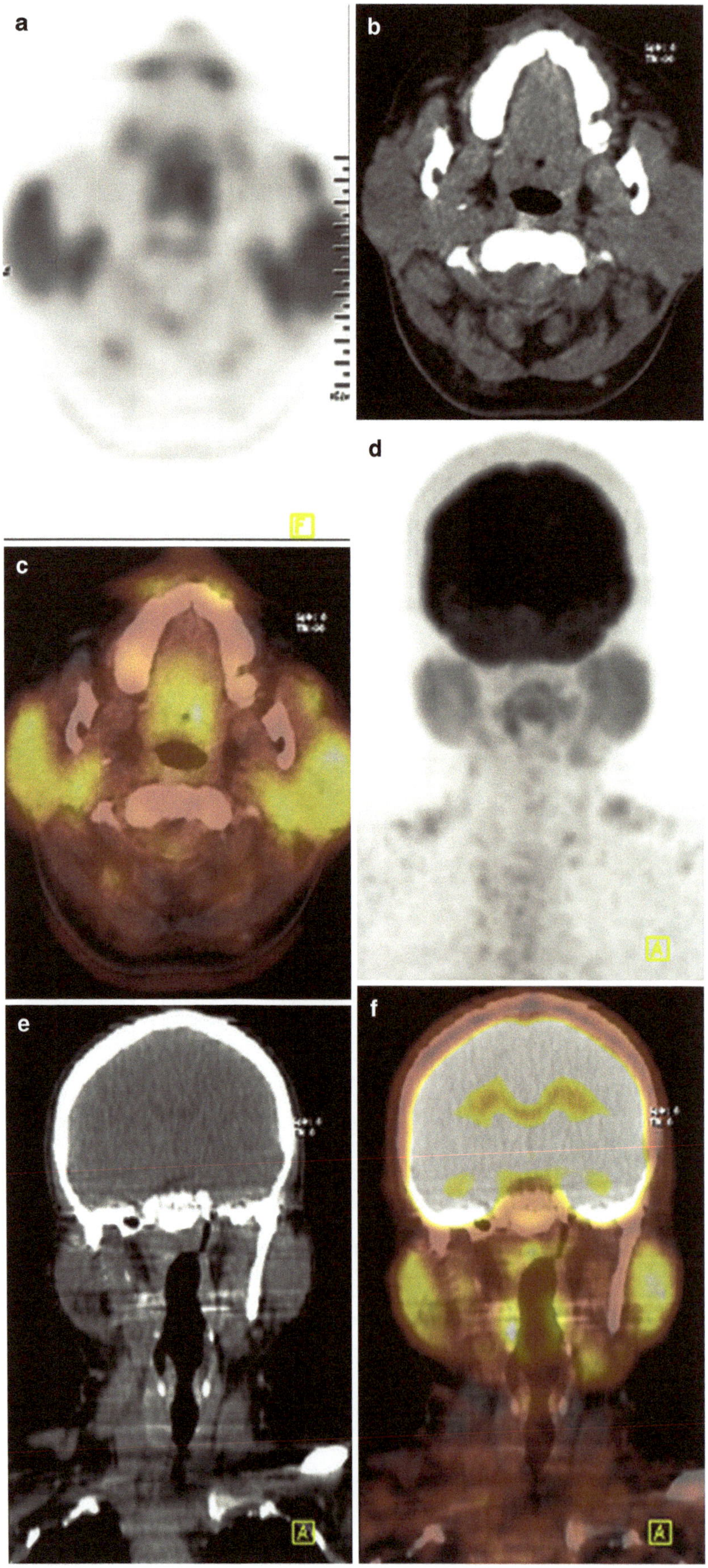

Fig. 2.12 Axial (**a**, **b**, **c**) and coronal (**d**, **e**, **f**) images showing increased FDG uptake at both parotid glands due to Sjögren's syndrome

Asymmetrical Uptake at Tongue Muscle

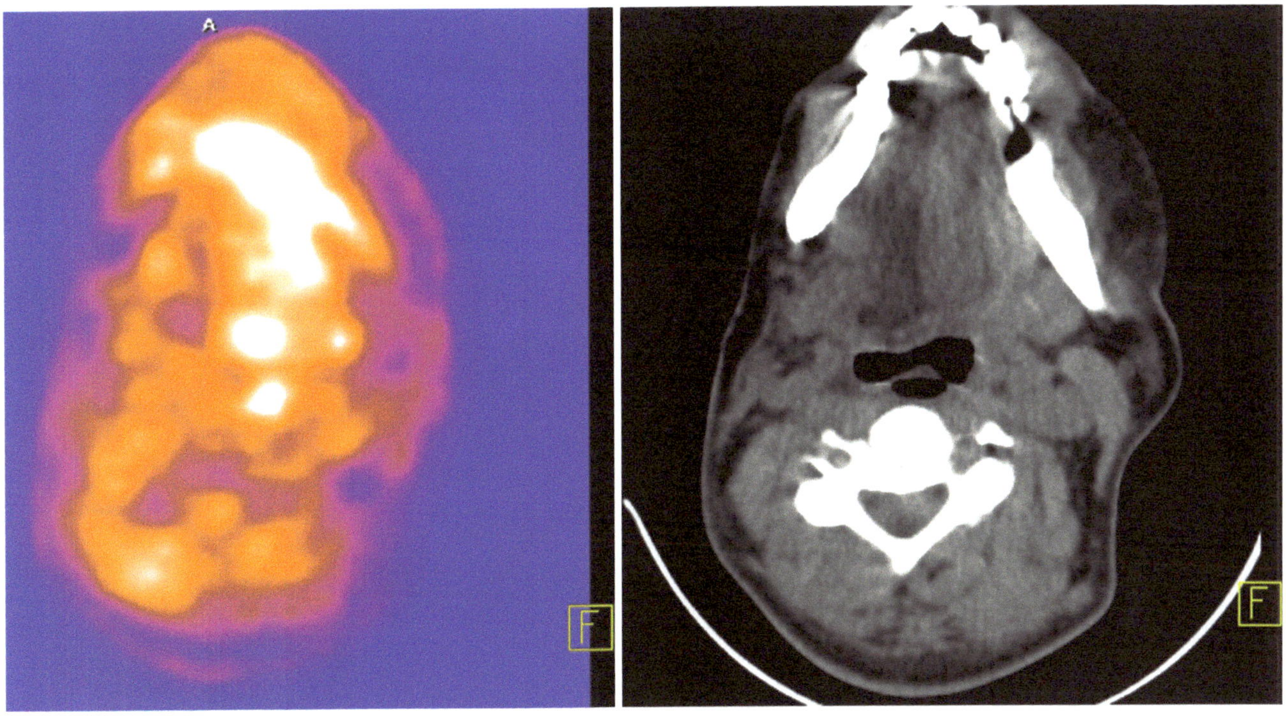

Fig. 2.13 A 55-year-old patient with nasopharynx carcinoma had right sided glossopharyngeal nerve paralysis which resulted in asymmetrical FDG uptake at left side of the tongue

Focal Infection at the Base of the Tongue

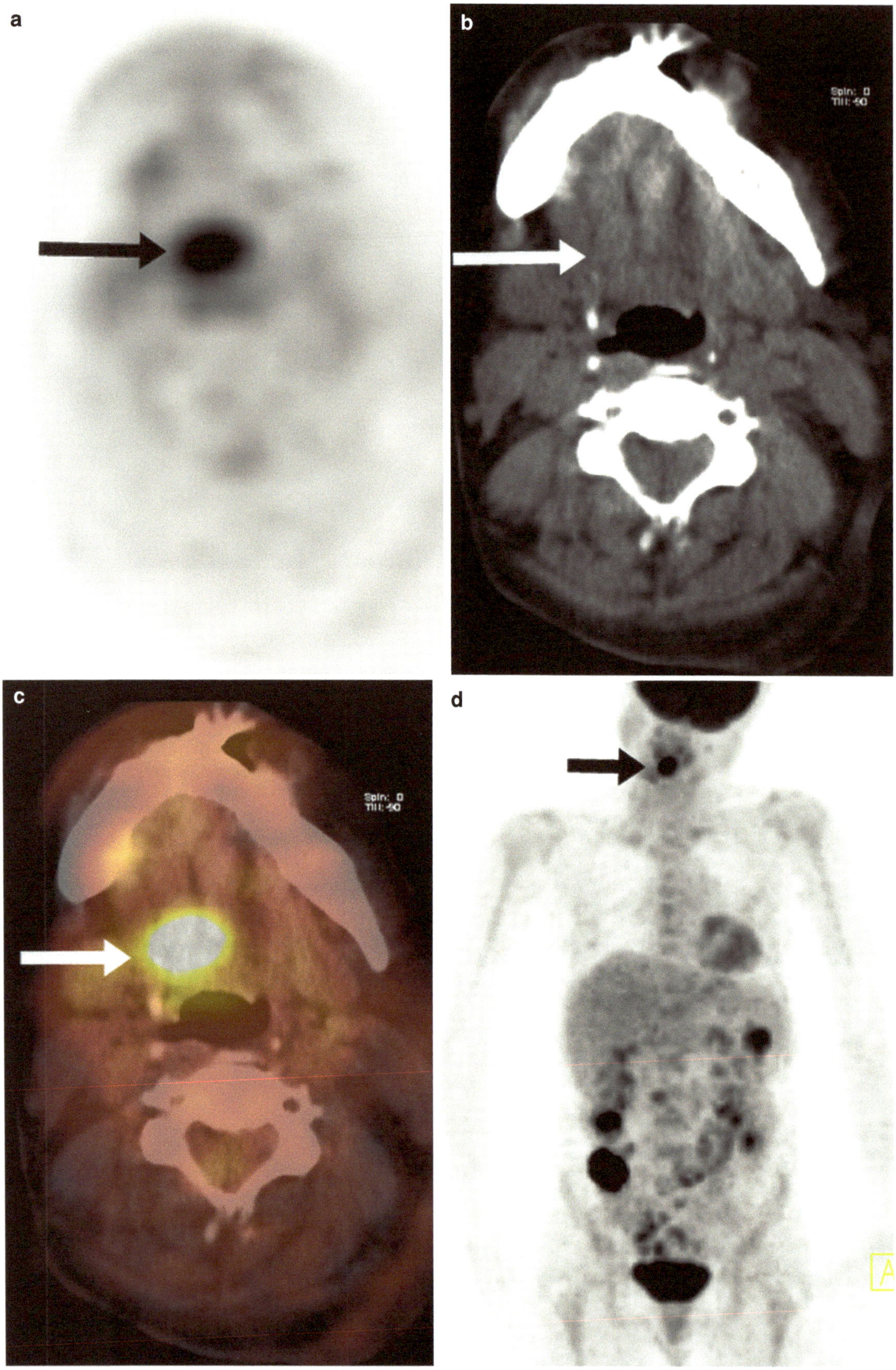

Fig. 2.14 Axial PET and CT (**a**, **b**), fusion and MIP (**c**, **d**) images showing focal increased FDG uptake at the base of the tongue consistent with focal infection (*arrows*)

Osteonecrosis at Mandibula

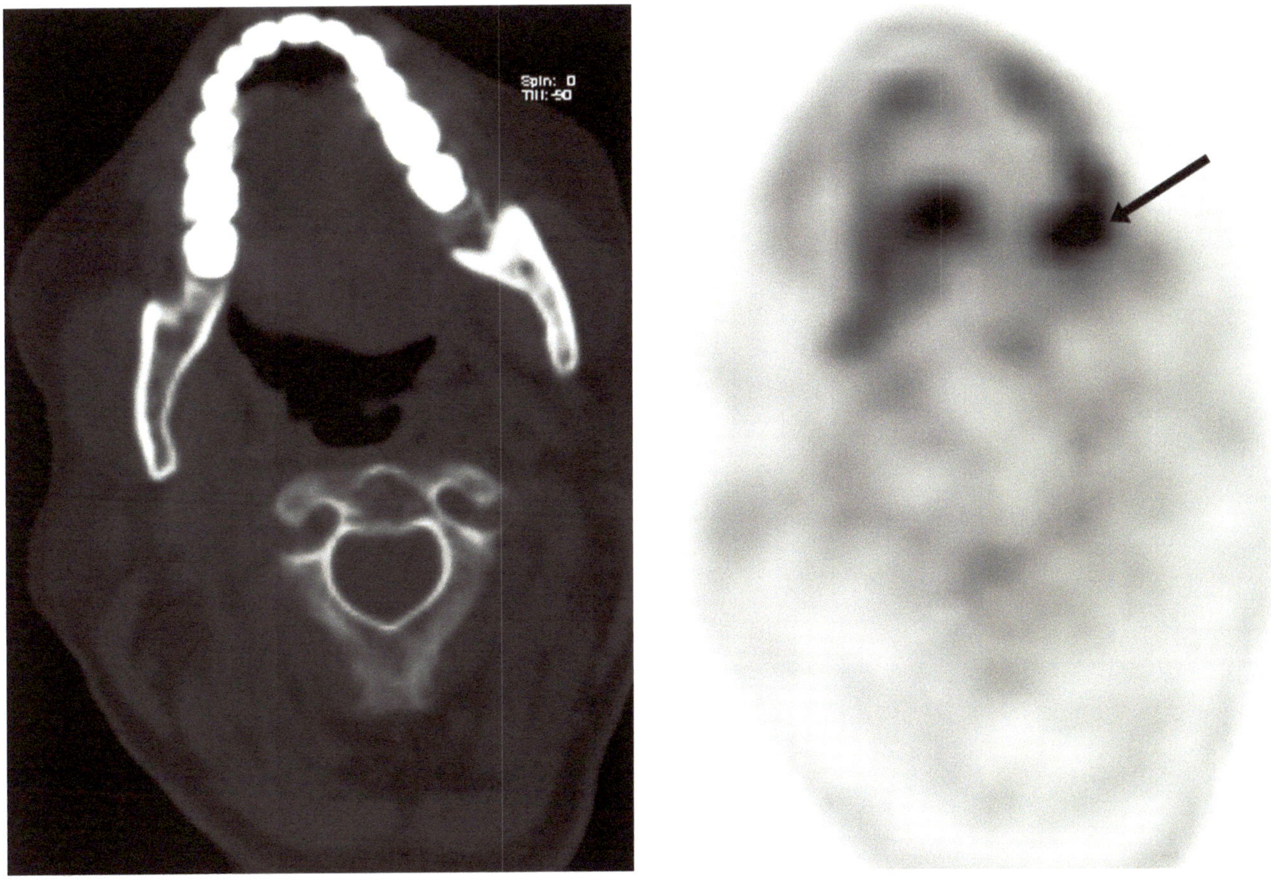

Fig. 2.15 Axial CT and PET images showing focal increased FDG uptake at left retromolar trigone due to osteonecrosis (*arrow*)

Cord Vocal Paralysis

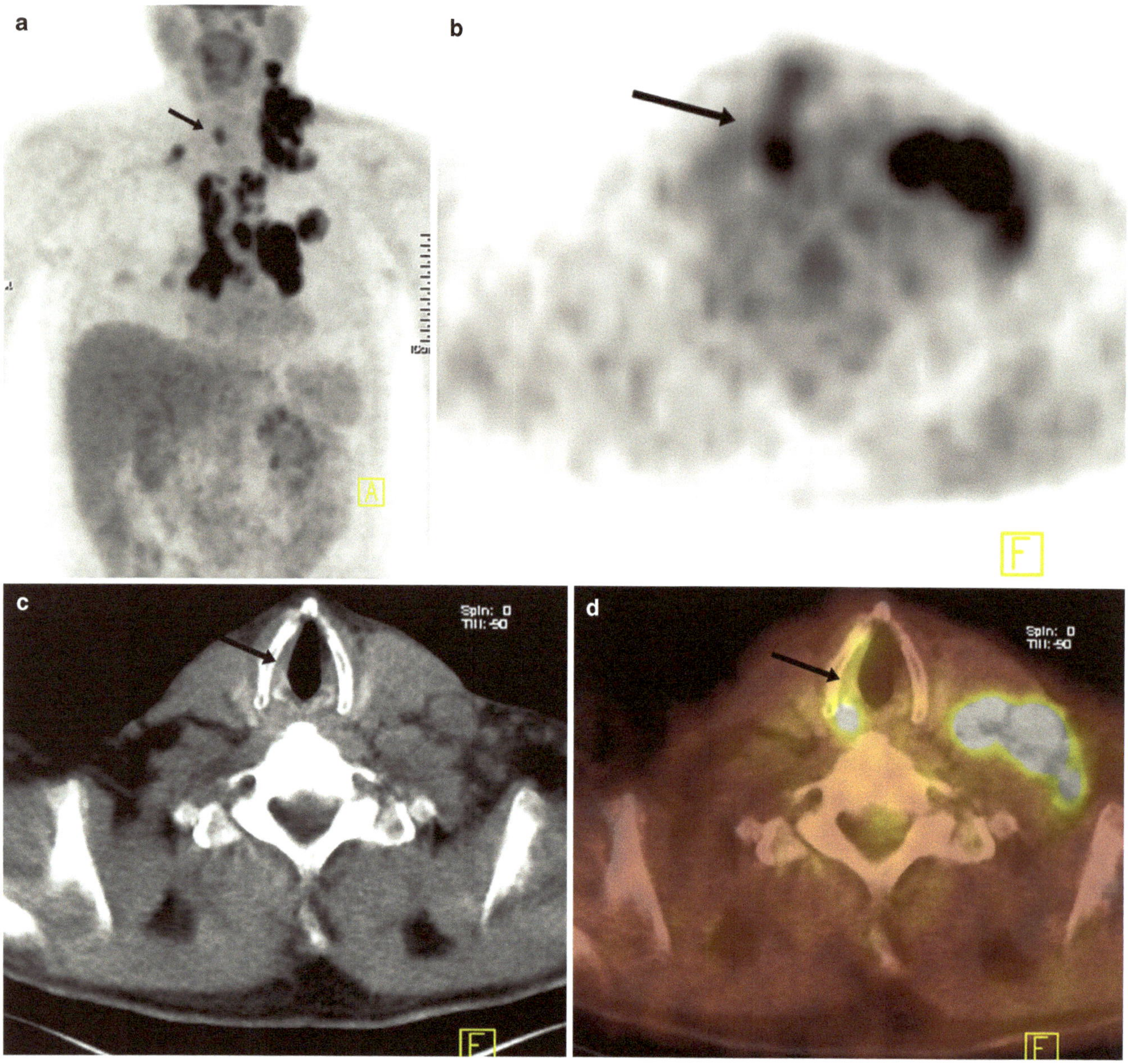

Fig. 2.16 MIP image shows intensely increased FDG uptake at left hilar mass lesion, right mediastinal and left cervical lymph nodes (**a**), axial PET, CT, and fusion images (**b–d**) show asymmetrically increased FDG uptake at right vocal cord (*arrows*). Compression of the recurrent laryngeal nerve by the mass lesion at hilar region leads to ipsilateral vocal cord paralysis. Unusual asymmetrical FDG uptake is detected due to excessive muscle activity of the functional vocal cord as it compensates for paralysis of the contralateral vocal cord

Increased Vocal Cord Uptake

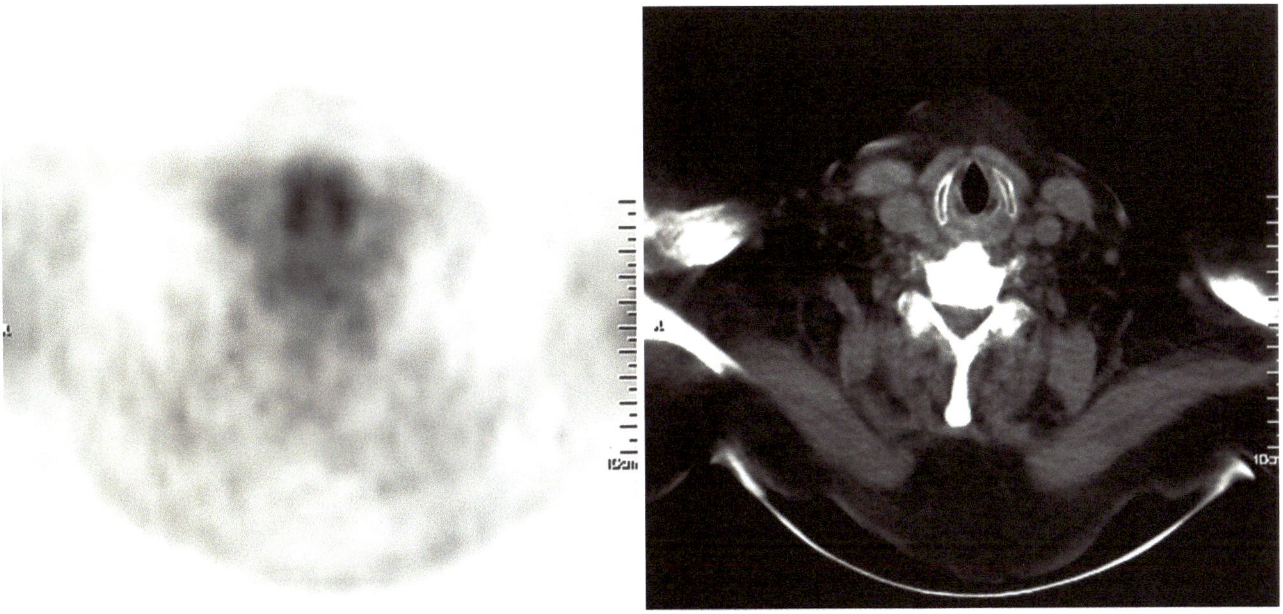

Fig. 2.17 Patient was shouting during the uptake phase that followed injection of the tracer

Incidentally Found Thyroid Nodule

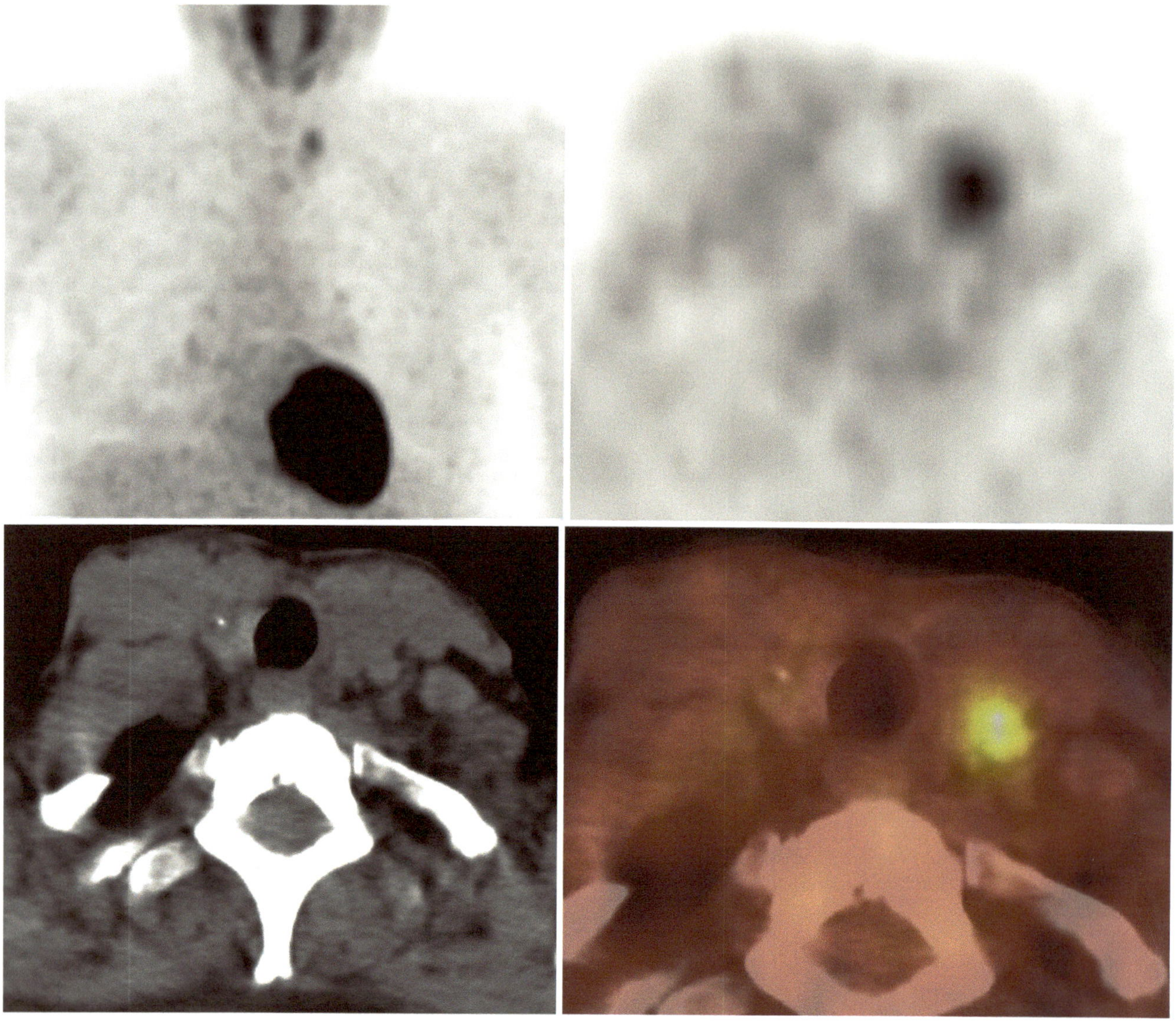

Fig. 2.18 Focal ^{18}F-FDG uptake at left lobe of thyroid gland in a thyroid nodule found incidentally. Lesion turned out to be benign colloid nodule. Focal high uptake of ^{18}F-FDG in the thyroid as an incidental finding occurs in approximately 1 % of the patients undergoing PET/CT examination. One third of these lesions are malignant in nature

Chronic Thyroiditis

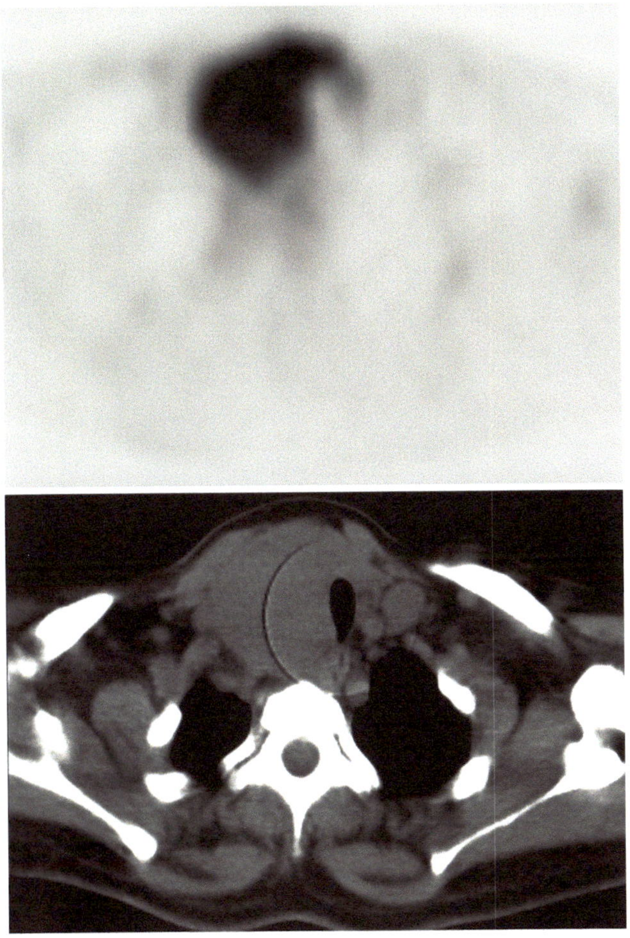

Fig. 2.19 Axial PET and CT images show diffuse intense FDG uptake at both thyroid lobes being more prominent at right. Chronic thyroiditis may cause intense and FDG uptake, unlike the focal uptake of nodules

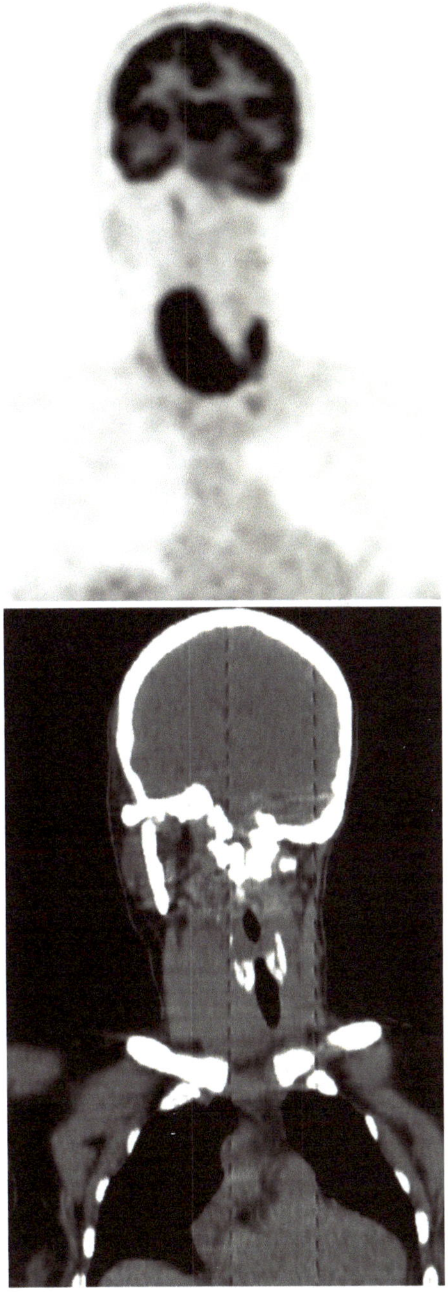

Fig. 2.20 Coronal PET and CT images

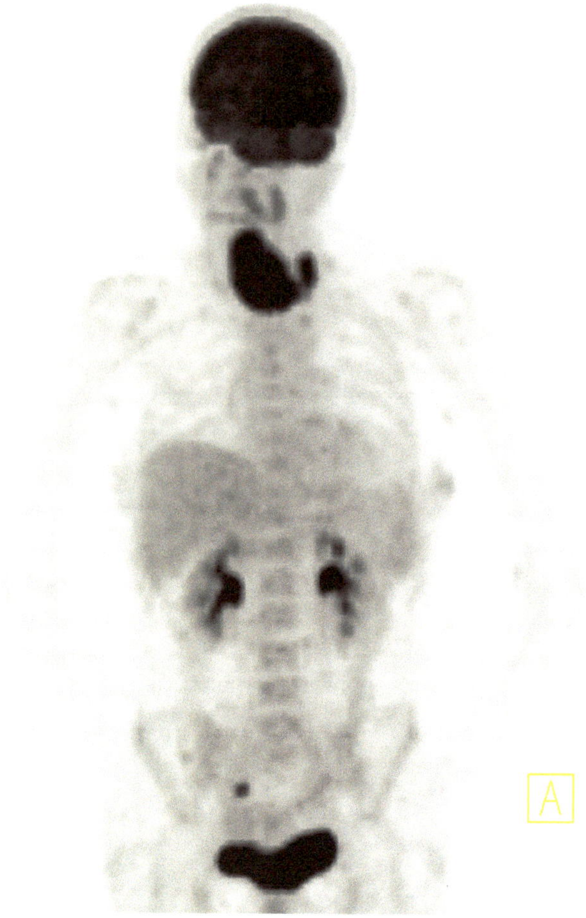

Fig. 2.21 MIP image

Discoid Lupus Erythrematosus

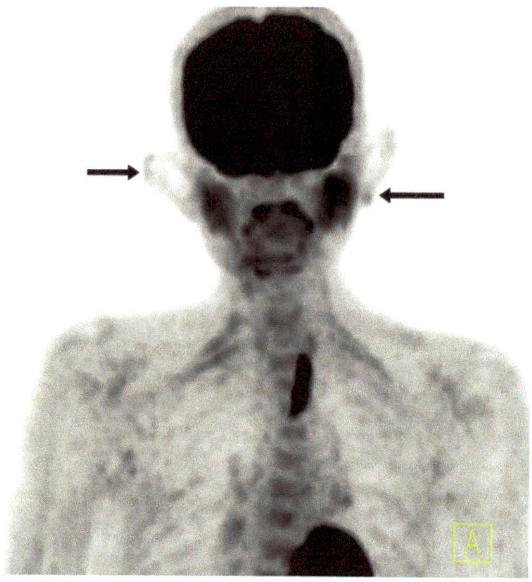

Fig. 2.22 A 55-year-old male patient with unusual FDG uptake at both ears due to inflammation secondary to discoid lupus erythrematosus (*arrows*)

2.2 Thorax

Physiologically Increased Uptake at Lactating Patient with Breast Cancer

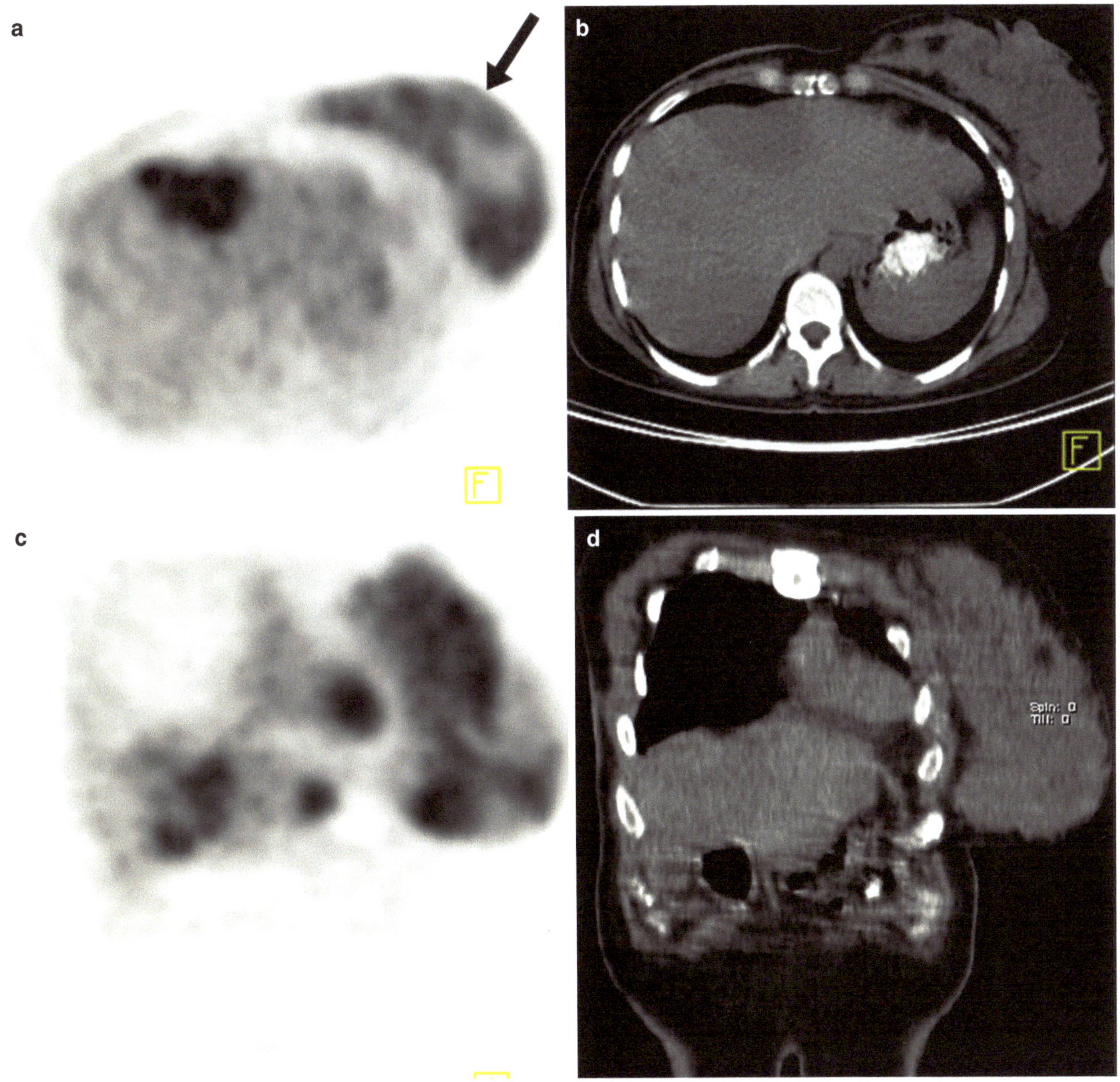

Fig. 2.23 A 38-year-old woman underwent right mastectomy for breast cancer. ^{18}F-FDG PET/CT is performed 1 month after she gave birth to a baby and while she was lactating. Axial (**a**, **b**) and coronal (**c**, **d**) PET and CT images show metastatic hypermetabolic lesions at left lobe of liver and diffuse physiologically increased uptake at left breast (*arrow*)

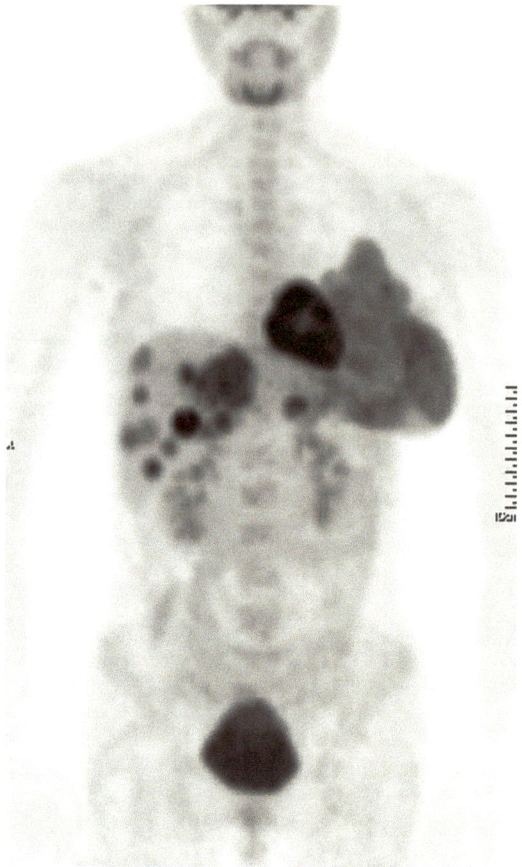

Fig. 2.24 MIP image of patient

Physiologically Increased Uptake at Lactating Breast

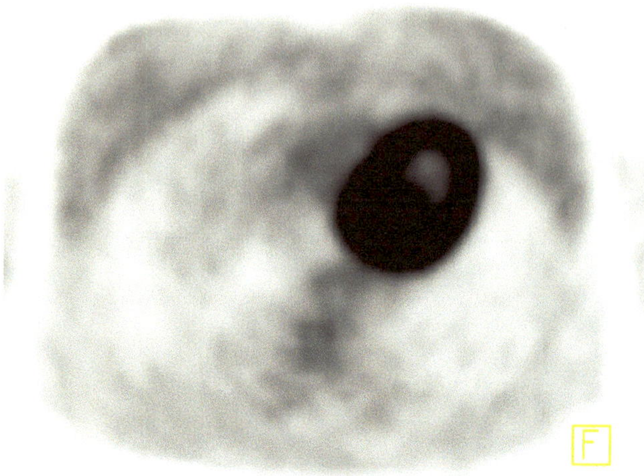

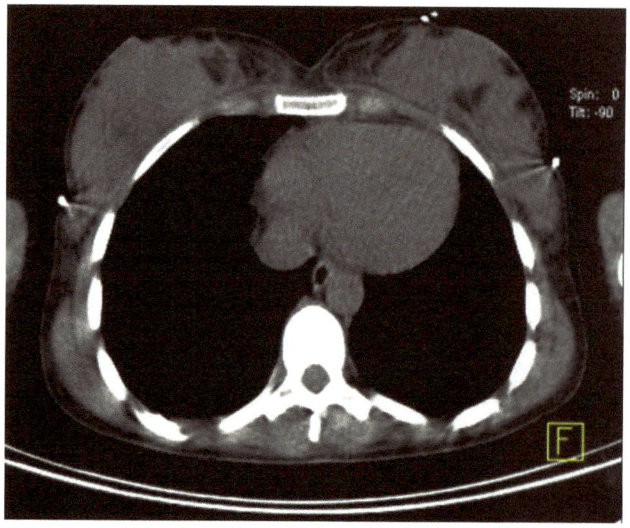

Fig. 2.25 Axial PET and CT images of a 28-year-old female patient display physiologically increased uptake at both breasts while she was lactating

Seroma After Breast Surgery

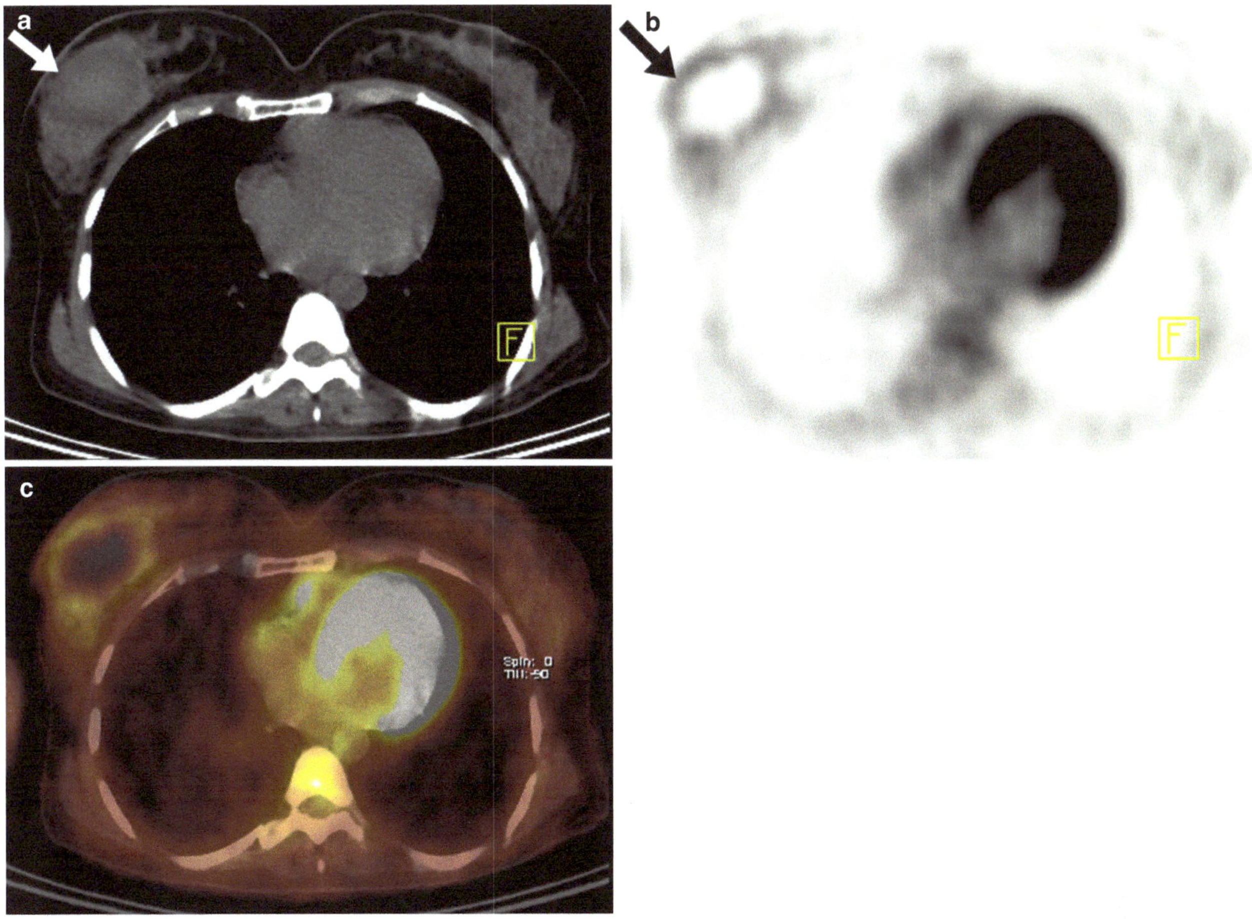

Fig. 2.26 Axial CT, PET, and fusion images of a female patient who underwent lumpectomy for a mass lesion at right breast (**a**–**c**). Hypodense lesion on CT is consistent with fluid collection at surgery site. PET image shows circumferentially increased FDG uptake at seroma (*arrows*)

Thymic Uptake

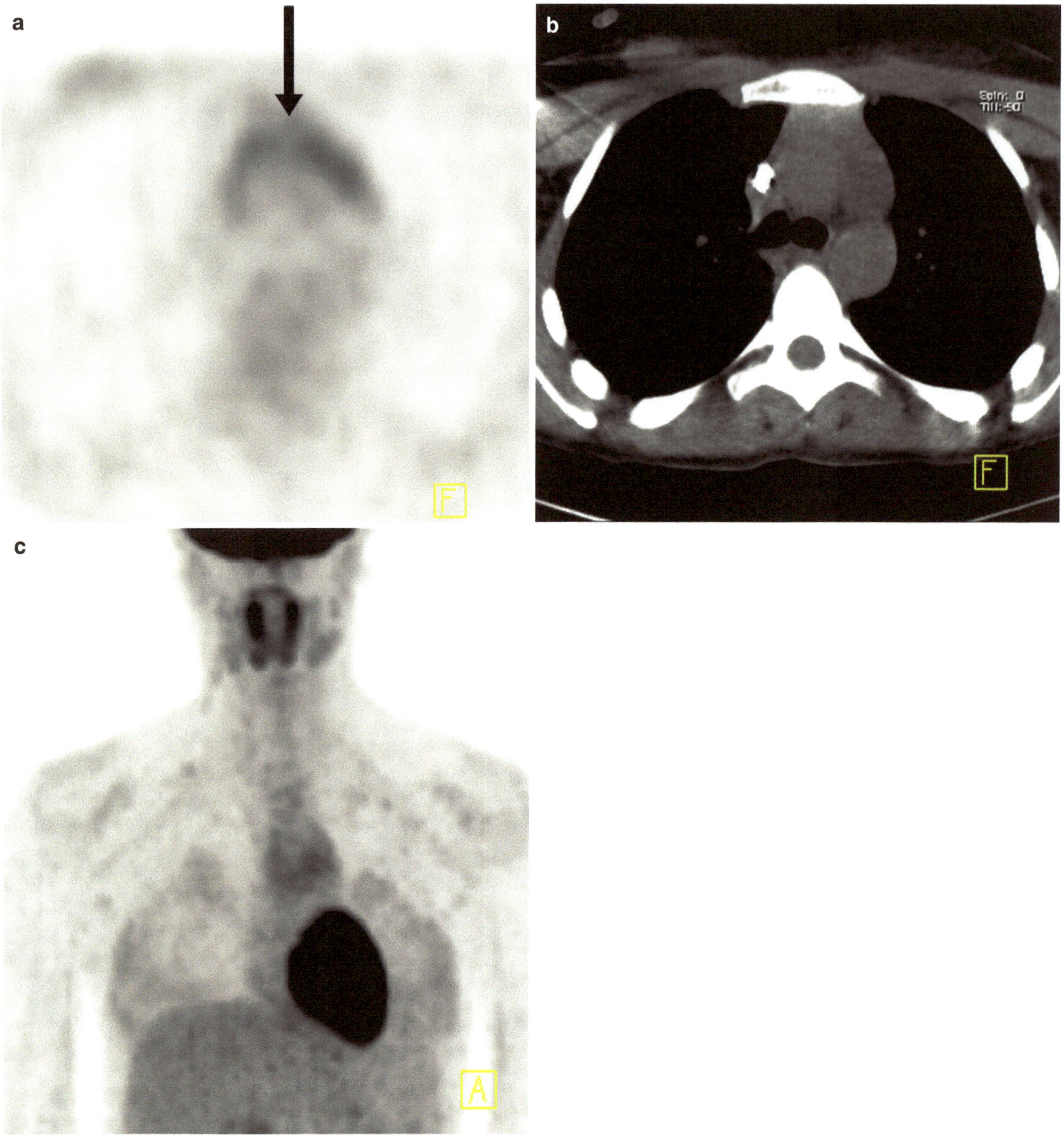

Fig. 2.27 A 20-year-old female with lymphoma underwent ^{18}F-FDG PET/CT scan for recurrence detection. Minimally increased physiological FDG uptake (SUVmax 3.8) at thymus is noted *(arrow)* (**a**–**c**). Increased thymic ^{18}F-FDG uptake may represent normal physiologic uptake but may also indicate the presence of thymic hyperplasia, lymphomatous infiltration, primary thymic neoplasm, or metastatic disease. It may be seen in post chemotherapy patients as a result of rebound hyperplasia

Hamartoma

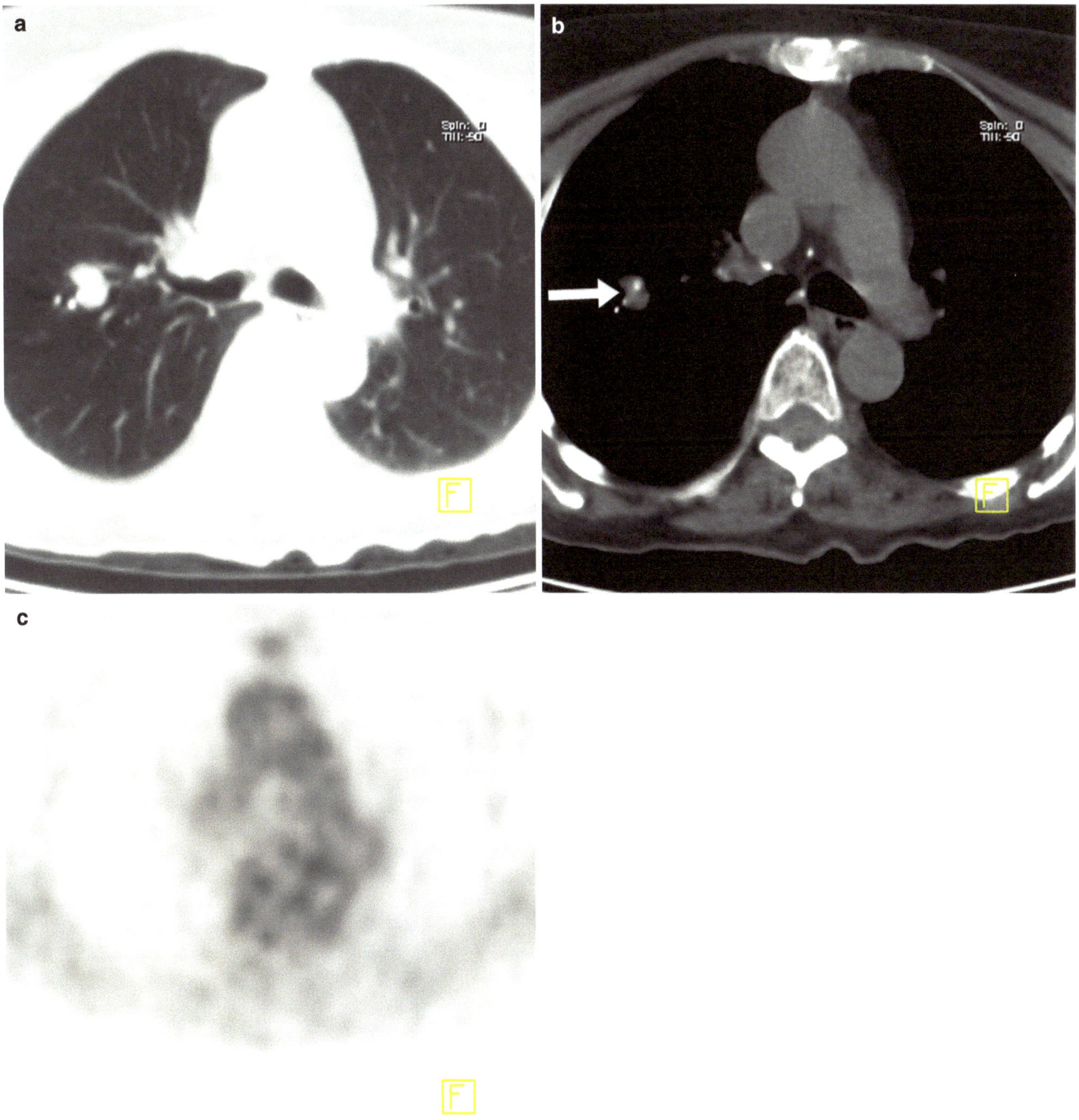

Fig. 2.28 Solid lesion with lobulated contours and a focus of calcification on CT (*arrow*) is consistent with hamartoma (**a**, **b**). The lesion does not show any corresponding FDG uptake (**c**). A pulmonary hamartoma is a benign neoplasm composed of cartilage, connective tissue, muscle, fat, and bone. Hamartomas rarely show FDG uptake

Pneuomothorax

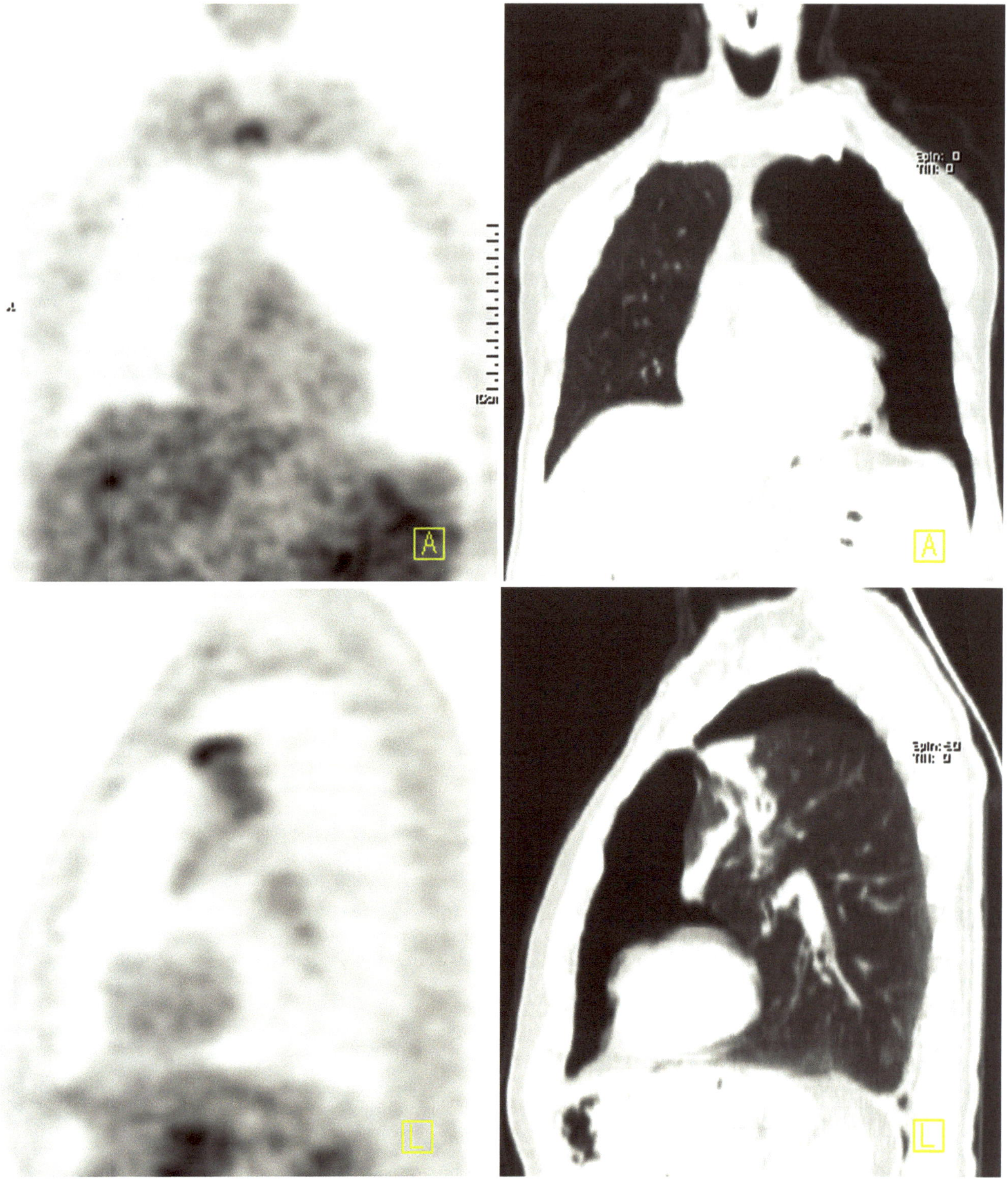

Fig. 2.29 Coronal and sagittal PET and CT images of a patient who is being staged for lung carcinoma show pneumothorax developed following a lung biopsy

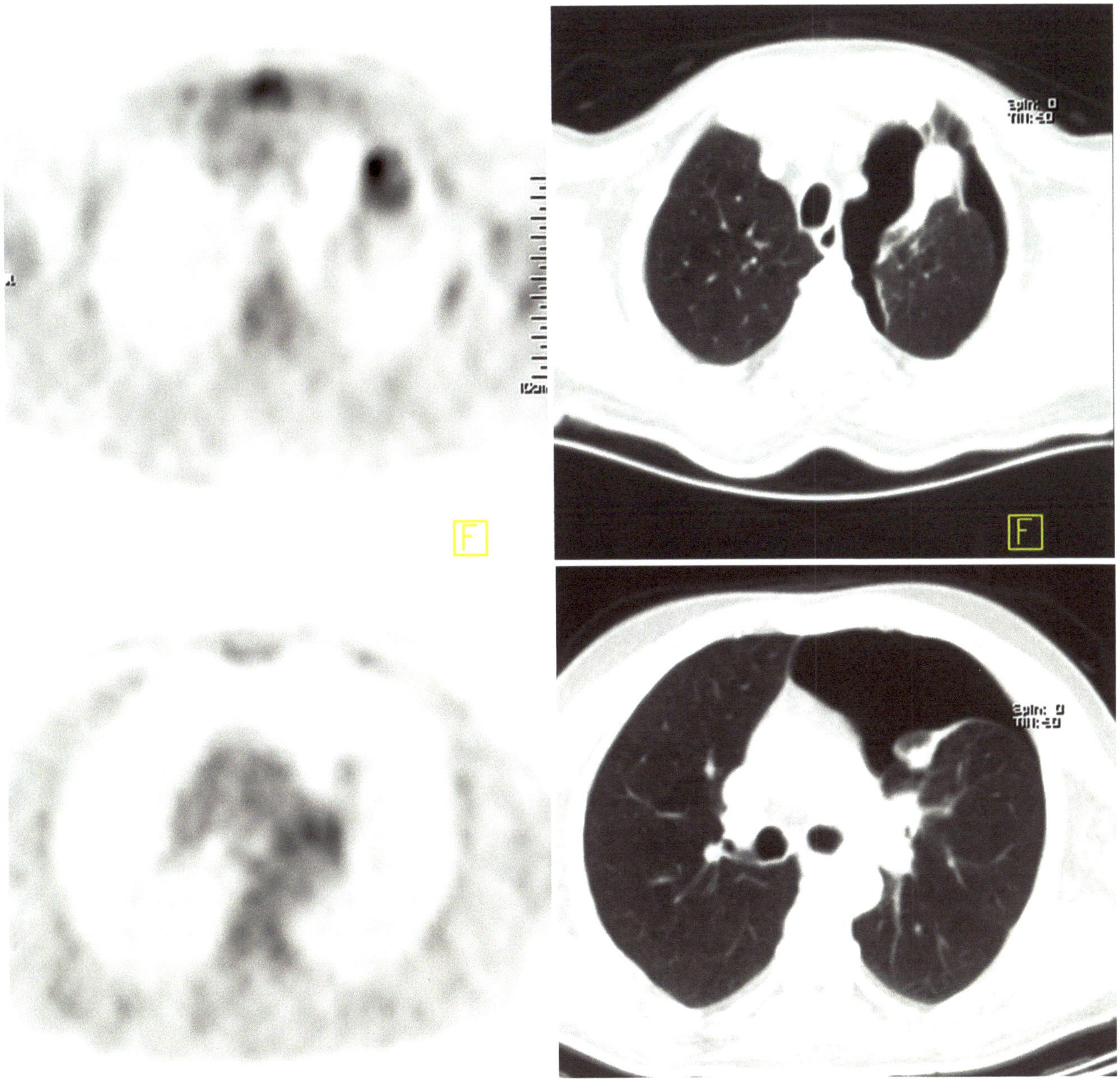

Fig. 2.30 Axial PET and CT images of the patient

Postradiotherapy Inflammation

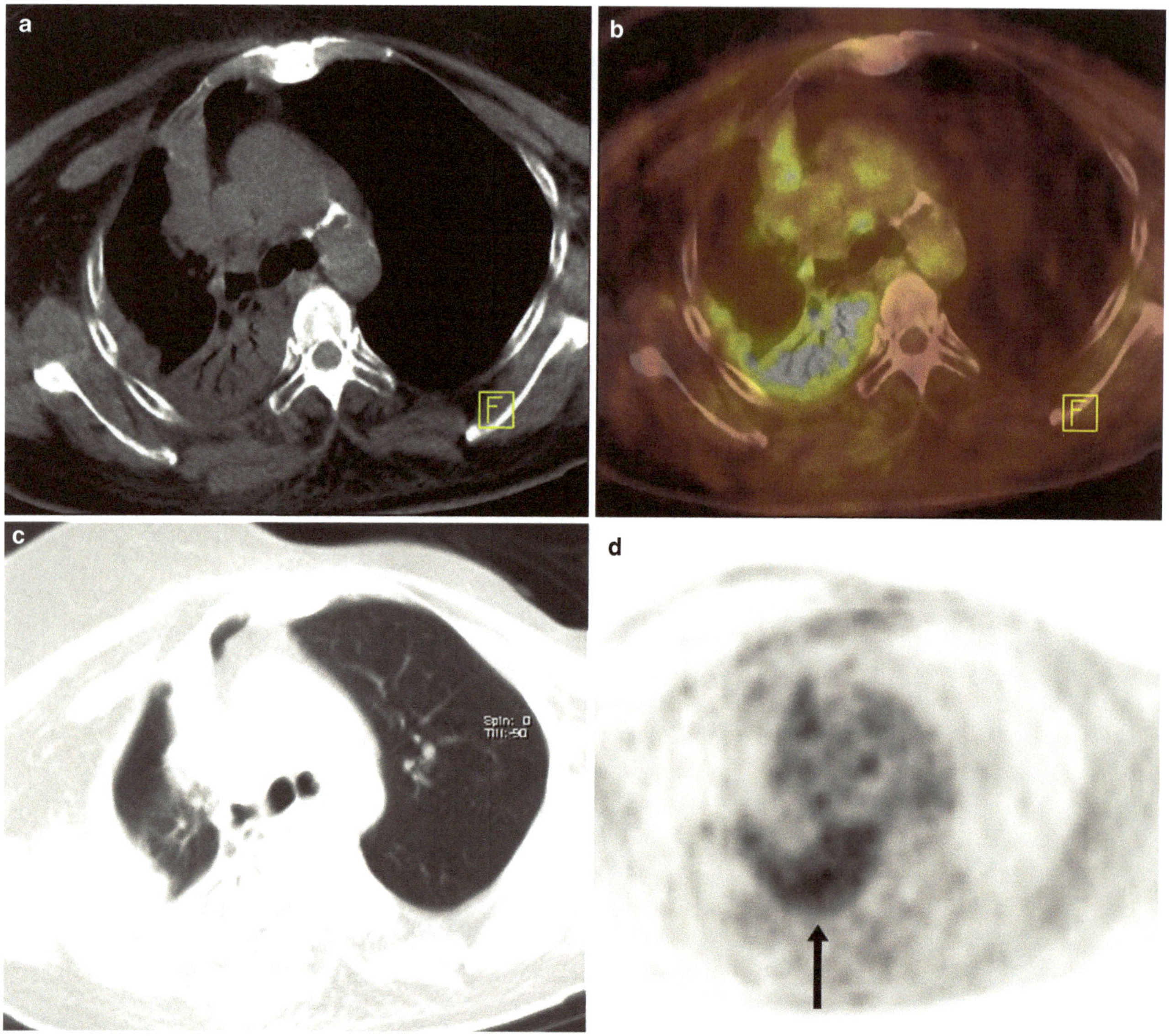

Fig. 2.31 A 63-year-old female patient underwent external beam radiotherapy (EBRT) for lung cancer. ^{18}F-FDG PET/CT is performed for evaluation of therapy response. Axial CT (**a**, **c**), fusion (**b**), and PET (**d**) images display mildly increased diffuse FDG uptake at the consolidation area with air bronchogram, representing postradiotherapy inflammation (*arrow*)

Pulmonary Infection After Chemotherapy

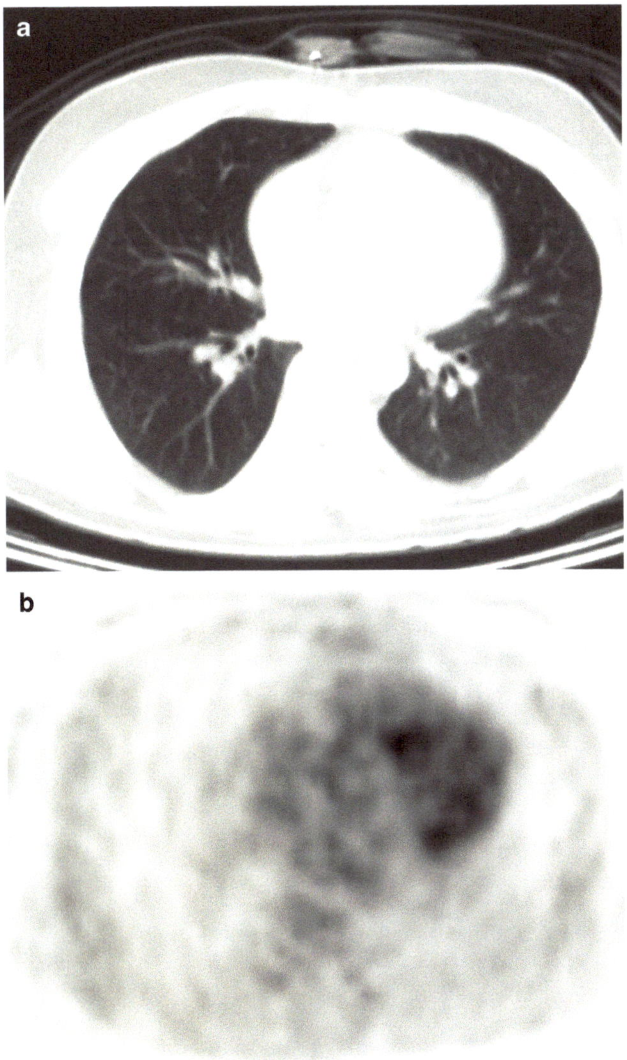

Fig. 2.32 A 32-year-old male patient with testicular carcinoma underwent ^{18}F-FDG PET/CT scan. Axial CT and PET images does not show any pathology (**a**, **b**)

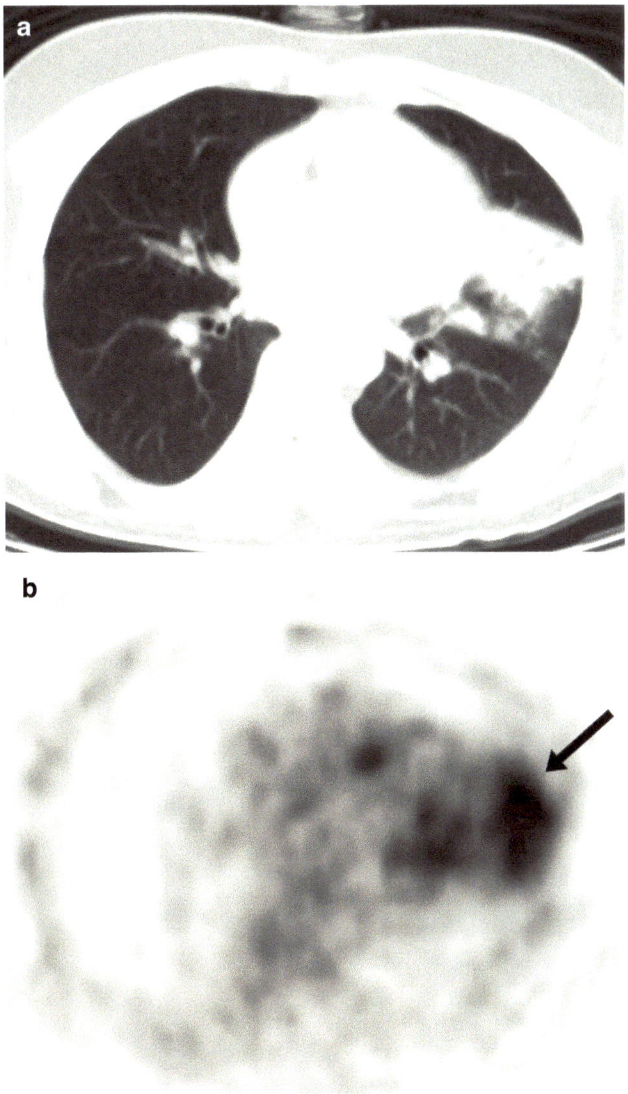

Fig. 2.33 ^{18}F-FDG PET/CT was repeated after the patient had chemotherapy, and mildly hypermetabolic infiltration at left lung compatible with infection was detected (*arrow*) (**a**, **b**)

Pneumonic Consolidation

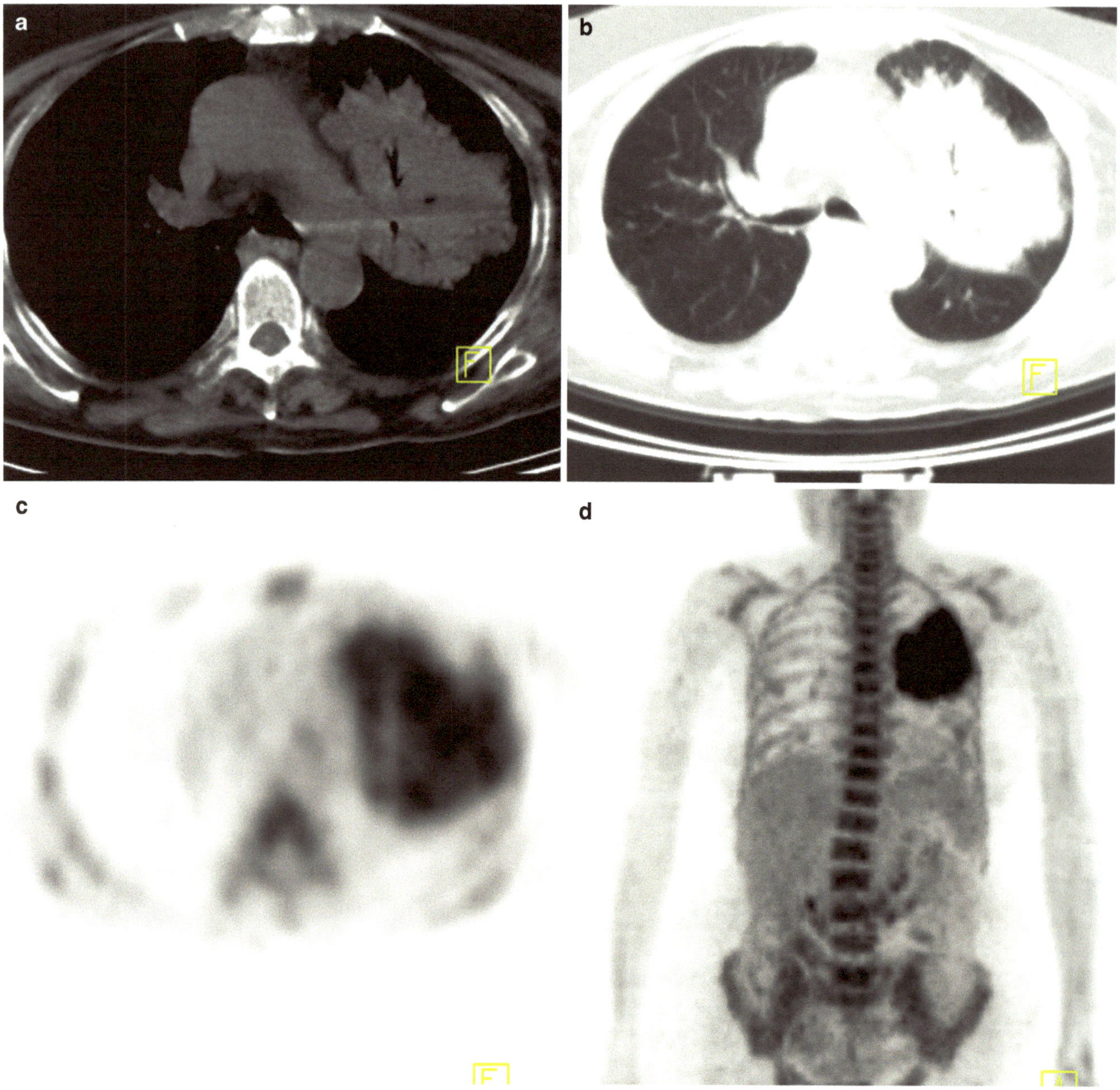

Fig. 2.34 A 74-year-old patient underwent ^{18}F-FDG PET/CT for oncologic workup. Axial CT (**a**, **b**), PET (**c**) and MIP (**d**) images show pneumonic consolidation area with high FDG uptake at left lung

Pulmonary Tuberculosis

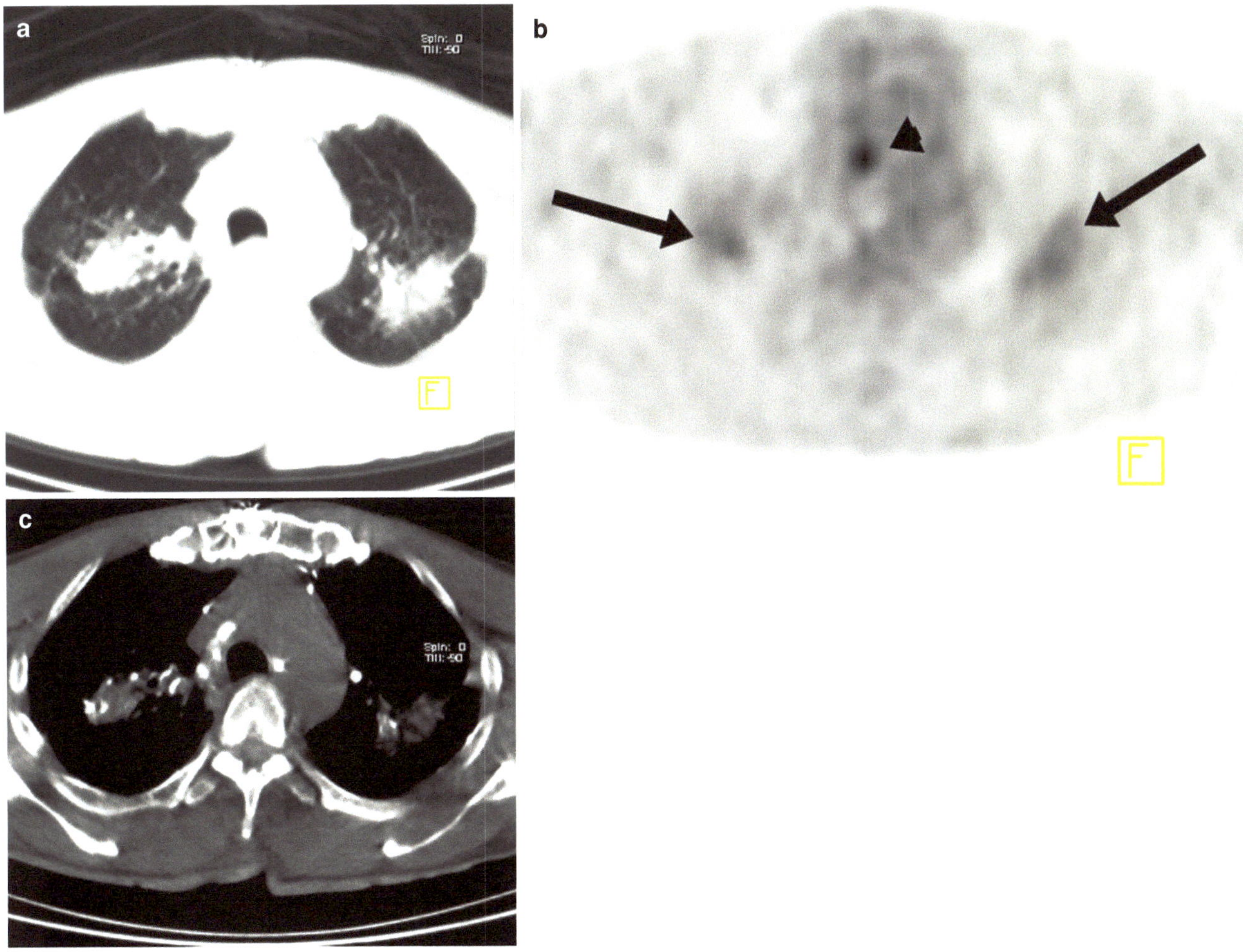

Fig. 2.35 A 50-year-old patient who had pulmonary tuberculosis (TB) underwent ^{18}F-FDG PET/CT scan. Consolidation areas at upper zones of both lungs including foci of calcifications are detected on CT (**a**, **c**). Mildly increased FDG uptake at the consolidation areas is consistent with inflammation (*arrow*) (**b**). There is also a focal increased FDG uptake representing a right upper tracheal lymph node showing reactive hyperplasia (*arrow head*). While performing FDG PET/CT for oncologic workup, TB is encountered as a common pathology simulating cancer and producing uptake patterns that are sometimes being hard to distinguish from that of malignant lesions

Pneumoconiosis

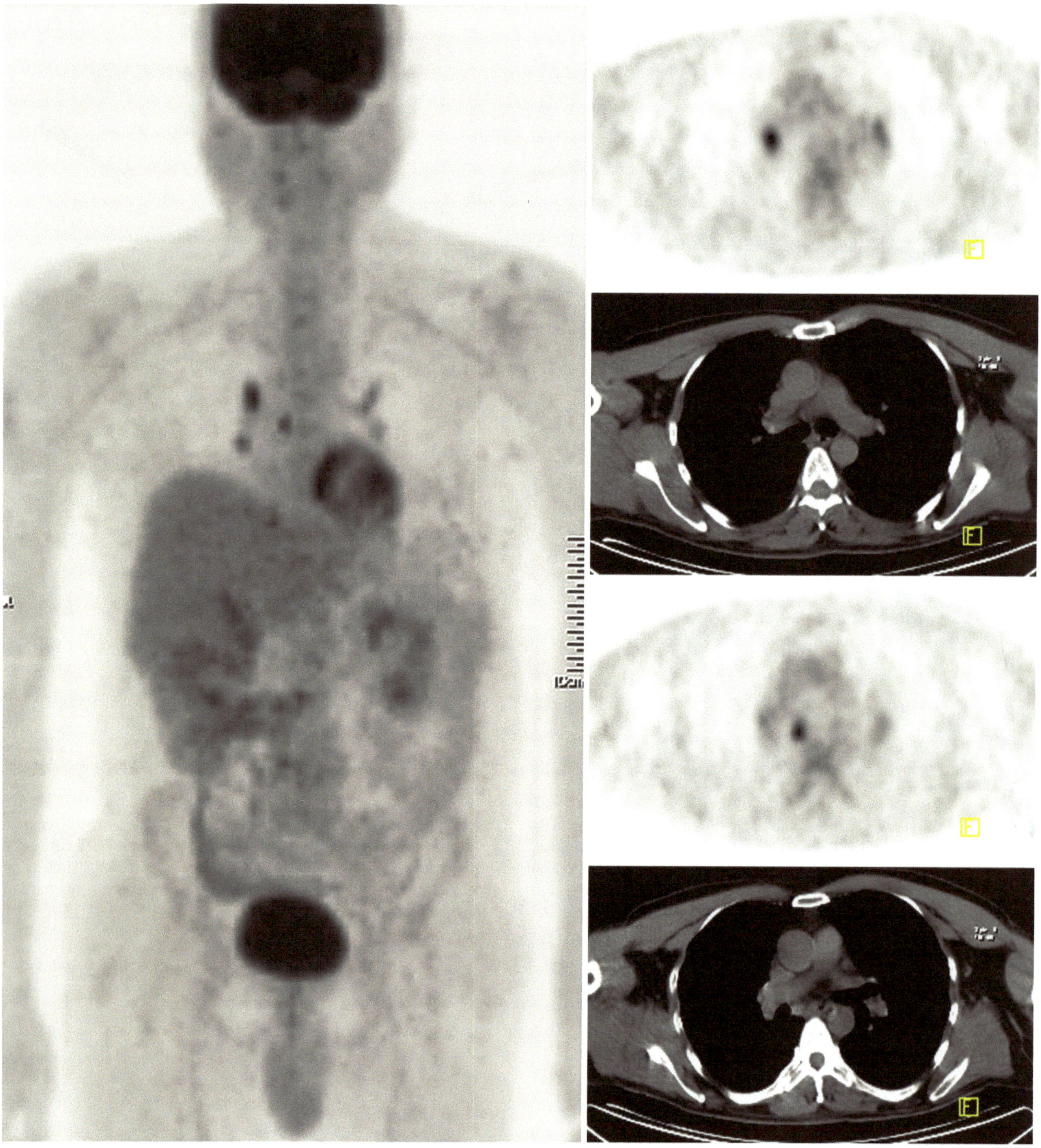

Fig. 2.36 Mediastinal lymph node enlargement that is moderately hypermetabolic on ^{18}F-FDG PET/CT. Histopathological findings of anthracotic pigment accumulation in mediastinal lymph nodes led to diagnosis of anthracotic pneumoconiosis

Sarcoidosis

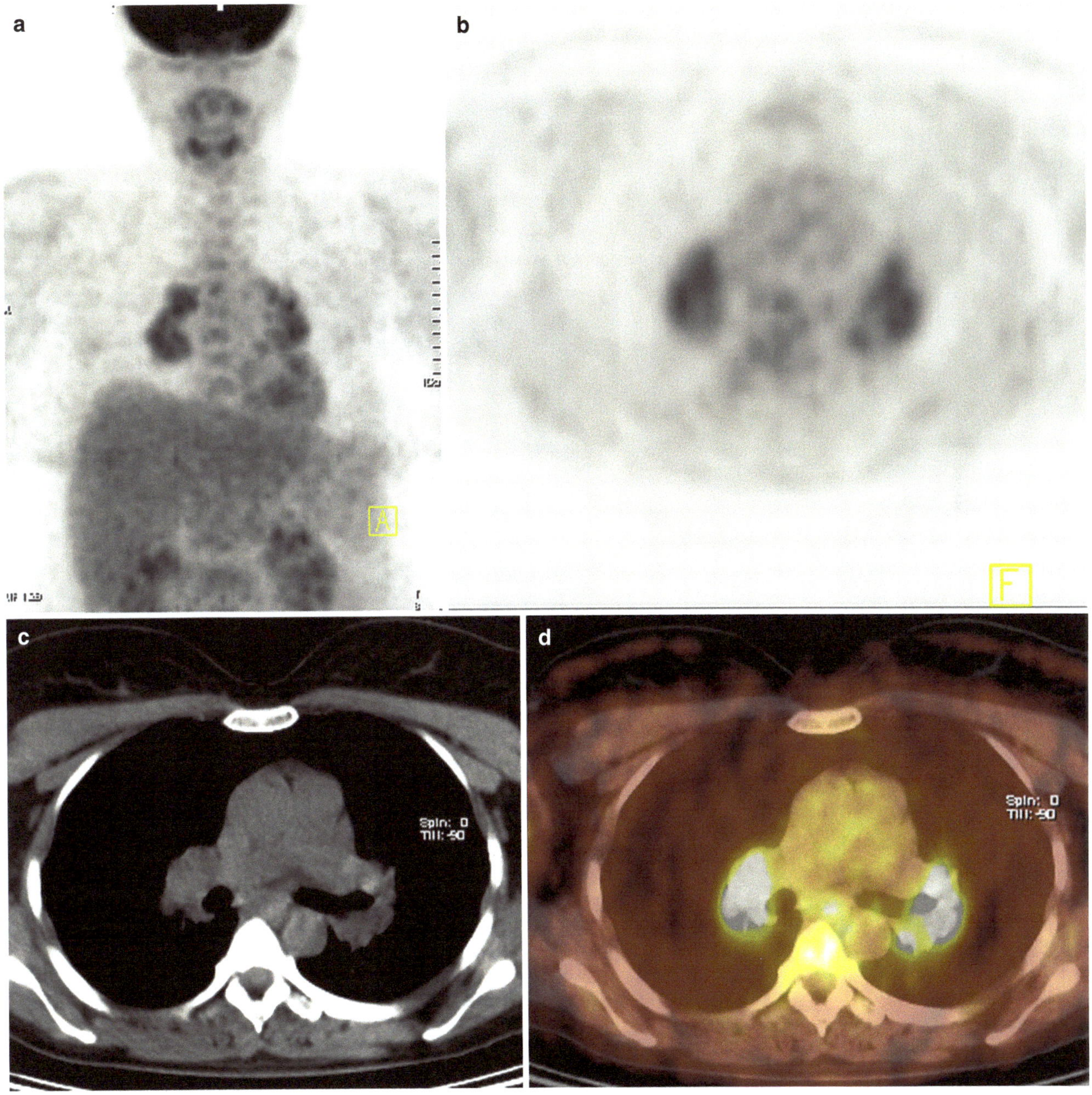

Fig. 2.37 MIP (**a**), axial PET, CT, and fusion images (**b–d**) show bilateral hilar enlarged lymph nodes with moderately increased FDG uptake (SUVmax 4.7) consistent with sarcoidosis. ^{18}F-FDG PET/CT scans can make contribution in the diagnosis of sarcoidosis and might also be used to monitor therapy response

Sarcoidosis

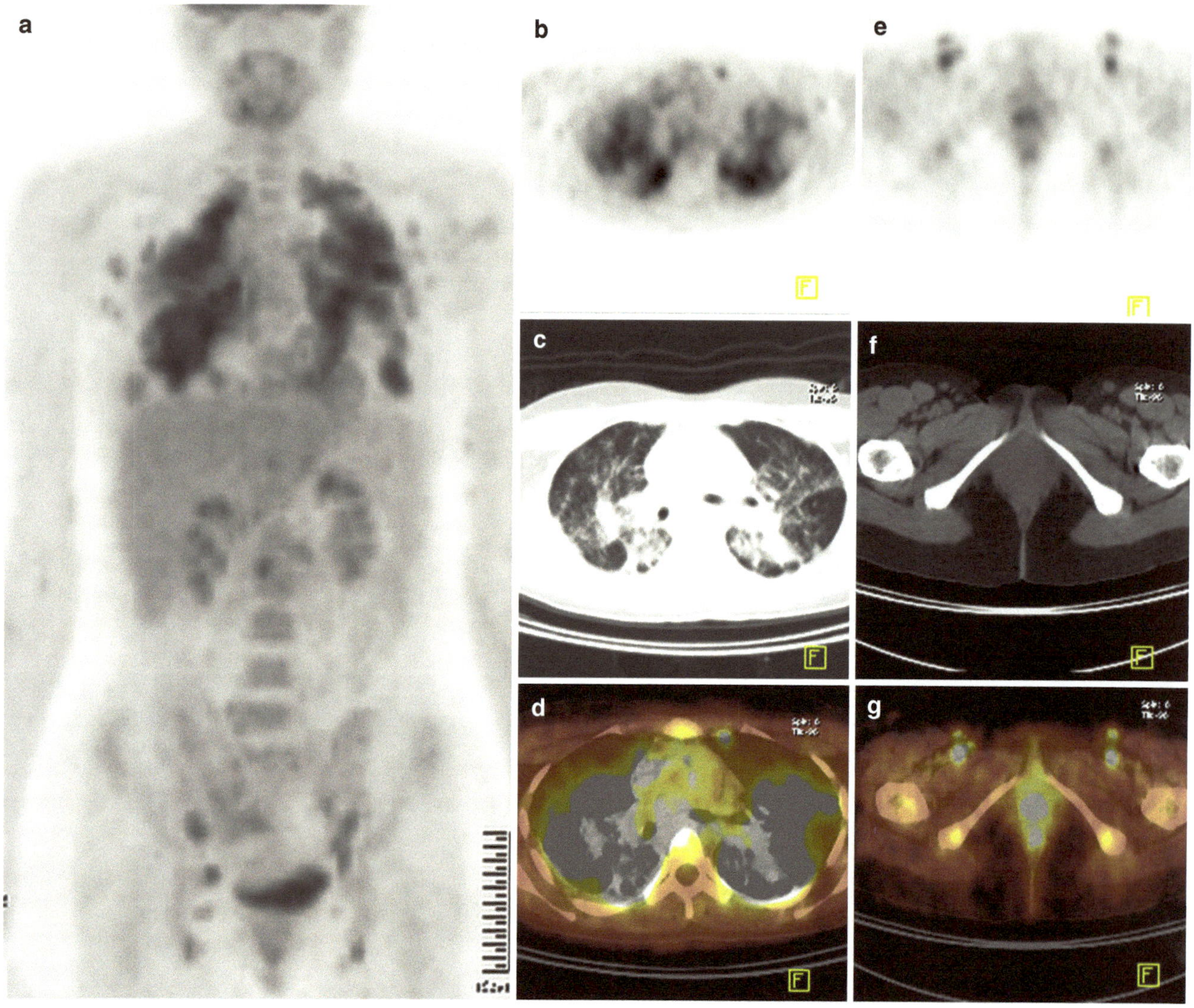

Fig. 2.38 MIP image (**a**), axial PET, CT, and fusion images (**b–d**) showing bilateral hilar enlarged lymph nodes and reticulonodular opacities at both lungs parenchyma with moderately increased FDG uptake (SUVmax 6.6). Axial fusion, PET, and CT images of pelvis (**e–g**) show bilateral hypermetabolic inguinal lymph nodes (SUVmax 2.2). All these lesions are compatible with sarcoidosis

Talc Pleurodesis

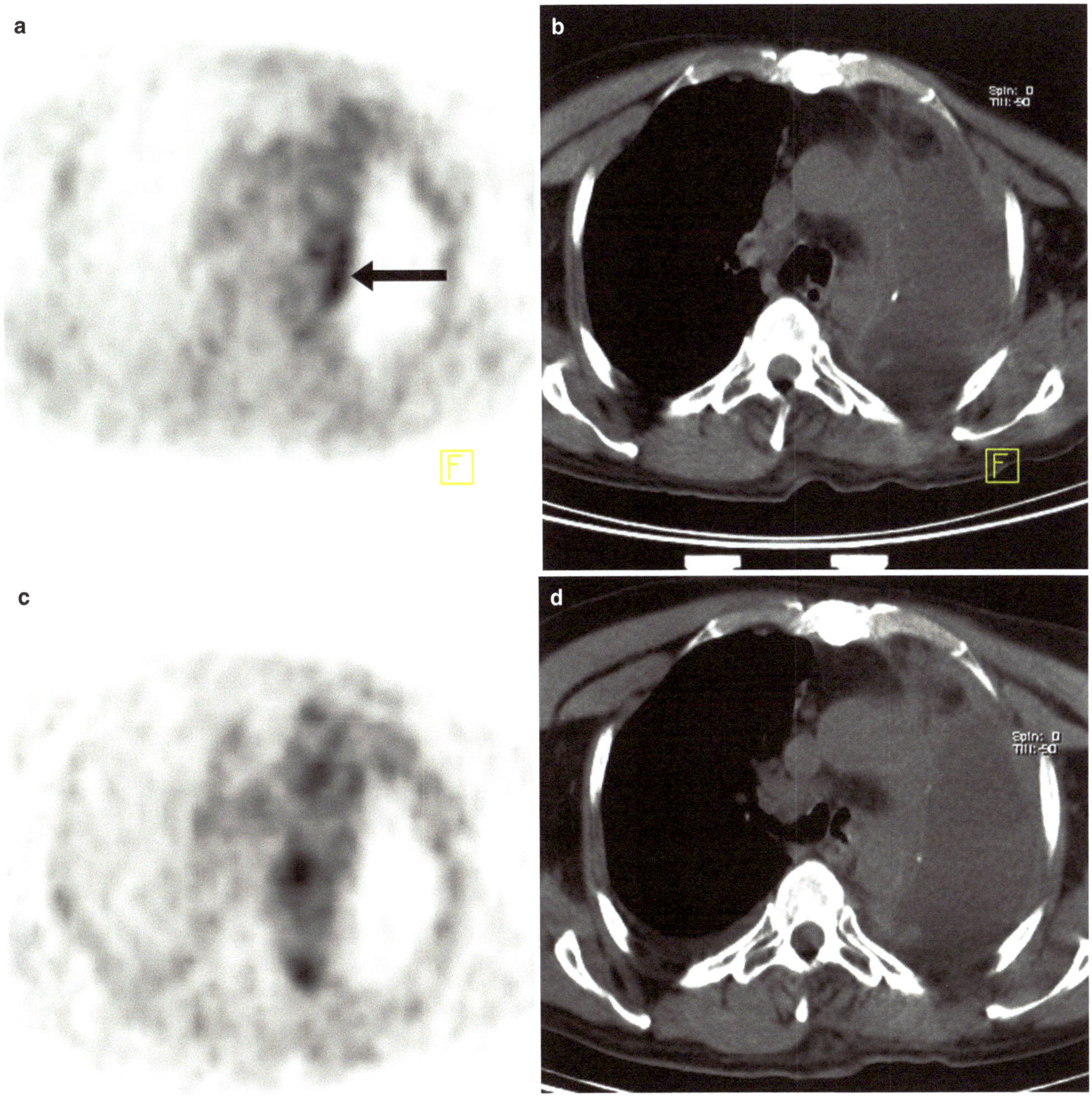

Fig. 2.39 A 56-year-old male patient with lung carcinoma was treated with talc pleurodesis. ^{18}F-FDG PET/CT scan performed after application of talc pleurodesis showed increased FDG uptake at mediastinal pleural thickening consistent with talc deposit (*arrow*) (**a**, **b**). ^{18}F-FDG PET/CT applied 4 months later displayed the clearance of pathological FDG uptake that was detected in the previous study, confirming the benign pathology. Two foci of newly developed FDG uptake possibly representing metastatic lymph nodes is also seen (**c**, **d**). Talc deposits in the pleura produce areas of increased uptake on PET study that correspond to the areas of high density pleural thickening on CT. These PET findings should be carefully evaluated in correlation with CT to distinguish this benign inflammatory process from malignancy

Pleural Tuberculosis

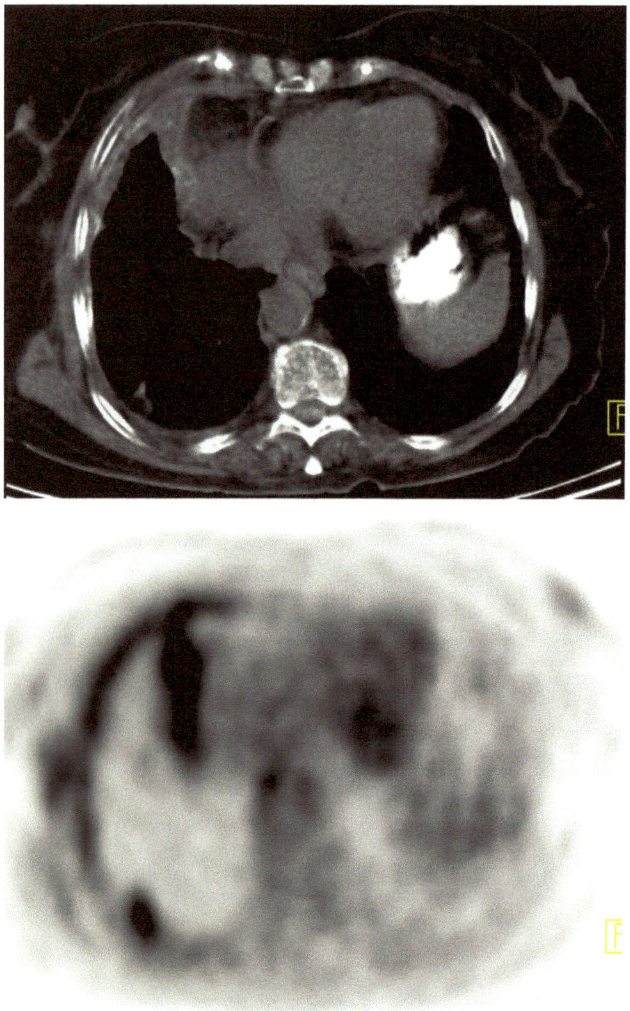

Fig. 2.40 Axial slices of CT and PET images show thickenings at costal and mediastinal pleura with corresponding increased FDG uptake, compatible with pleural tuberculosis

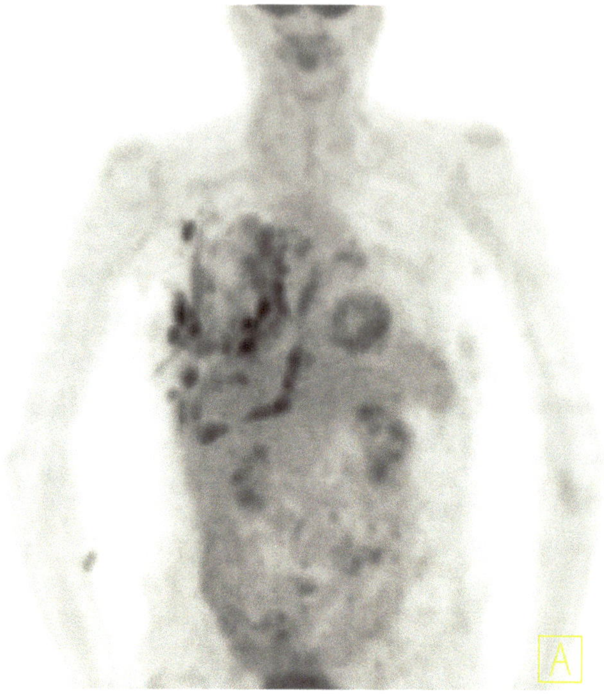

Fig. 2.41 MIP image

Diminished Myocardial Uptake in Fasting

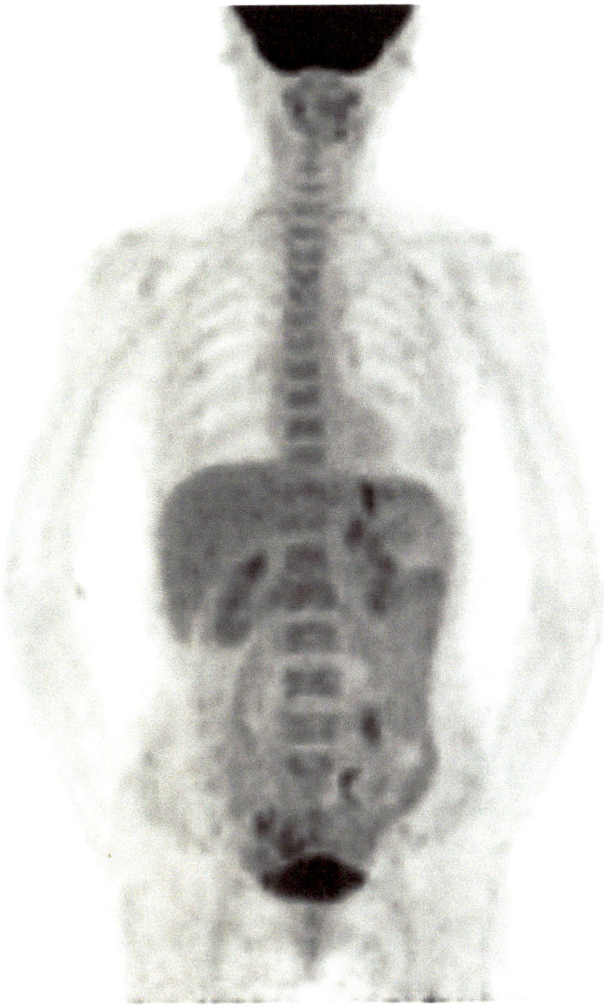

Fig. 2.42 MIP image of ^{18}F-FDG PET/CT scan of a female patient, who had a prolonged fasting of 20 h before acquisition. Myocardial uptake is not seen, because myocardium metabolizes free fatty acids instead of glucose in case of fasting

Esophagitis

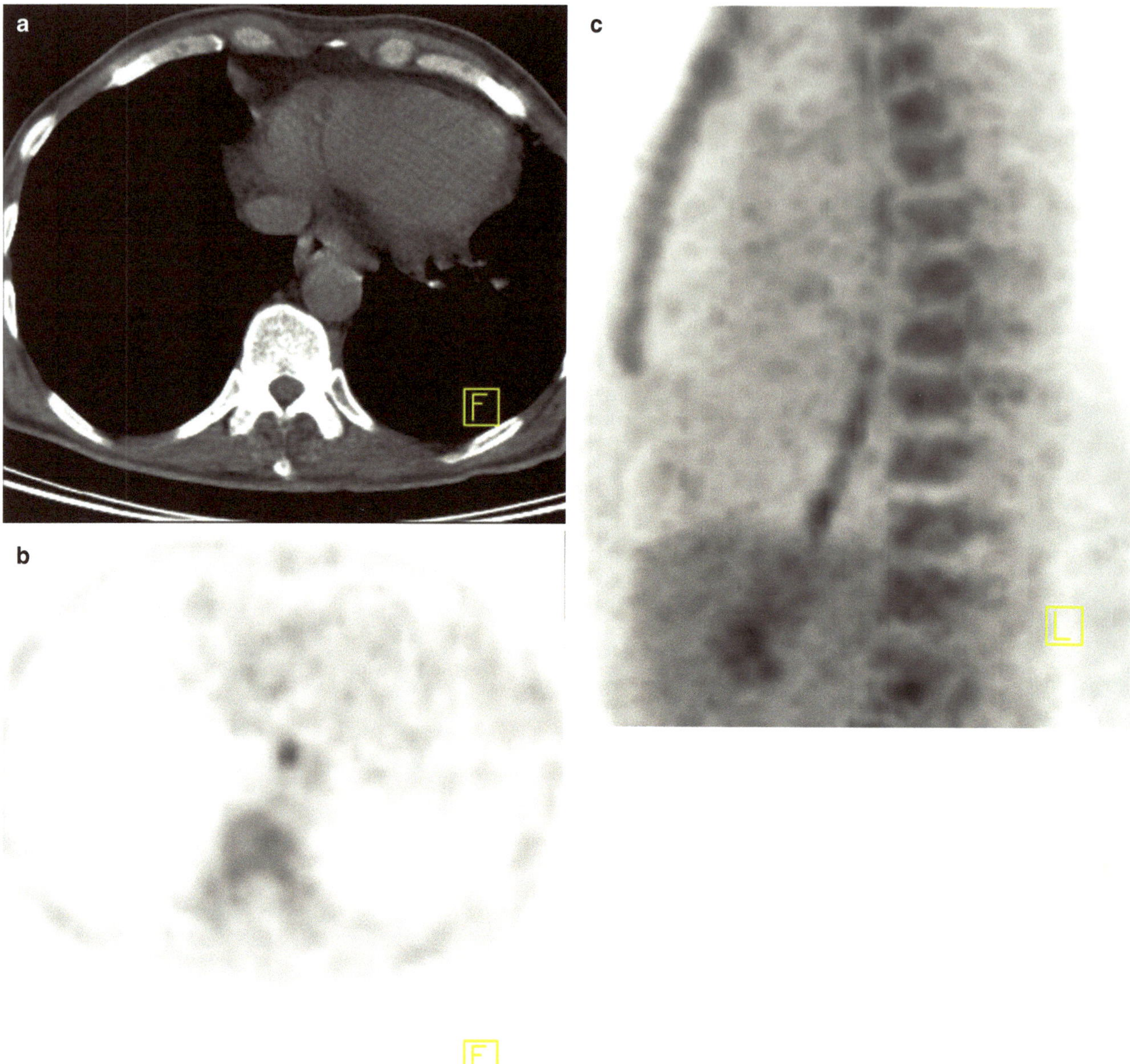

Fig. 2.43 Axial CT and PET (**a**, **b**) and sagittal MIP (**c**) images show increased FDG uptake at esophagus due to esophagitis

2.3 Abdomen

Herniated Stomach

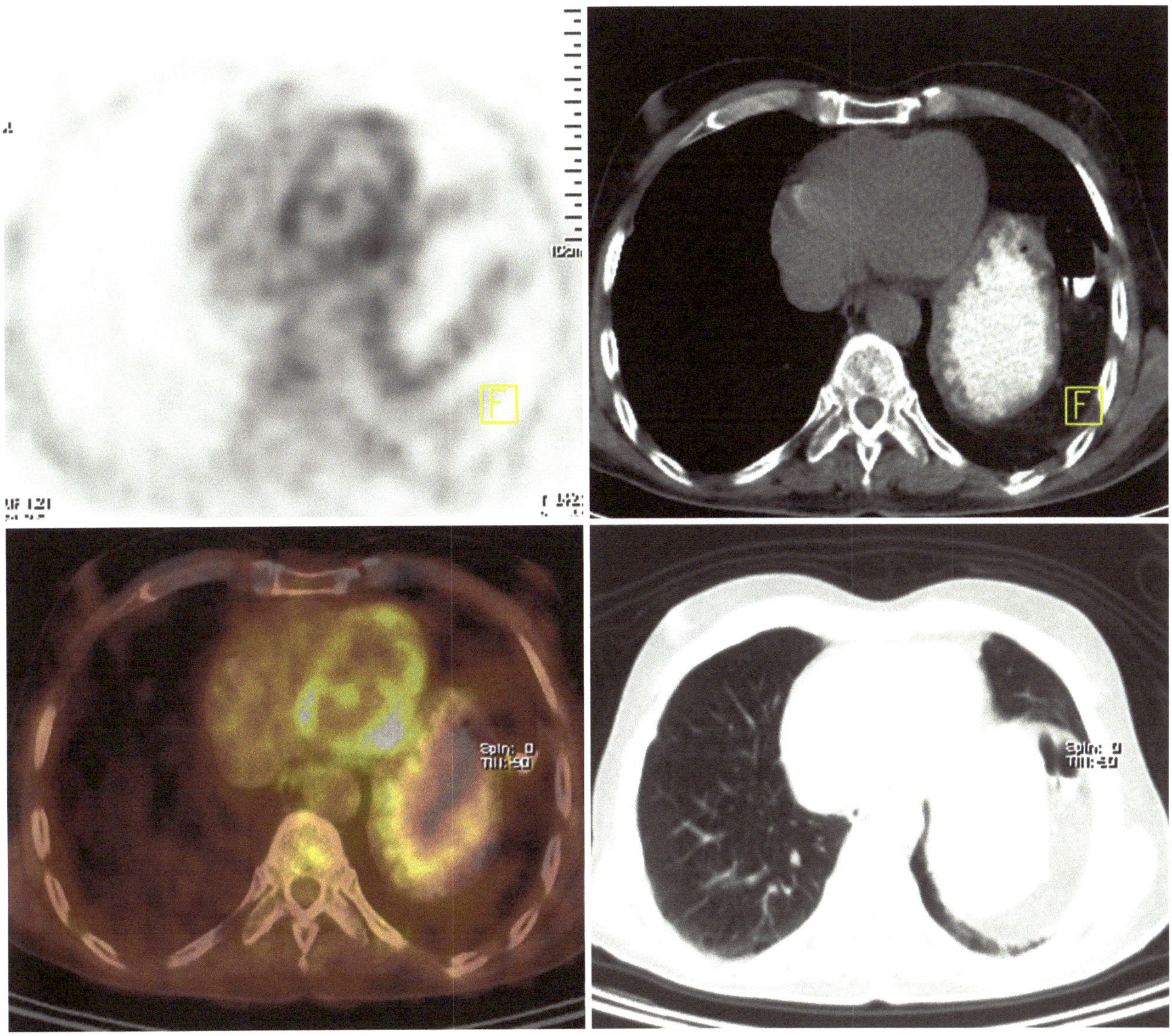

Fig. 2.44 Stomach herniated into thorax

Hiatal Hernia

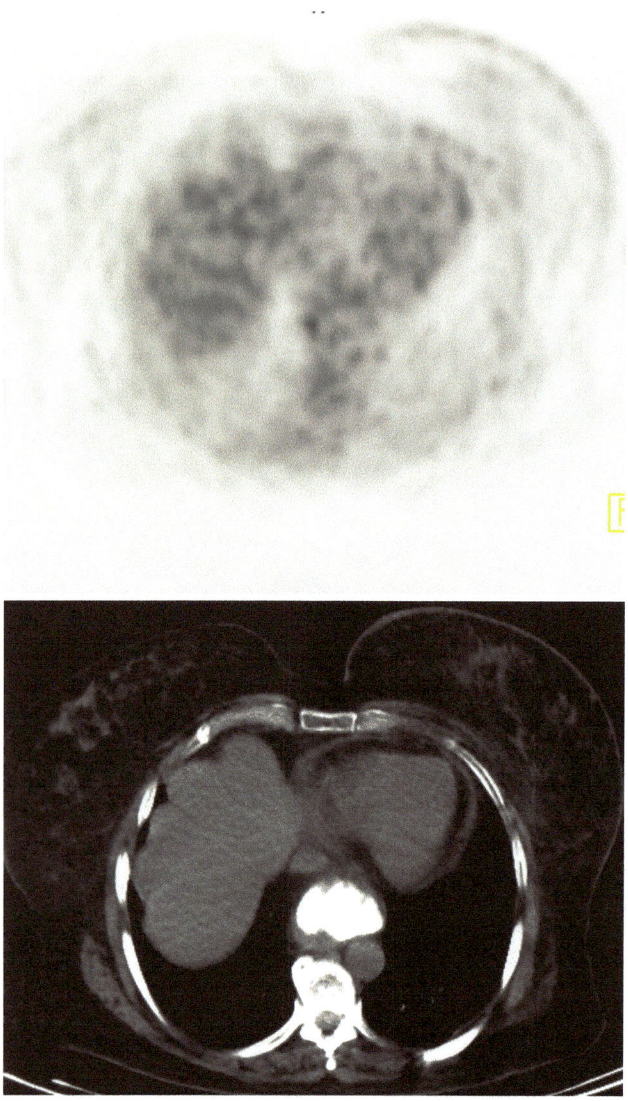

Fig. 2.45 Axial PET (**a**) and CT (**b**) images show a sliding hernia; the GE junction and a portion of the stomach slides upward into the mediastinum

Chilaiditi Syndrome

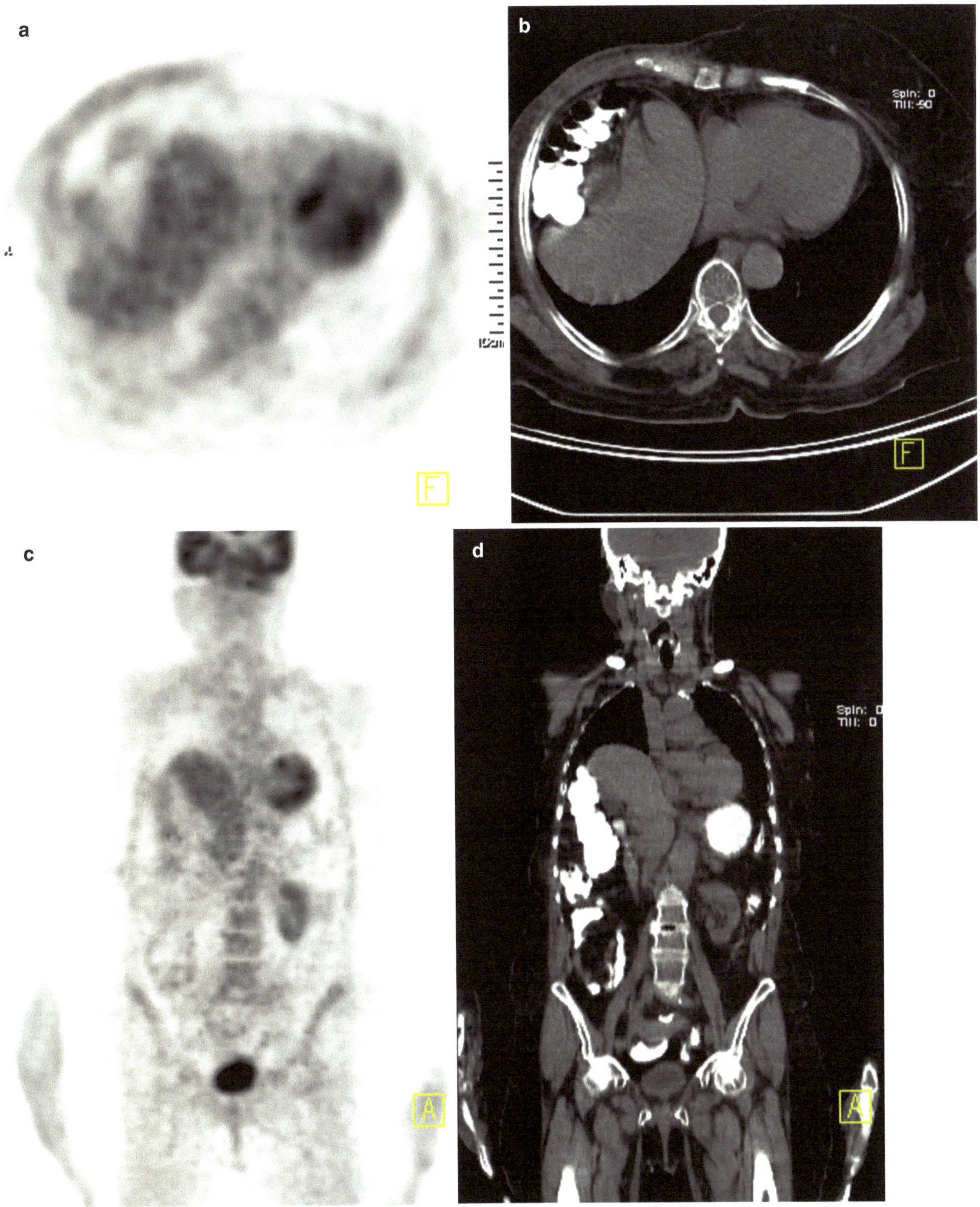

Fig. 2.46 Axial (**a**, **b**) and coronal (**c**, **d**) PET and CT images show interposition of the colon segment between the liver and the right hemidiaphragm

Gastritis

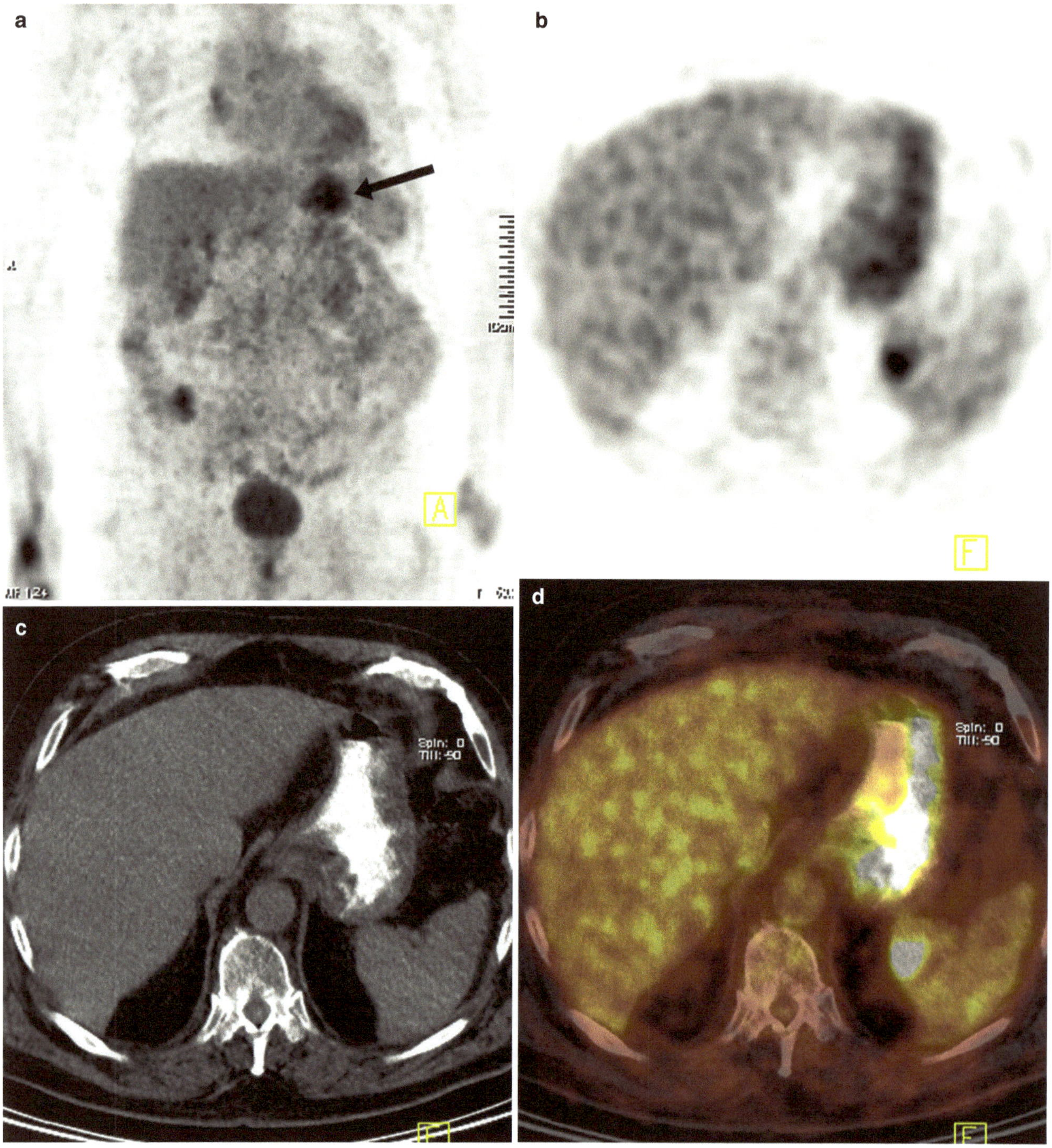

Fig. 2.47 MIP (**a**); axial PET, CT, and fusion (**b–d**) images show increased tracer uptake at thickened gastric wall (*arrow*). This patient is diagnosed to have gastritis but sometimes diffuse intense FDG uptake due to gastritis may mimic malignancy. Repeating imaging of gastric region after drinking water may show resolution of FDG uptake confirming its benign nature

Lipoma in Duodenum

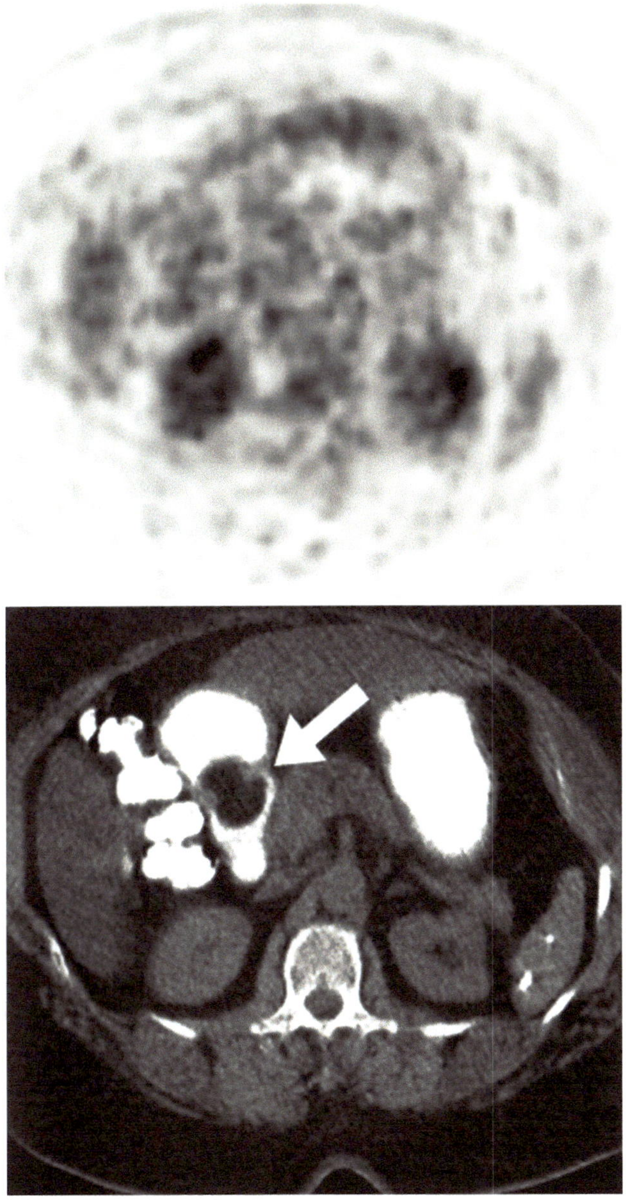

Fig. 2.48 Focal filling defect in duodenum on CT image does not exhibit any FDG uptake on corresponding PET image and it is consistent with lipoma (*arrow*)

Metformin

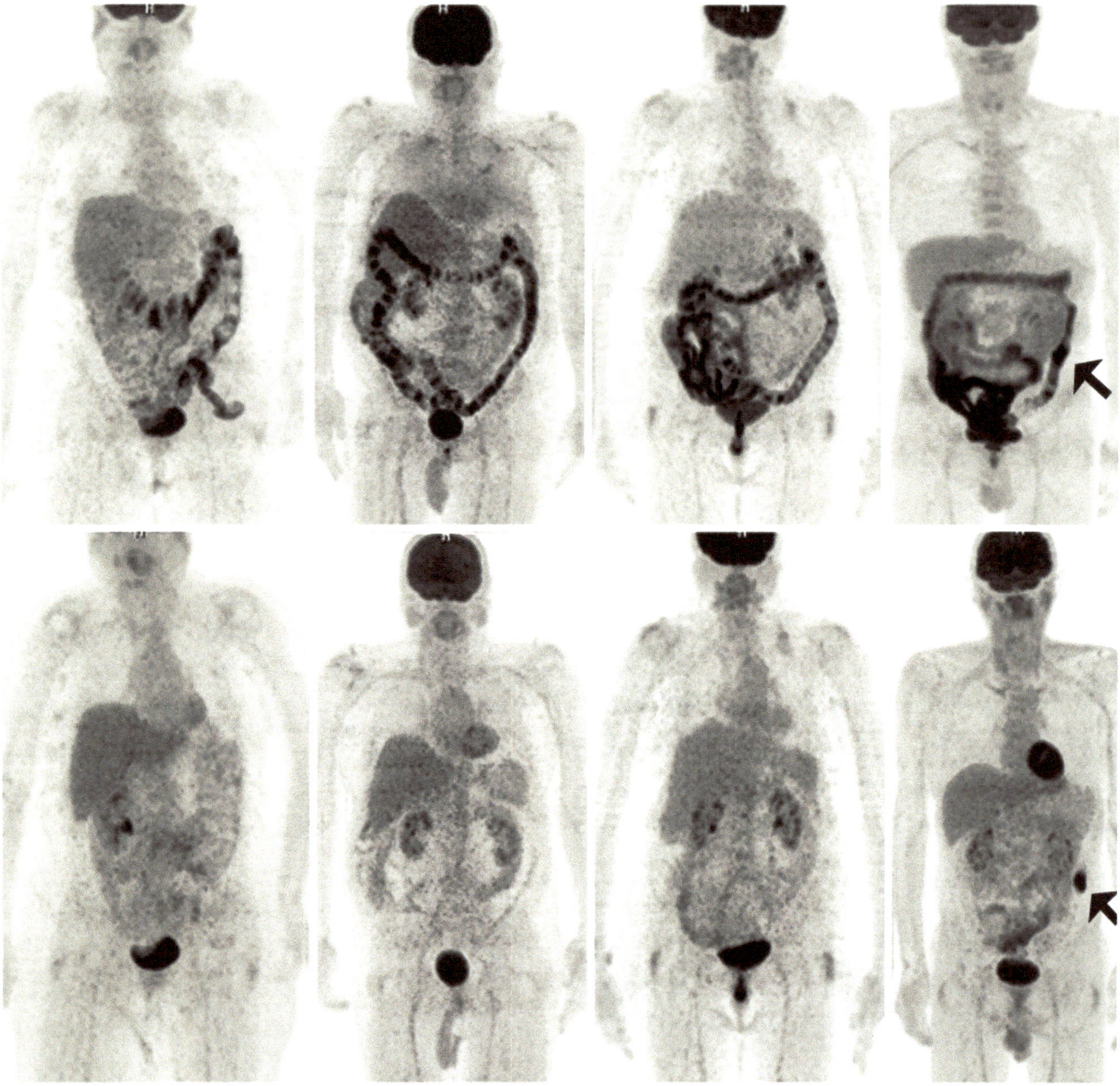

Fig. 2.49 ^{18}F-FDG PET/CT MIP images in patients while taking metformin (*upper row*) and corresponding images after stopping metformin (*lower row*). Intense and diffuse uptake in the bowel segments is seen while taking metformin, and clearance of FDG uptake from the bowel segments is seen after stopping metformin. Note the better visualization of a lesion located in the left colon after clearance of activity (*arrow*)

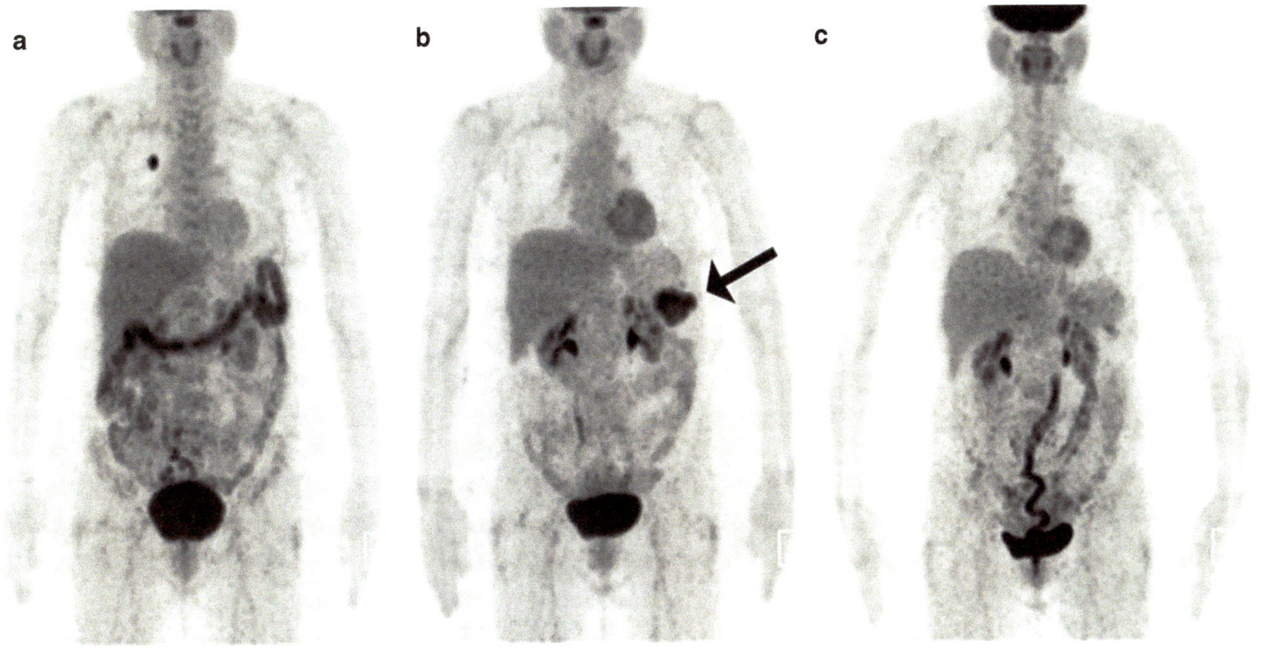

Fig. 2.50 ^{18}F-FDG PET/CT MIP images in a patient with ovarian carcinoma: image obtained while taking metformin shows intense and diffuse FDG uptake in bowel segments (**a**), image obtained 3 months after the first study after stopping metformin shows a mass lesion with intense FDG uptake in the left upper quadrant (*arrow*) (**b**), image obtained after six courses of chemotherapy shows disappearance of the lesion confirming the malignant nature of the lesion (**c**)

Physiological Intestine Uptake

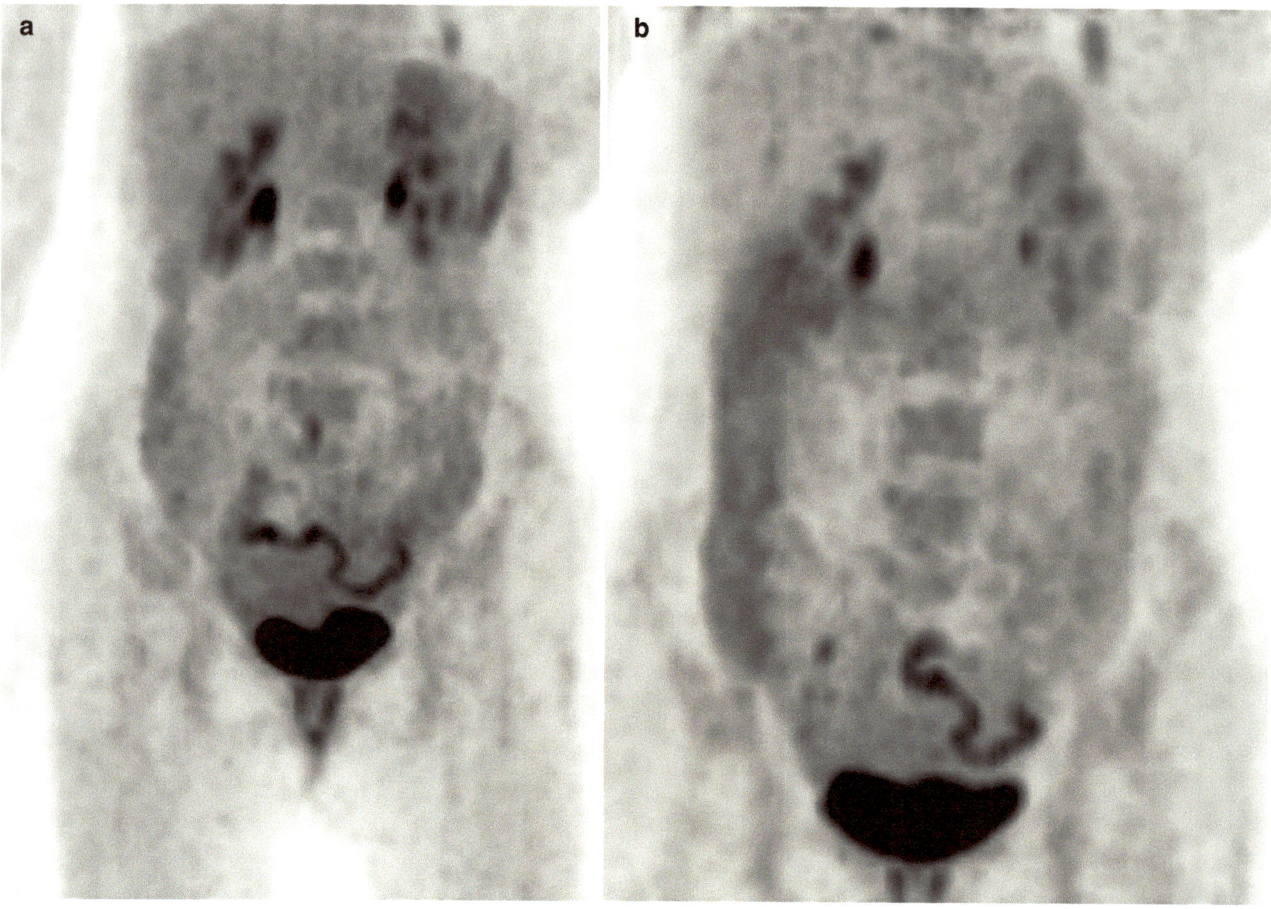

Fig. 2.51 MIP image (**a**) shows segmental bowel uptake which is suspicious for inflammatory bowel disease, but on delayed image (**b**) the activity in the bowel moved distally, proving physiological nature of this uptake

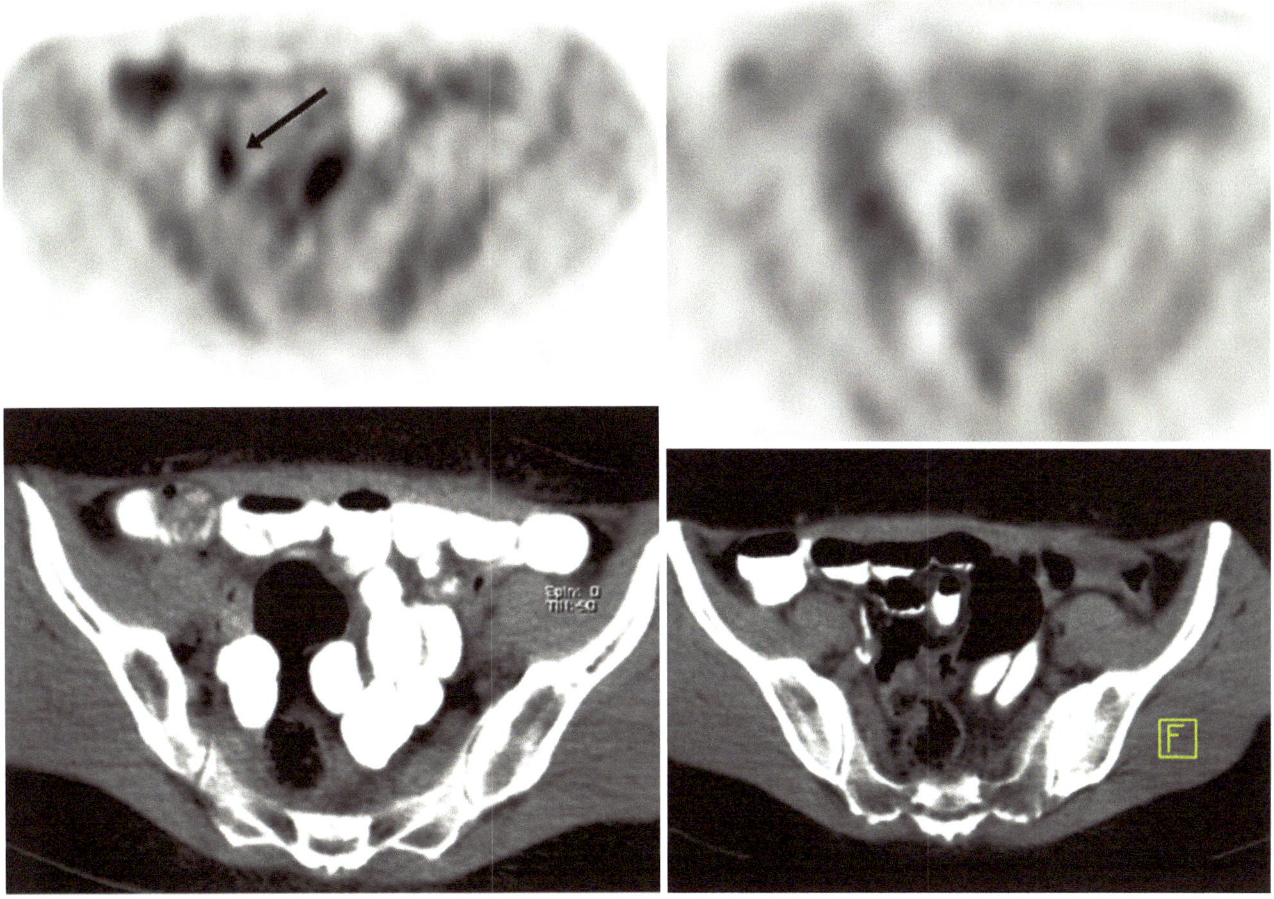

Fig. 2.52 Axial slices of PET and CT images of the previous patient show focal physiological FDG uptake (*arrow*) which is disappeared at late images

Inguinal Hernia

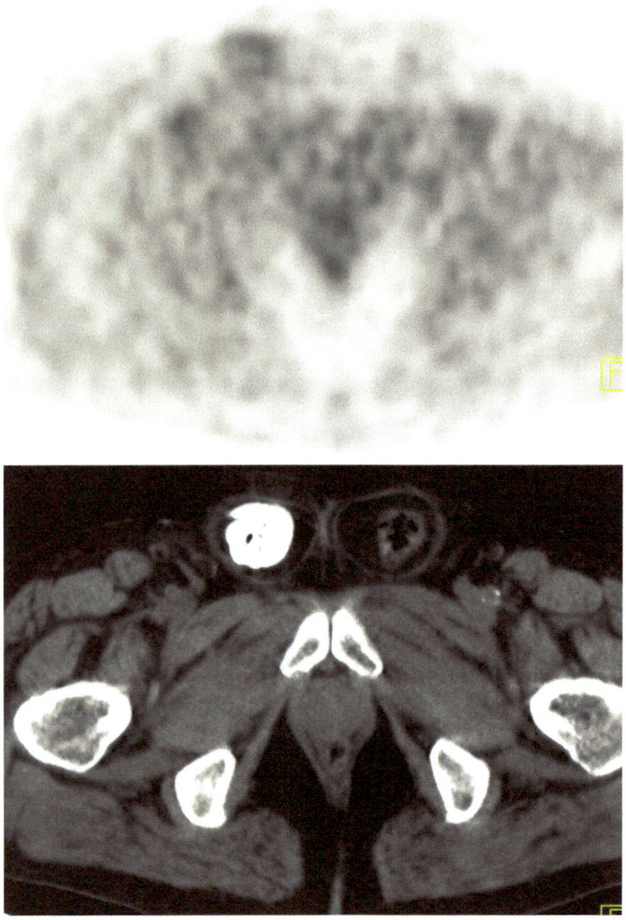

Fig. 2.53 Bilateral inguinal hernia is seen on axial CT image. Increased tracer uptake is noticed at right inguinal region on PET corresponding to the hyperdense contrast in the bowel

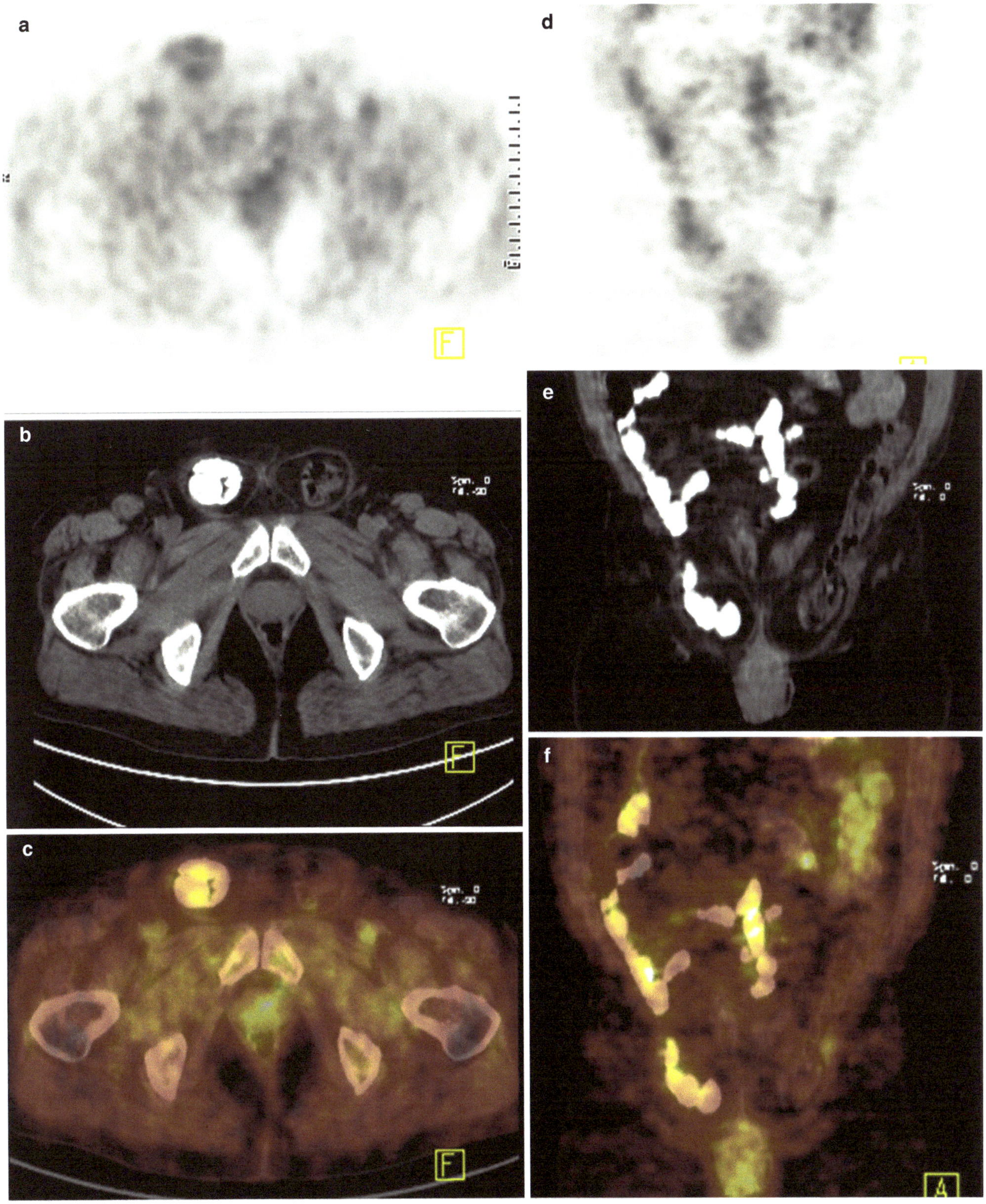

Fig. 2.54 Axial PET, CT, and fusion images (**a**–**c**), and coronal PET, CT and fusion images (**d**–**f**)

Radiation Proctitis

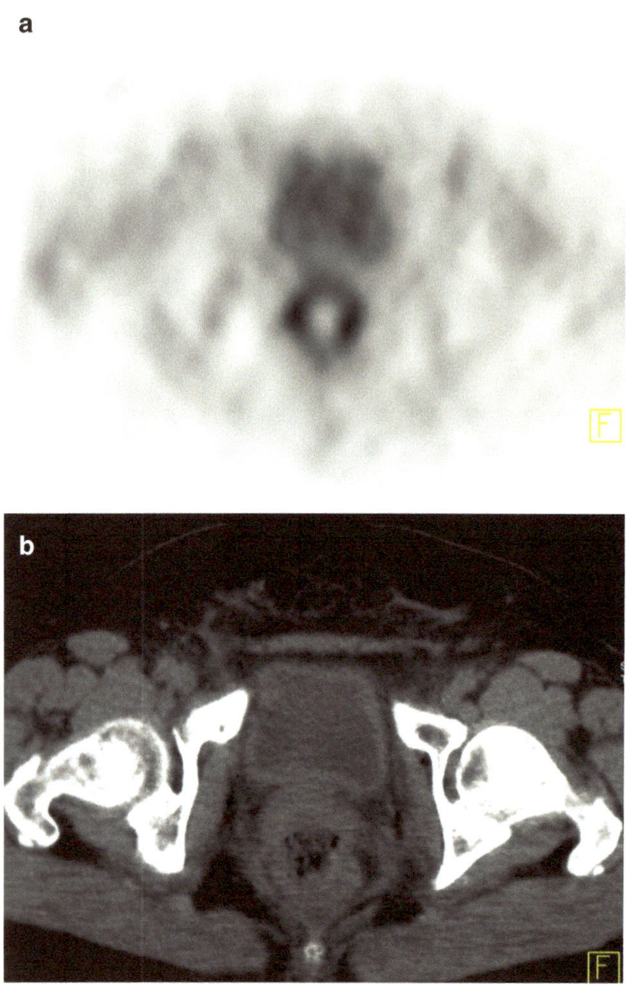

Fig. 2.55 Axial PET and CT (**a**, **b**) images

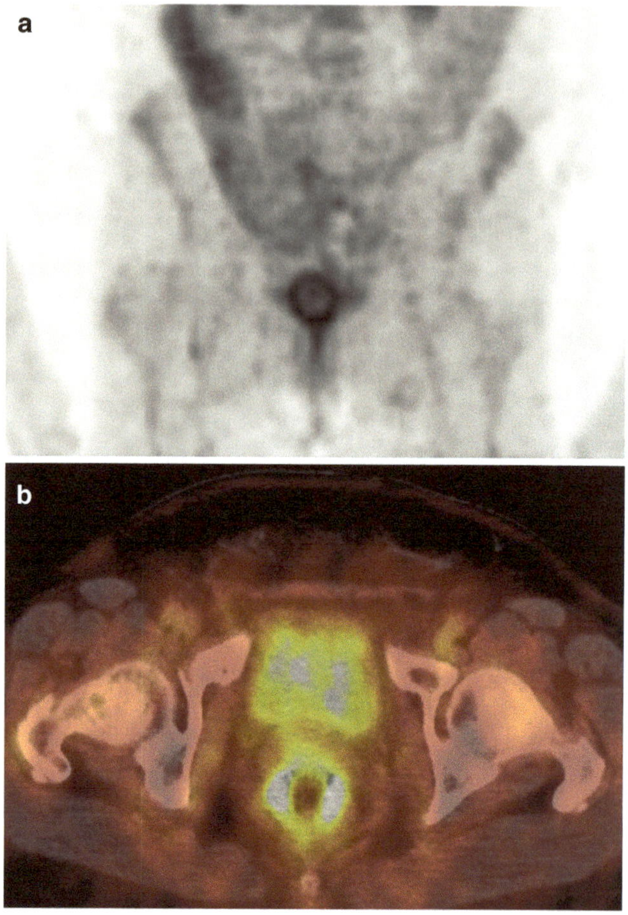

Fig. 2.56 MIP and axial fusion (**a**, **b**) images show circular FDG uptake at rectum due to inflammation from external radiotherapy given for cervix carcinoma

Presacral Fibrotic Tissue

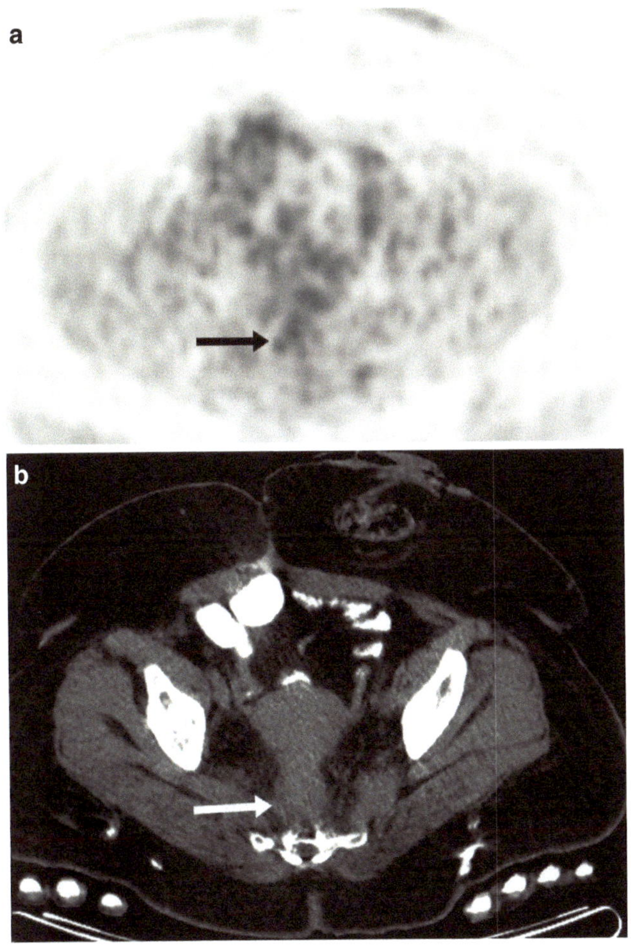

Fig. 2.57 A 62-year-old female patient who had been operated for rectum carcinoma and received EBRT underwent ^{18}F-FDG PET/CT scan for detection of recurrence. On CT images, solid lesion in soft tissue density at presacral region (**a**) which is suspicious for local recurrence does not show any pathological FDG uptake on PET image (**b**) (*arrows*). This lesion represents benign fibrotic tissue and malignancy is ruled out by ^{18}F-FDG PET/CT scan

Pilonoidal Sinus

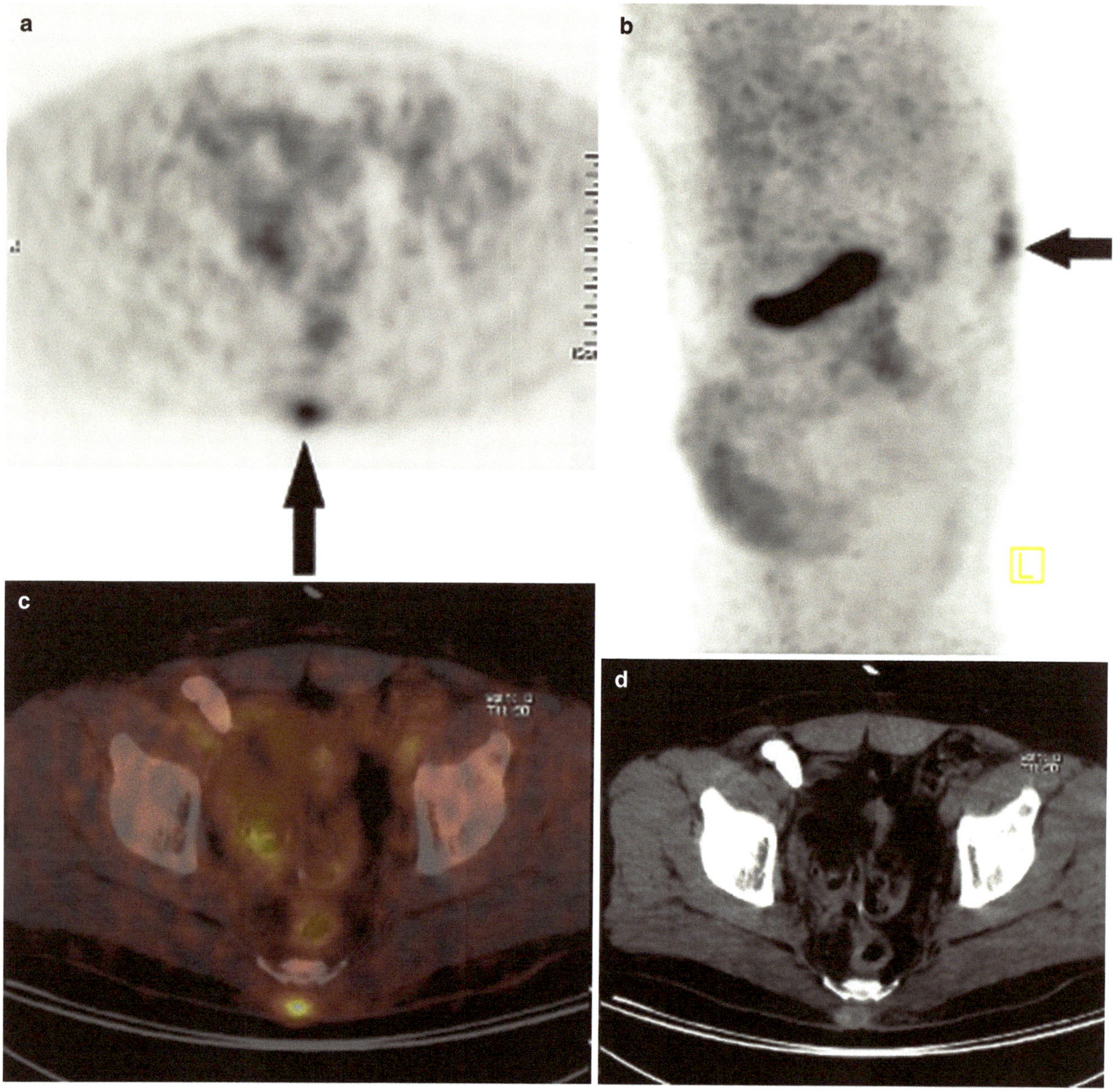

Fig. 2.58 Pilonoidal sinus located posteriorly to coccyx show mildly increased FDG uptake (*arrows*) (**a–d**)

Diffuse Fatty Infiltration of the Liver

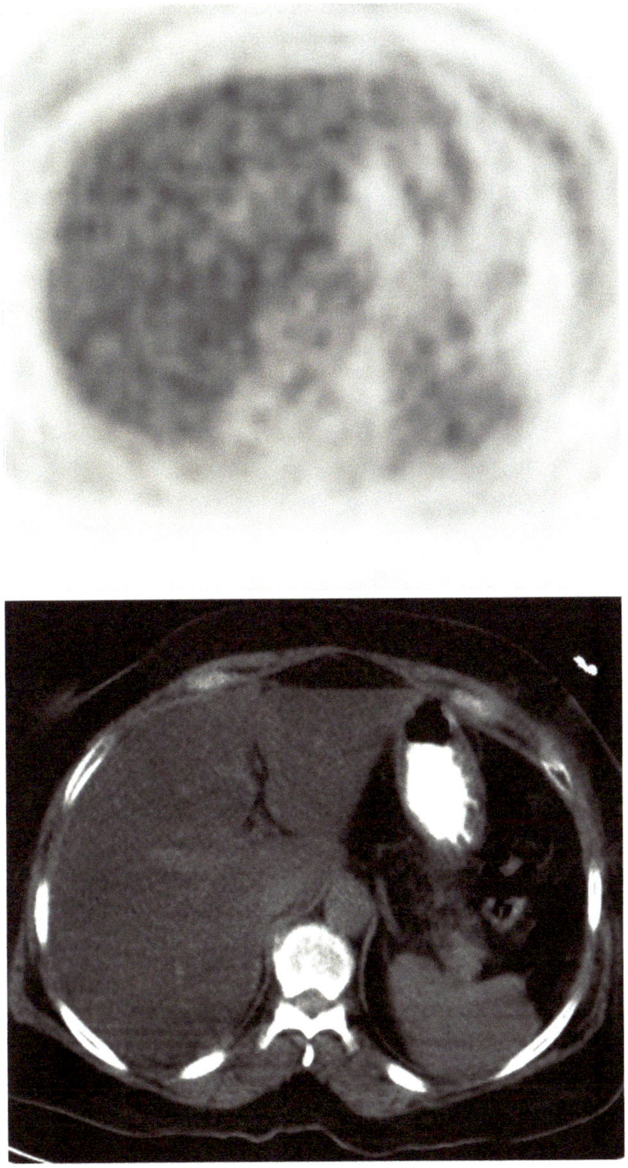

Fig. 2.59 Axial image of a patient shows hypodense appearance of liver with an attenuation (in Hounsfield units) less than that of the spleen. This pattern is compatible with fatty infiltration of liver. Liver shows homogeneous and normal level of FDG uptake with SUVmax 3.2, while the spleen has a SUVmax of 2.9. According to a recent study, no clinically important correlation between liver attenuation at CT and SUVmax is detected. In addition, SUV max measurements in the patients with evidence of diffuse fatty infiltration of the liver were not significantly different from those in the healthy control subjects

Fatty Liver with a Fat Spared Area

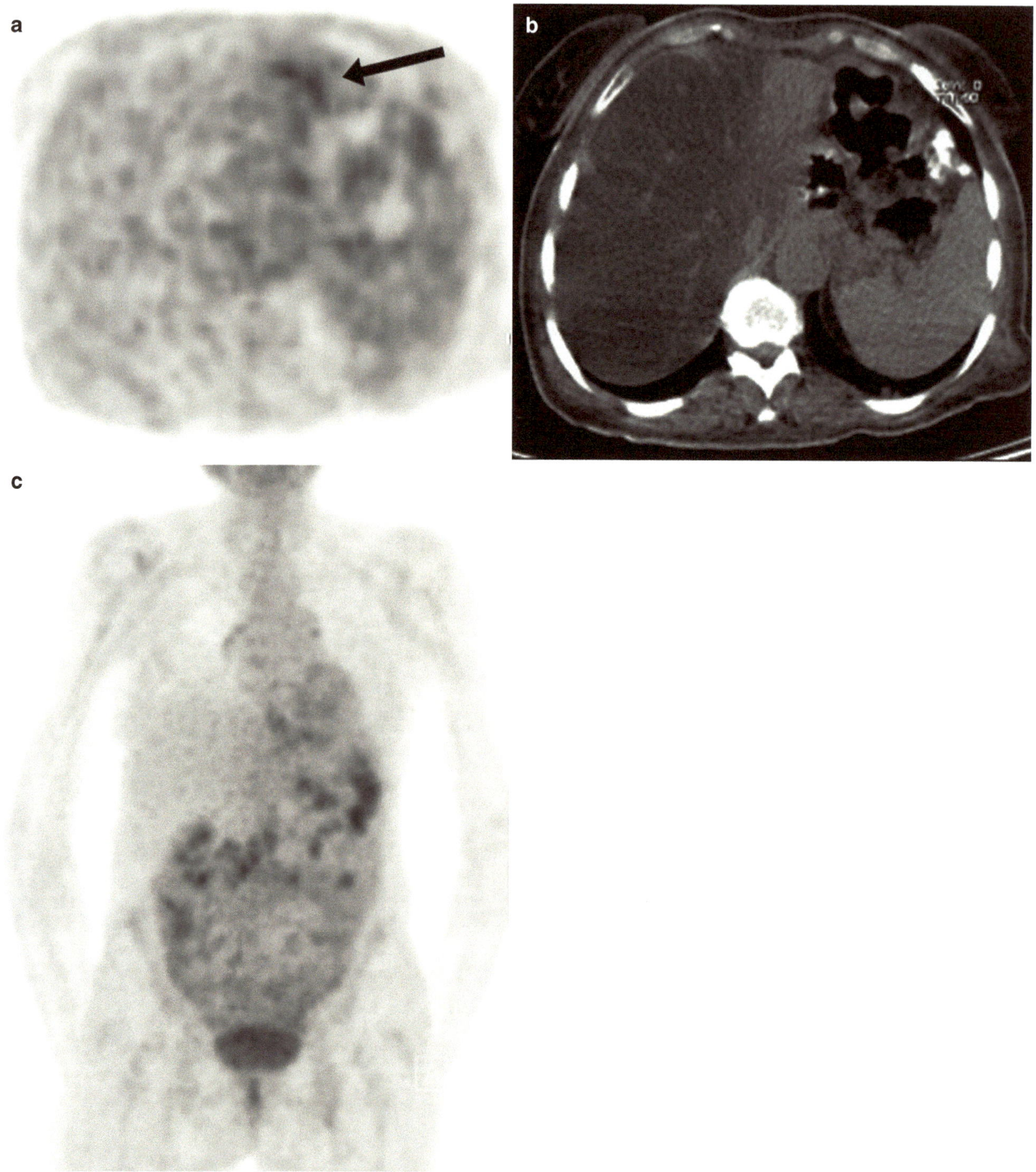

Fig. 2.60 Liver is hypodense on CT except a small area at left lobe which shows higher FDG uptake compared to the rest of the liver. Fat spared area of liver may appear as focal areas of elevated FDG uptake on a PET scan and mimic metastases (*arrow*) (**a**–**c**)

Liver Abscess Due to Yersiniae Bacteremia

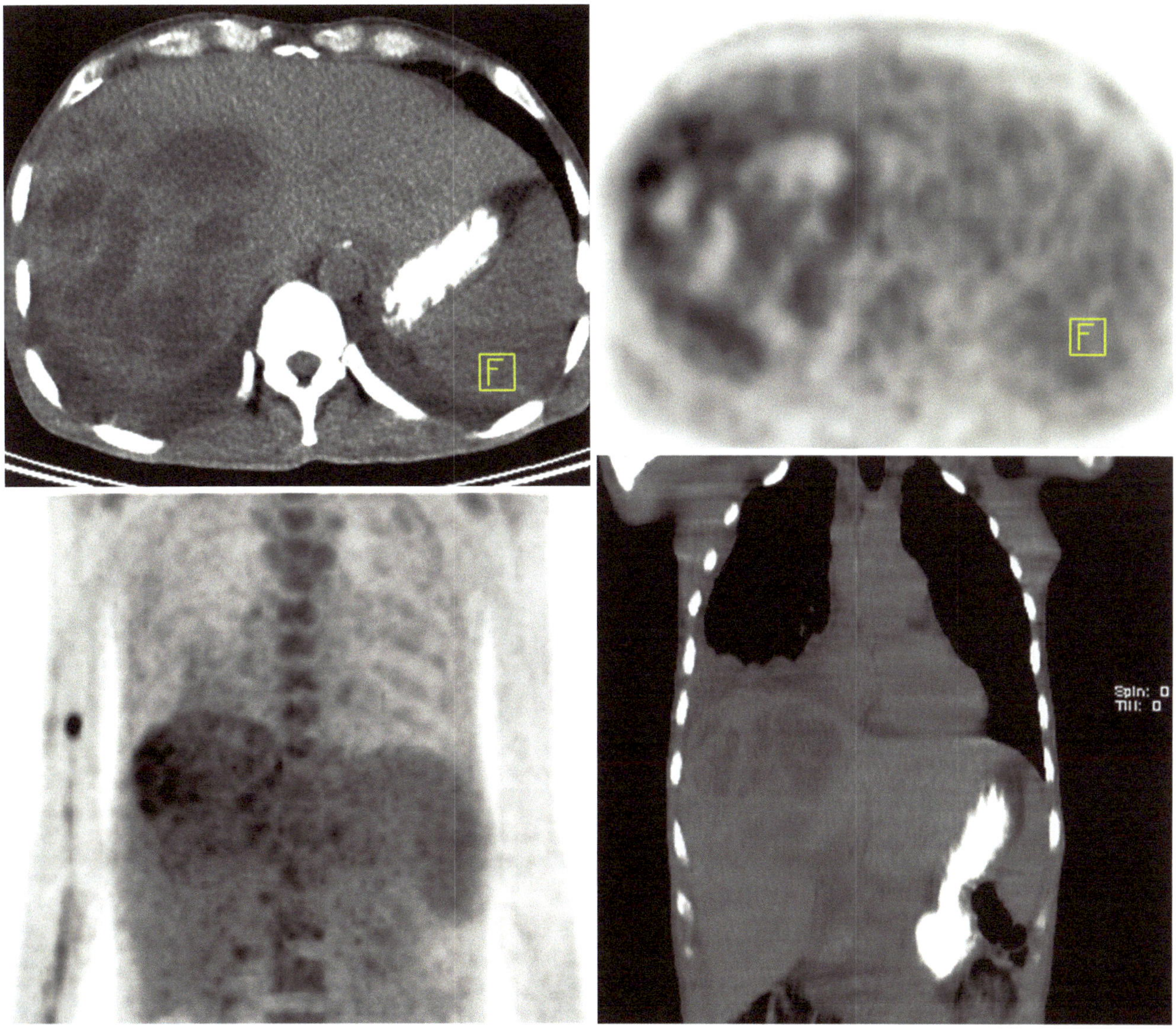

Fig. 2.61 ^{18}F-FDG PET/CT scan showed minimally increased ^{18}F-FDG uptake with hypometabolic regions inside the liver corresponding to a mass lesion with septations in CT. The lesion in liver is consistent with abscess caused by *Yersinia enterocolitica*

Liver Cyst

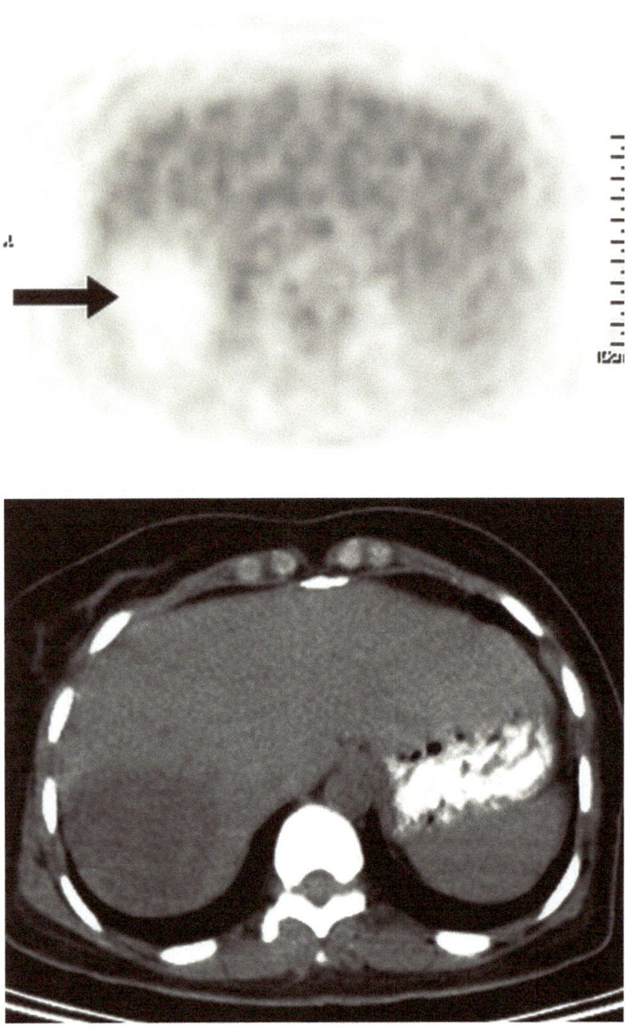

Fig. 2.62 Hypodense lesion on CT without corresponding FDG uptake on PET image (*arrow*), consistent with liver cyst

Hydatid Cyst

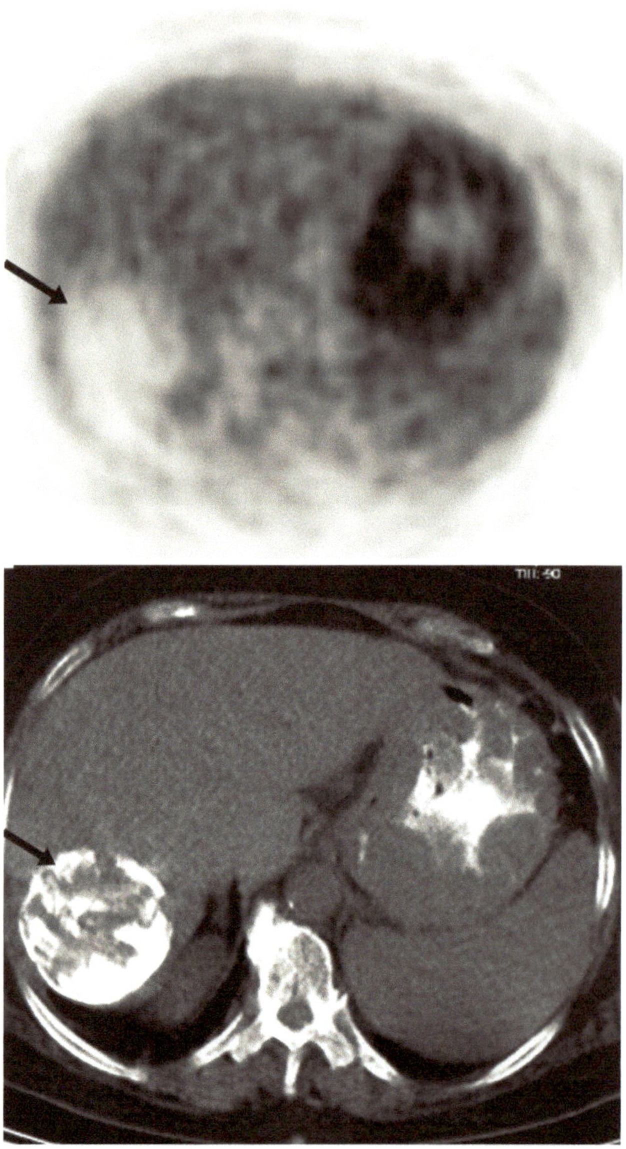

Fig. 2.63 Calcified mass lesion of hydatid cyst at right lobe of liver on CT image does not show any FDG uptake on corresponding PET image (*arrows*). Hydatid cyst lesions may also exhibit FDG uptake and mimic metastatic lesions so it should be considered in differential diagnosis while evaluating ^{18}F-FDG PET/CT images in countries where zoonotic infections are relatively common

Liver Hemangioma

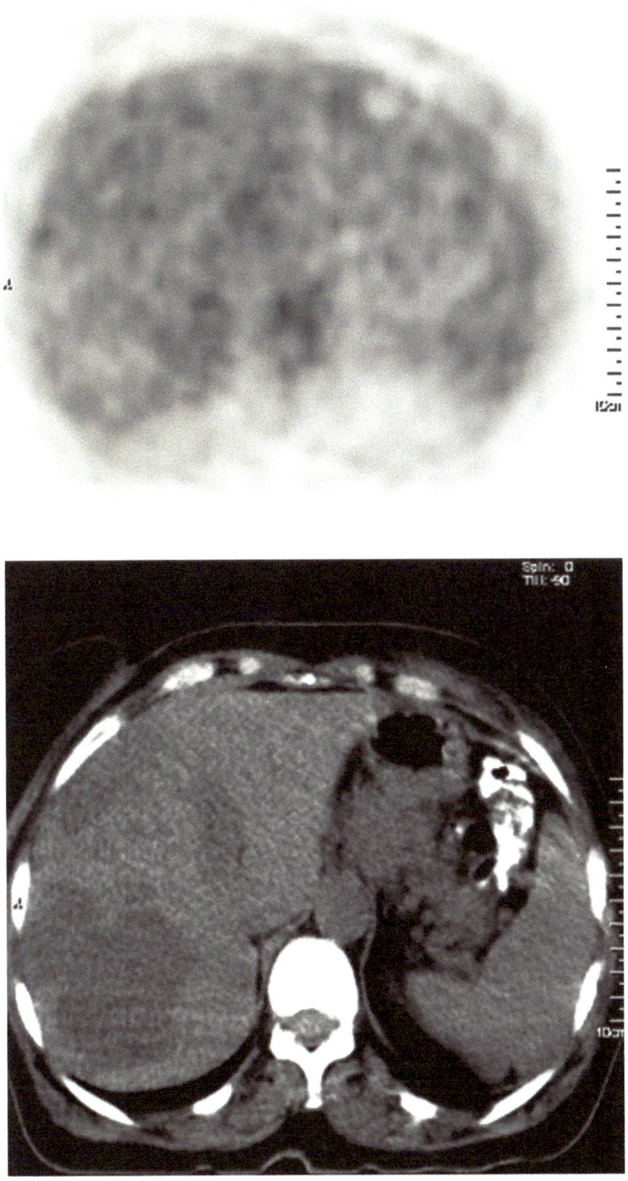

Fig. 2.64 Axial PET and CT images display multiple hypodense lesions at both lobes of liver without any significant FDG uptake, which are proved to be hemangiomas

Acute Cholecystitis

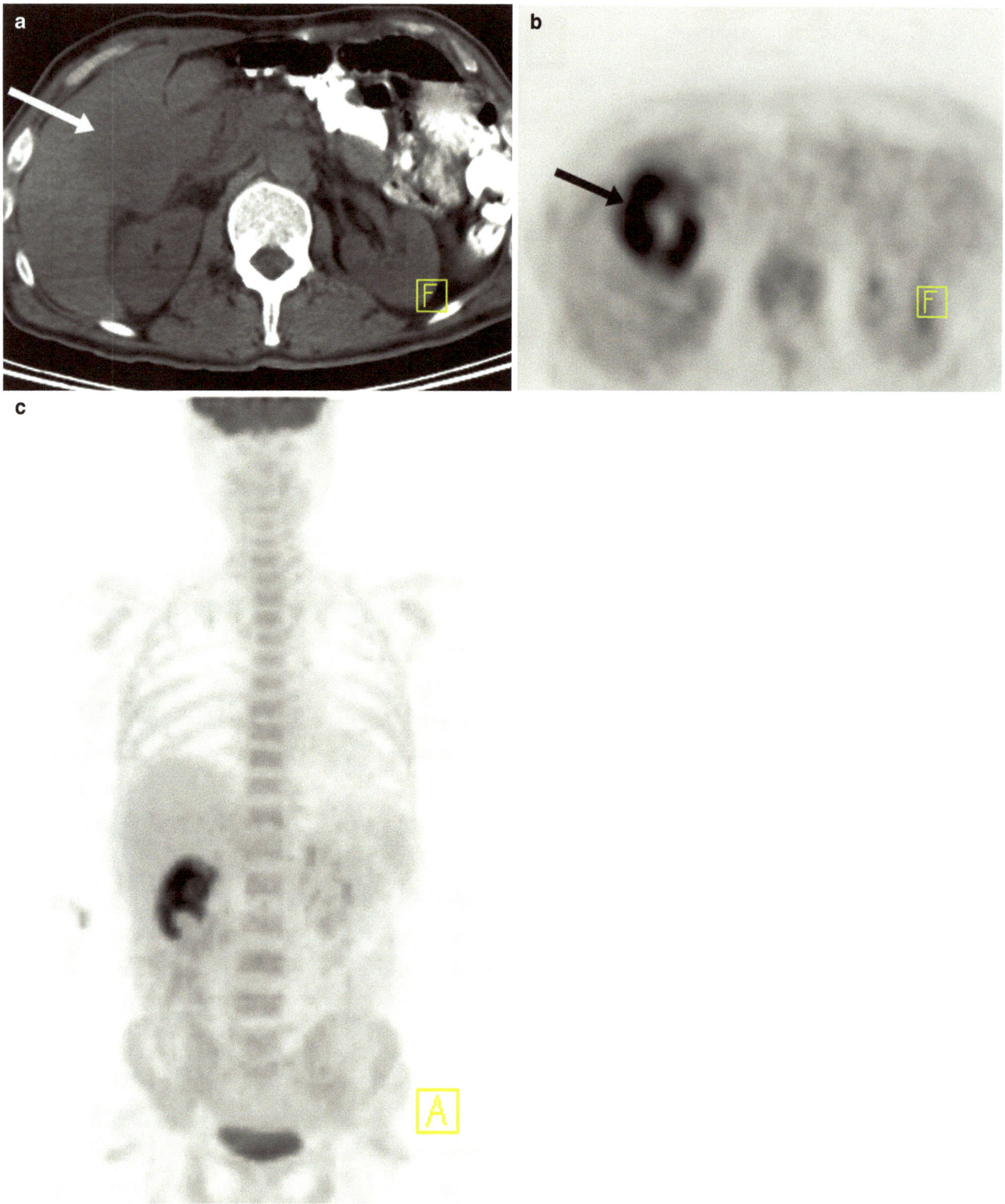

Fig. 2.65 Axial CT (**a**), PET (**b**), and MIP (**c**) images show enlarged gallbladder with increased radiotracer uptake in the gallbladder wall with a central photopenic area, which is indicative of acute cholecystitis (*arrow*)

Pancreas Cyst

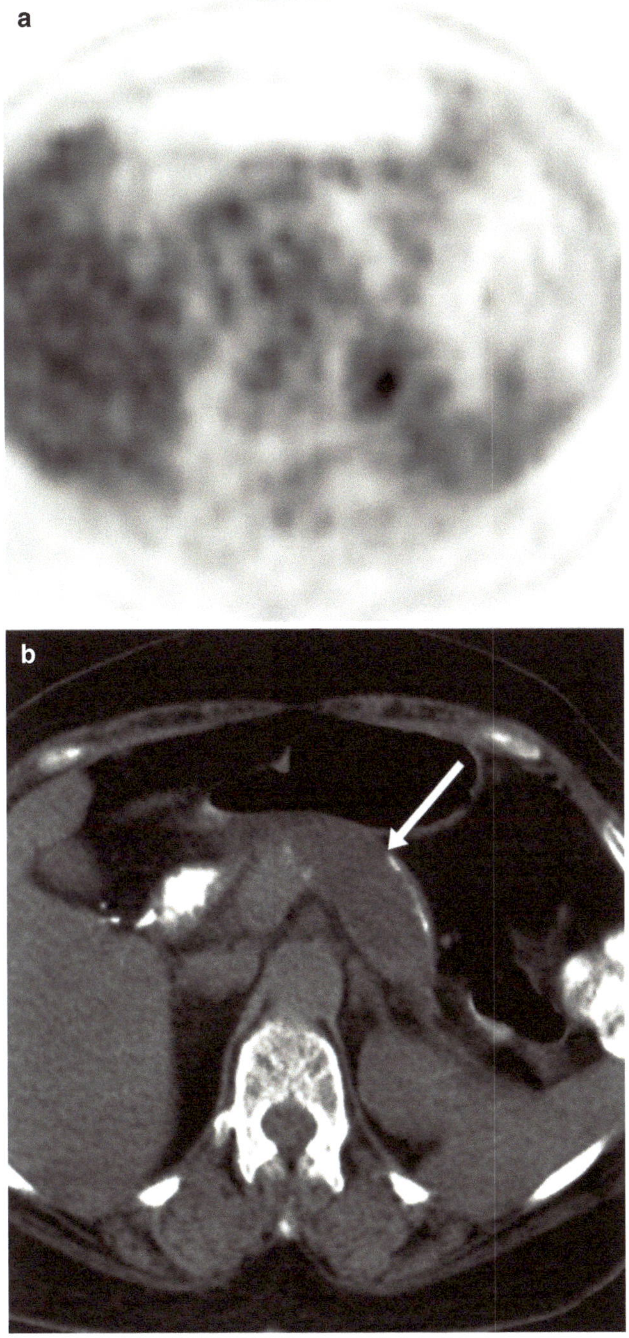

Fig. 2.66 Lesion occupying corpus and tail of pancreas which is hypodense on CT (*arrow*) (**a**) and not showing any corresponding uptake on PET images (**b**) is consistent with pancreas cyst

Surrenal Tuberculosis

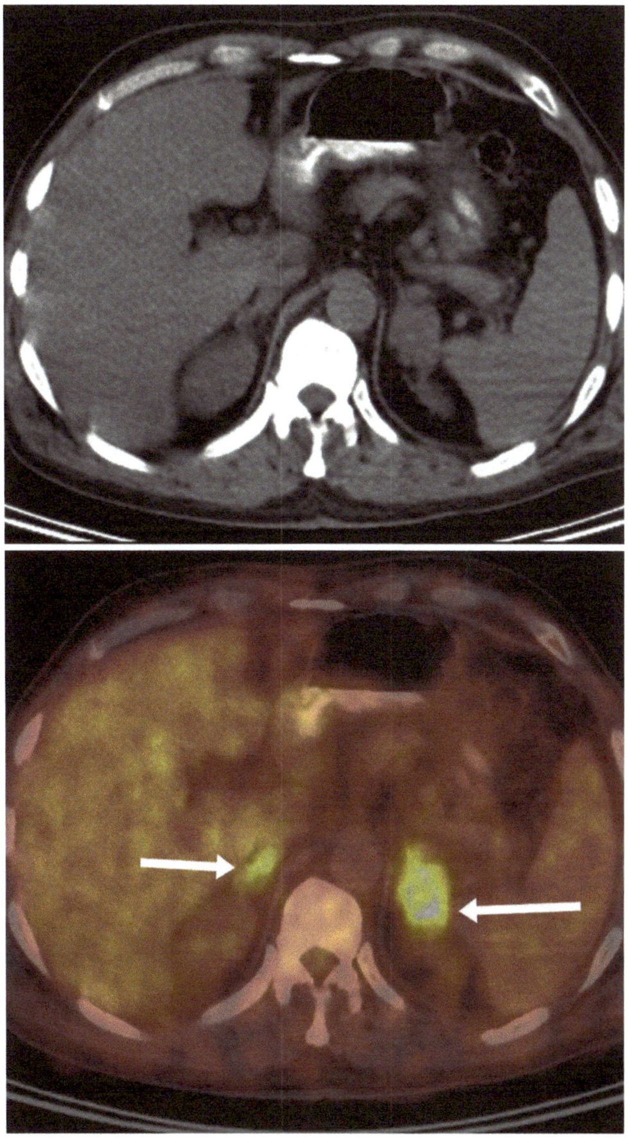

Fig. 2.67 A 42-year-old male patient underwent ^{18}F-FDG PET/CT study for metabolic characterization of the adrenal masses. Obvious ^{18}F-FDG uptake (SUVmax: 6.1) at the left adrenal mass and moderately increased ^{18}F-FDG uptake at the nodule in the right adrenal gland (*arrows*) (SUVmax: 5.1) is detected (*arrows*). The patient underwent a laparoscopic left adrenalectomy and histopathology revealed adrenal tuberculosis

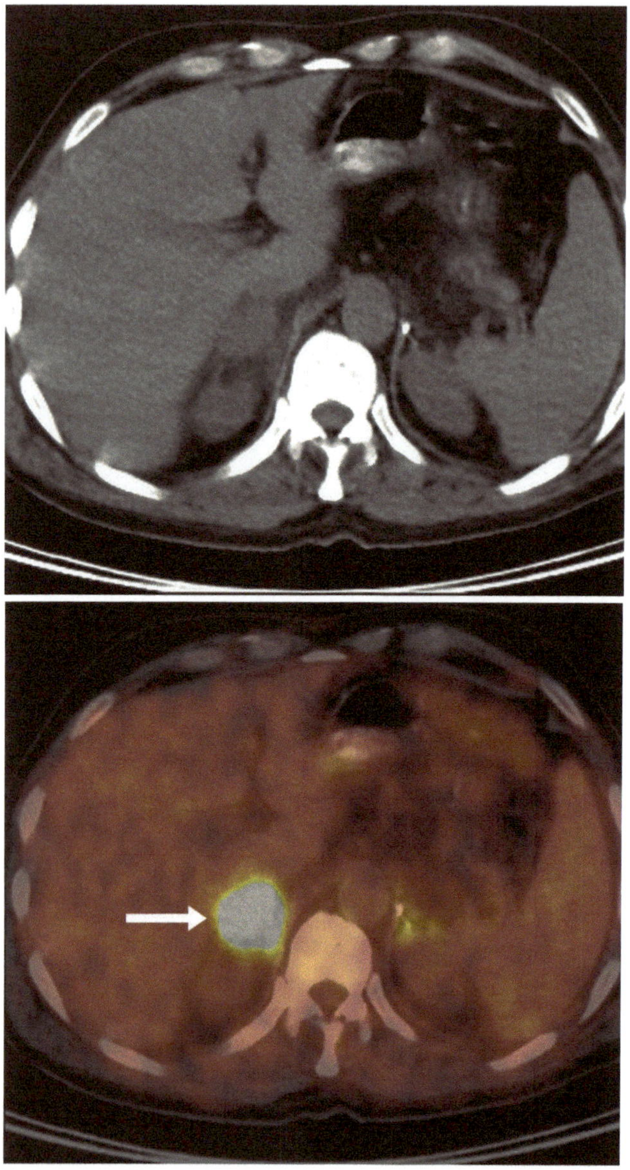

Fig. 2.68 ^{18}F-FDG PET/CT study was repeated 3 months later and the right adrenal nodule which had been detected on the first study, showed progression with further increased ^{18}F-FDG uptake (*arrow*)

Horseshoe Kidney

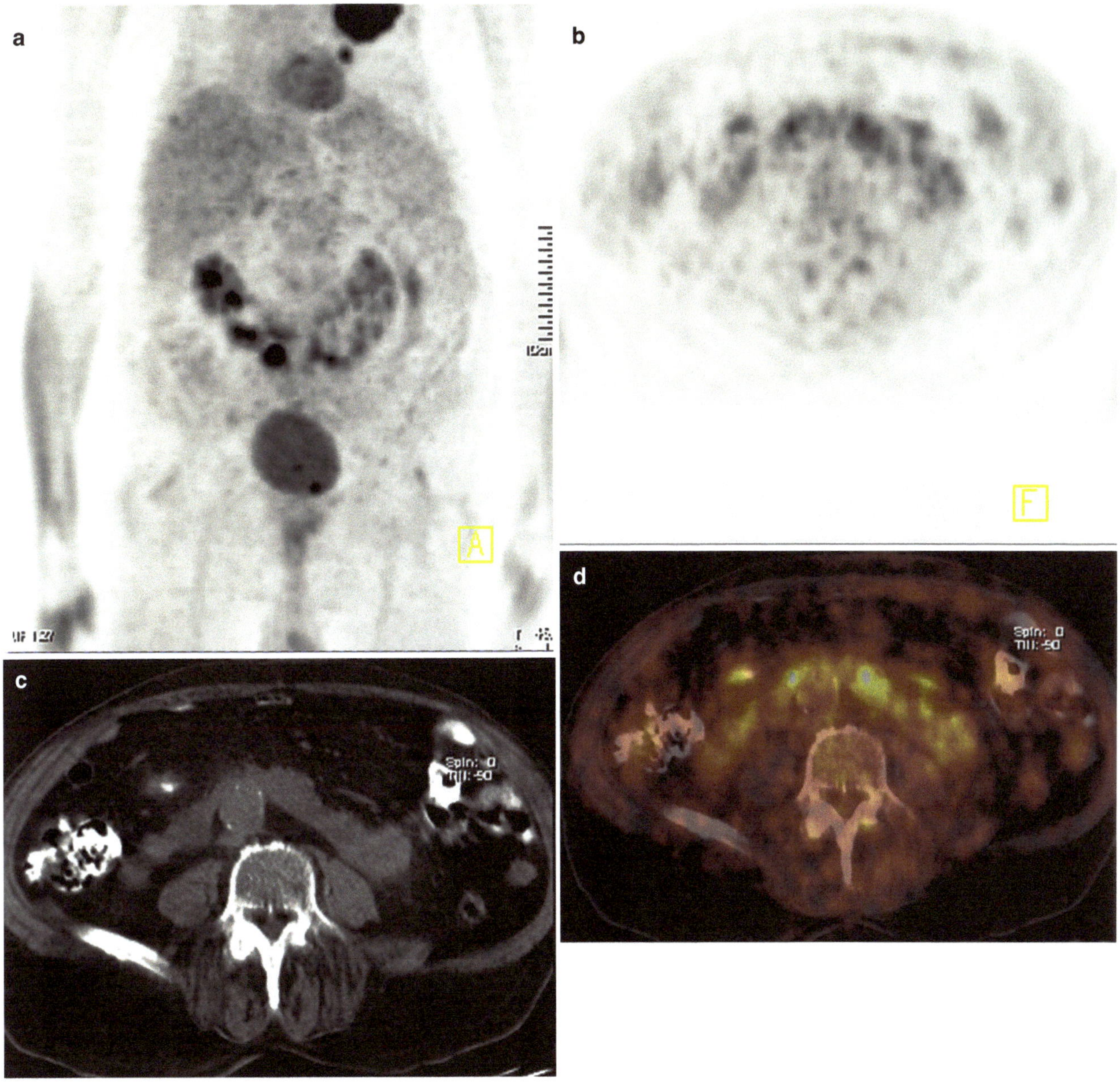

Fig. 2.69 MIP (**a**), axial PET, CT and fusion (**b**–**d**) images show horseshoe kidney

Pelvic Kidney

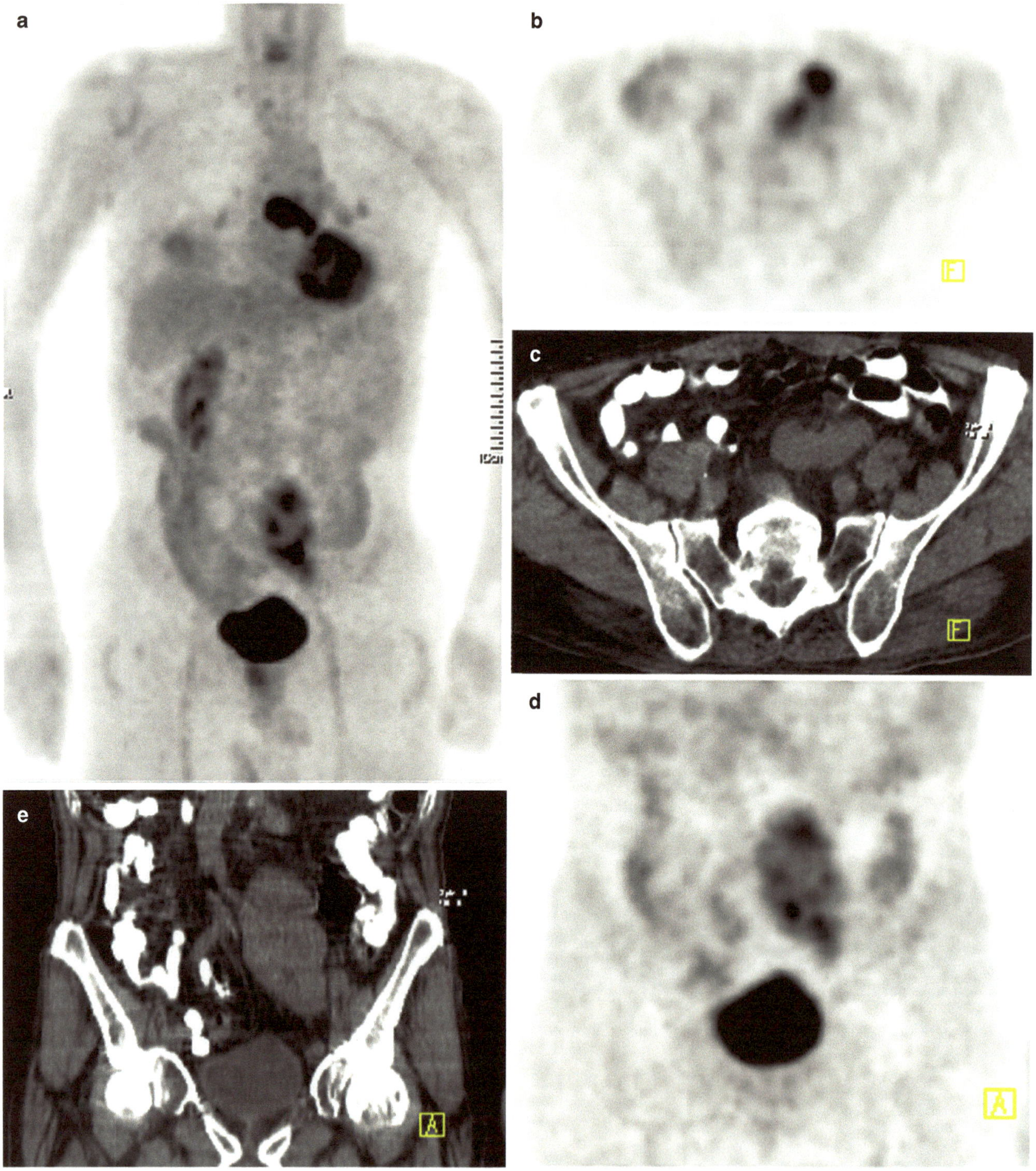

Fig. 2.70 MIP (**a**), axial (**b**, **c**), and coronal (**d**, **e**) PET and CT images show pelvic kidney

Cross Ectopic Fusion

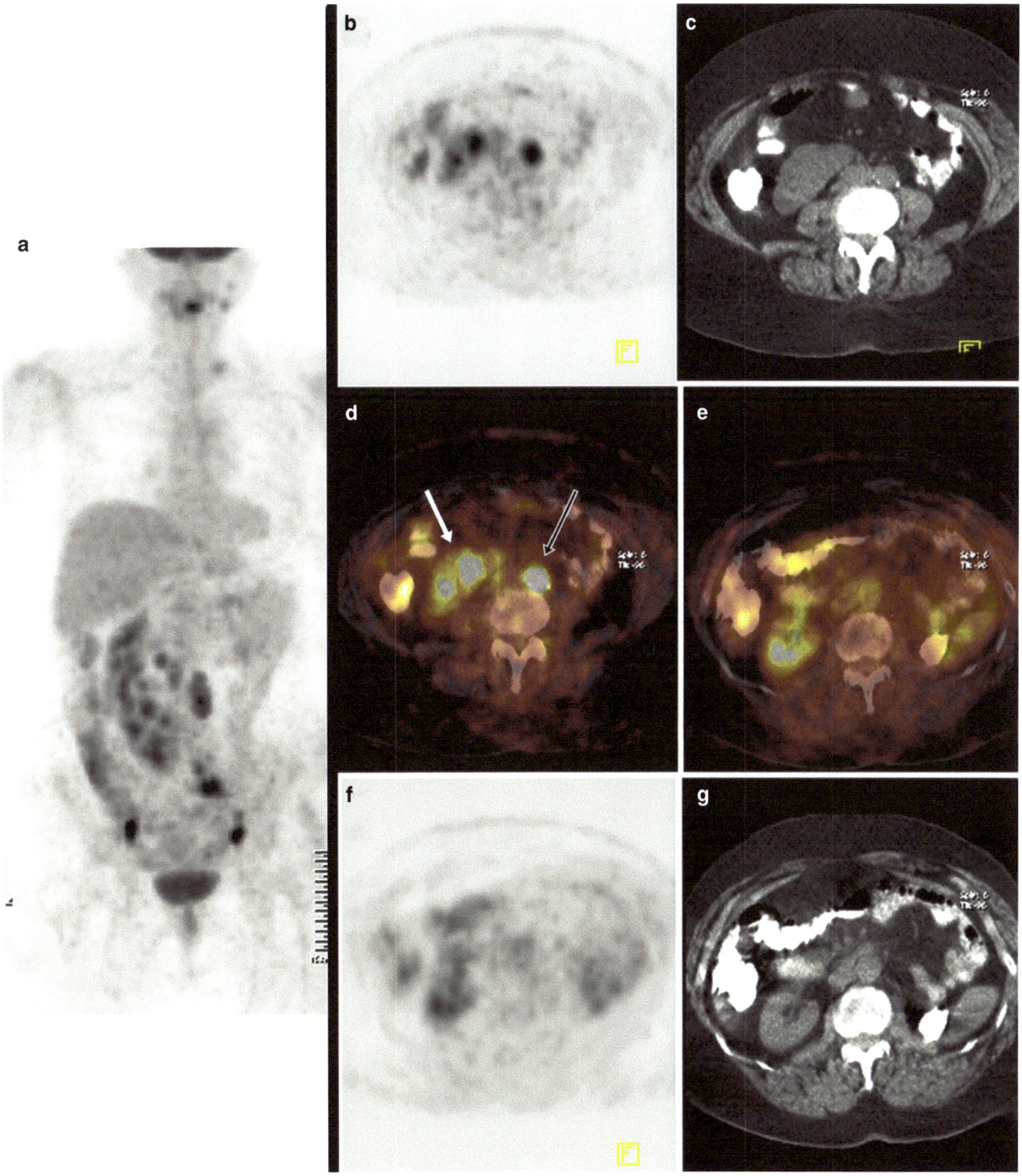

Fig. 2.71 MIP (**a**), axial PET, CT, and fusion images (**b–g**) show cross ectopic fusion anomaly at right side of abdomen (*white arrow*) and hypermetabolic lymph node at left paraaortic region (*empty arrow*)

Kidney Transplant Rejection

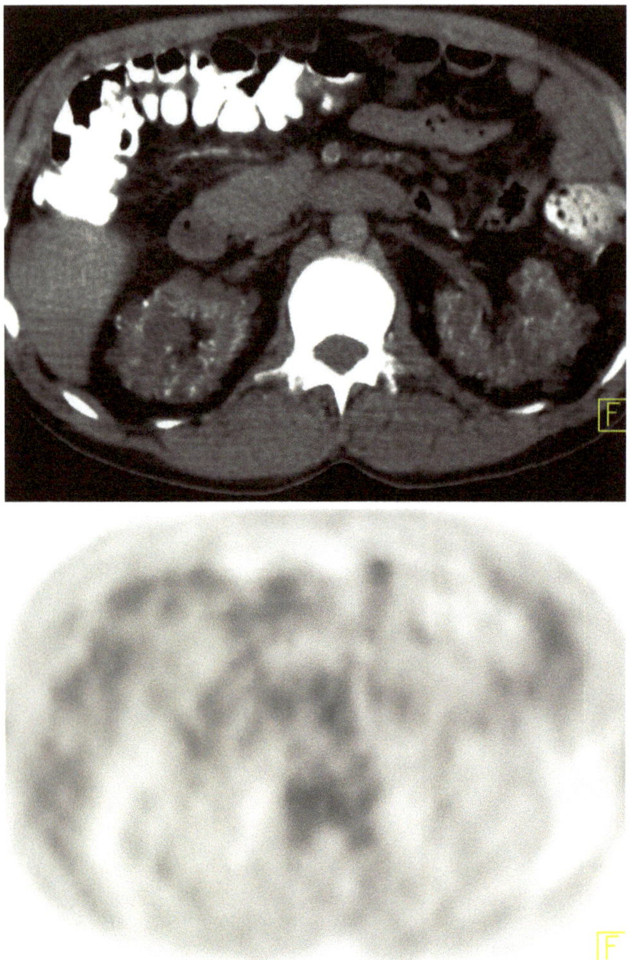

Fig. 2.72 Axial CT and PET images show absence of FDG uptake at both kidneys with end-stage renal disease

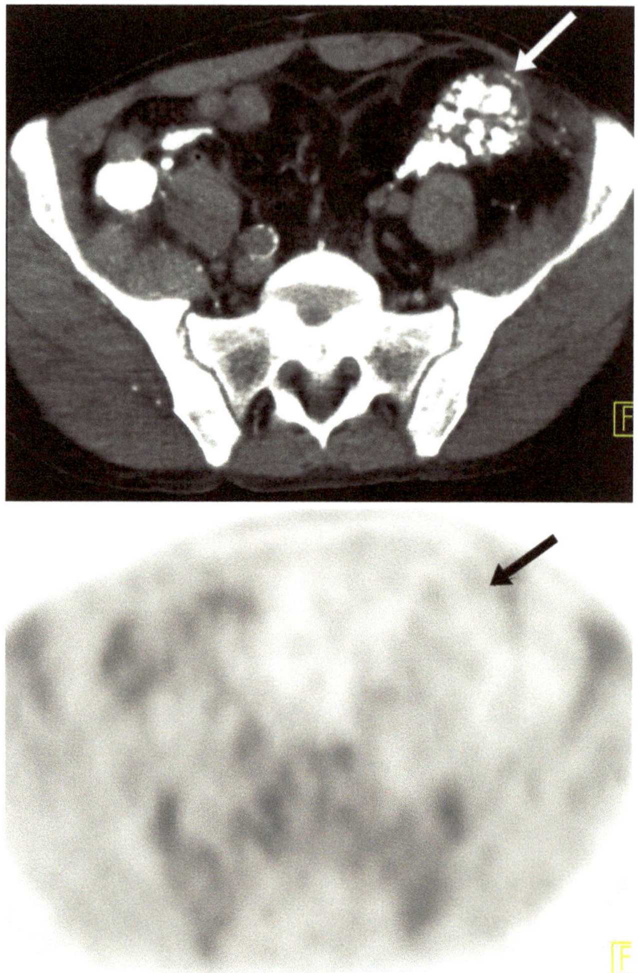

Fig. 2.73 Axial CT and PET images show rejected kidney transplant which does not have any FDG uptake (*arrow*)

Renal Cortical Cyst

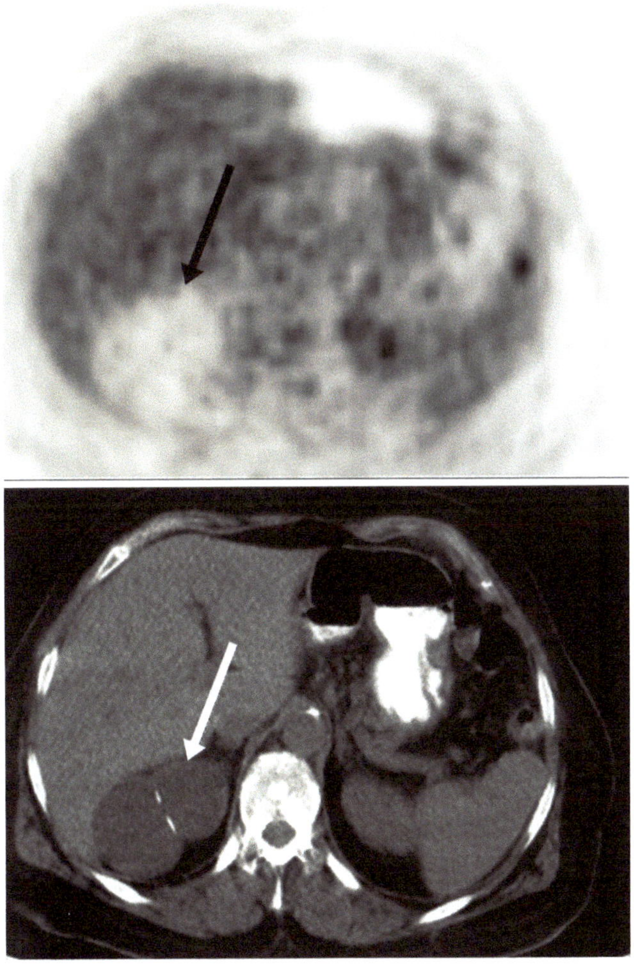

Fig. 2.74 Hypodense lesion which is ametabolic on PET image is consistent with renal cortical cyst (*arrows*)

Hydroureteronephrosis

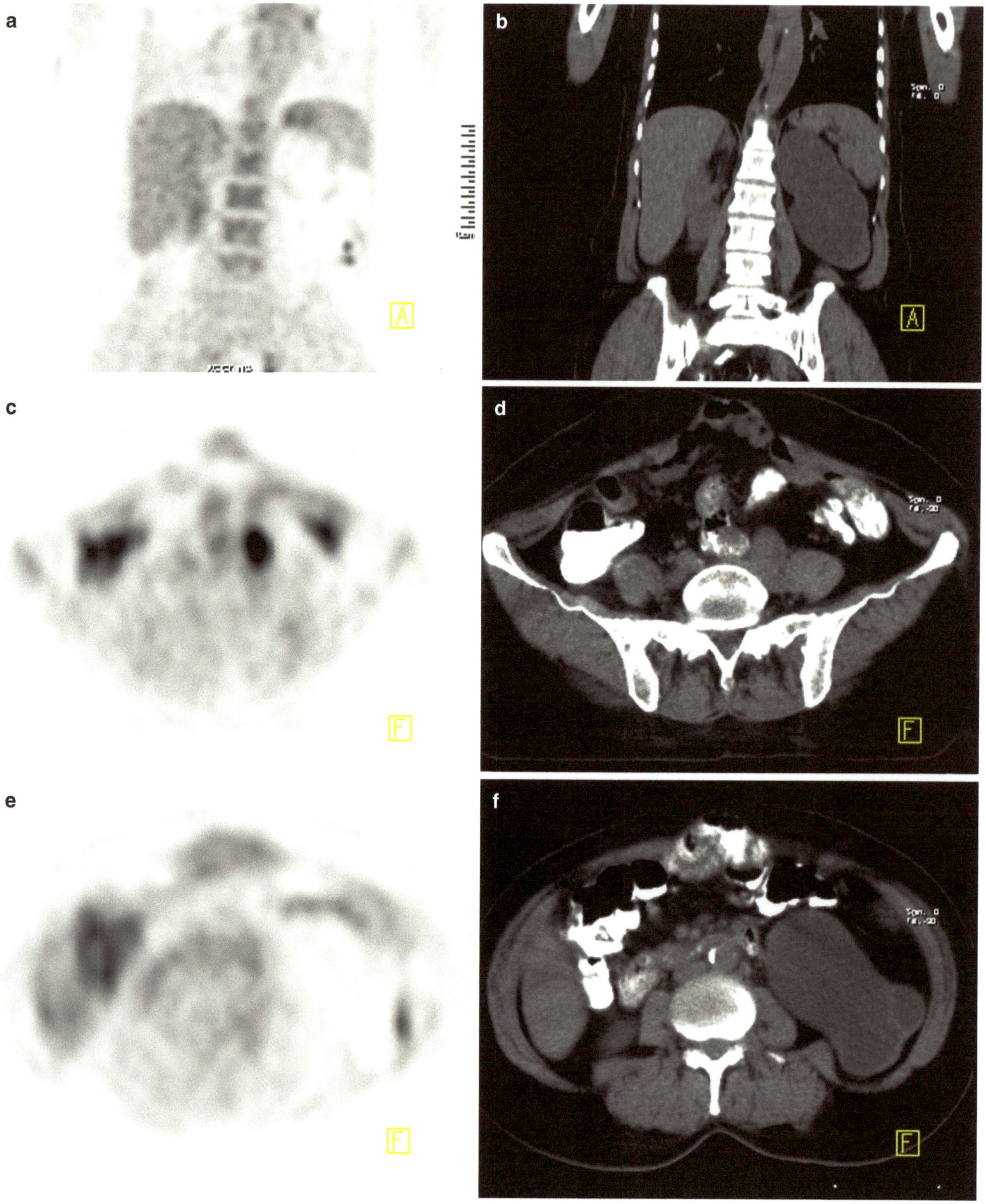

Fig. 2.75 Coronal (**a**, **b**) and axial (**e**, **f**) PET and CT images show hydronephrosis in left kidney which is ametabolic on PET images. Axial PET and CT images (**c**, **d**) show focal hypermetabolism at left common iliac area consistent with activity in dilated ureter

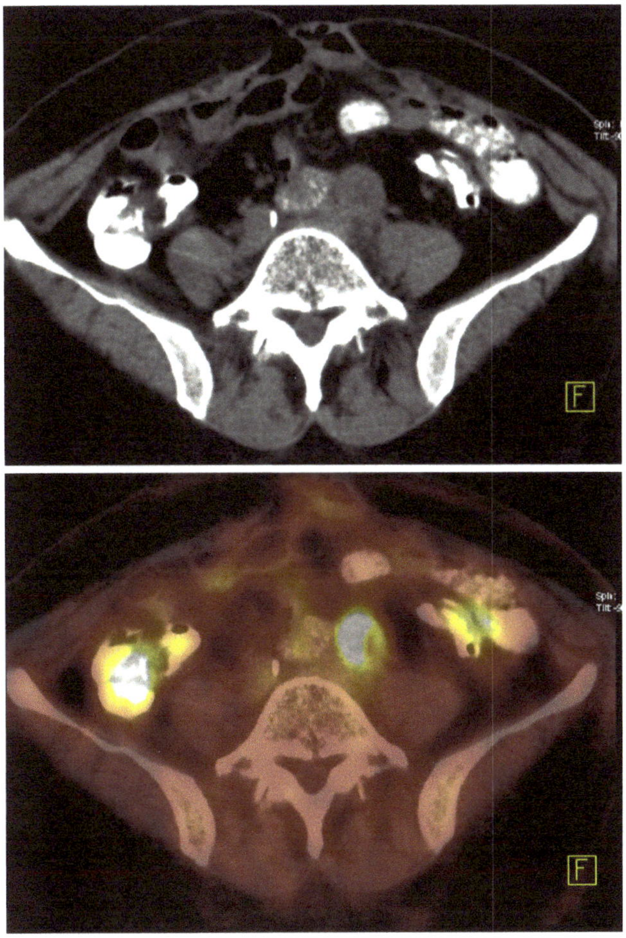

Fig. 2.76 Axial CT and fusion images show focal hypermetabolism at left common iliac area consistent with activity in dilated ureter. Evaluating the MIP image may be helpful in distinguishing this urinary activity from metastatic lymph node at this area

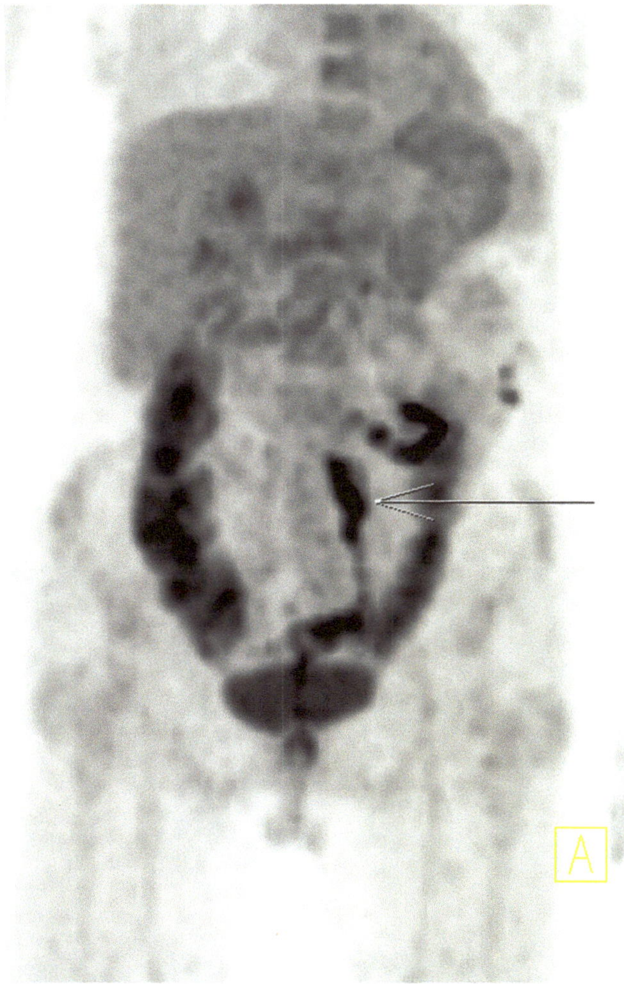

Fig. 2.77 MIP image show accumulation of activity at left ureter (*arrow*) in the patient with hydroureteronephrosis

Urinary Retention After TUR-P

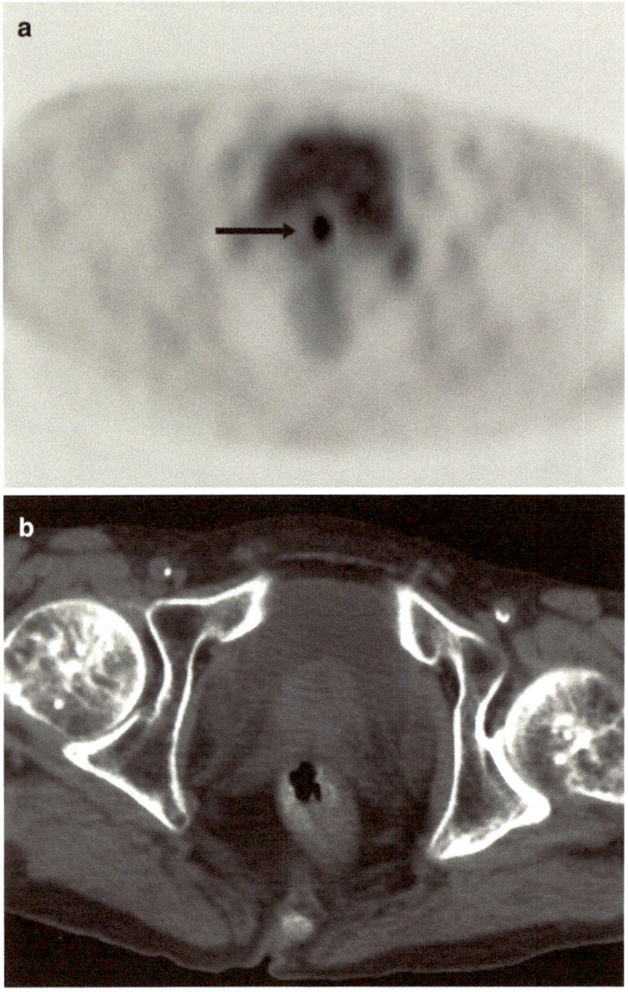

Fig. 2.78 There is focal increased FDG uptake at prostate (*arrow*), representing retention of urine following transurethral resection of the prostate (TUR-P) (**a**, **b**)

Bladder Diverticula

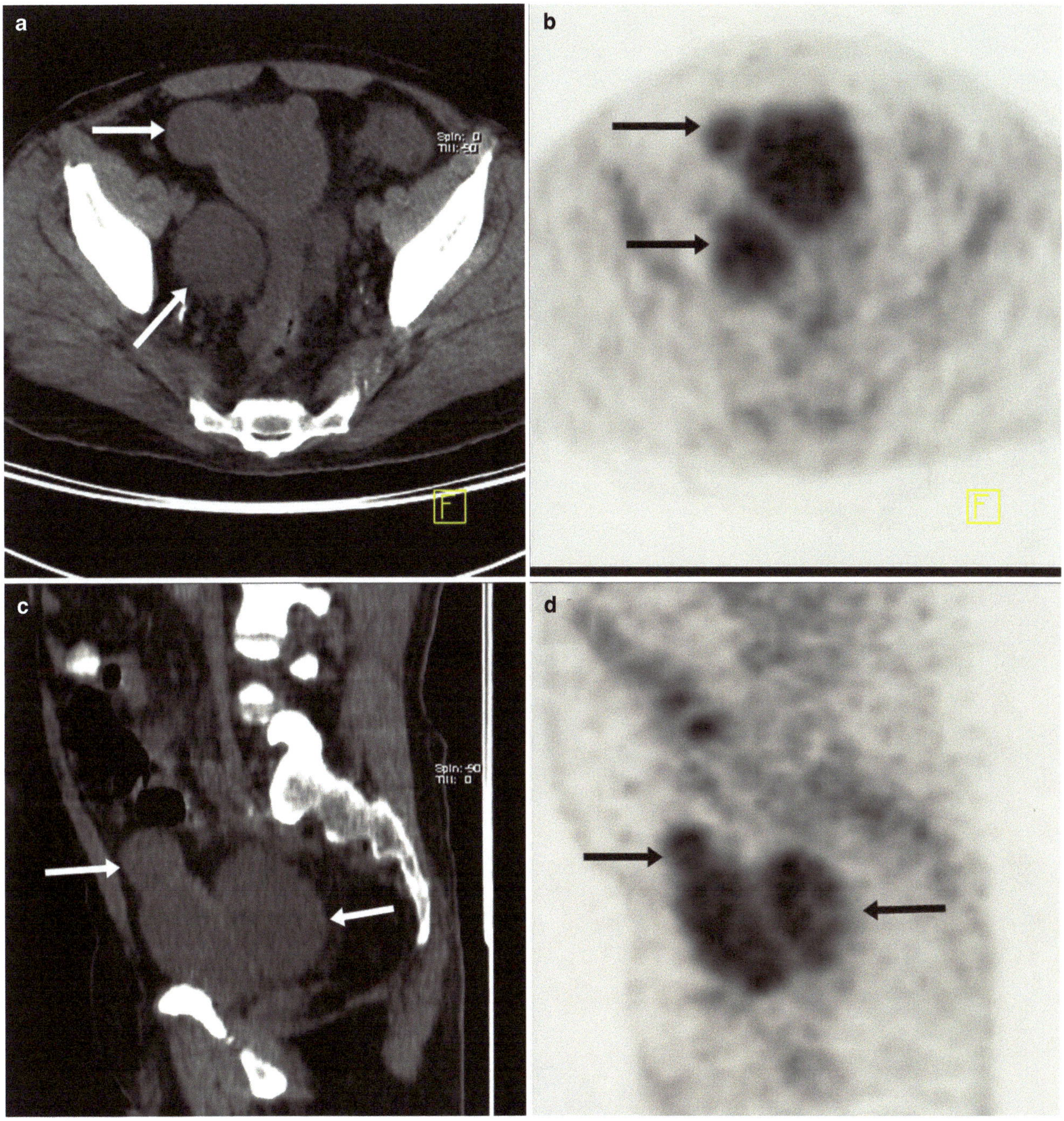

Fig. 2.79 Axial (**a**, **b**) and sagittal (**c**, **d**) slices of ^{18}F-FDG PET/CT study showing focal intense FDG accumulations on PET images, localized at bilateral anterolateral and posterolateral aspects of bladder (*black arrows*) and corresponding circular hypodensities on CT images with well-defined margins (*white arrows*) consistent with diverticula

Herniated Bladder

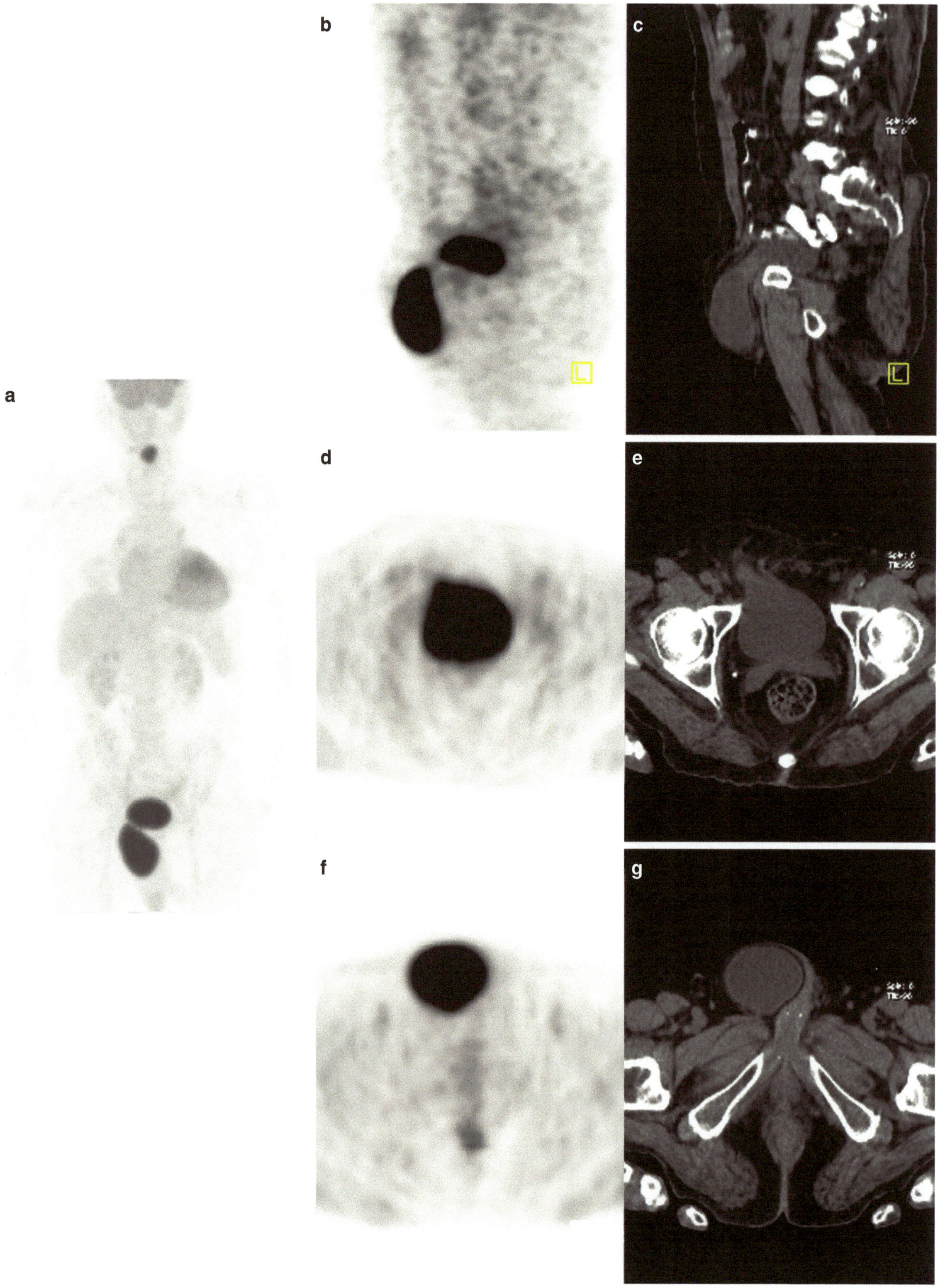

Fig. 2.80 MIP (**a**), sagittal (**b**, **c**), and axial (**d**–**g**) images display herniation of bladder

Bladder Calculus

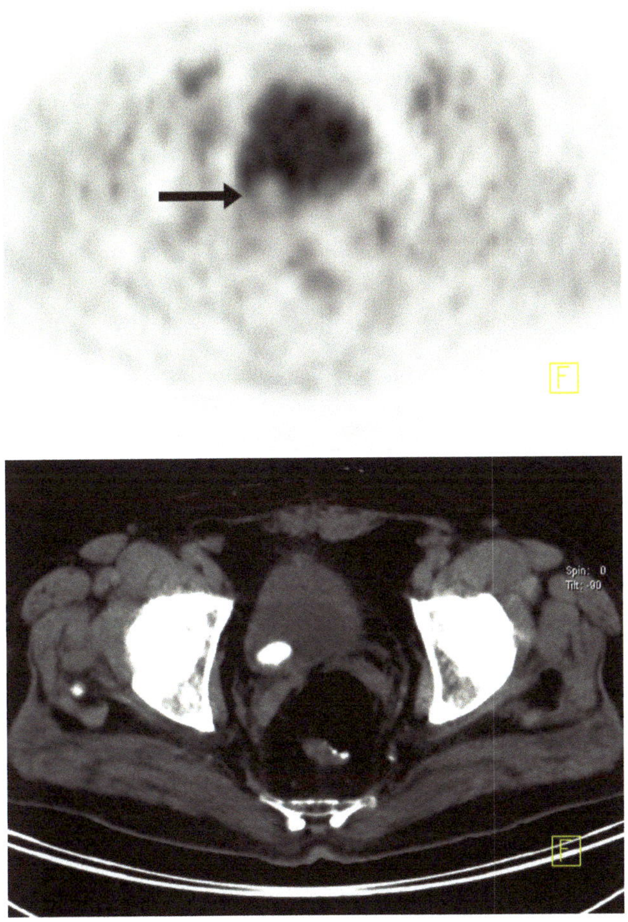

Fig. 2.81 Bladder calculus at right posterolateral aspect of bladder presenting as photopenic focus on PET image (*arrow*)

Neobladder

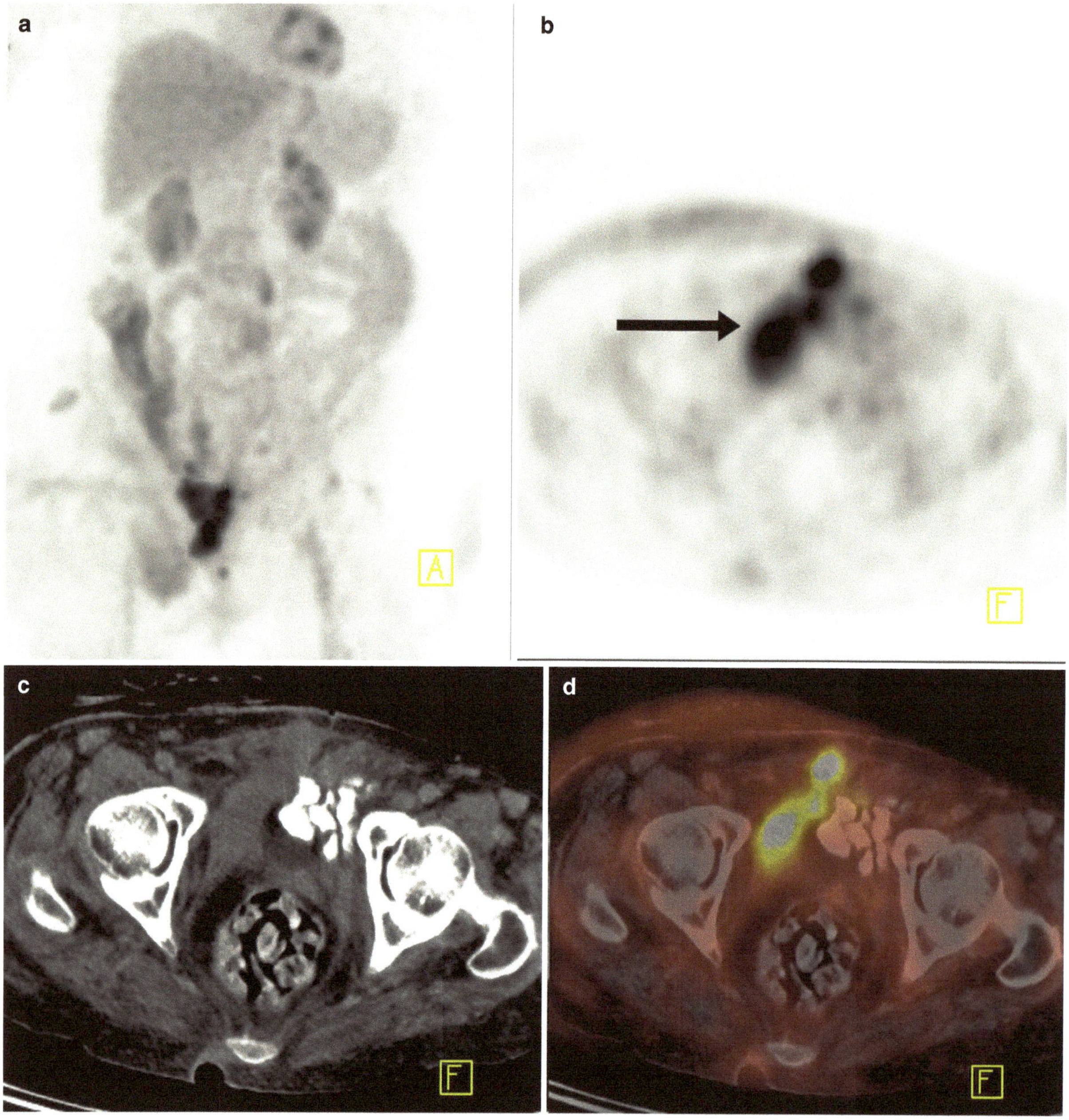

Fig. 2.82 Patient underwent radical cystectomy and a neobladder is created out of a piece of bowel. High concentration of ^{18}F-FDG in neobladder is seen representing physiological urinary excretion (*arrow*) (**a**–**d**)

Testicular Hydrocele

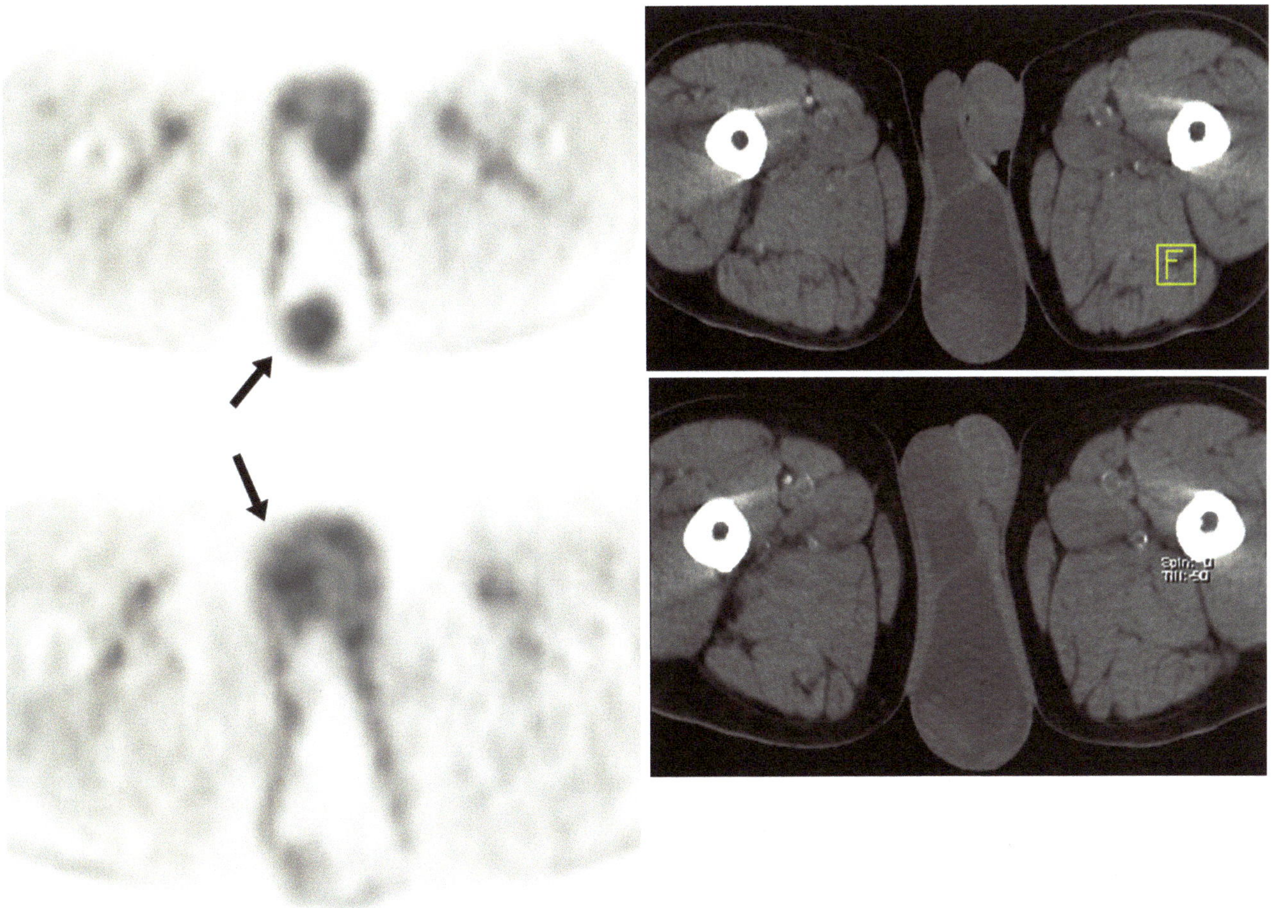

Fig. 2.83 Axial slices of PET and CT showing large testicular hydrocele. Testicles are pushed anteriorly and posteriorly (*arrows*) due to collection of fluid in scrotum

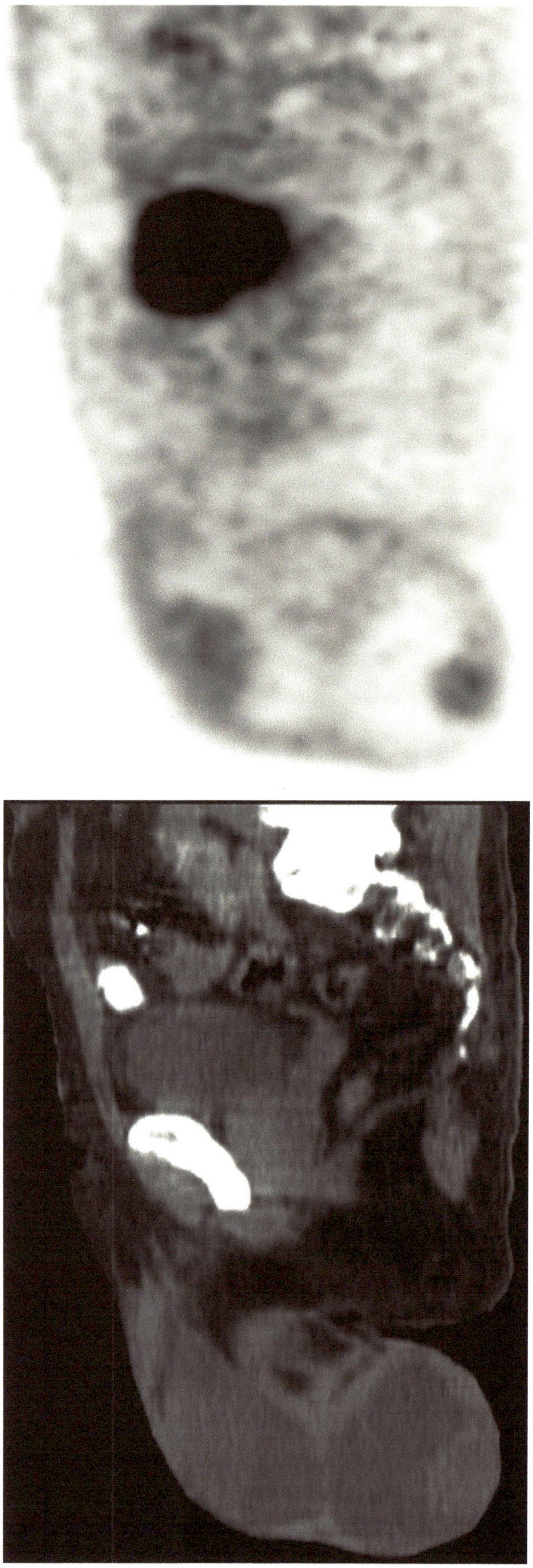

Fig. 2.84 Sagittal slices of PET and CT showing large testicular hydrocele

Follicular Ovarian Cyst

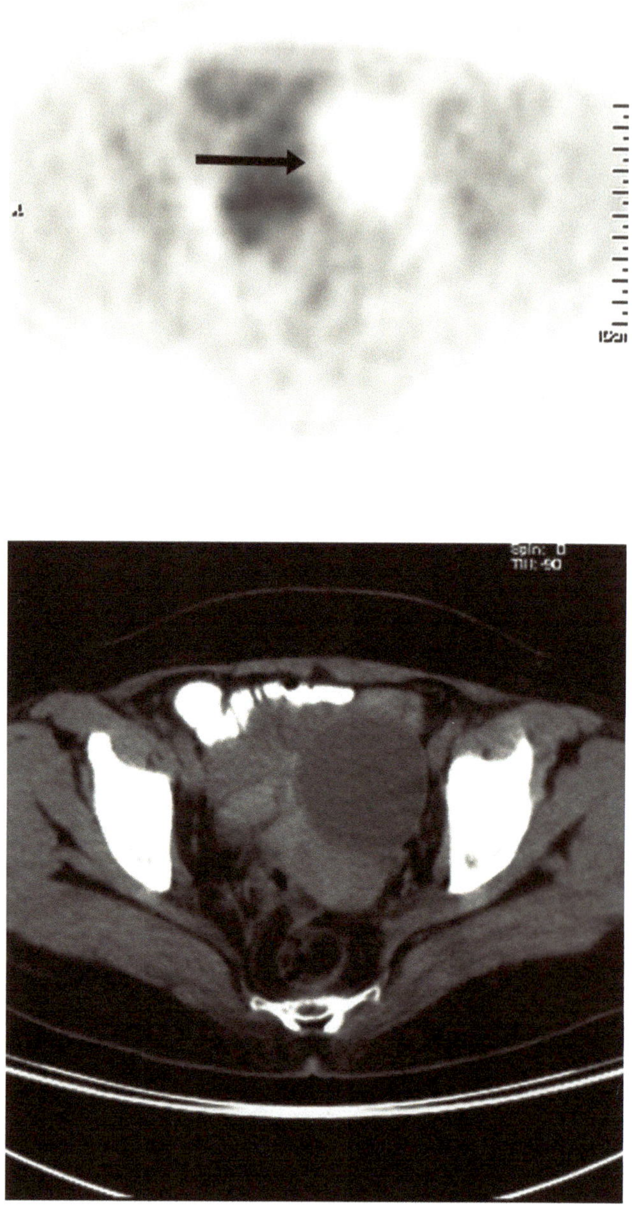

Fig. 2.85 Follicular ovarian cyst which does not show any FDG uptake (*arrow*) displaces the bladder

Calcified Myomatous Lesion

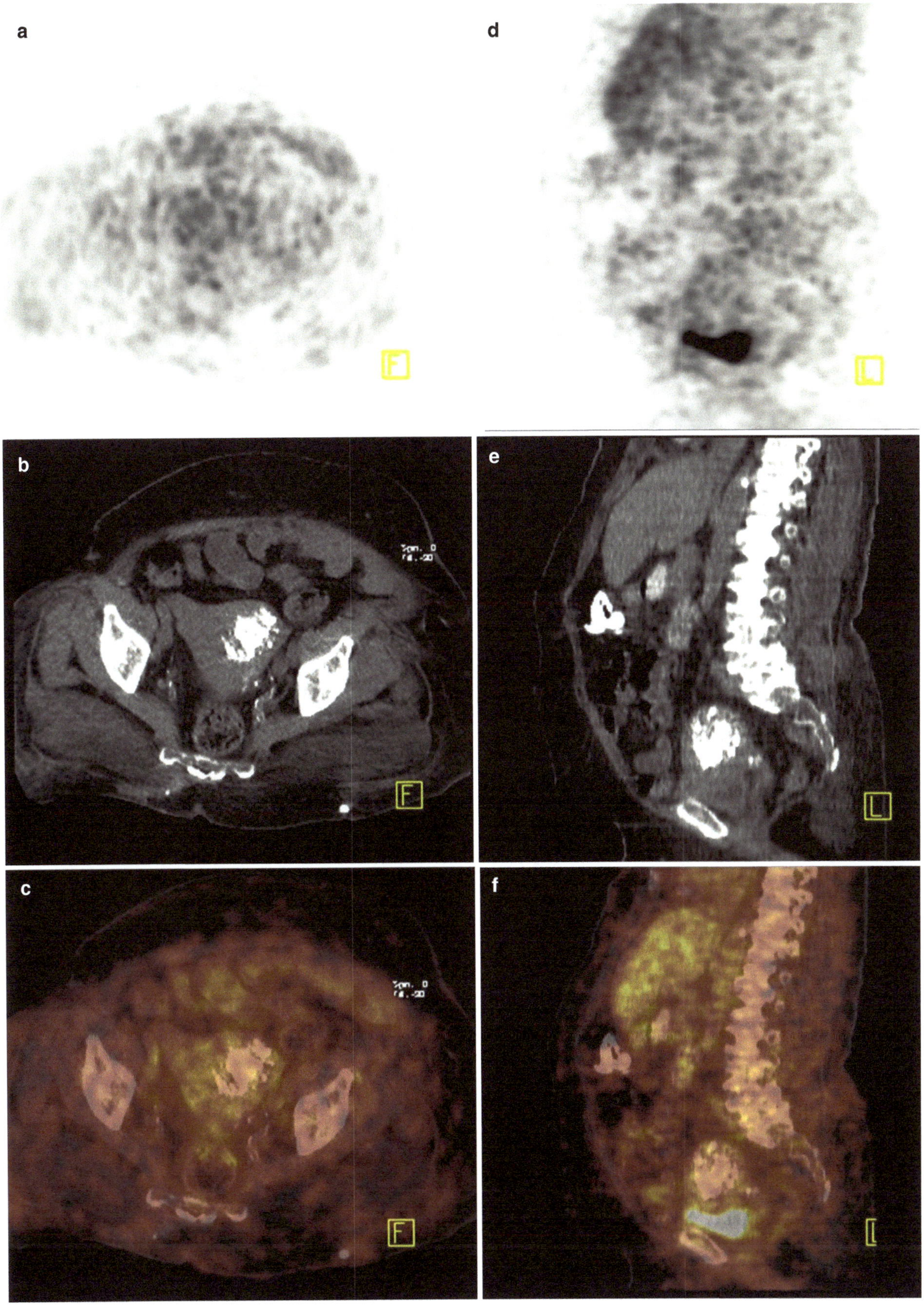

Fig. 2.86 Axial (a–c) and sagittal (d–f) PET, CT fusion images display calcified lesion at uterus without significant corresponding FDG uptake on PET, consistent with calcified myomatous lesion at uterus

Physiologically Increased FDG Uptake at Endometrium and Ovaries

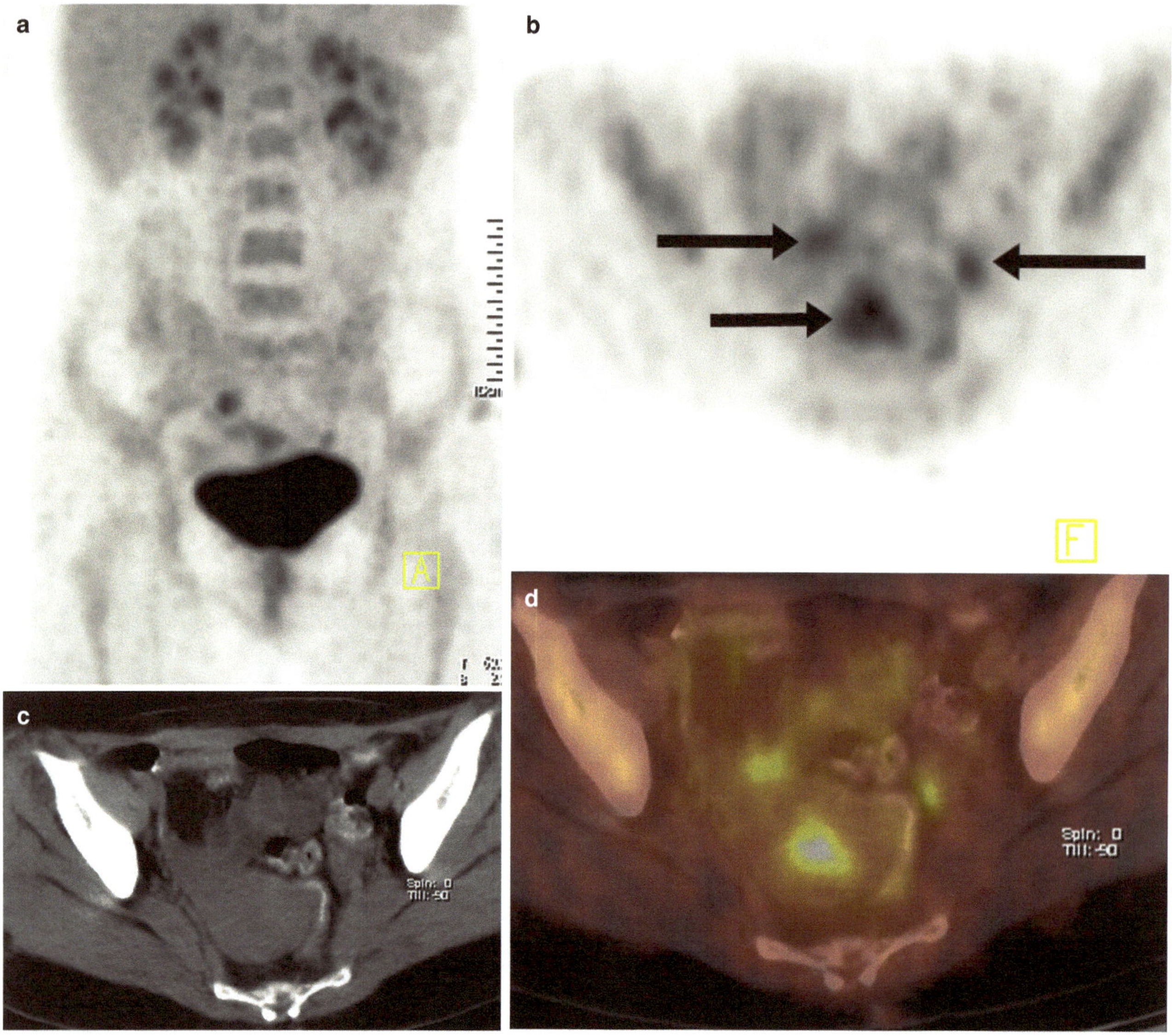

Fig. 2.87 MIP (**a**), axial PET, CT, and fusion (**b**, **c**, **d**) images of a female patient during menstruation shows physiologically increased FDG uptake at endometrium and ovaries (*arrows*)

Retroperitoneal Fibrosis

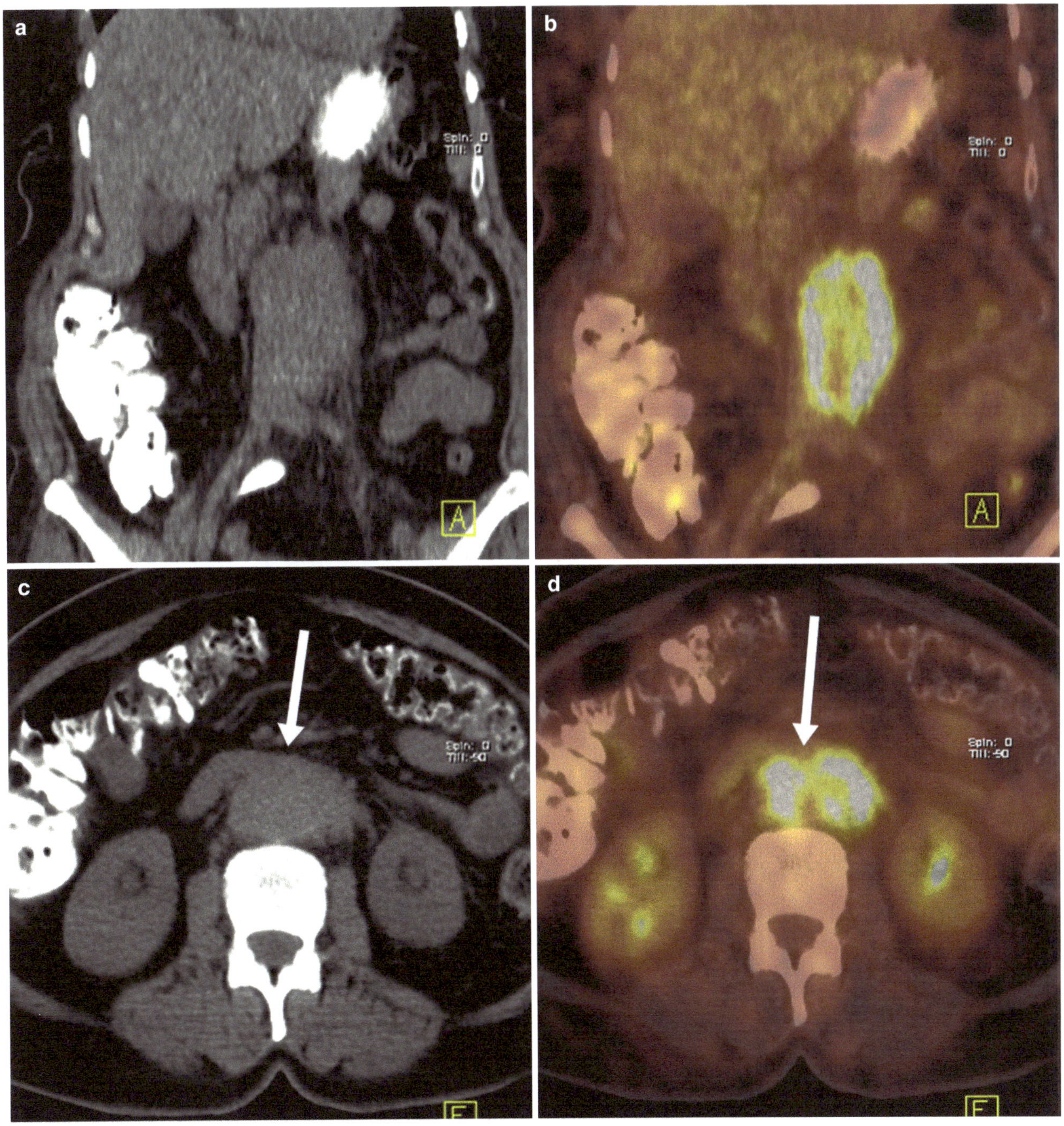

Fig. 2.88 A 48-year-old man with colorectal carcinoma underwent ^{18}F-FDG PET/CT scan. Circumferential soft-tissue thickening around the distal aorta showing diffuse intense FDG uptake on PET image (*arrows*) is consistent with retroperitoneal fibrosis (RPF) (**a**–**d**). RPF is mostly idiopathic, and although its etiology is unknown, an immune-mediated response to severe atherosclerosis is a proposed mechanism. Etiology of other secondary RF refers to medications (drug-induced RPF), infections, traumas, surgery, radiation therapy, and malignancies

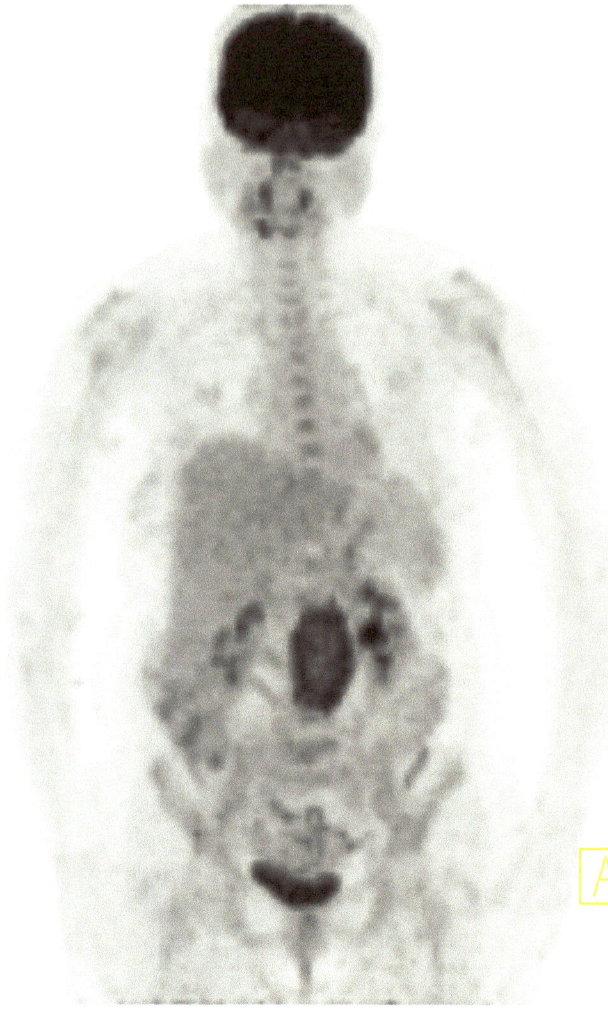

Fig. 2.89 MIP image

Aortic Mural Thrombus

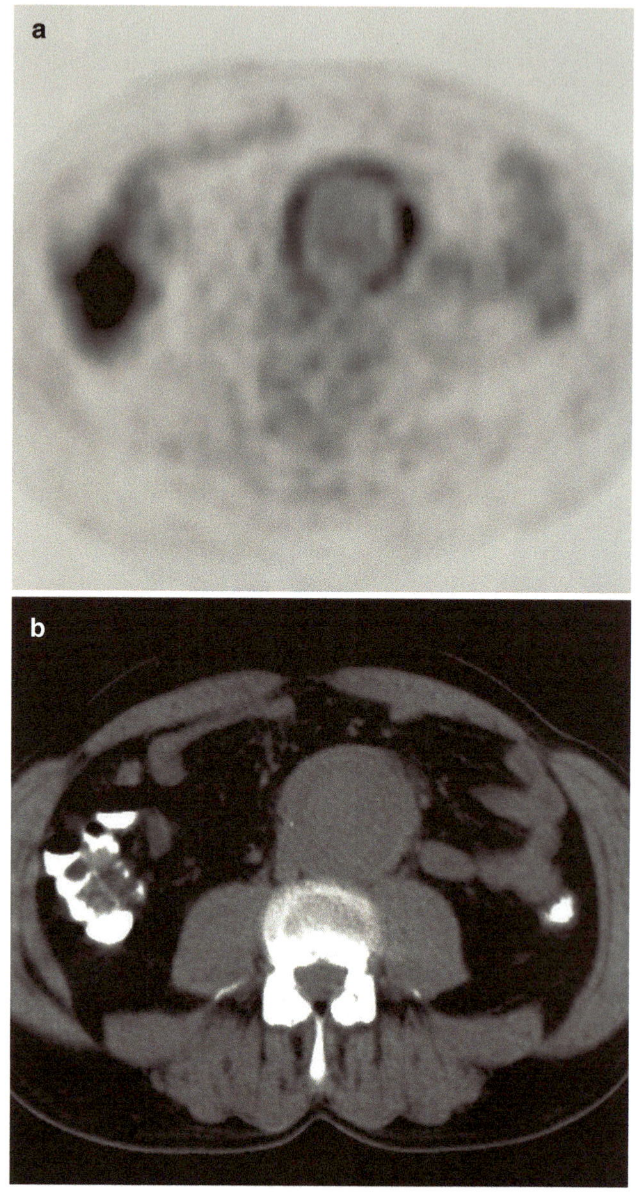

Fig. 2.90 Axial PET and CT and images (**a**, **b**) showing mass lesion at abdominal aorta with central photopenia and a mildly hypermetabolic rim which is consistent with eccentric aortic mural thrombus

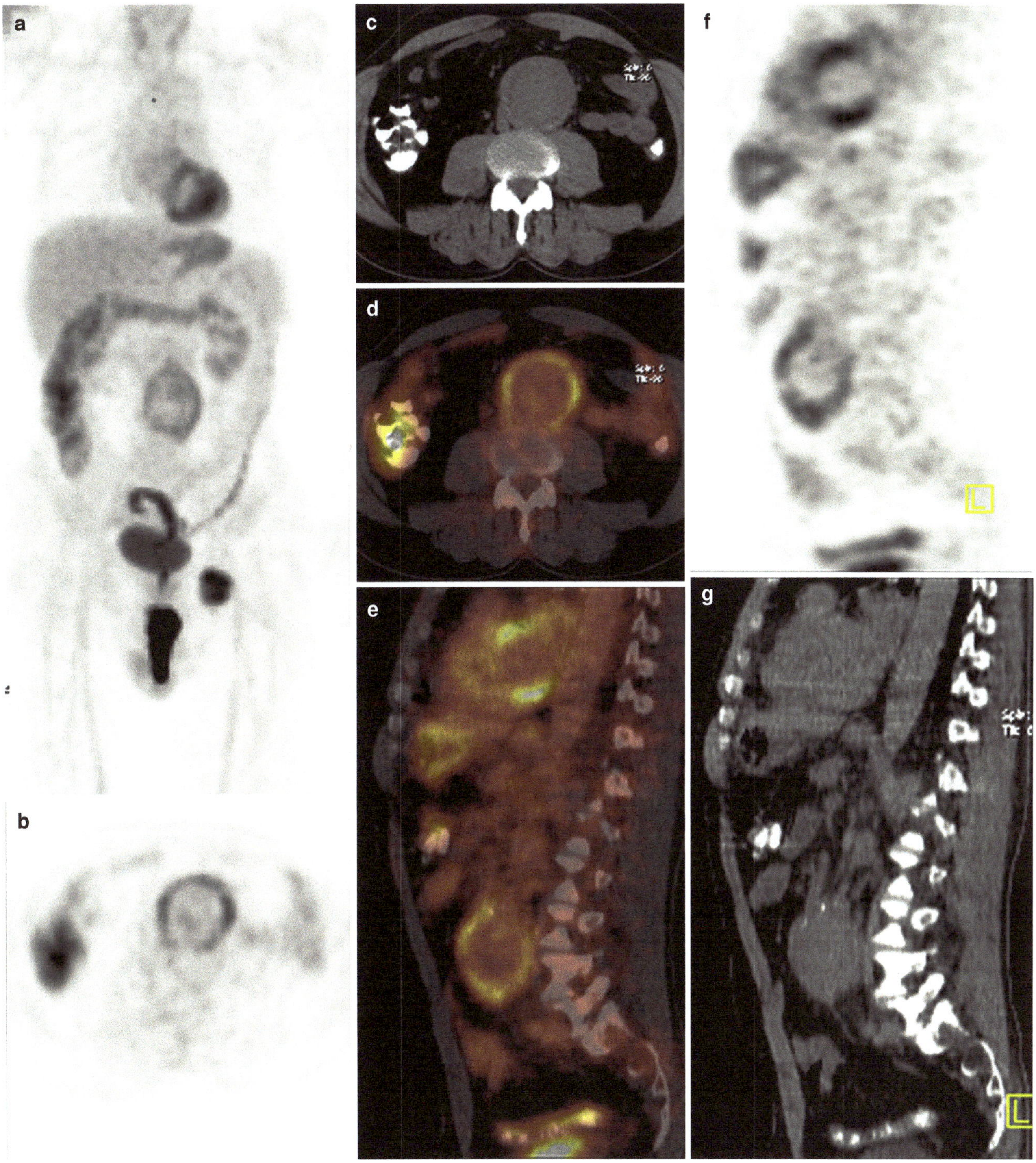

Fig. 2.91 MIP image (**a**), axial PET, CT, and fusion images (**b–d**), sagittal fusion, PET, and CT images (**e–g**)

Abdominal Aortic Aneurysm

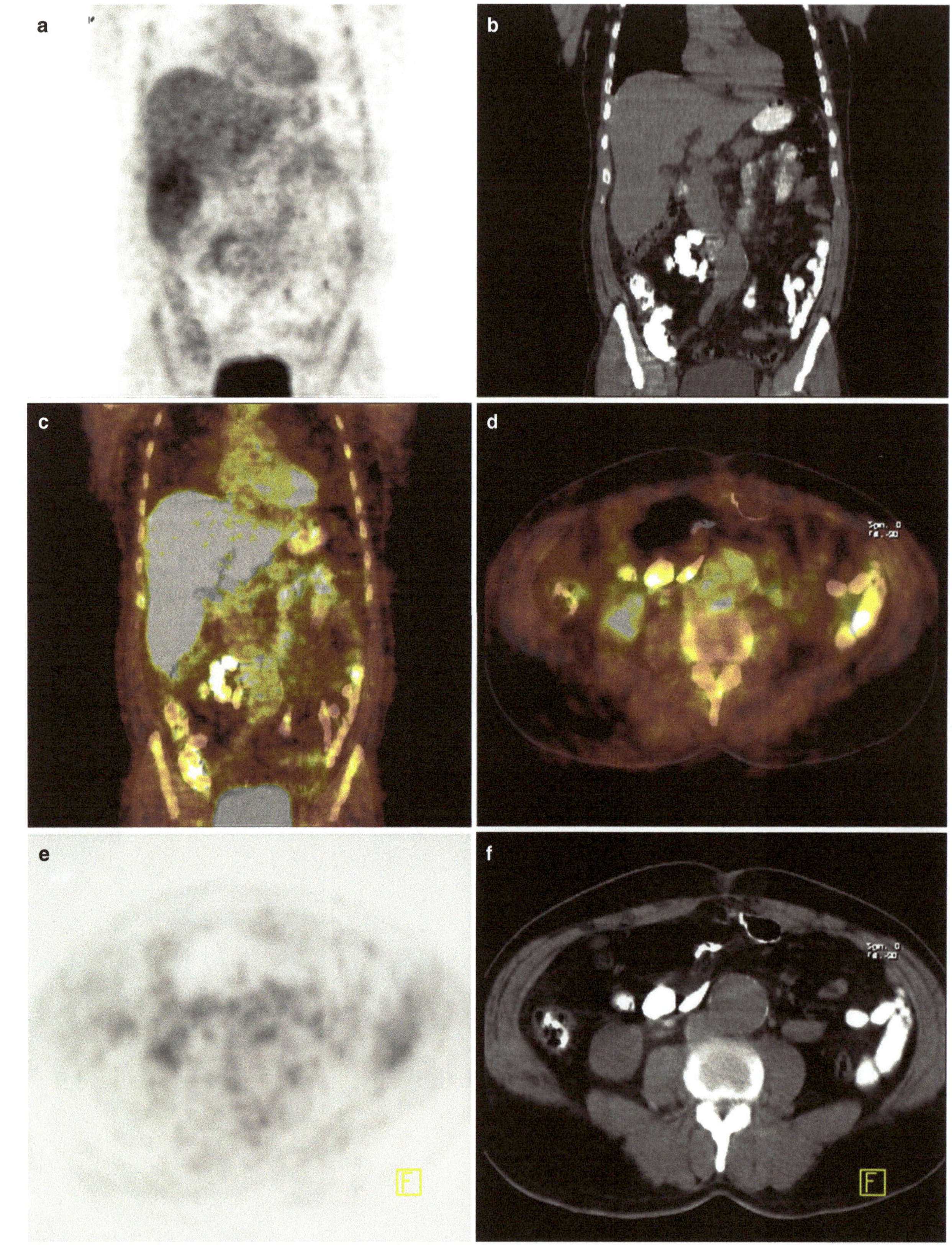

Fig. 2.92 Coronal PET, CT, and fusion images (**a–c**), axial fusion, PET, and CT images (**d–f**) show dilatation of abdominal aorta with a diameter reaching 40 mm at the largest part, consistent with abdominal aortic aneurysm (AAA). There is not any remarkable pathological FDG uptake at AAA on corresponding PET images. The AAA diameter is the most usual predictive factor for the risk of rupture and surgery is recommended when the maximum diameter is greater than 55 mm. So it must be pointed out when it is detected on ^{18}F-FDG PET/CT scan. Increased FDG uptake at the aneurysm may also be predictive of rupture

Abdominal Aortic Aneurysm

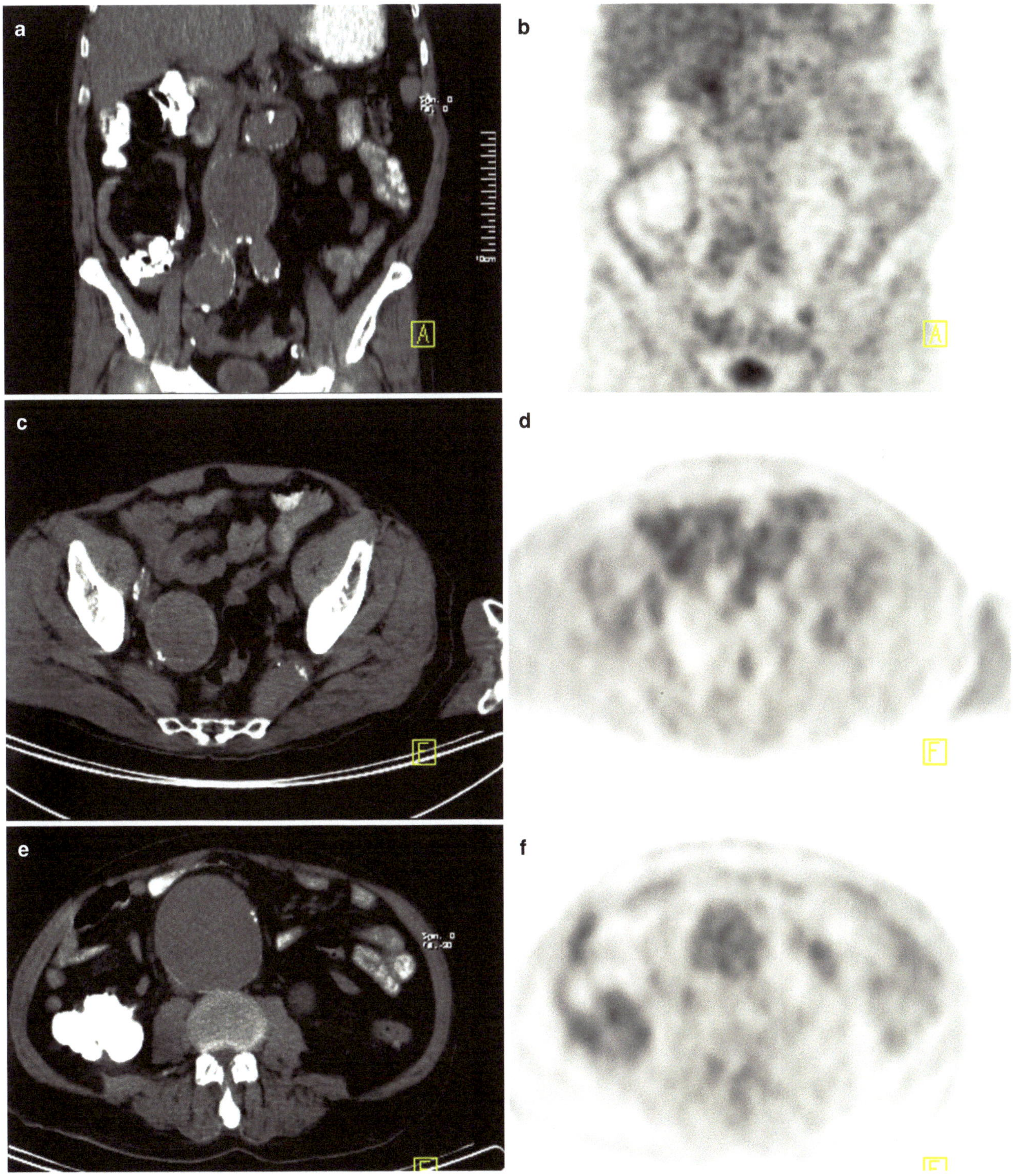

Fig. 2.93 Coronal (**a**, **b**) and axial (**c**, **d**, **e**, **f**) CT and PET images show aneurysmal dilatation at abdominal aorta and both common iliac arteries

Fat Necrosis

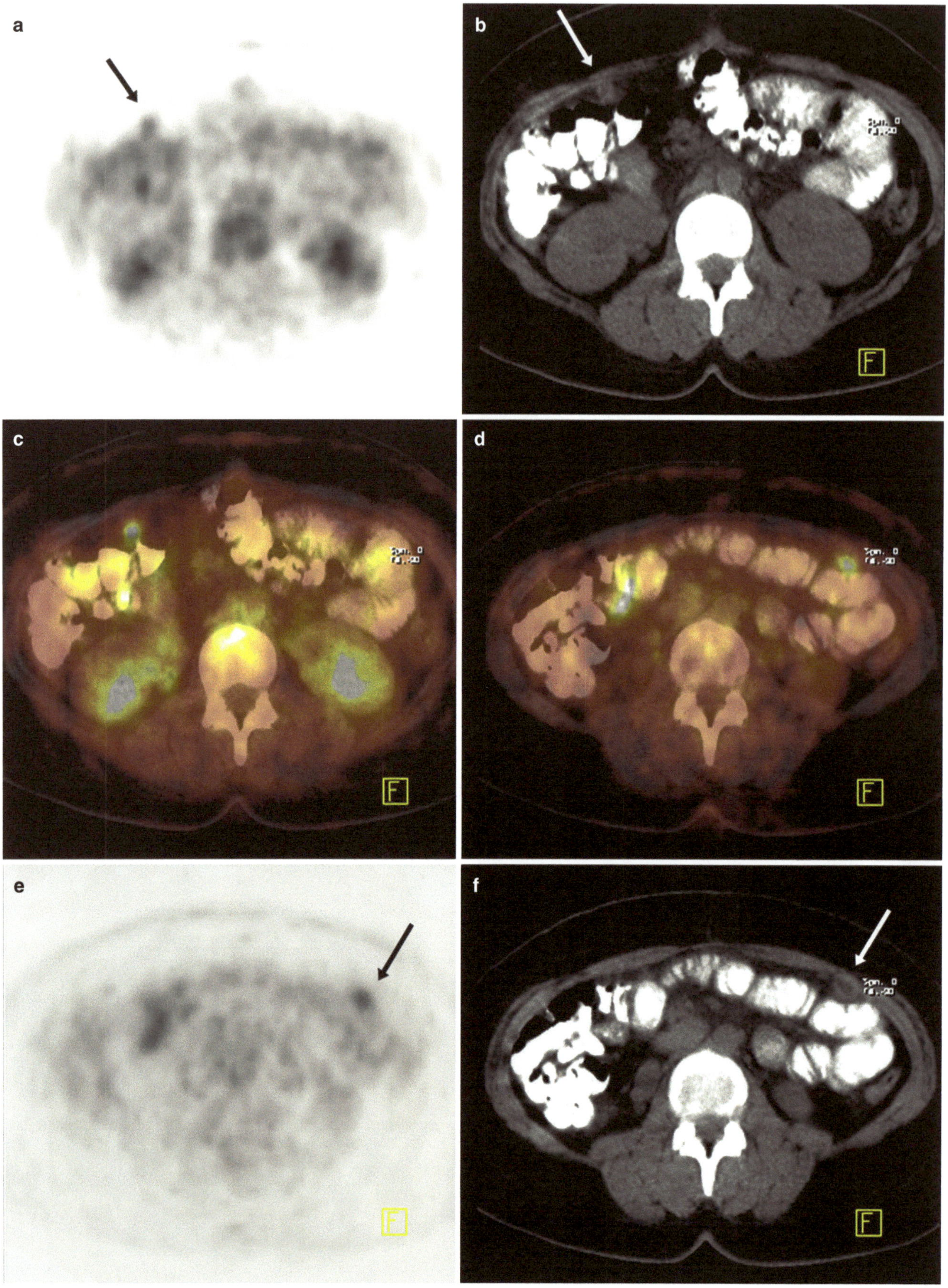

Fig. 2.94 Axial PET, CT, and fusion images (**a**–**c**) and axial fusion, PET, and CT images (**d**–**f**) display mild increased FDG uptake at omental fat necrosis areas (*arrows*)

FDG Uptake at Injection Site

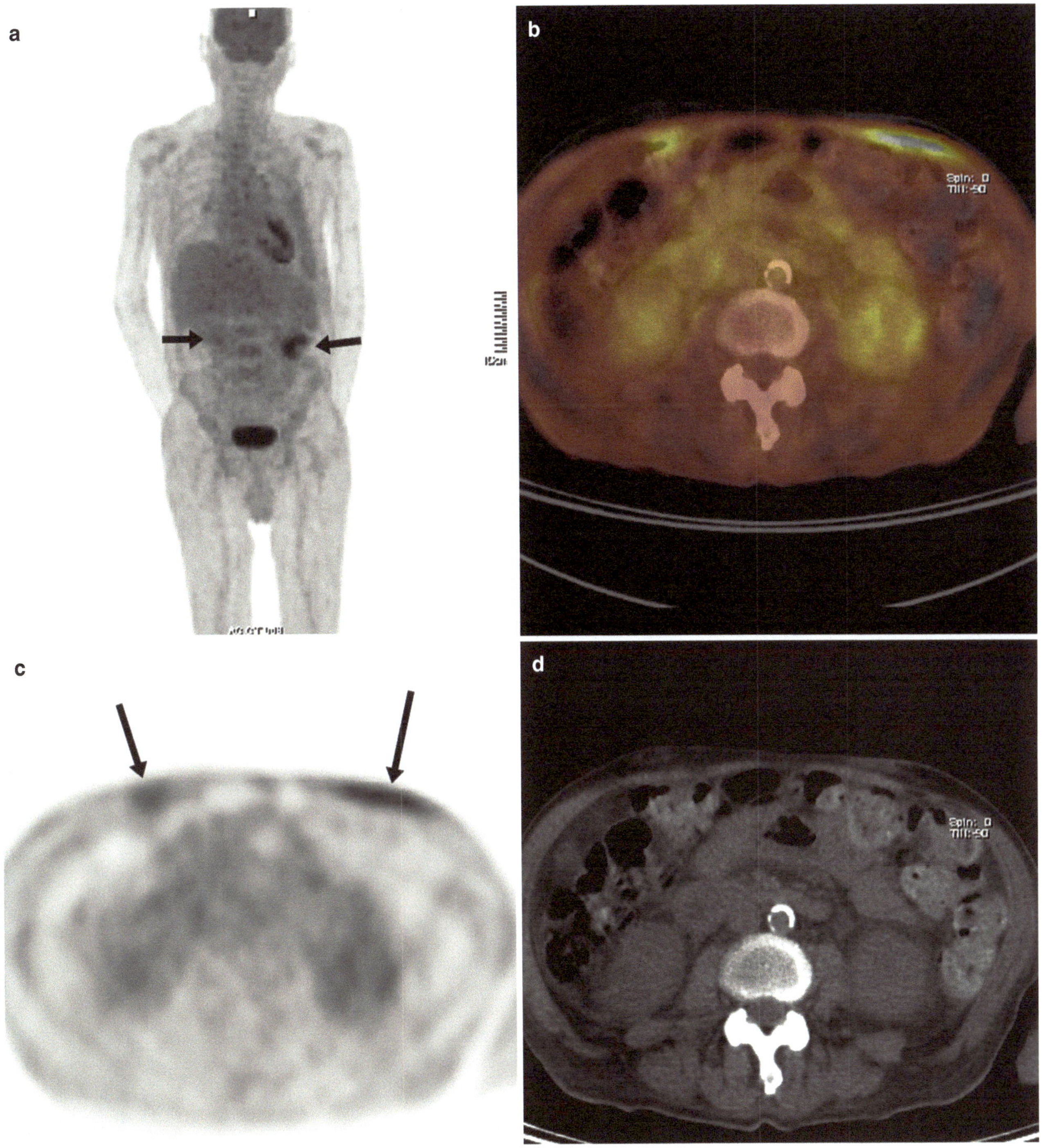

Fig. 2.95 Increased FDG uptake at subcutaneous tissues of anterior wall of abdomen due to inflammation occurred as a result of repetitive insulin injections (*arrows*) (**a**–**d**)

FDG Uptake Around Catheter

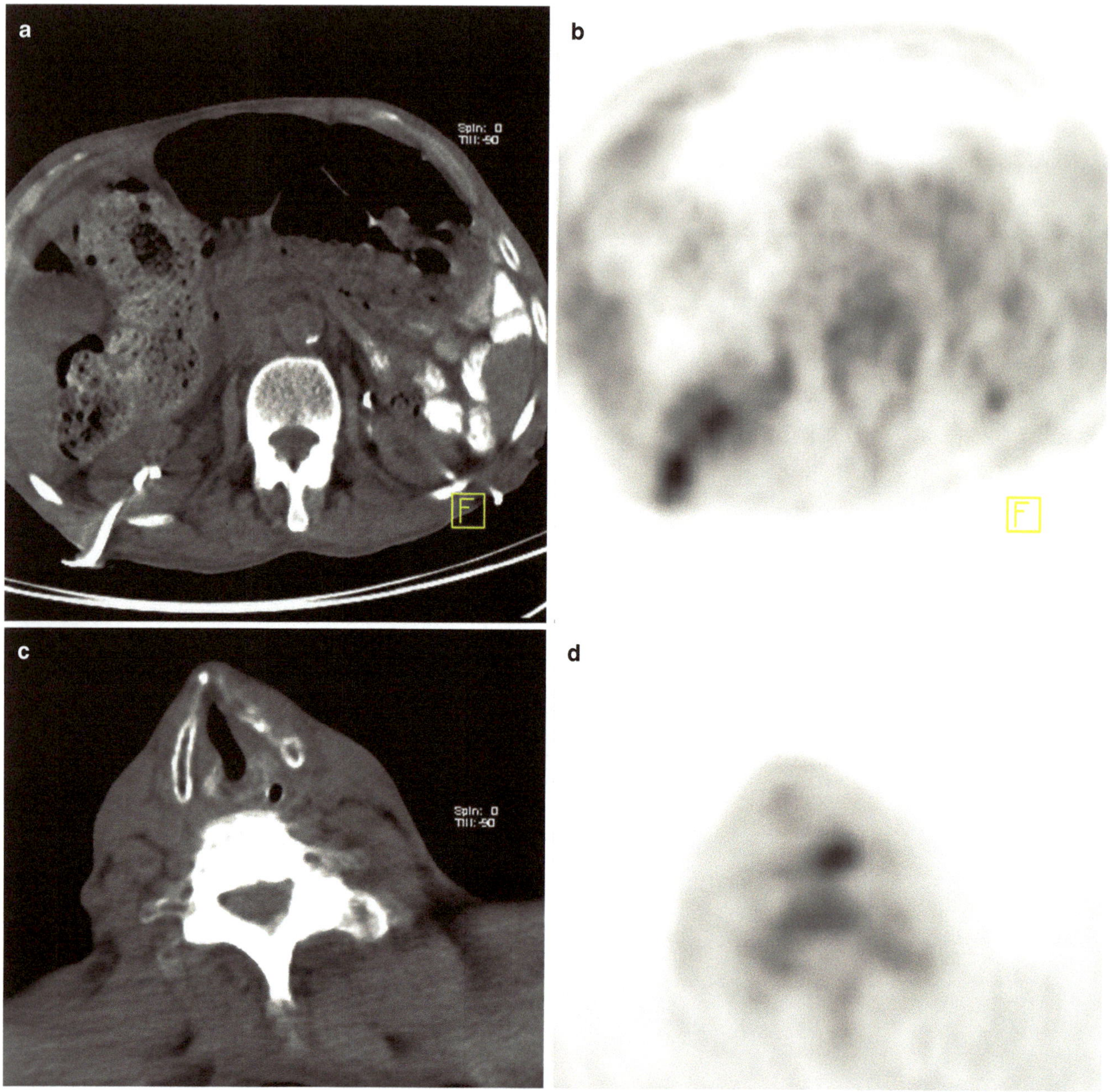

Fig. 2.96 FDG uptake at renal catheter due to urinary excretion and attenuation artifact (**a**, **b**), FDG uptake around nasogastric catheter due to inflammation (**c**, **d**)

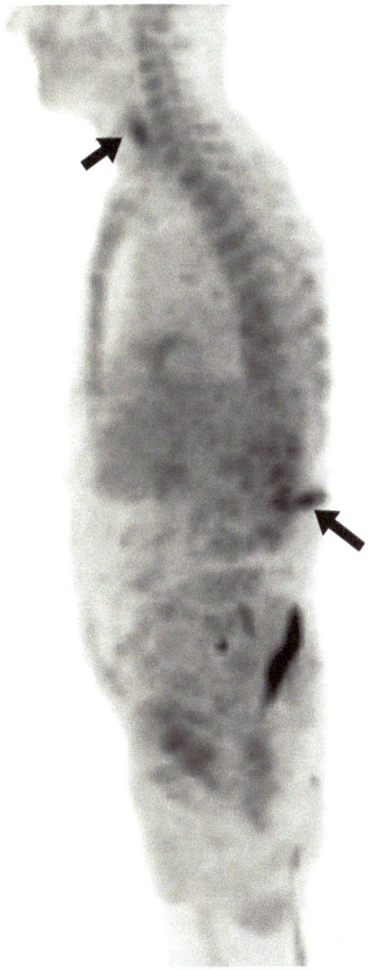

Fig. 2.97 MIP image shows hypermetabolism around nasogastric catheter (*short arrow*) and renal catheter (*long arrow*)

Catheter Balloon Artifact

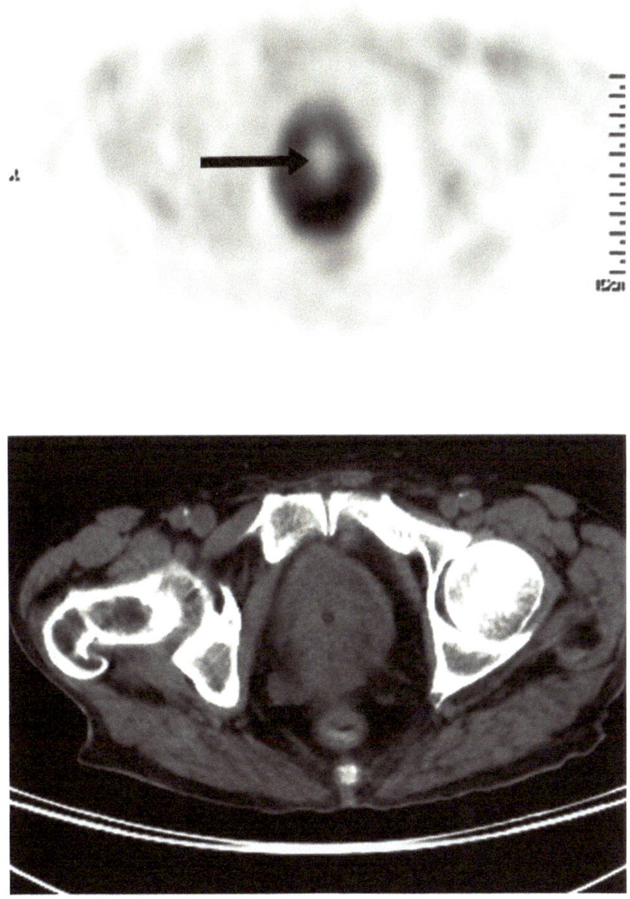

Fig. 2.98 Photopenic area representing catheter balloon in bladder (*arrow*)

2.4 Skeletal System and Soft Tissues

Clavicula Fracture

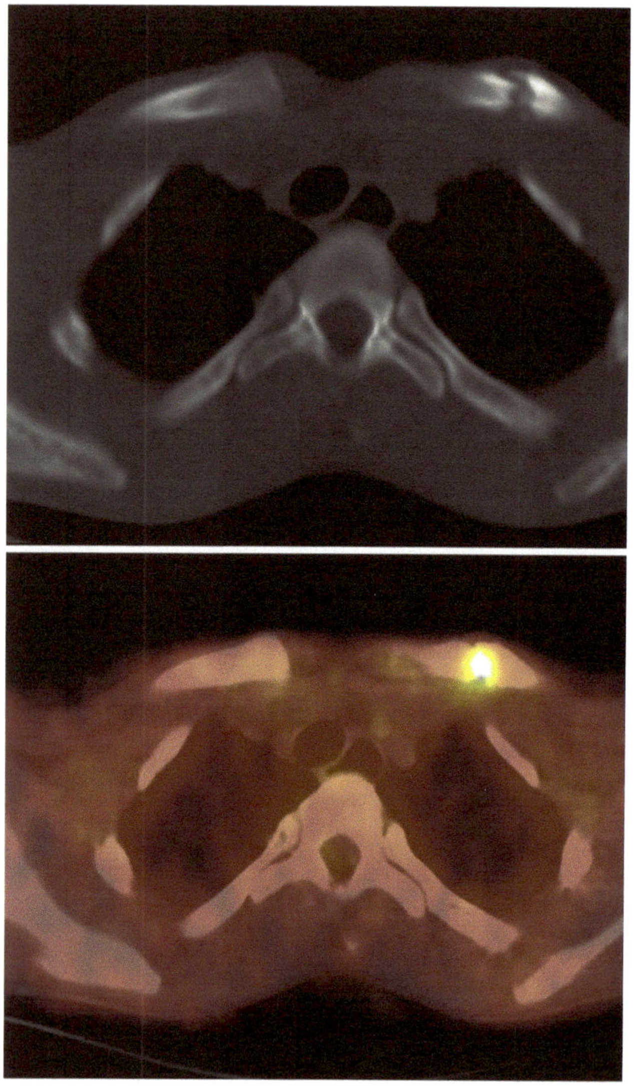

Fig. 2.99 Axial CT and fusion images show focal increased FDG uptake at fracture site at left clavicula

Multiple Costal Fractures

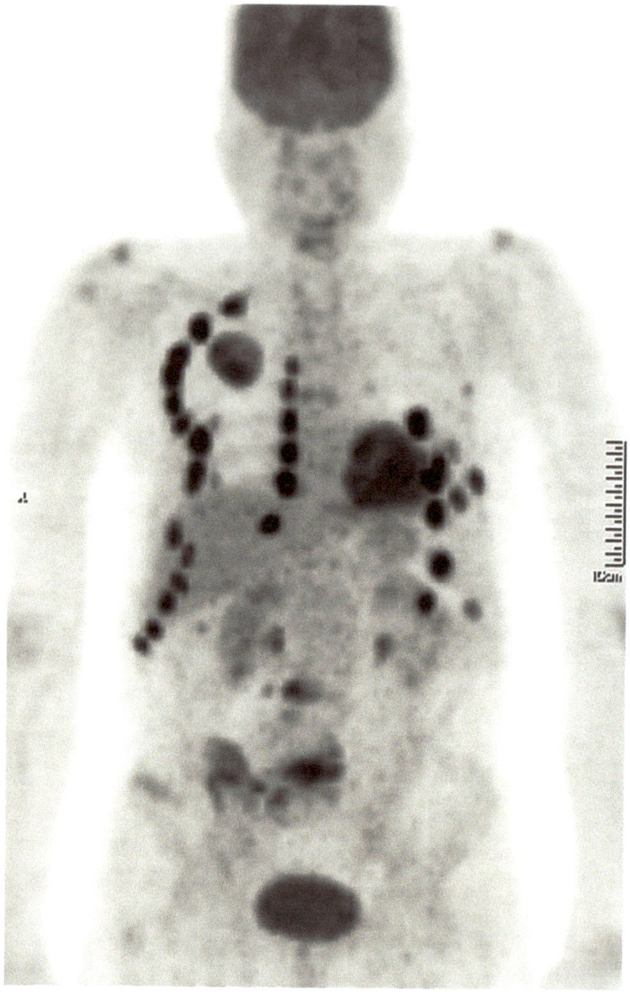

Fig. 2.100 MIP image shows increased tracer accumulation at rib fractures

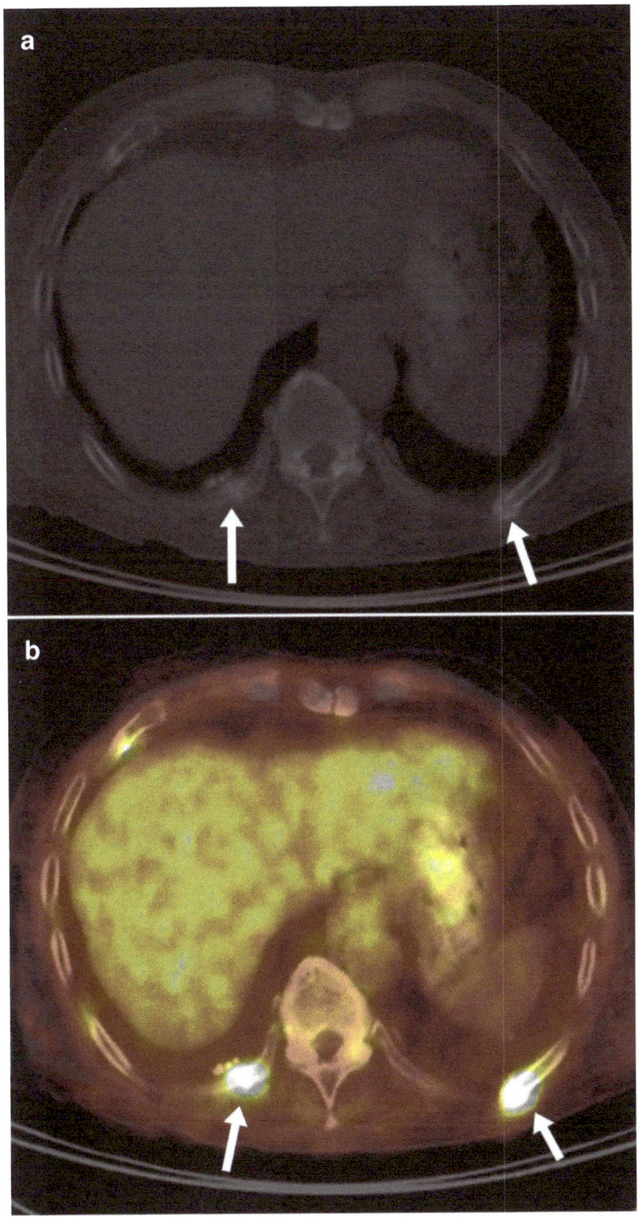

Fig. 2.101 Axial fusion and CT images (**a**, **b**). Hypermetabolism at fracture sites (*arrows*)

Compression Fracture

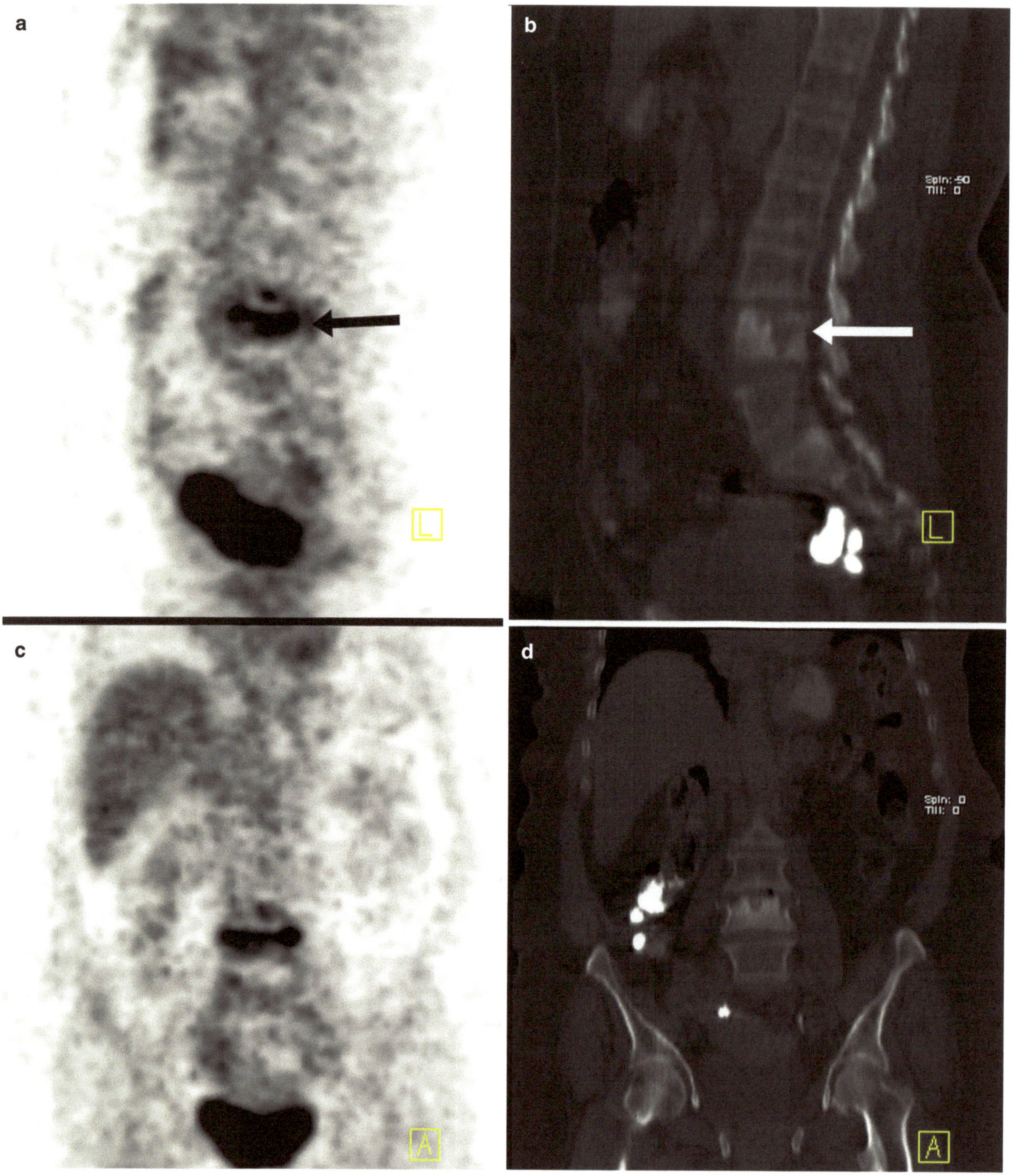

Fig. 2.102 Sagittal (**a**, **b**) and coronal (**c**, **d**) PET and CT images of a 75-year-old woman who is being followed up with the diagnosis of lymphoma. Intensely increased FDG uptake (SUVmax 12) at L4 vertebra corresponding the fracture on CT image is detected (*arrows*). Lesion turned out to be a benign compression fracture. ^{18}F-FDG PET/CT scan may be useful in distinguishing benign and malignant compression fractures. In one study sensitivity and specificity of FDG PET in differentiating benign from malignant compression fractures were 86 % and 83 %, respectively. In this case the lesion could be interpreted as malignant depending on the high FDG uptake, but when low FDG affinity of MALT lymphoma is concerned, the likelihood of benign compression fracture is higher

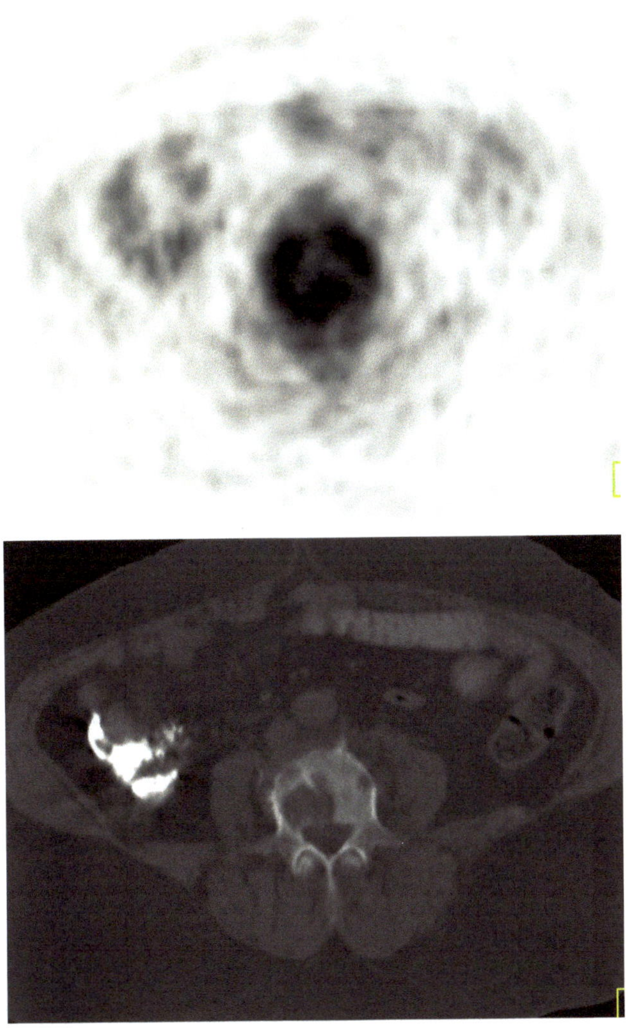

Fig. 2.103 Axial PET and CT images

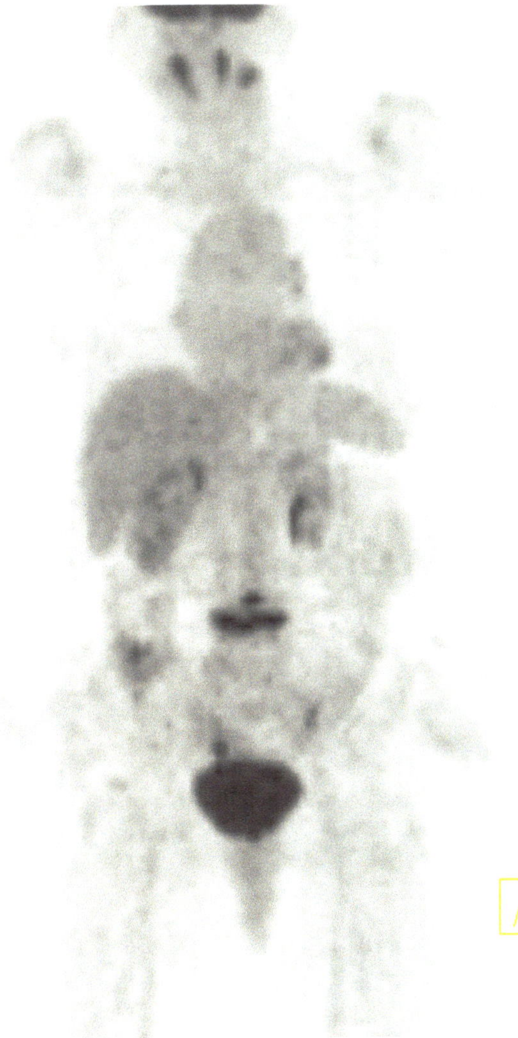

Fig. 2.104 MIP image

Sacral Fracture

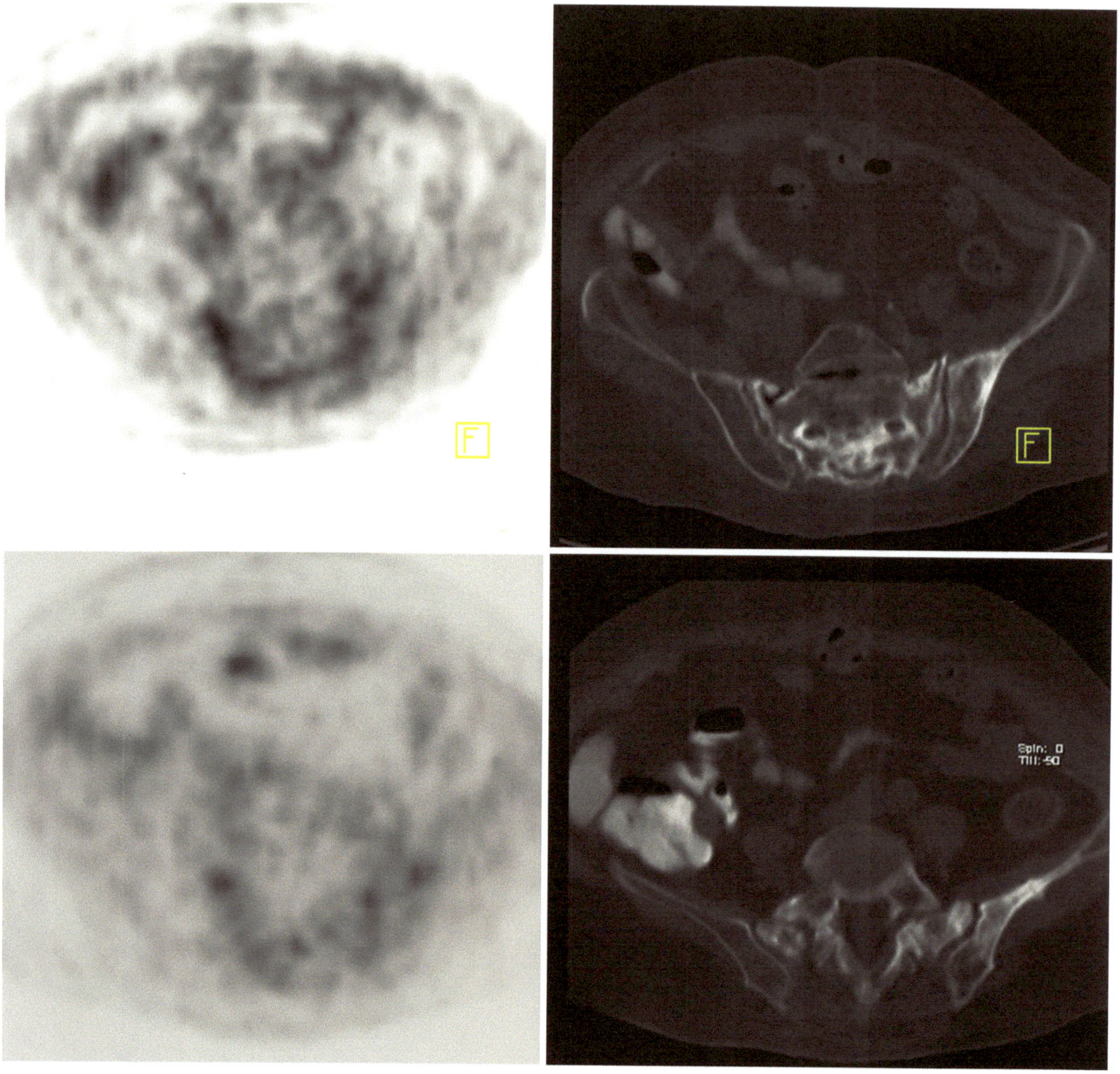

Fig. 2.105 Increased tracer uptake (SUVmax 3.4) at insufficiency fracture site at sacrum

Ruptured Tendon

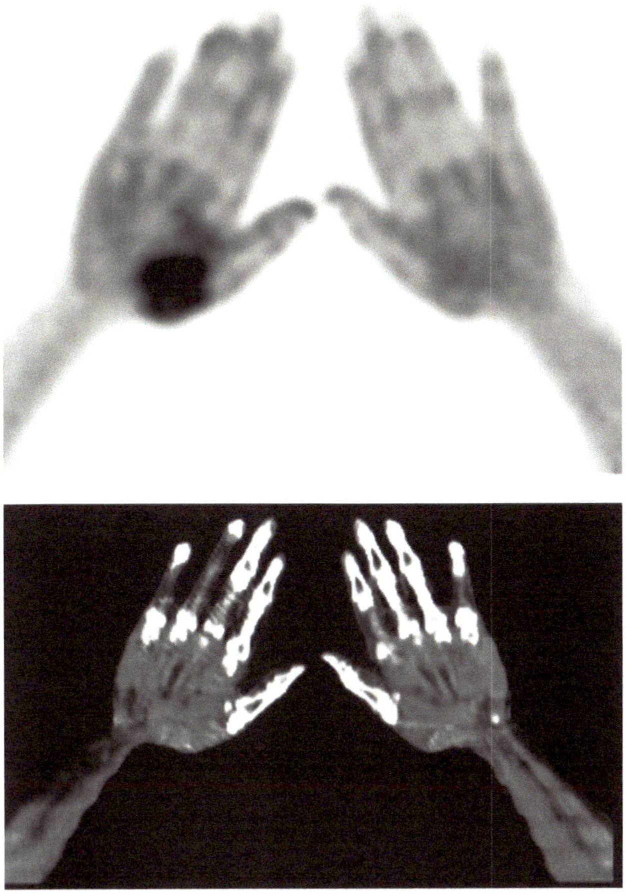

Fig. 2.106 Increased FDG uptake at tenar side of right hand represents inflammation due to ruptured tendon

Postoperative Inflammation

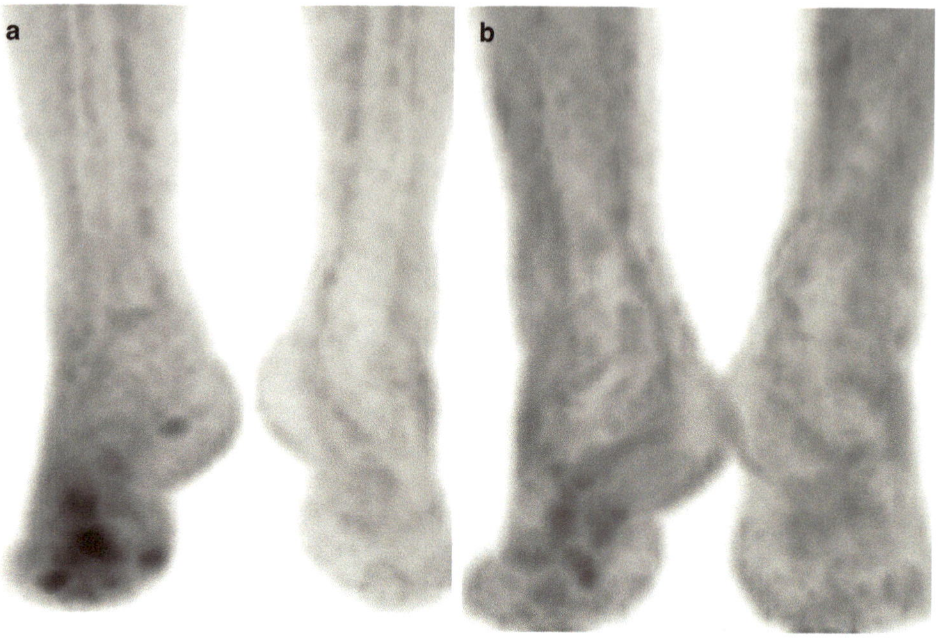

Fig. 2.107 The patient was operated for malignant melanoma at third digit of right foot and increased FDG uptake at this area is detected on $^{18F-FDG}$ PET/CT scan performed soon after the operation; MIP image (**a**), the clearance of the activity was observed on PET scan obtained 6 months after the operation (**b**) confirming that it was a benign inflammatory lesion

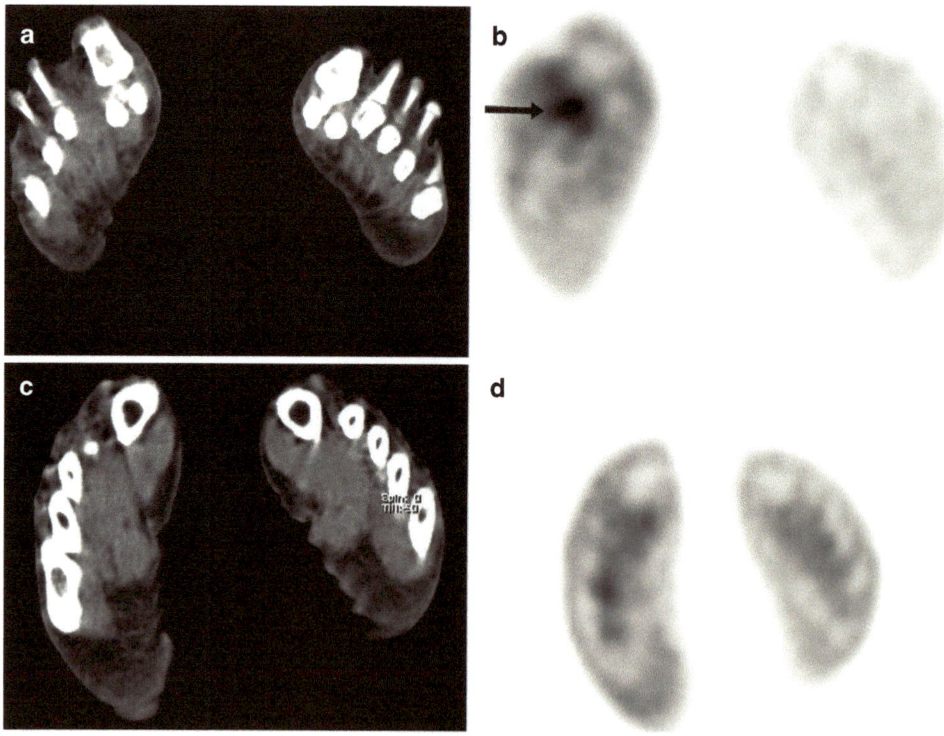

Fig. 2.108 Axial CT and PET images before (**a**, **b**) and after (**c**, **d**) the operation. Hypermatabolic focus at third digit of right foot (*arrow*) which is disappeared at follow up study is seen

Postoperative Inflammation

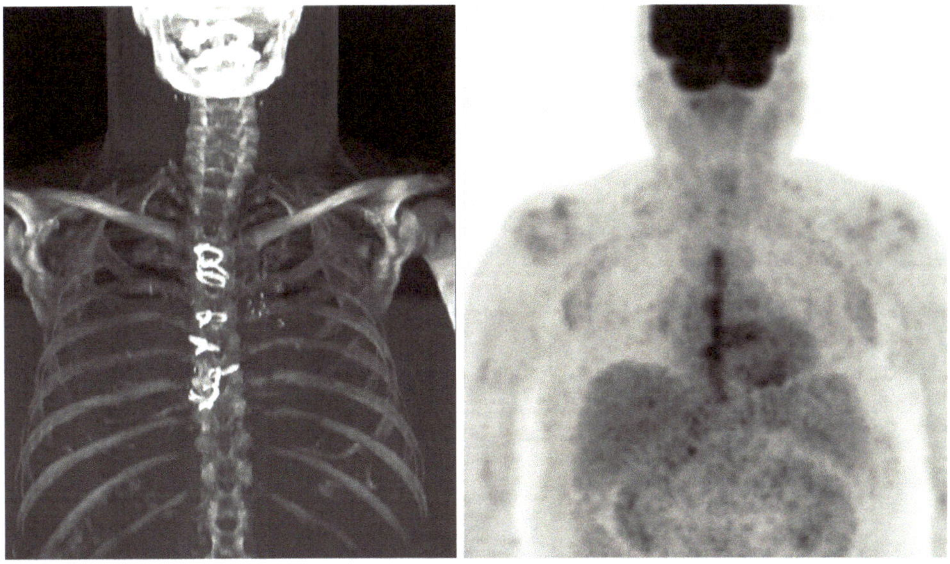

Fig. 2.109 The patient underwent by-pass operation 5 months ago. Coronal CT and PET images show increased FDG uptake at sternum due to postop inflammation

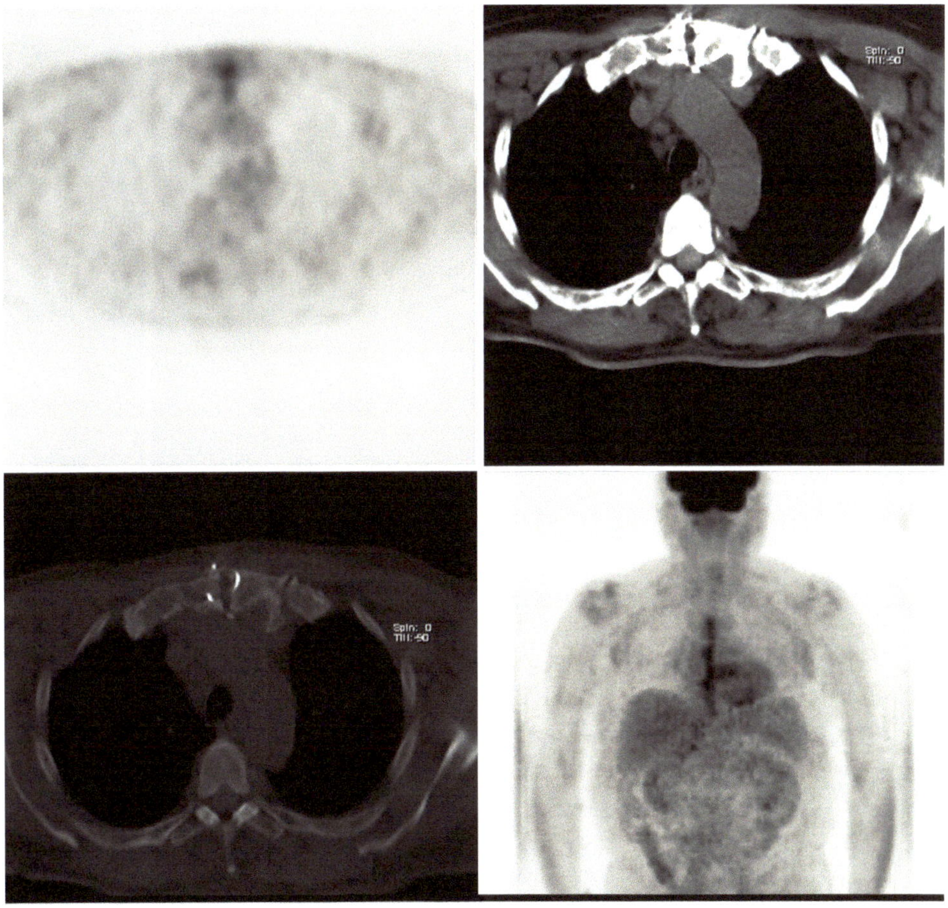

Fig. 2.110 Axial PET, CT, and MIP images

Osteophyte

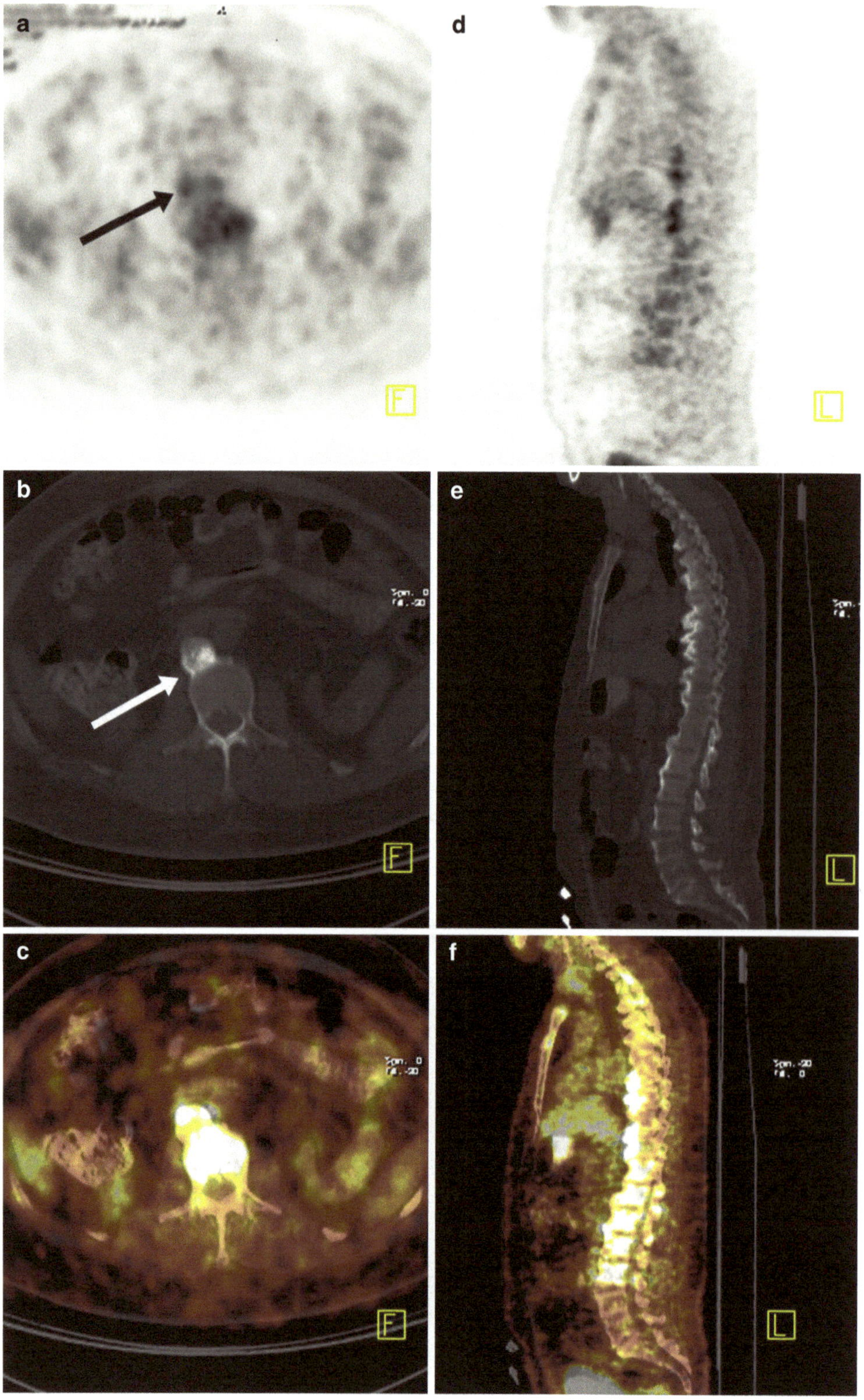

Fig. 2.111 Multiple osteophytes at vertebras showing increased FDG uptake (*arrows*), which is accounted for the inflammation at surrounding soft tissue (**a**–**f**)

Schmorl Nodule

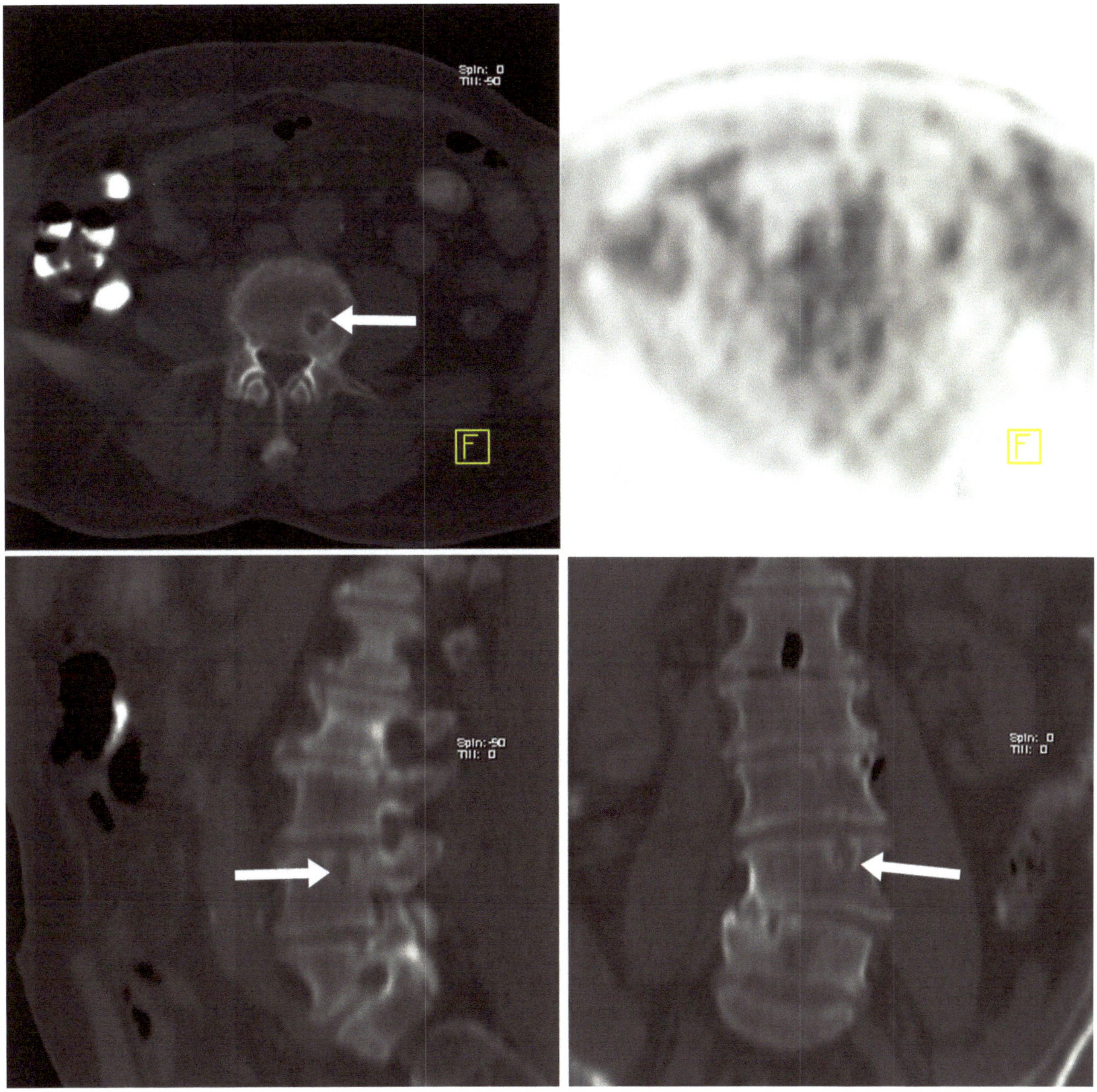

Fig. 2.112 Schmorl nodule without FDG uptake is seen (*arrow*). Schmorl nodule is an upward and downward protrusion of a spinal disk's soft tissue through end plate into the bony tissue of the adjacent vertebrae. They sometimes show FDG uptake and must be distinguished from malignant lesions

Schmorl Nodule with FDG Uptake

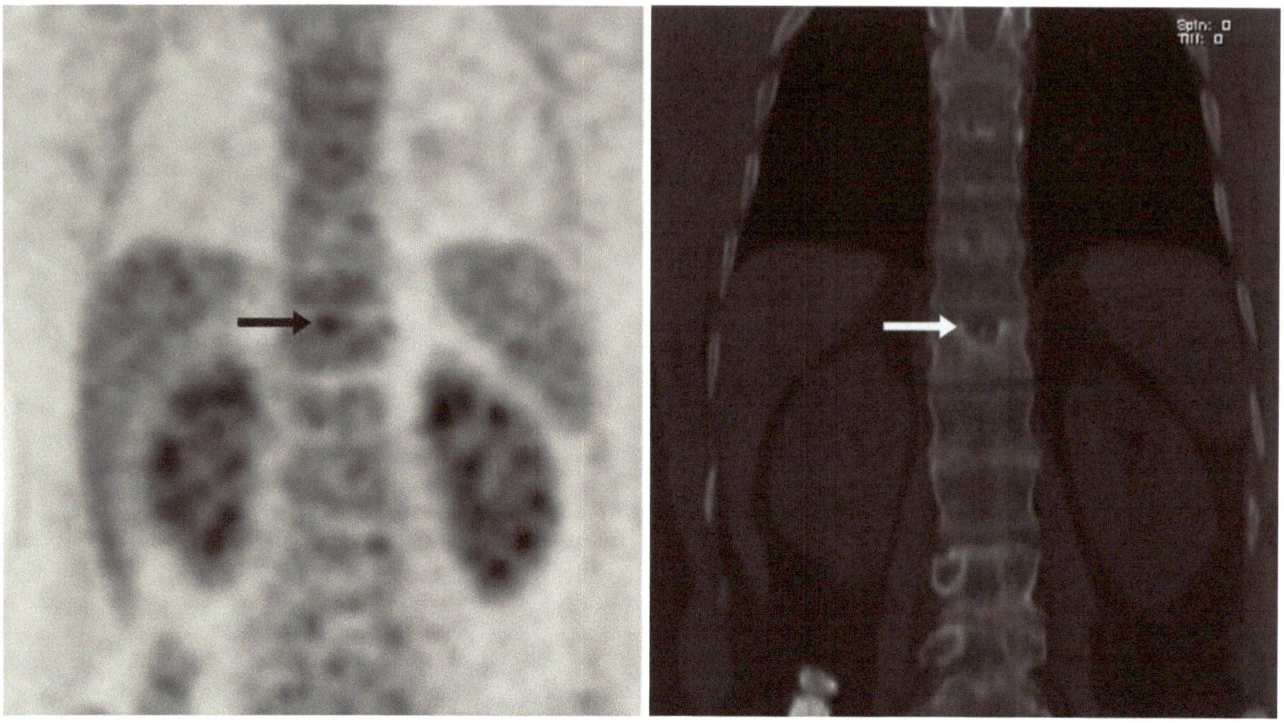

Fig. 2.113 Coronal PET and CT images show lytic lesion at corpus of D12 vertebra with corresponding FDG uptake (*arrow*). This lesion is consistent with Schmorl nodule

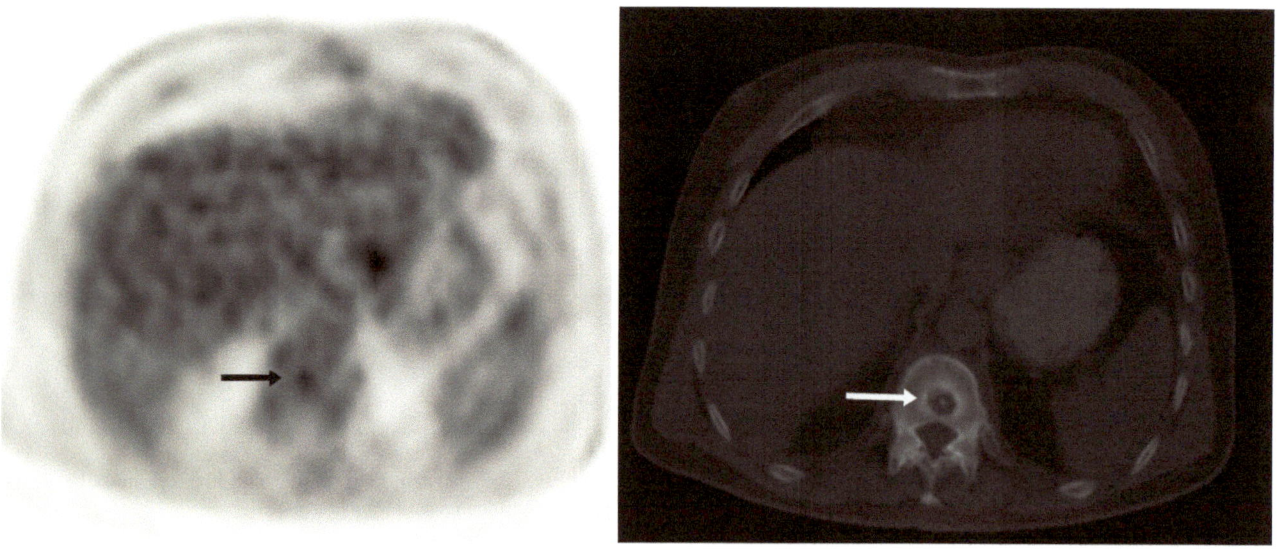

Fig. 2.114 Axial PET and CT images show lytic lesion at corpus of vertebra with corresponding FDG uptake (*arrow*)

Low FDG Uptake Following Radiotherapy

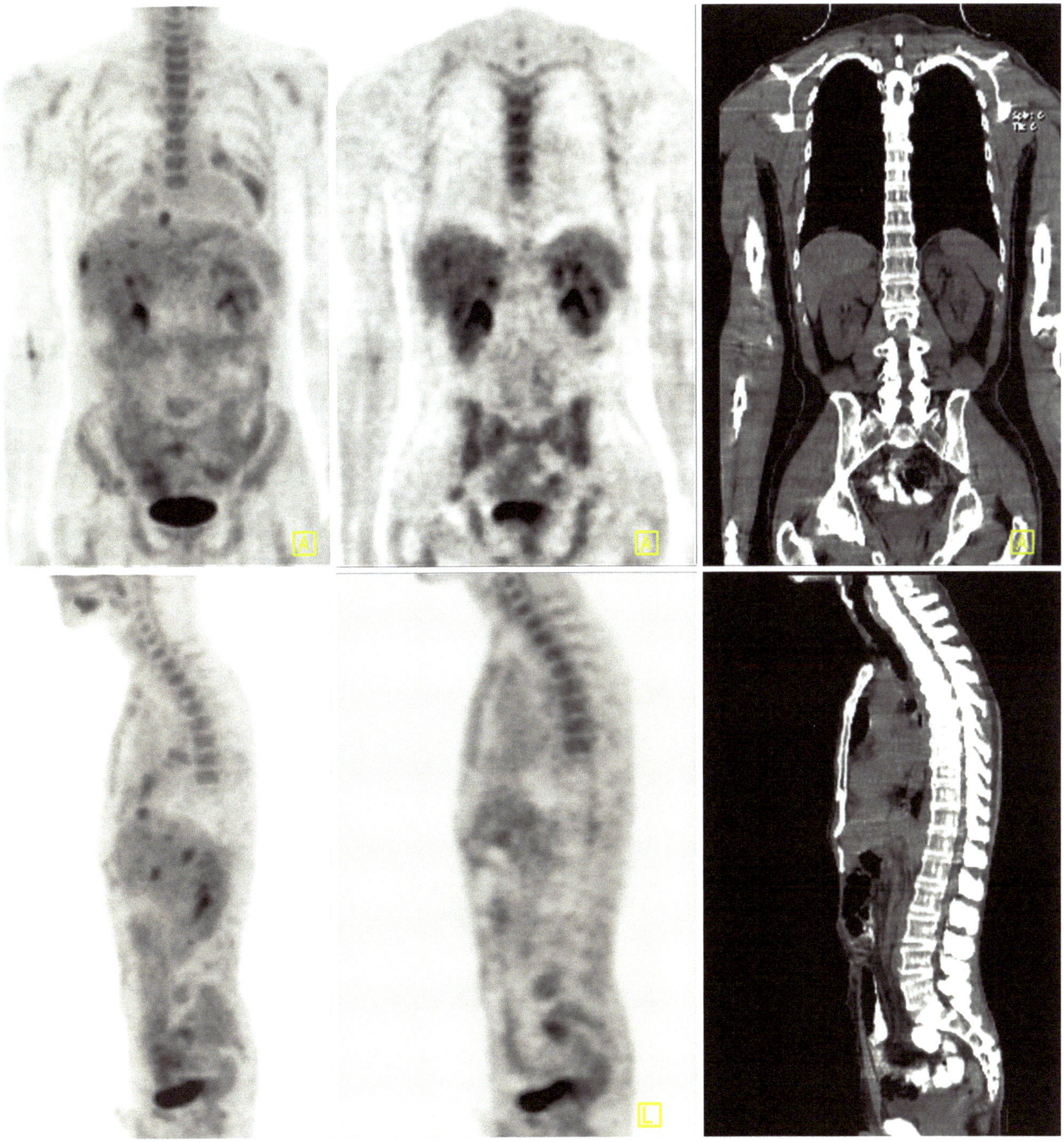

Fig. 2.115 Coronal (*upper row*) and sagittal images (*lower row*) show decreased FDG uptake at vertebra colon due to external radiotherapy

Paget Disease of Bone

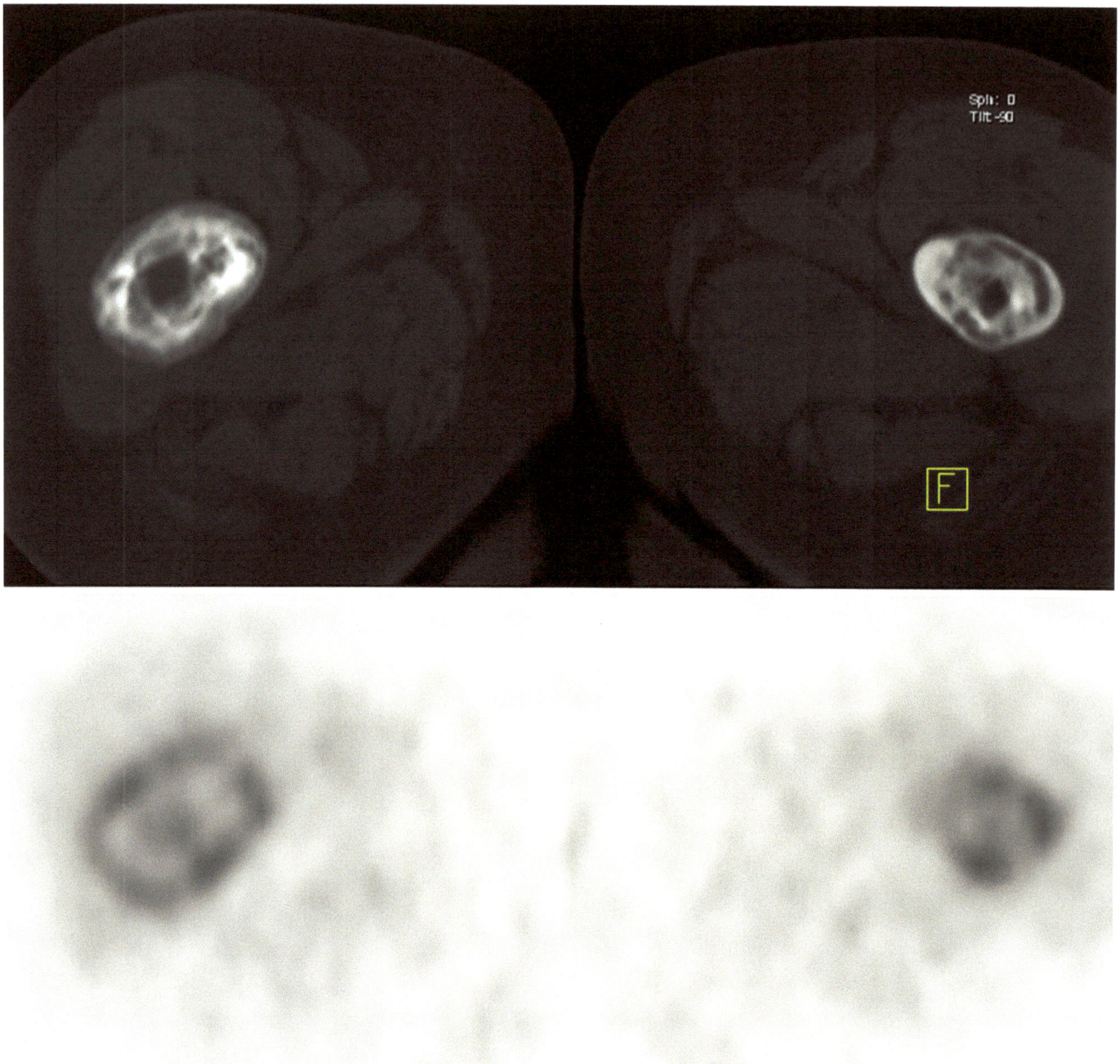

Fig. 2.116 A 49-year-old woman with breast cancer also had Paget disease of bone. Axial CT and PET images show increased FDG uptake at cortex of femur bilaterally, consistent with Paget disease

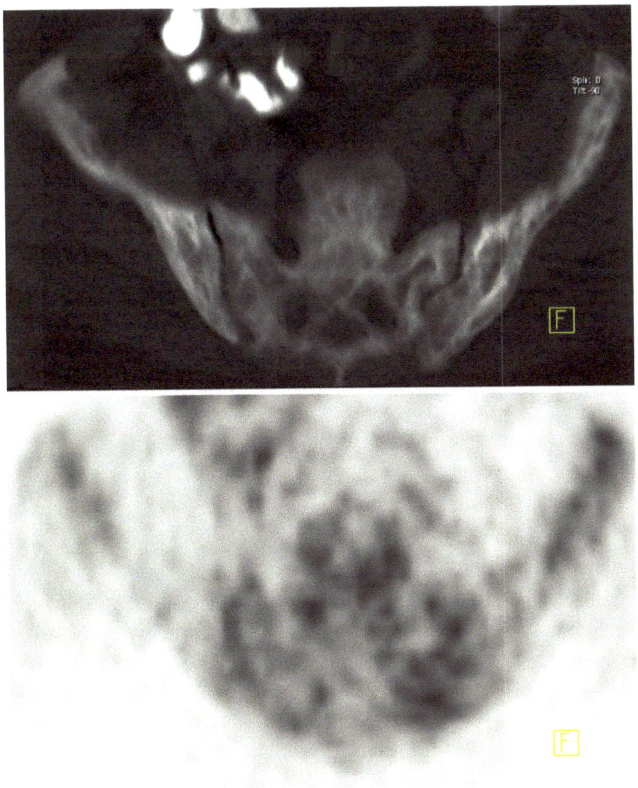

Fig. 2.117 Axial CT and PET images show increased FDG uptake at both iliac bones and sacrum

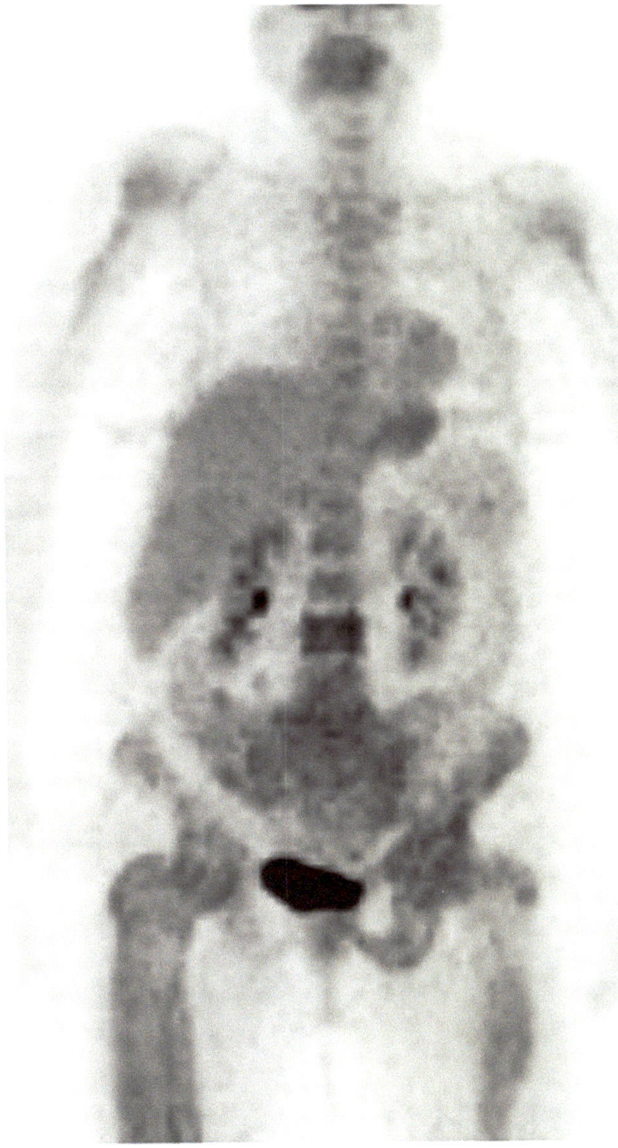

Fig. 2.118 MIP image

Paget Disease of Bone

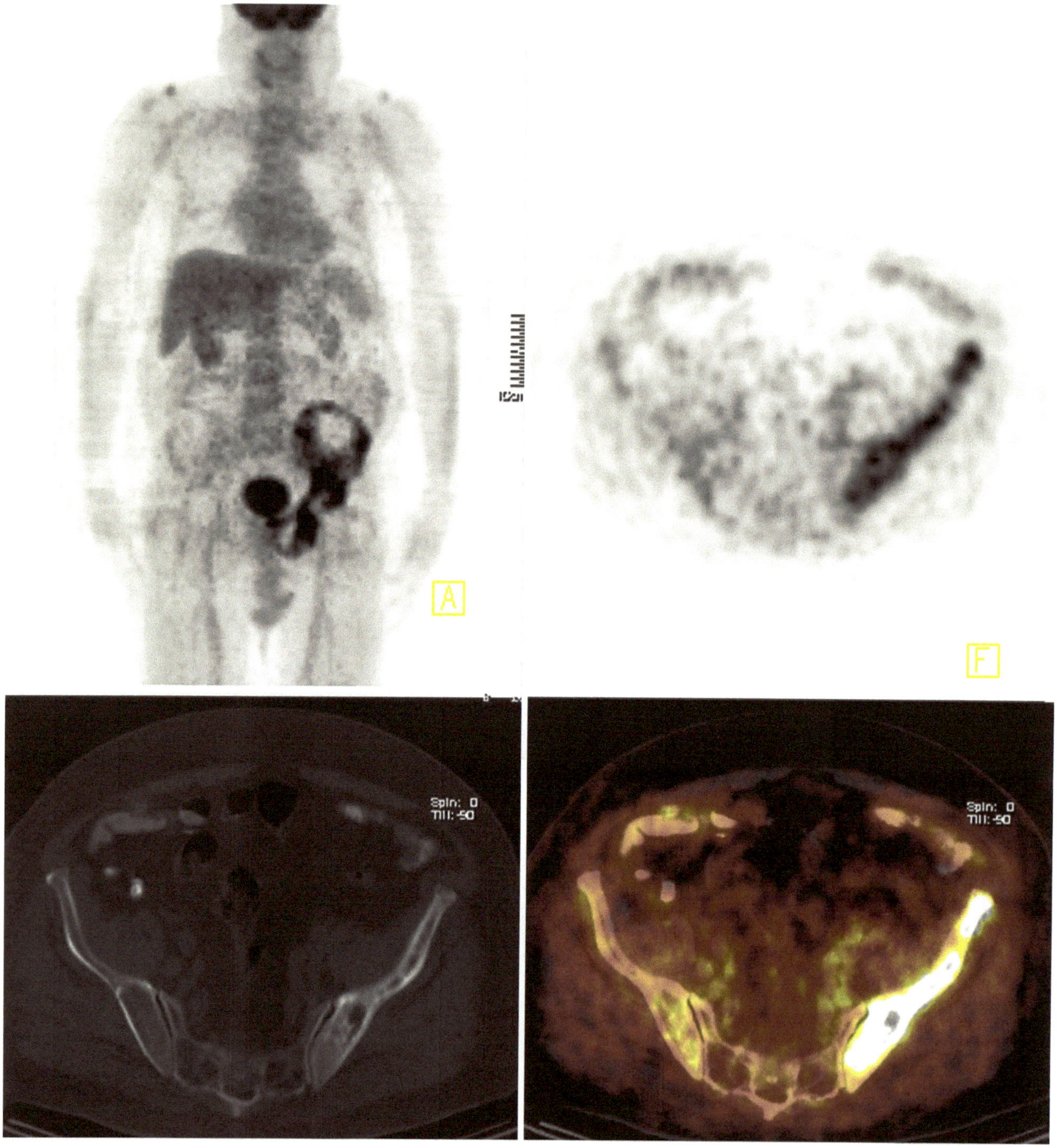

Fig. 2.119 ^{18}F-FDG PET/CT scan of a 73-year-old patient with lung carcinoma revealed intensely increased uptake at left hemipelvis. The patient had Paget disease of bone at left hemipelvis

Fibrous Dysplasia of Bone

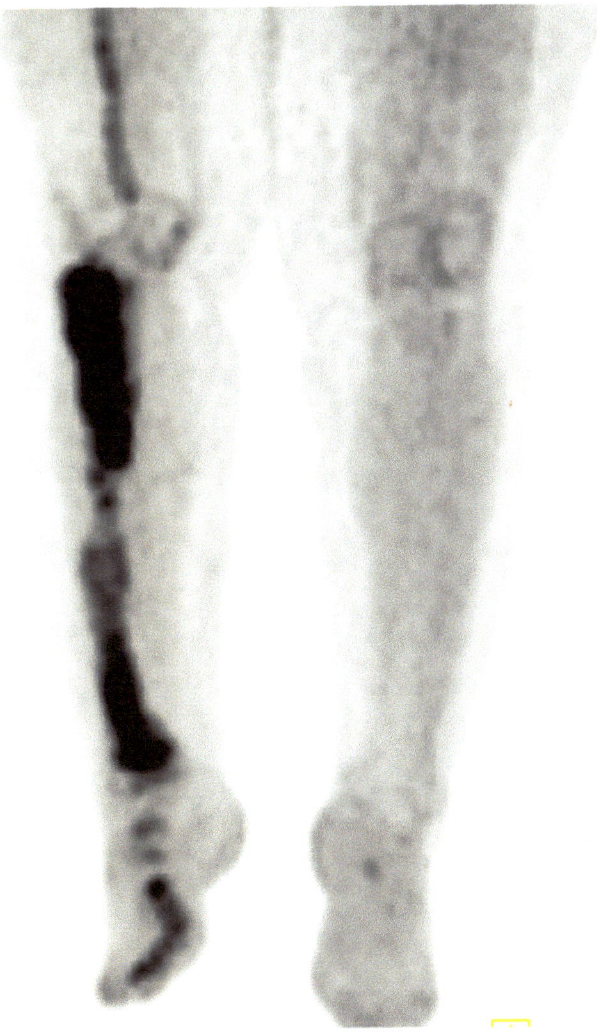

Fig. 2.120 MIP image of a patient with known fibrous dysplasia of bone shows intensely increased FDG uptake (SUVmax 8.6) at right tibia

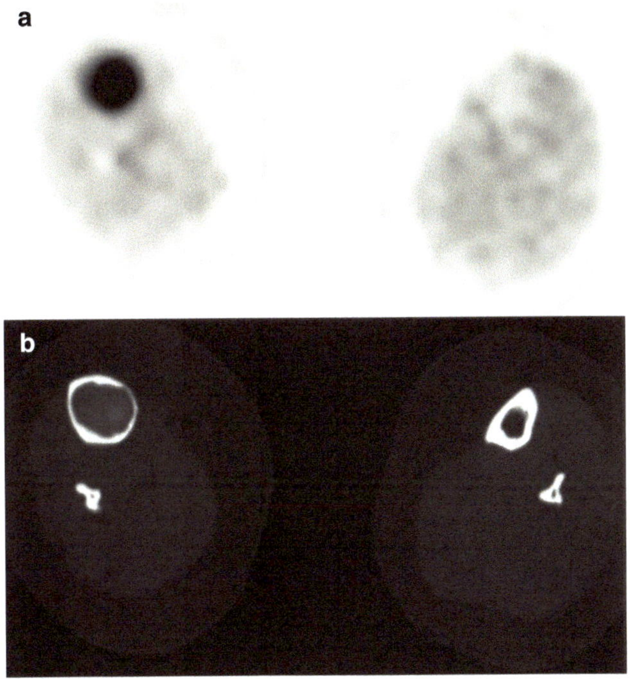

Fig. 2.121 Axial PET and CT images (**a**, **b**)

Fibrous Dysplasia of Bone

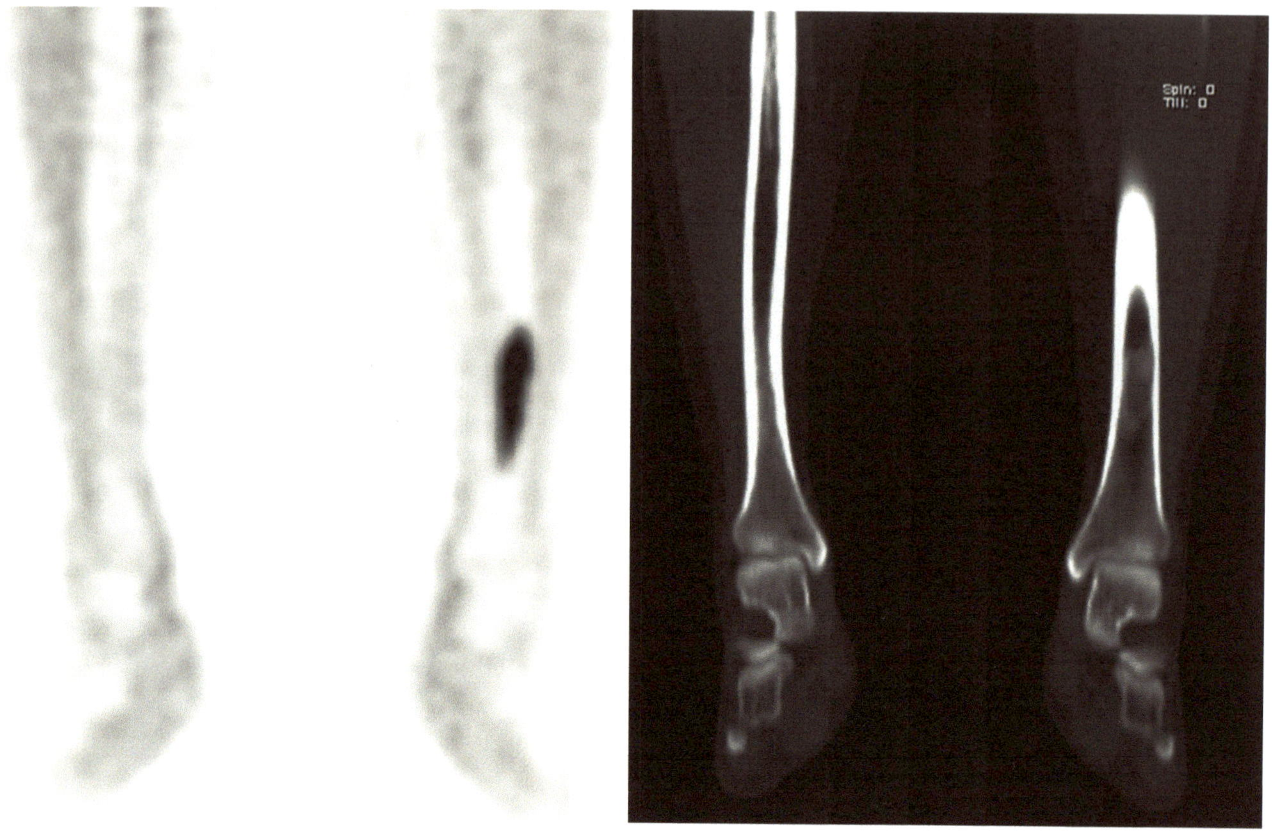

Fig. 2.122 ^{18}F-FDG PET CT scan of a 34-year-old female patient who was being followed up for breast carcinoma revealed intramedullary hypermetabolic lesion at left tibia diaphysis. The biopsy of the lesion was reported as fibrous dysplasia. MIP image shows significant FDG uptake at corresponding intramedullary lesion on CT. The lesion has sclerotic margins on CT and shows ground-glass appearance which are characteristic features of fibrous dysplasia

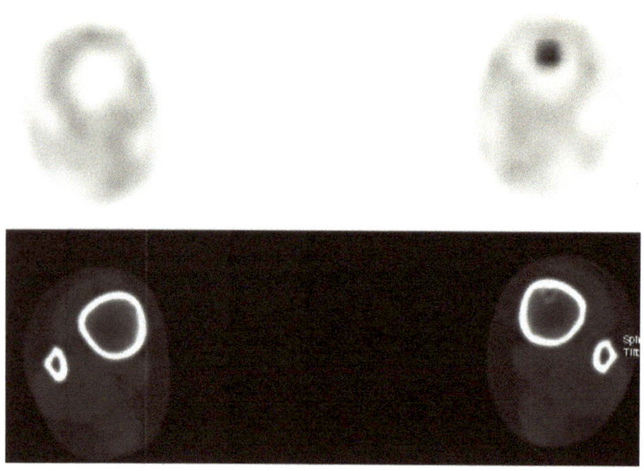

Fig. 2.123 Axial slices of PET and CT images show intramedullary increased FDG uptake at the lesion with sclerotic margins

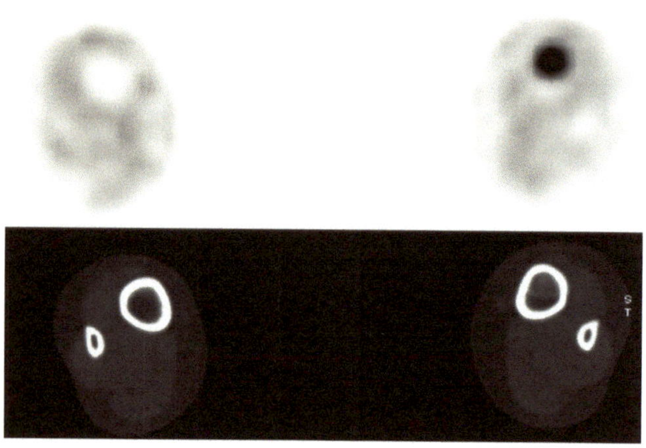

Fig. 2.124 Axial slices of PET and CT images

Fibrous Cortical Defect

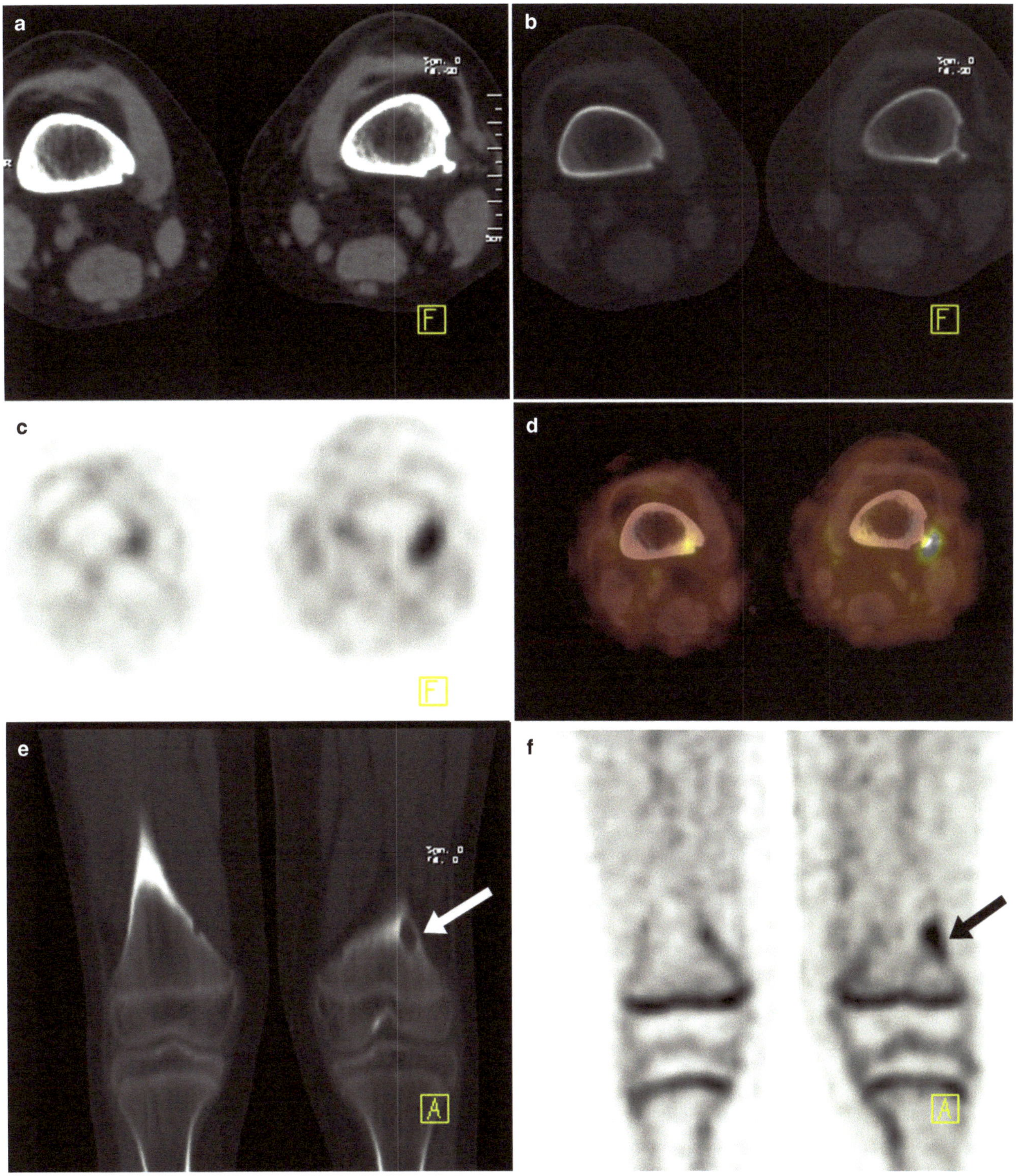

Fig. 2.125 A 15-year-old boy underwent ^{18}F-FDG PET/CT for malignant melanoma. Lucent intracortical defects at distal metaphysis of left femur showing mild FDG uptake (*arrows*), are consistent with fibrous cortical defect (**a–f**)

Hematopoietic Activation Due to Anemia

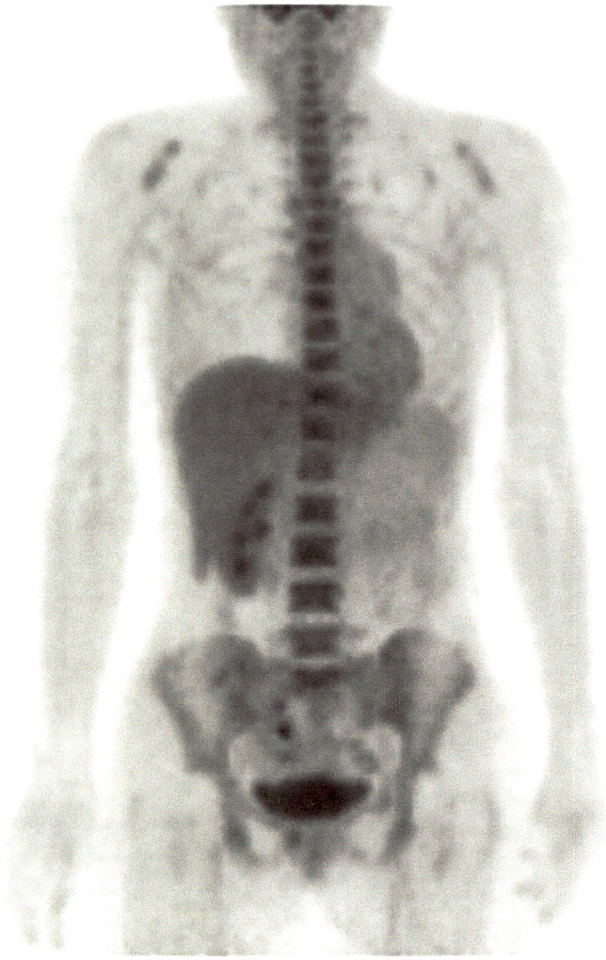

Fig. 2.126 MIP image of ^{18}F-FDG PET/CT scan of a patient with renal cell carcinoma. Diffuse increased FDG uptake at bone marrow of vertebral colon and pelvic bones is due to hematopoietic activation as a reaction to anemia. Differentiation of this phenomenon from metastatic infiltration can be done with the heterogenous uptake seen in the latter

Aplastic Anemia

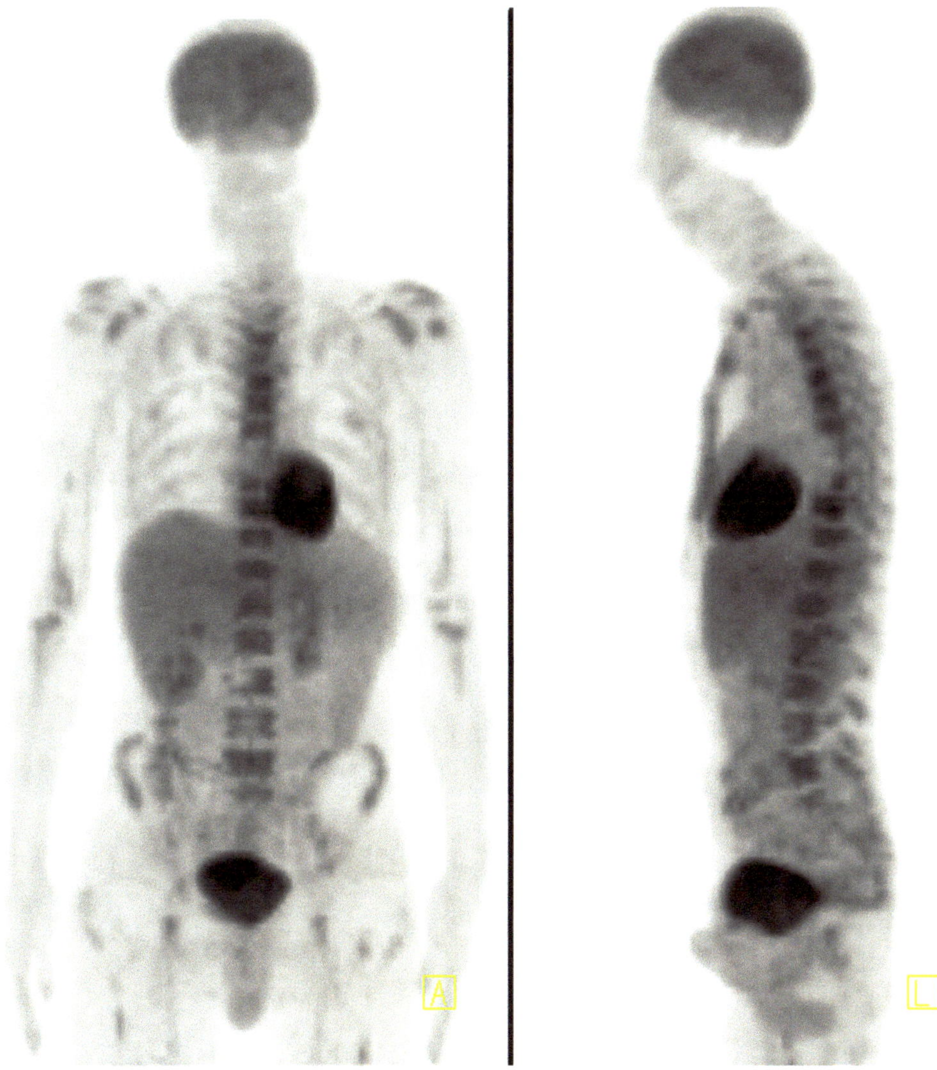

Fig. 2.127 ^{18}F-FDG PET/CT scan of a 45-year-old patient with aplastic anemia. MIP image showed a patchy uptake pattern in bone marrow, indicating residual compensatory hypercellular marrow

Neupogen Induced Bone Marrow Uptake

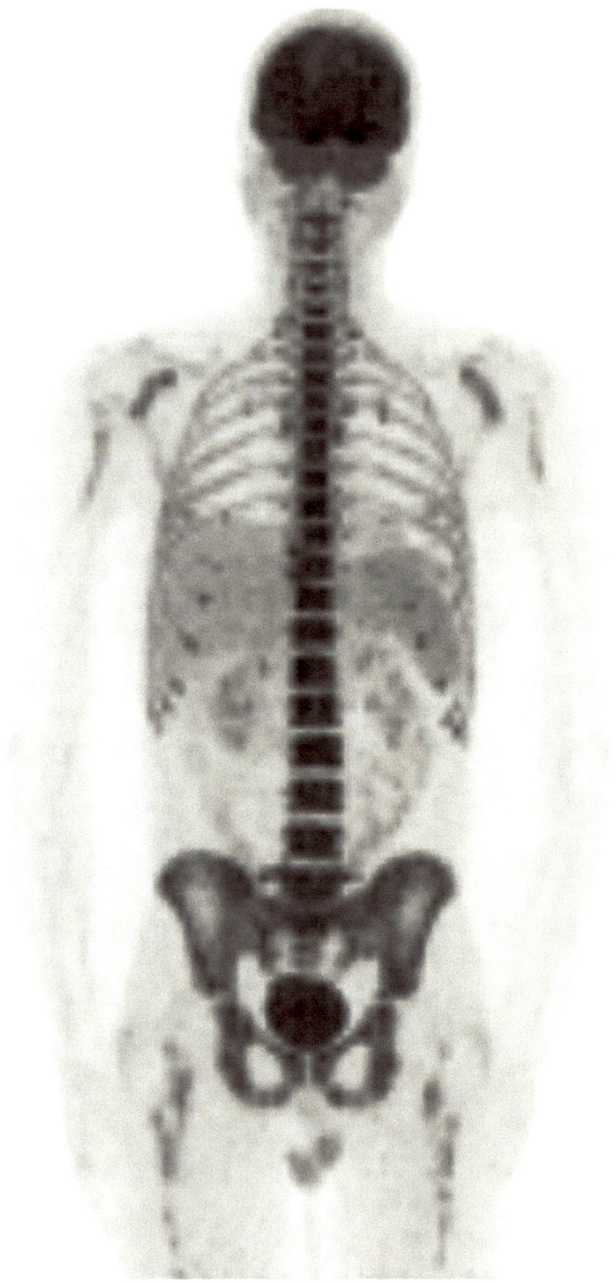

Fig. 2.128 Diffuse homogeneous bone marrow FDG uptake reflecting hyperplastic bone marrow secondary to colony-stimulating factor (neupogen) administration. The time interval between the cessation of Neupogen and ^{18}F-FDG PET/CT scan should be 5–30 days in order to avoid this unwanted uptake

Brucella Infection

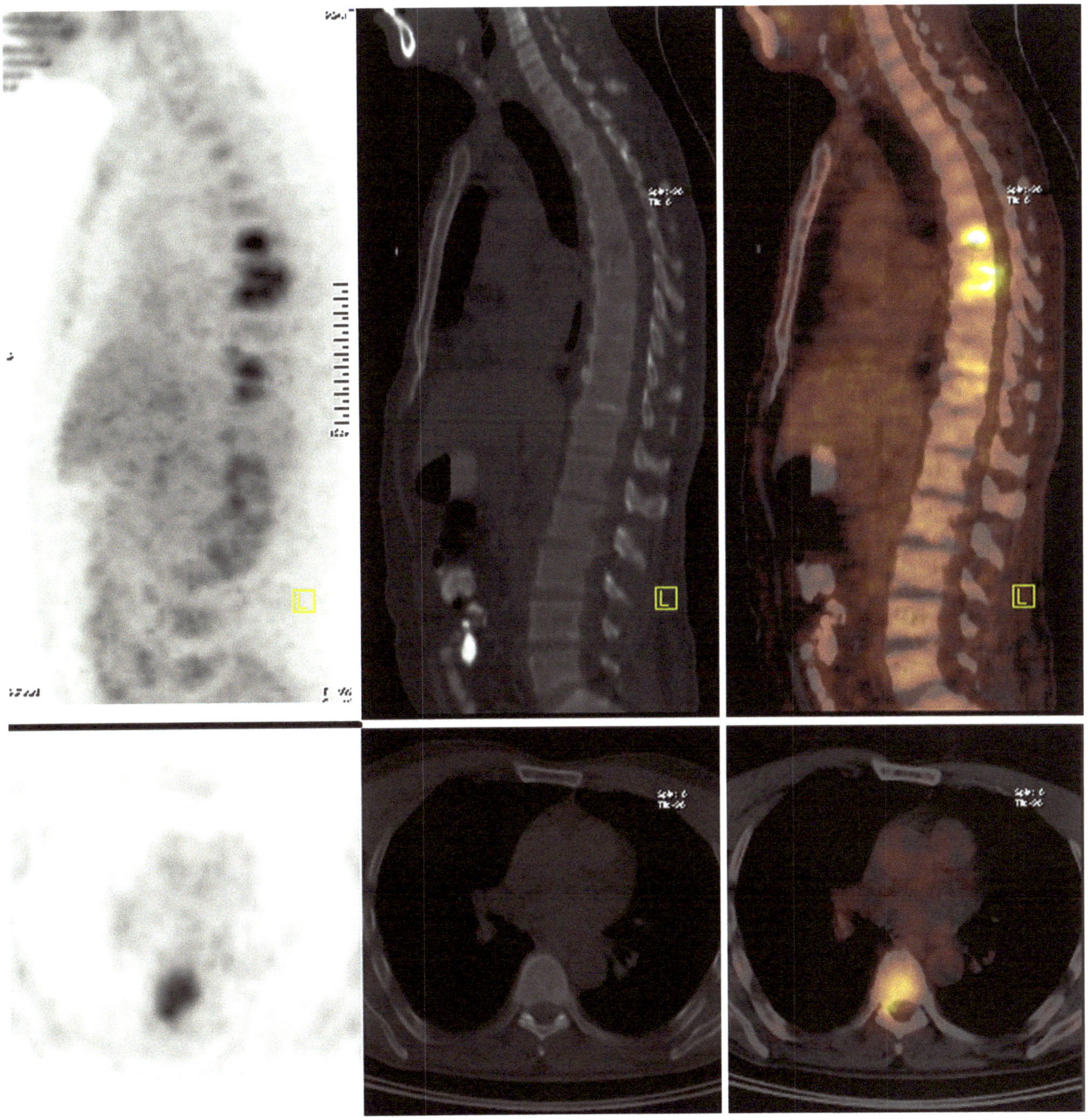

Fig. 2.129 A 58-year-old patient was being evaluated for identification of primary malignancy after suspicious metastatic lesions at dorsal vertebrae were detected on CT and bone scan images. Sagittal (*upper row*) and axial (*lower row*) slices of PET, CT, and fusion images display intensely increased FDG uptake (SUVmax 11.8) at D6, D7, D8, D10, and D11 vertebrae and there was not any other pathologically increased FDG uptake at other sites of the body to be evaluated as primary malignancy. On histopathology, the lesions at vertebrae turned out to be involvement with *Brucella* infection

Rheumatoid Arthritis

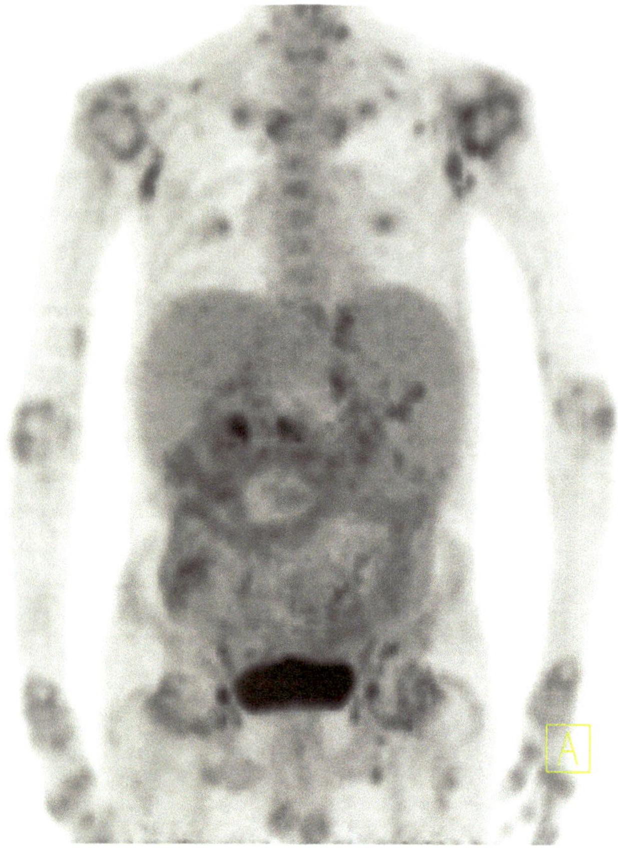

Fig. 2.130 A 48-year-old patient underwent ^{18}F-FDG PET/CT scan. MIP image show increased FDG uptake at shoulder, elbow, wrist, interphalangeal, and coxofemoral joints due to rheumatoid arthritis

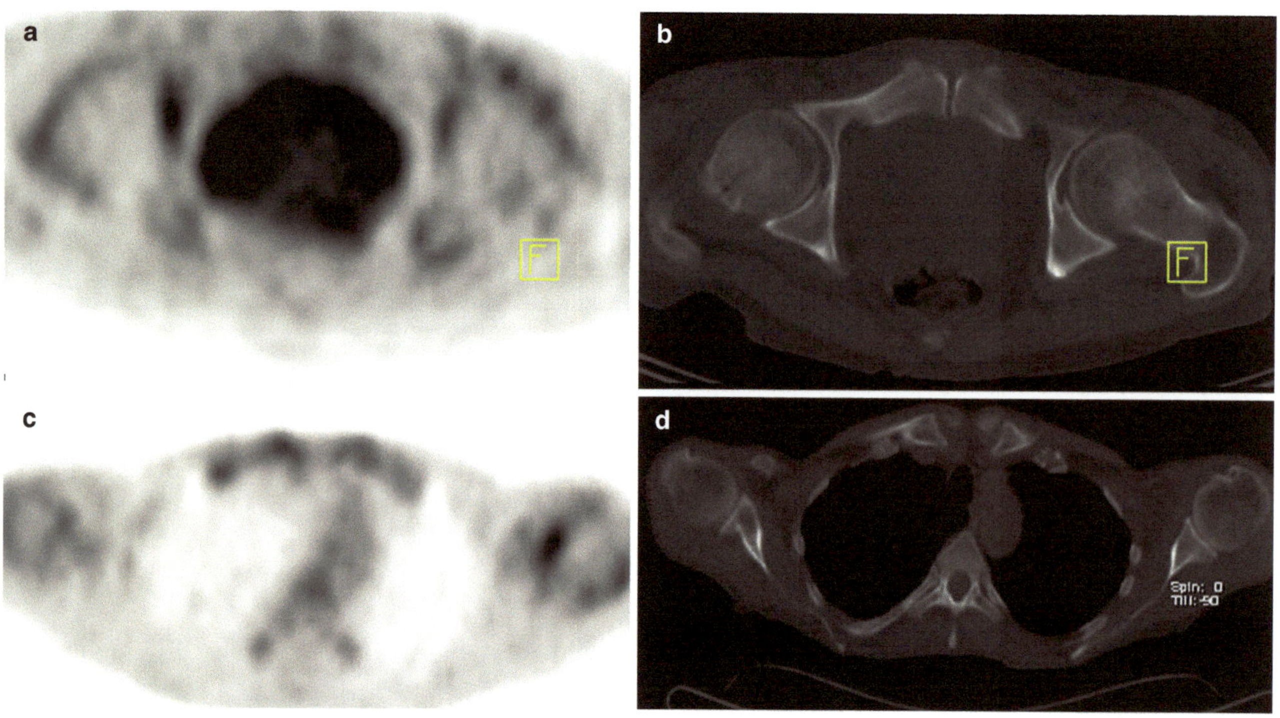

Fig. 2.131 Axial slices of PET and CT images (**a**–**d**)

Gout Arthropathy

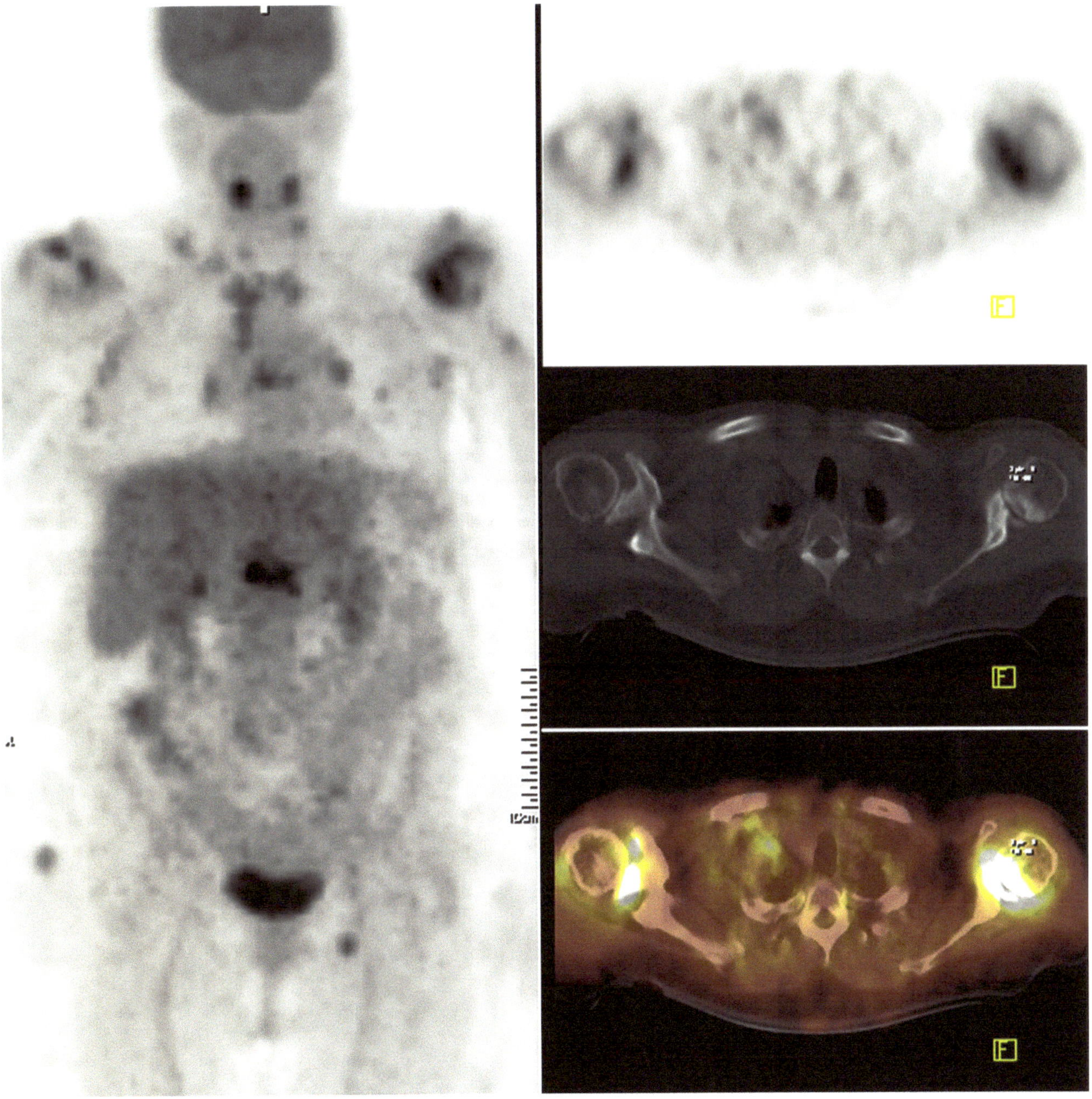

Fig. 2.132 Hypermetabolism detected at bilateral shoulder joints is consistent with gout arthropathy

Lentigo Simplex

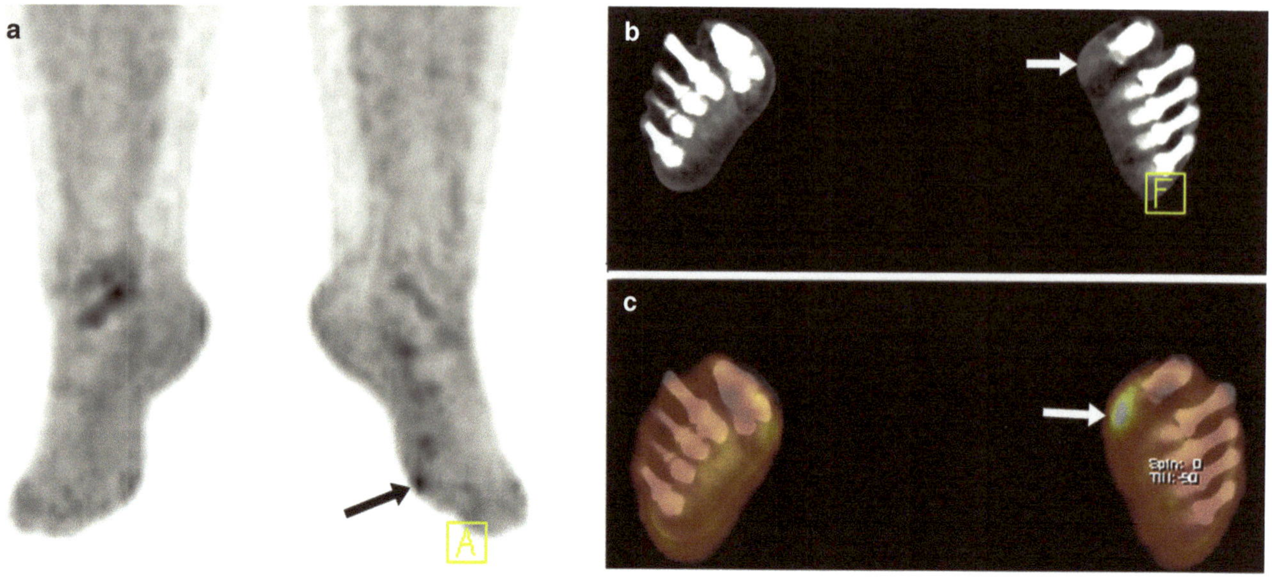

Fig. 2.133 A 63-year-old woman who is being followed up for malignant melanoma underwent ^{18}F-FDG PET/CT scan and focal increased FDG uptake at plantar surface of first toe is detected (*arrows*) (**a**–**c**). The lesion was suspicious for metastasis but histopathology revealed lentigo simplex. Lentigo simplex lesions are benign lesions that cause no harm. However, their appearance sometimes may mimic melanomas or other cancerous lesions so they need to be taken into account

Diabetic Ulcer

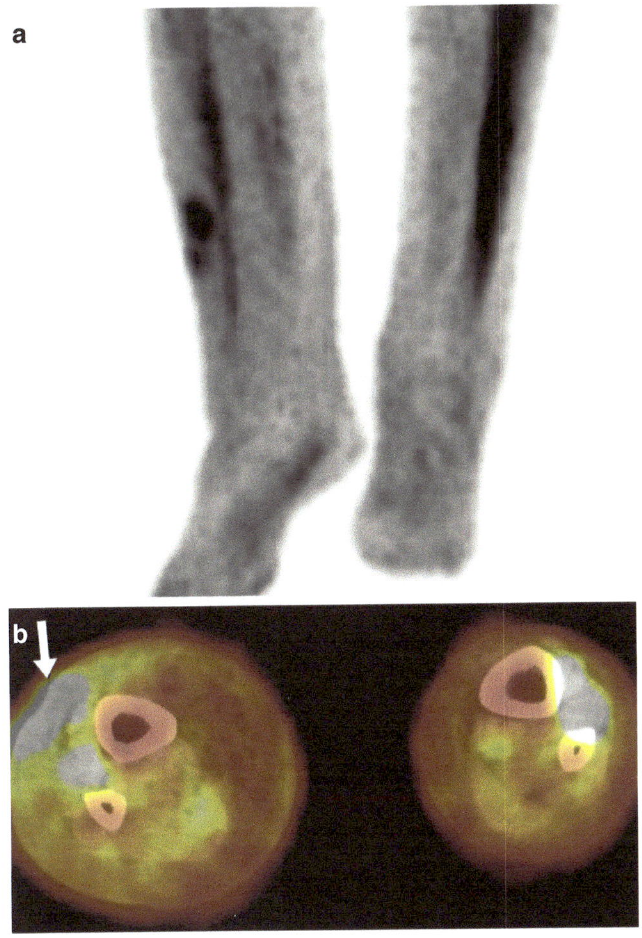

Fig. 2.134 A 89-year-old woman who is being followed up for endometrium carcinoma recurrence underwent ^{18}F-FDG PET/CT scan. The patient also had diabetes mellitus and MIP (**a**) and axial fusion (**b**) images show focal increased FDG uptake at skin and subcutaneous tissues at right anterolateral cruris, which is consistent with diabetic ulcer

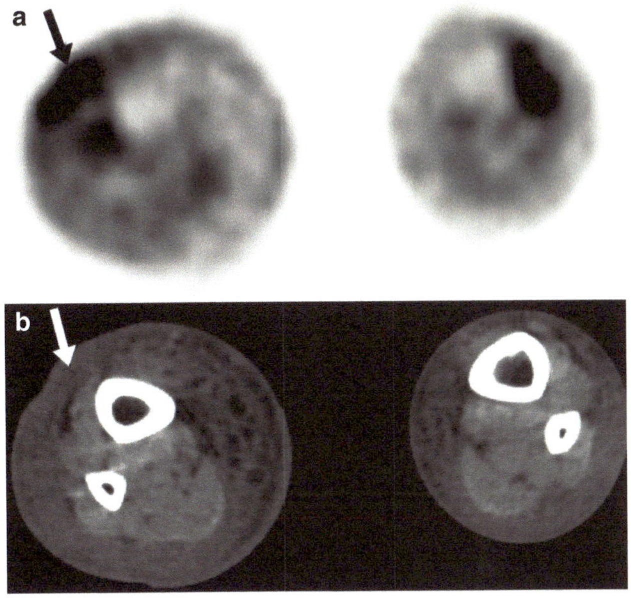

Fig. 2.135 Axial PET (**a**) and CT (**b**) images show hypermetabolism at skin and subcutaneous tissues at right anterolateral cruris (*arrows*)

Fat Necrosis

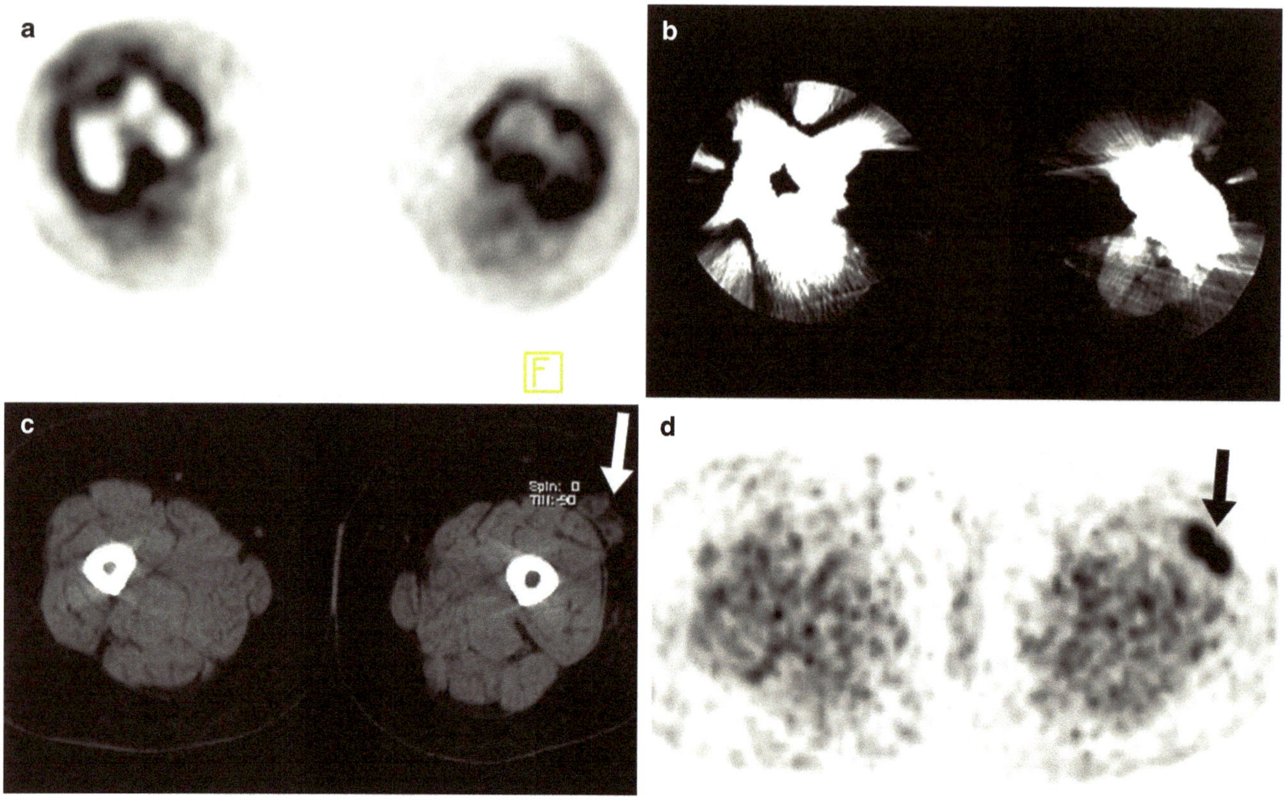

Fig. 2.136 Axial PET and CT images (**a**, **b**) images show increased FDG uptake around bilateral knee prosthesis suggestive of loosening but this activity might also be due to attenuation correction artifact. Axial CT and PET images (**c**, **d**) of same patients show focal subcutaneous FDG accumulations at anterolateral aspect of left cruris consistent with fat necrosis (*arrows*)

Fat Necrosis

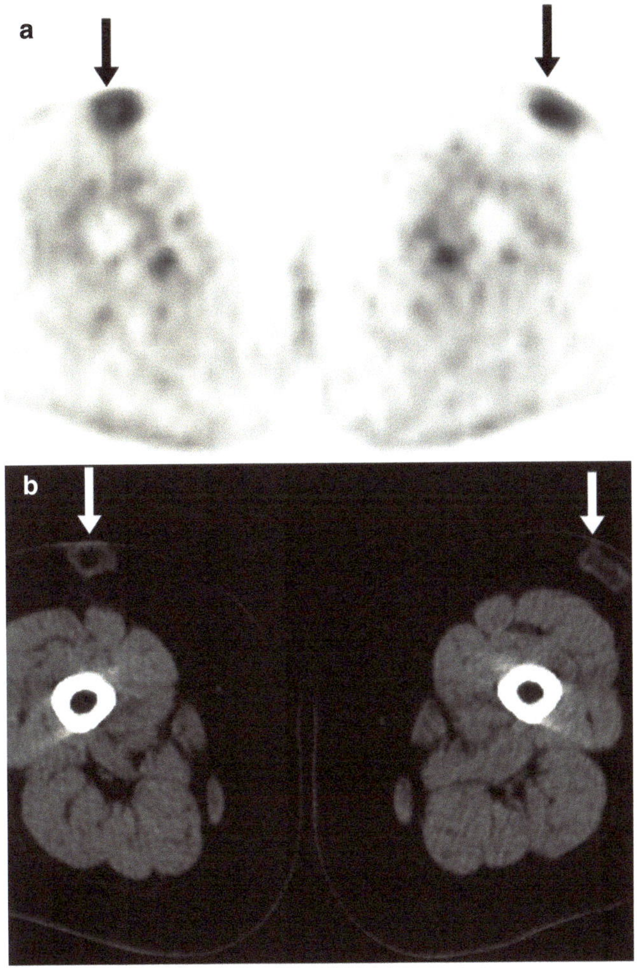

Fig. 2.137 Subcutaneous lesions with central hypodense region at bilateral anterior thigh on axial CT image is associated with increased FDG uptake on axial PET image (*arrows*) (**a**, **b**). These lesions are compatible with fat necrosis

Fat Necrosis in Bone Marrow

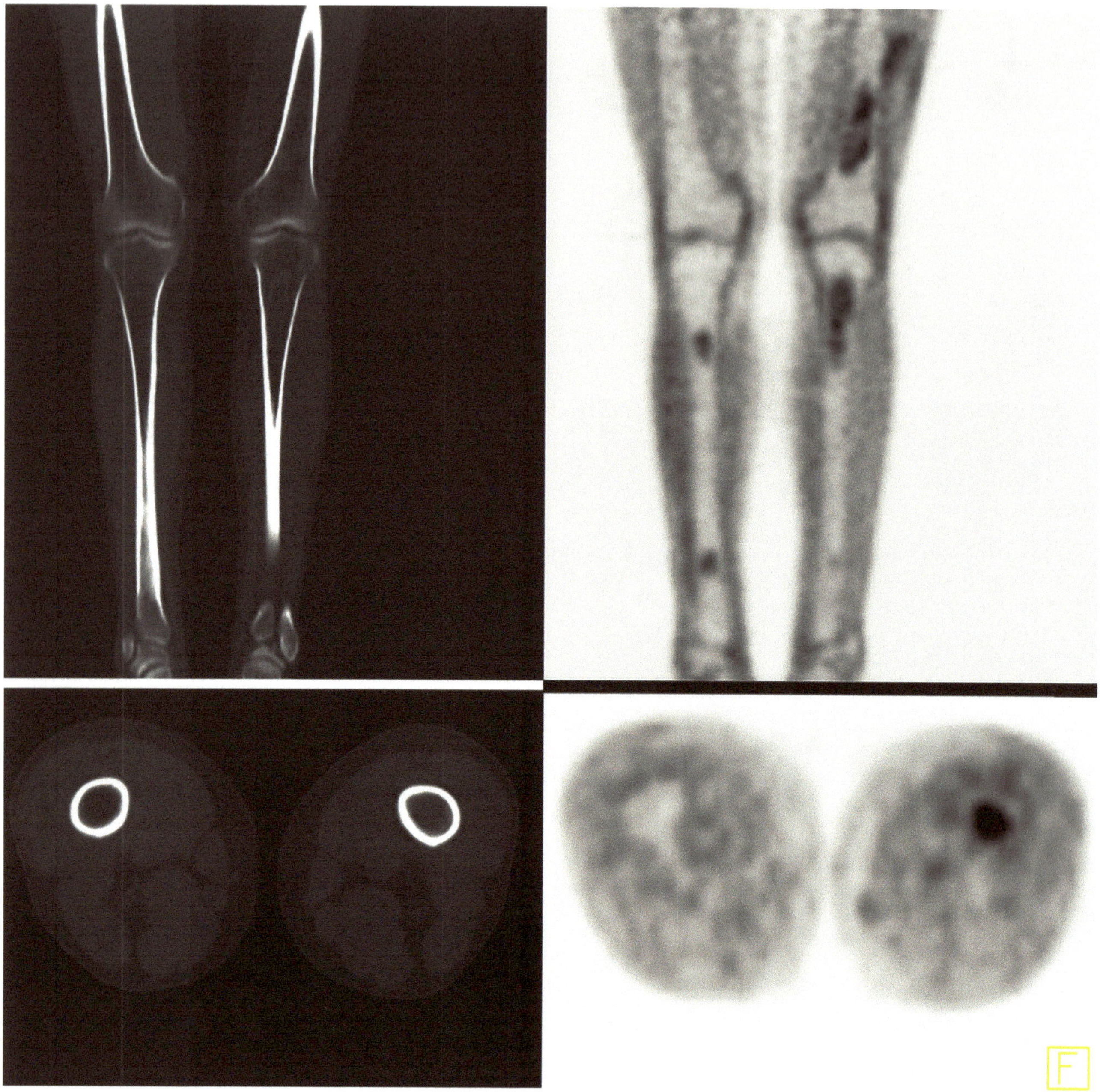

Fig. 2.138 A 40-year-old patient who was being followed-up with the diagnosis of HL underwent ^{18}F-FDG PET/CT. Intramedullary focal increased FDG accumulations are noticed at left distal femur, left proximal tibia, right proximal, and distal tibia. The lesions exhibit a central fat density surrounded by a soft tissue density giving a doughnut appearance. Biopsy of the lesions revealed fat necrosis

Lipoma

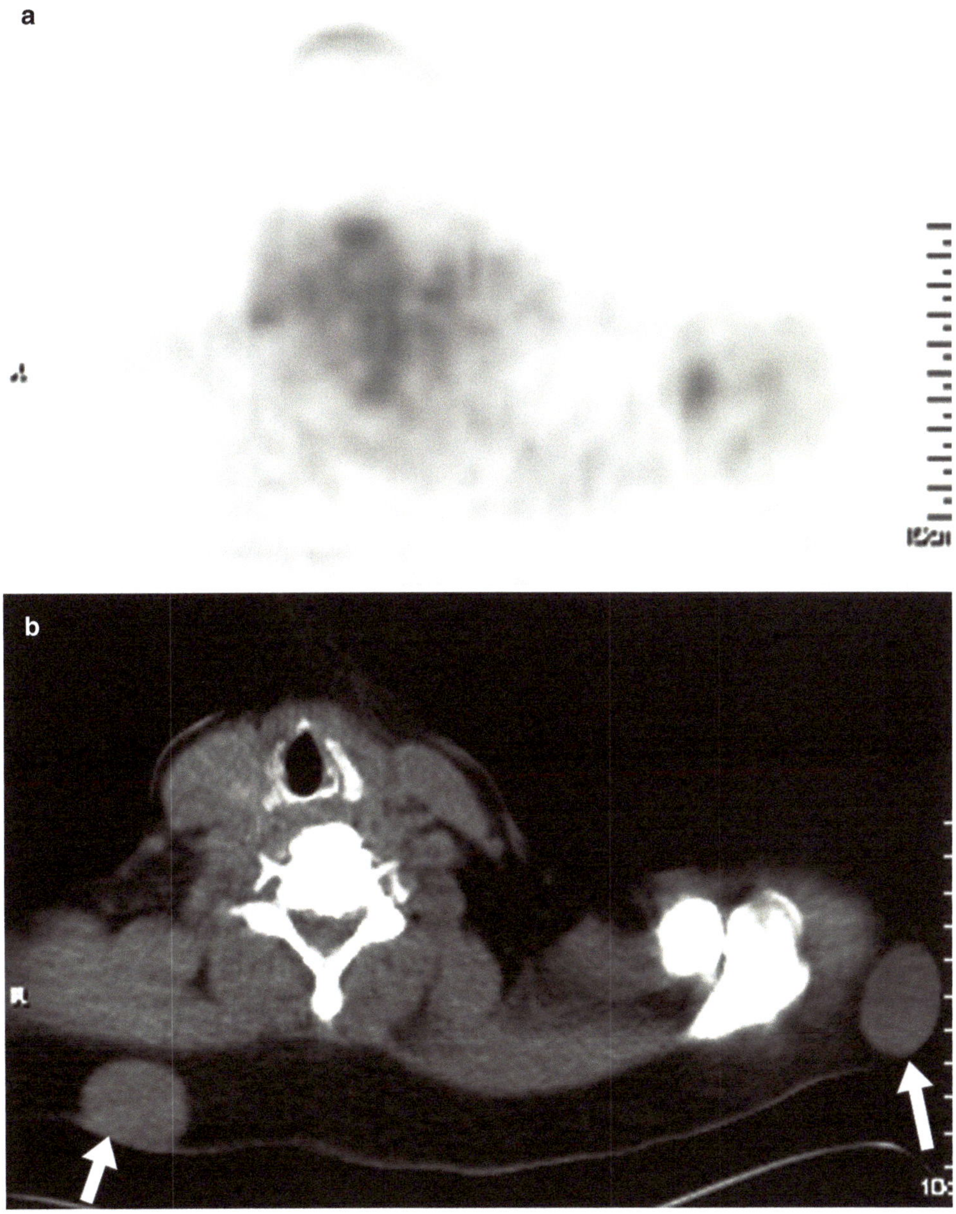

Fig. 2.139 Subcutaneously located lesions in soft tissue density at right dorsal area of thorax (**a**) do not show any significant FDG uptake on PET image (**b**) and they are consistent with lipoma (*arrows*)

Exertional Dyspnea

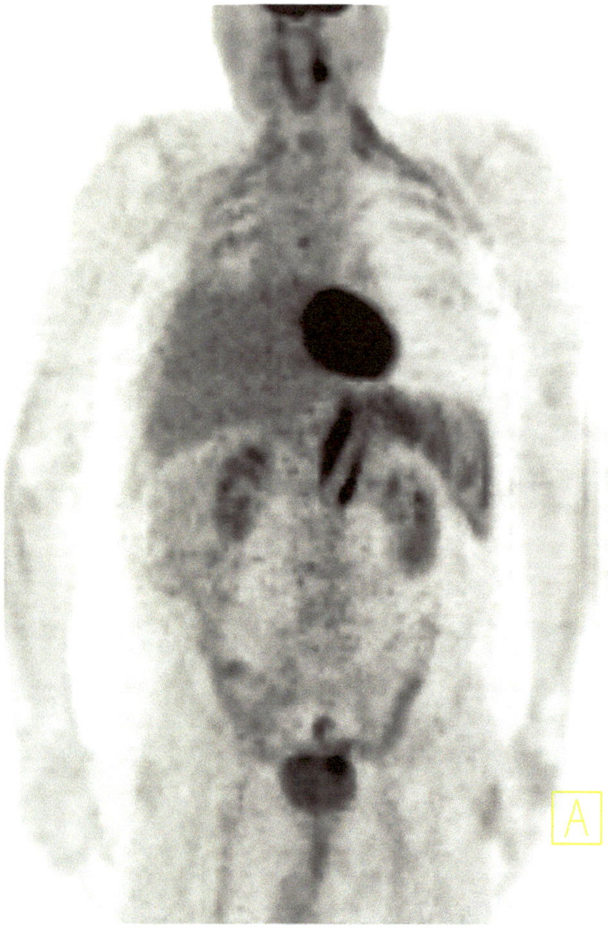

Fig. 2.140 MIP image exhibit increased ^{18}F-FDG uptake in the respiratory muscles (diaphragm, intercostal muscles, and scalene muscles) due to exertional dyspnea

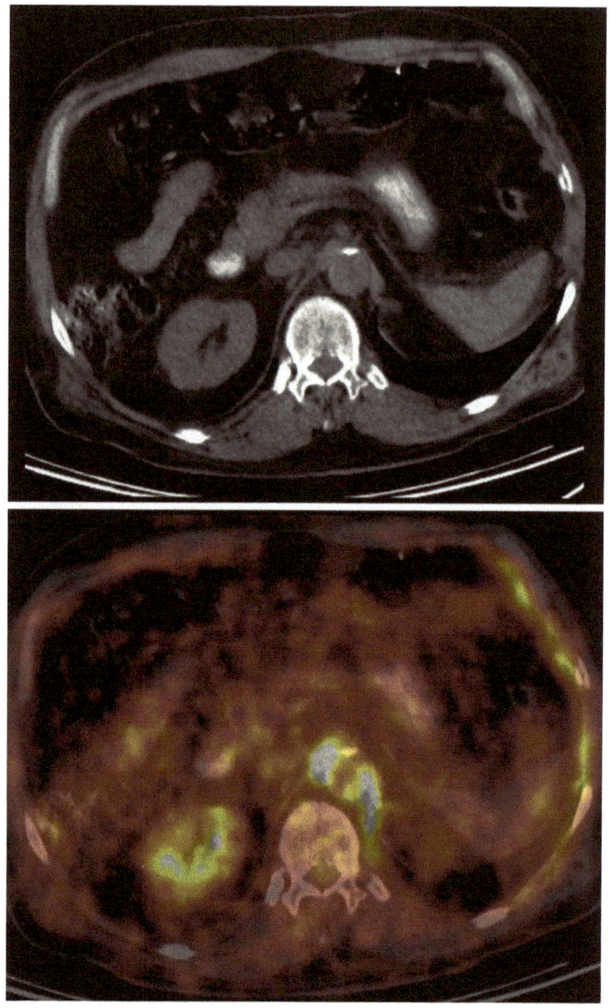

Fig. 2.141 Axial CT and fusion images show hypermetabolism at diaphragm crus and intercostal muscles

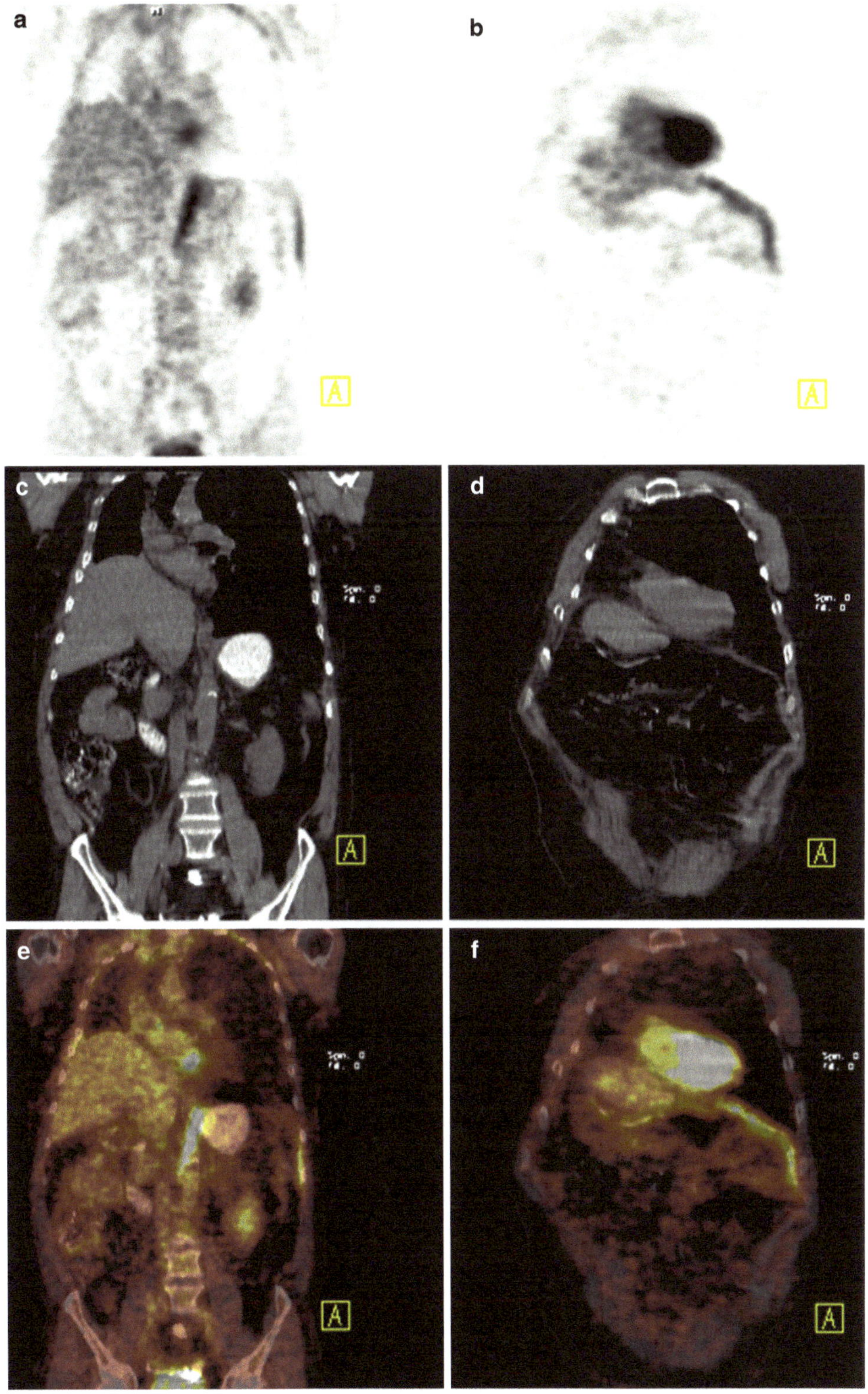

Fig. 2.142 Coronal and sagittal PET, CT, and fusion images show linear uptake at diaphragm which could be misinterpreted as focal uptake at axial images (**a**–**f**)

2.5 Artifacts

Beam Hardening

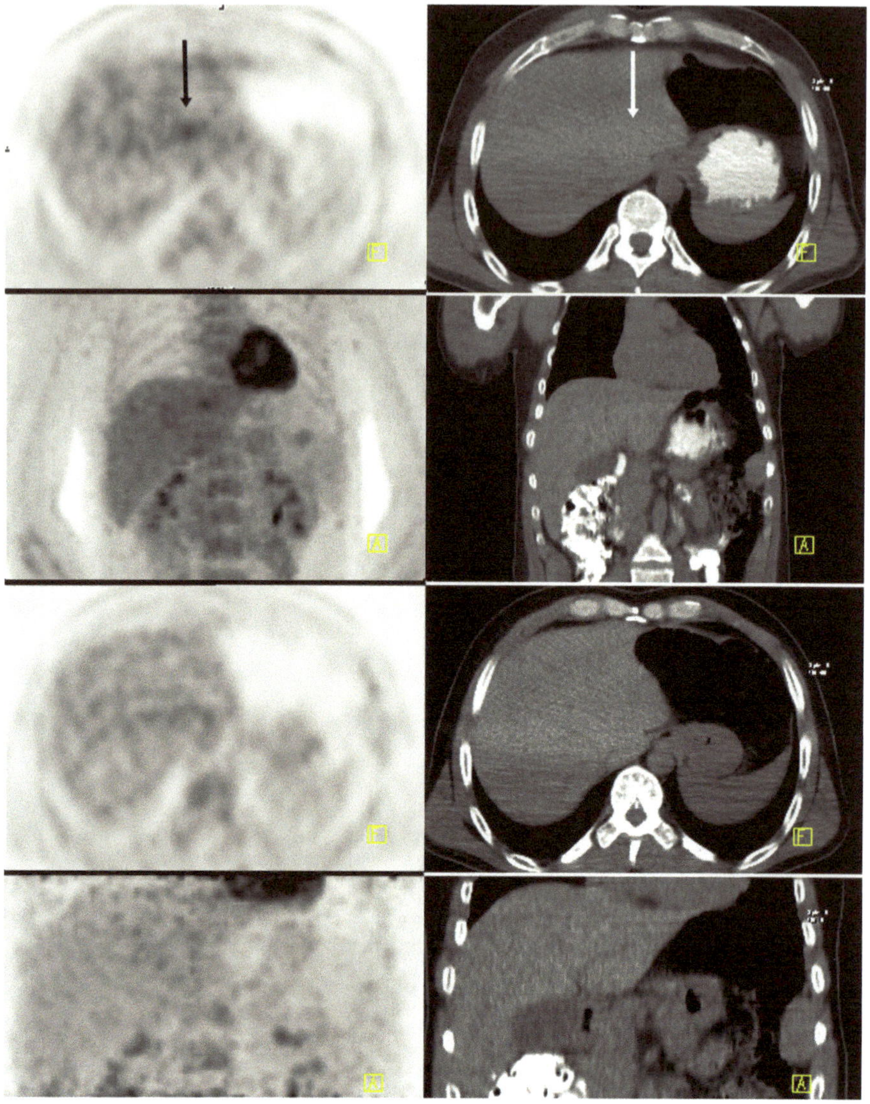

Fig. 2.143 Artificially increased FDG uptake at liver extending from right to left is an attenuation artifact due to beam hardening effect (*arrow*). Beam hardening is seen with polychromatic X-ray sources. As the X-ray passes through the body, low energy X-ray photons are attenuated more easily, but the remaining high energy photons are not attenuated as easily producing dark streaks between two high attenuation objects, such as metal, bone, iodinated contrast, or barium. Since the CT data have artificially higher HU due to beam hardening, CT-corrected PET images show artificial activity in these pixels

Beam Hardening

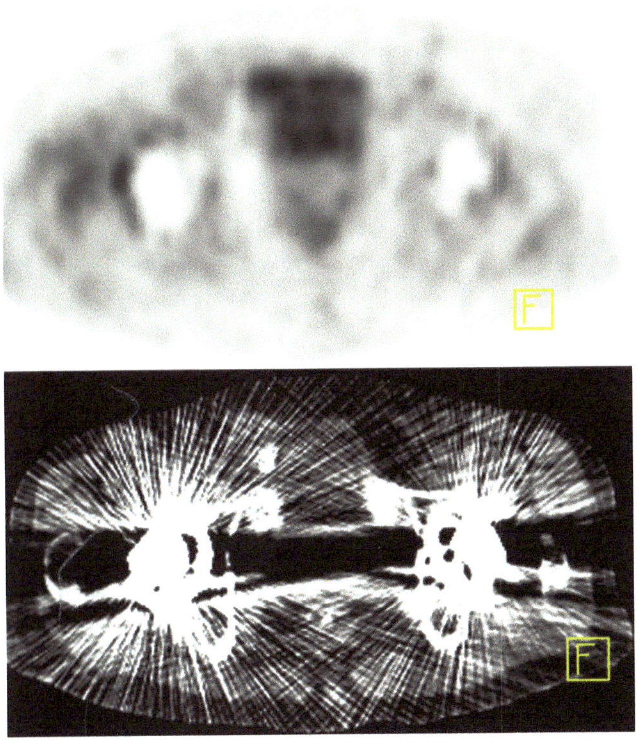

Fig. 2.144 Bilateral metal prostheses at coxofemoral joints cause beam hardening and increased scatter resulting in image distortions. CT-corrected PET images show artificial activity around prostheses which might be interpreted as infection or inflammation by mistake

Attenuation Artifact

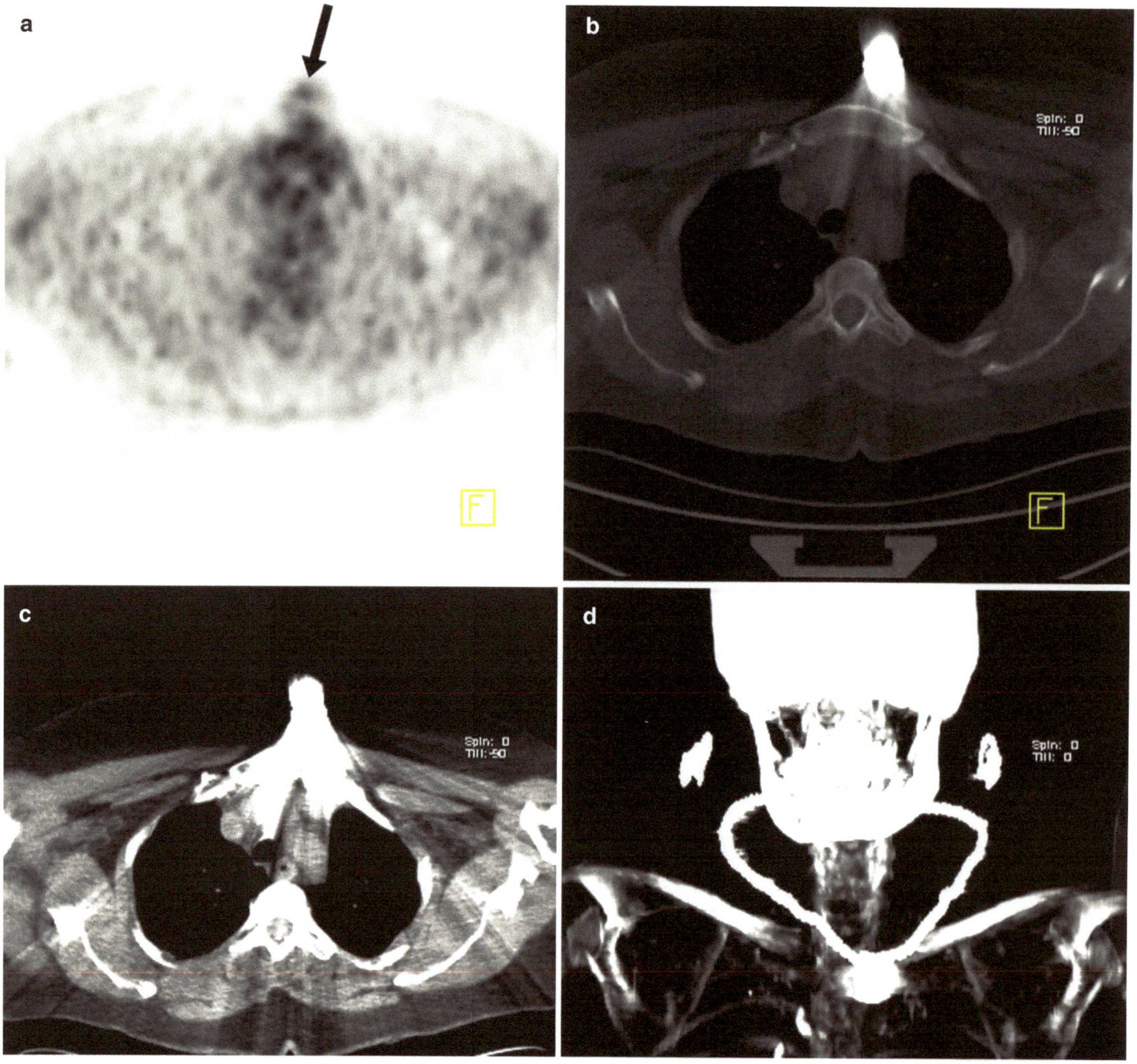

Fig. 2.145 Necklace of the patient causes artificially increased uptake at neck region due to attenuation correction (*arrow*) (**a–d**)

Resolution of Attenuation Artifact at Uncorrected Image

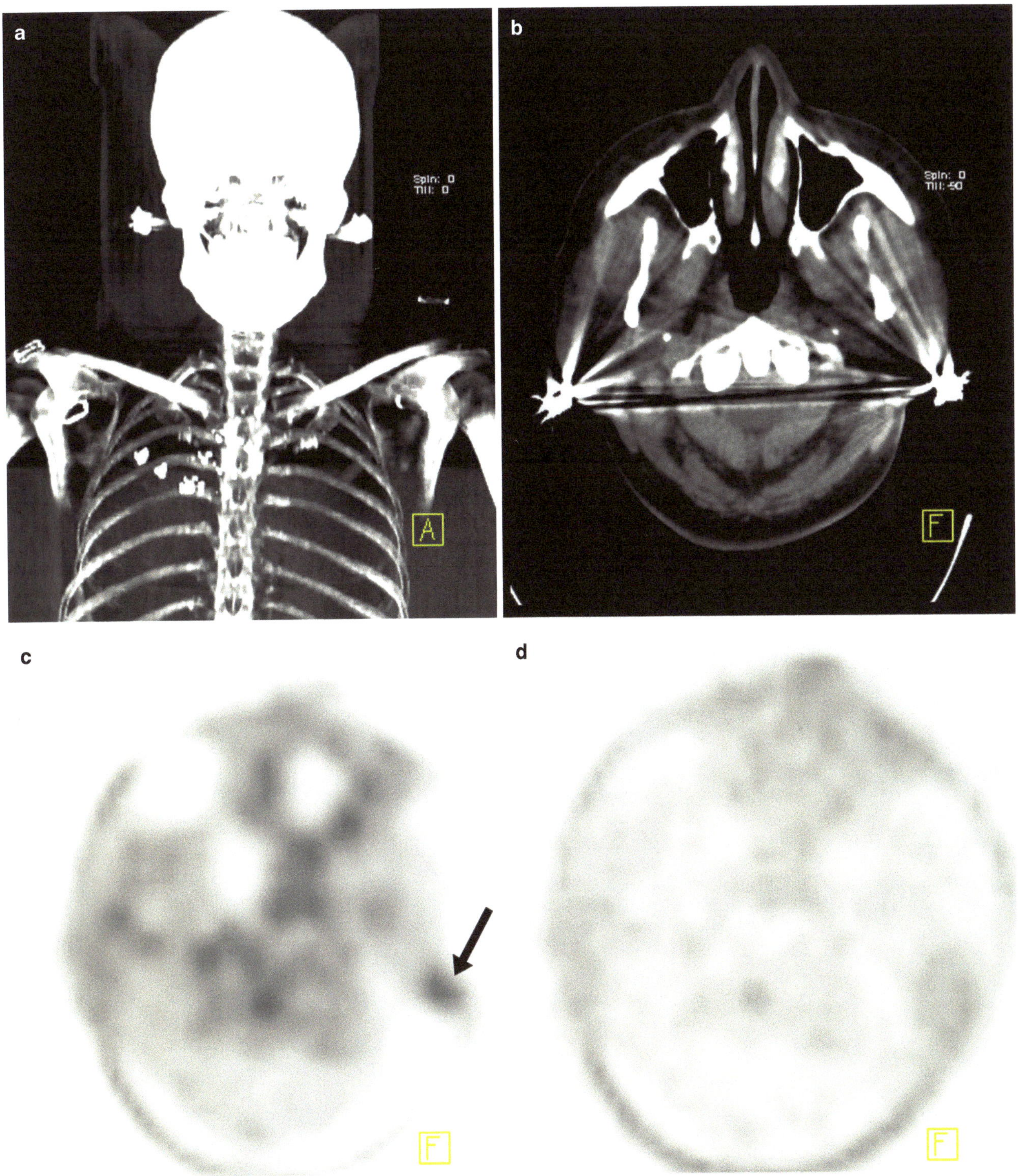

Fig. 2.146 Ear rings of the patient cause beam hardening artifact on CT images (**a**, **b**), artificially increased FDG uptake at left ear due to attenuation correction (*arrow*) (**c**), resolution of this activity in uncorrected images (**d**)

Iatrogenic FDG Pulmonary Embolus

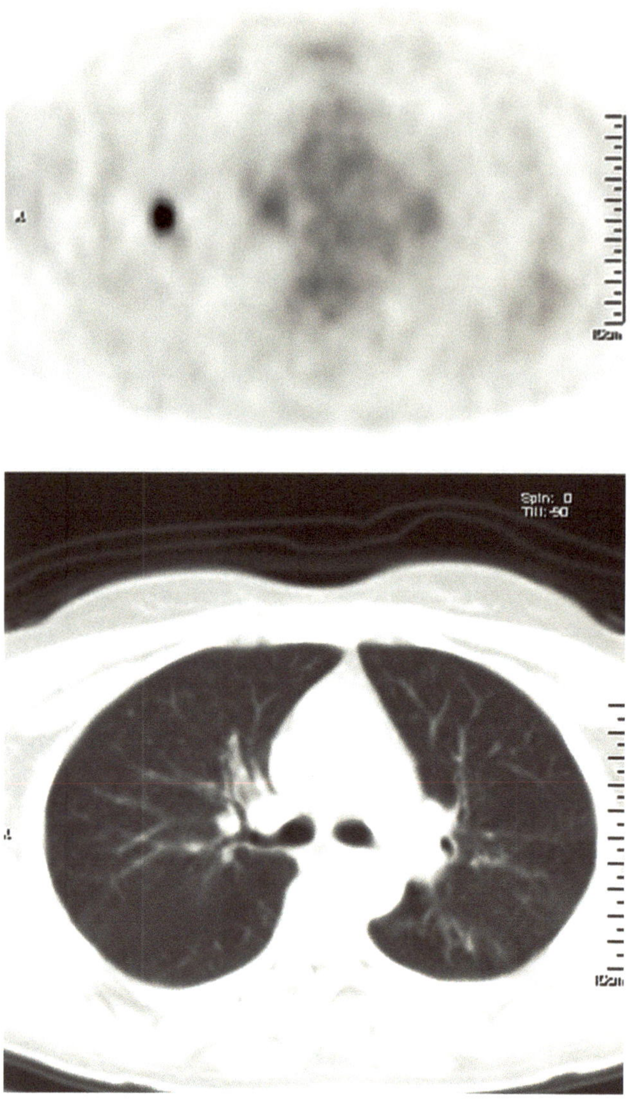

Fig. 2.147 Intense focus of ^{18}F-FDG pulmonary uptake on PET image without detectable lesions on CT is suggestive of FDG microembolus

2.6 Others

Situs Inversus

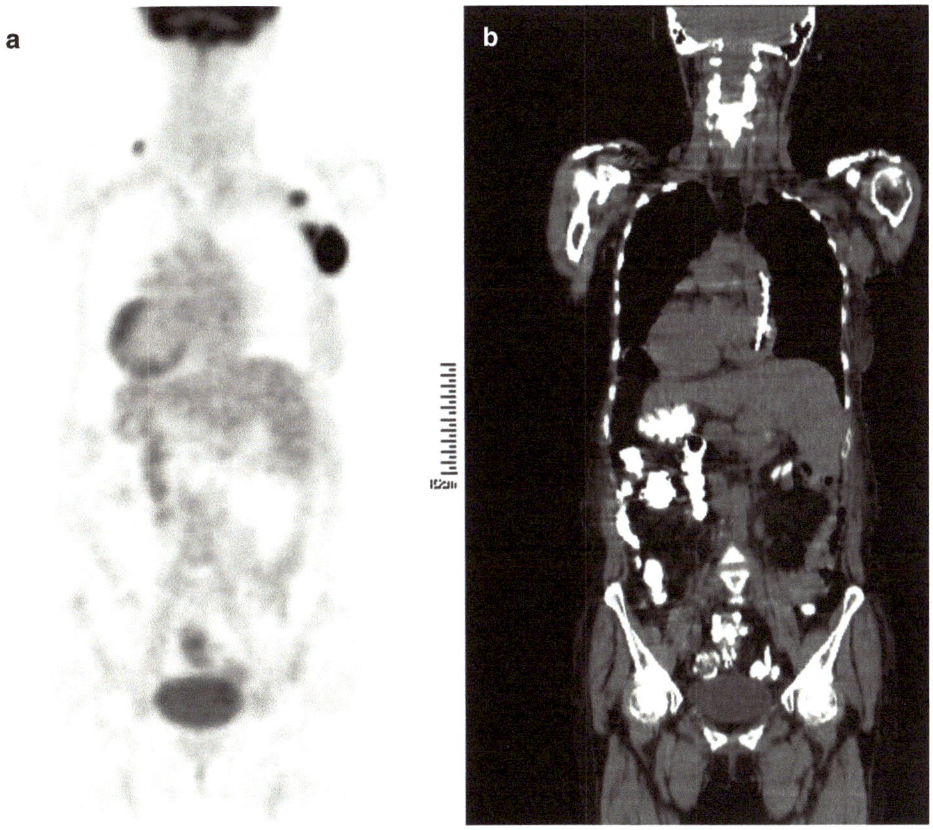

Fig. 2.148 Coronal PET and CT images (**a**, **b**) display situs inversus totalis with myocardium at right hemithorax and liver at left side of abdomen. Note the pathologically increased FDG uptake at left axillar fossa and right lower cervical region

Oral FDG Administration

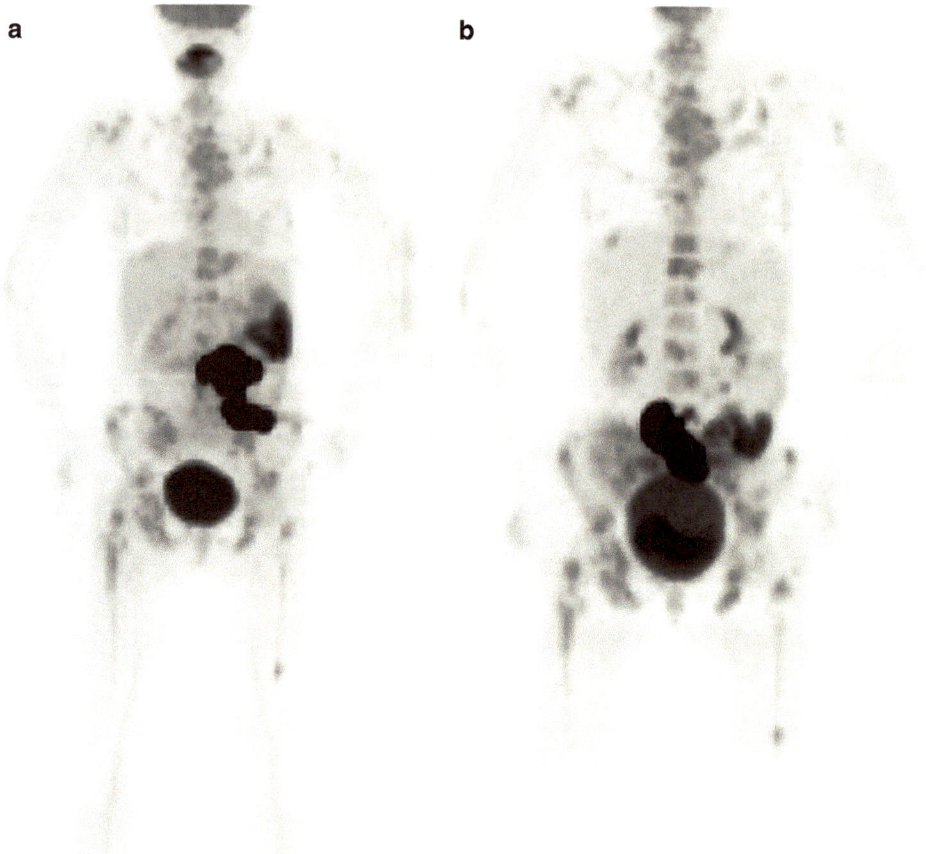

Fig. 2.149 MIP image (**a**) of ^{18}F-FDG PET/CT scan performed following the oral administration of FDG show significant uptake at gastrointestinal system. Ninety minutes after the first acquisition, PET scan was repeated and FDG uptake at metastatic bone lesions is identified; MIP image (**b**)

Brown Adipose Tissue

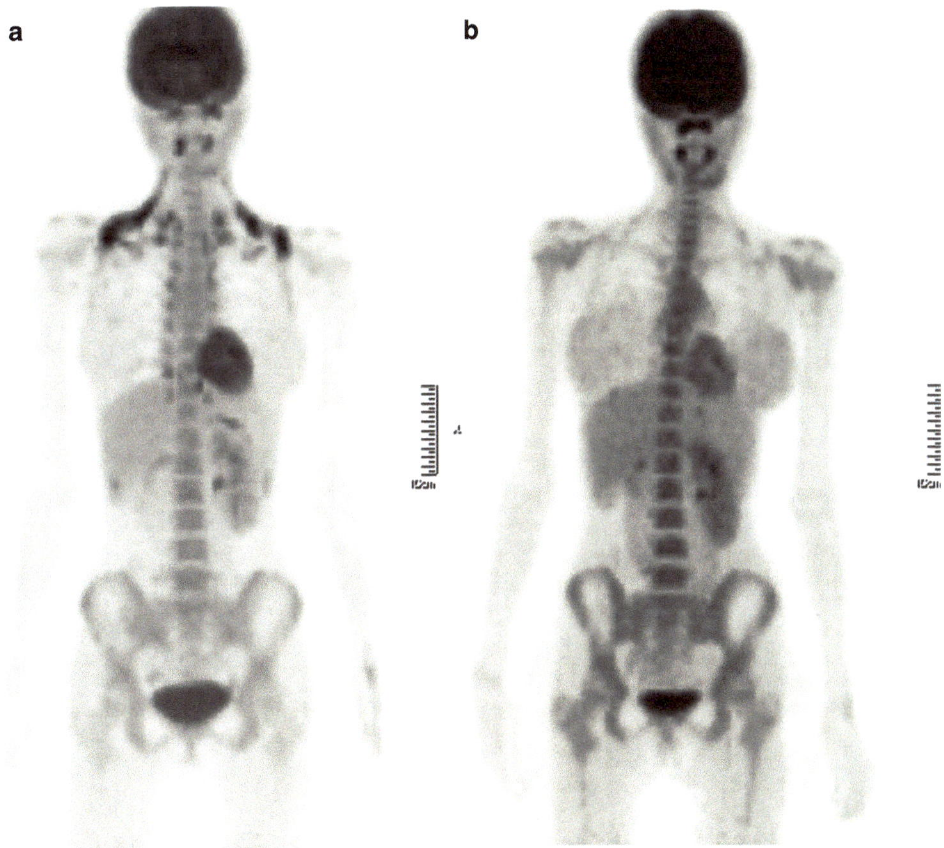

Fig. 2.150 A 15-year-old girl who is being followed up with the diagnosis of lymphoma underwent ^{18}F-FDG PET/CT scan. MIP image of PET scan (**a**) displays increased FDG uptake at deep cervical, supraclavicular, interscapular, and paravertebral regions representing increased FDG uptake at BAT. BAT has the capacity to generate heat. When the sympathetic nervous system is activated by cold stimulation, glucose uptake at brown fat increases. MIP image of PET scan (**b**) performed after the patient was kept warm show the clearance of this physiological uptake

Effect of Insulin Release

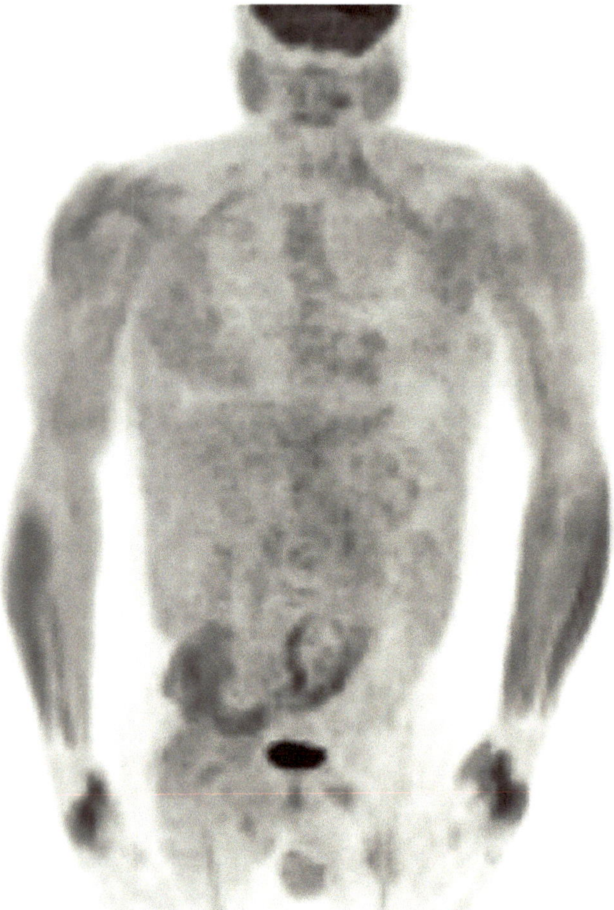

Fig. 2.151 The patient who is being followed up with the diagnosis of lymphoma ate 2 h before FDG administration and consequent release of insulin made the injected FDG accumulate at muscles. The patient should not have eaten during the 4–6 h before the study

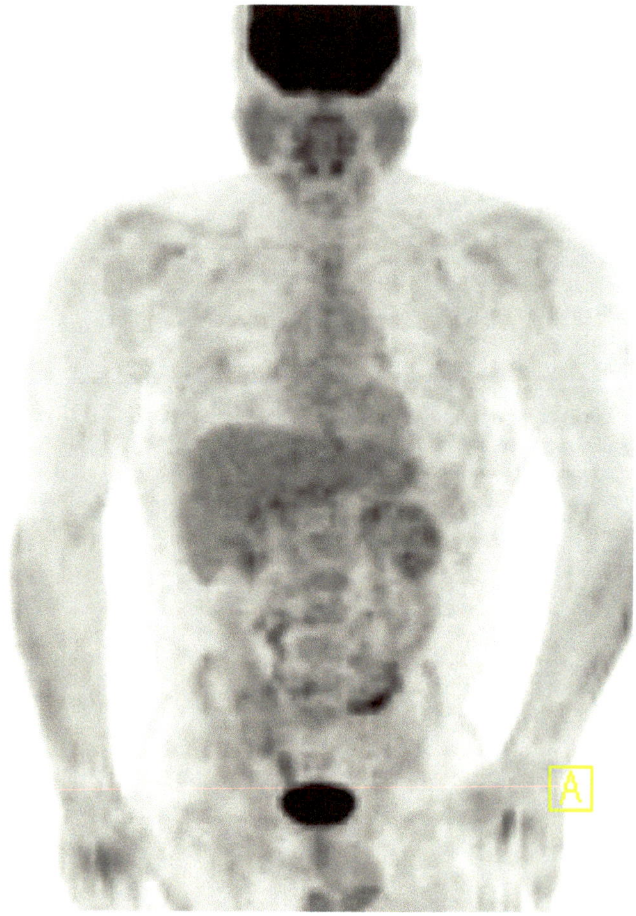

Fig. 2.152 MIP image of PET/CT repeated after fasting shows normal distribution

Extravasation of Radionuclide

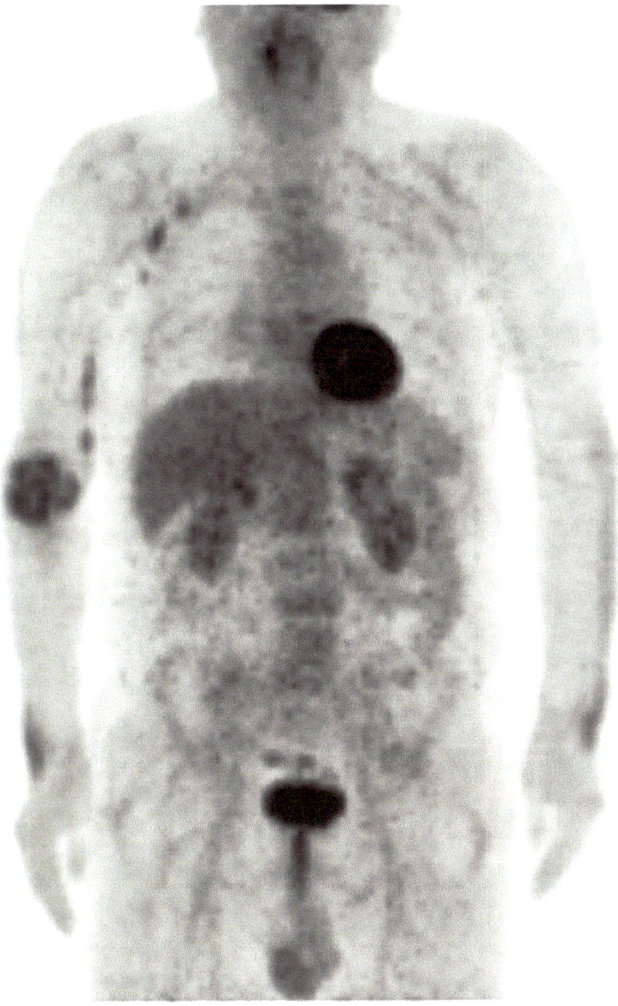

Fig. 2.153 MIP image shows right axillary lymph node visualization after subcutaneous infiltration of ^{18}F-FDG is seen

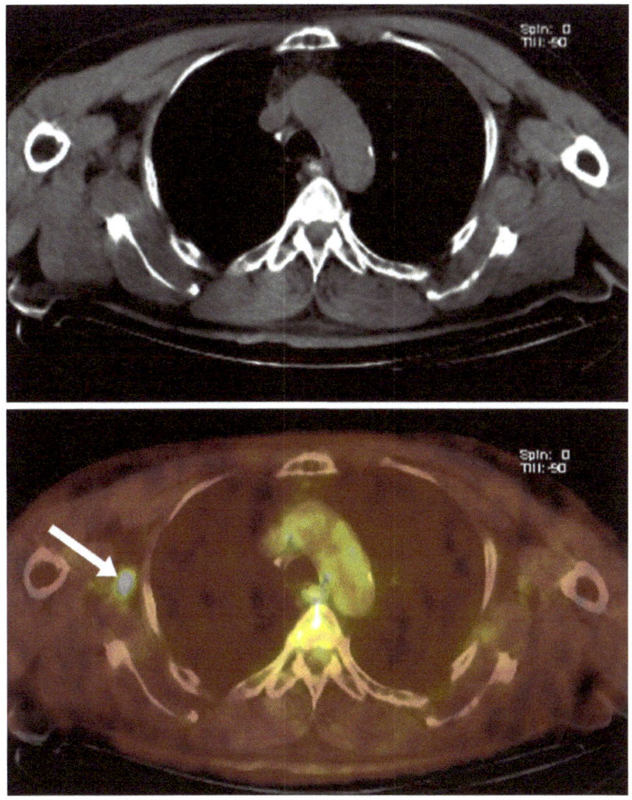

Fig. 2.154 Axial CT and fusion images show hypermetabolic lymph node at right axillary fossa (*arrow*)

Extramedullary Hematopoiesis

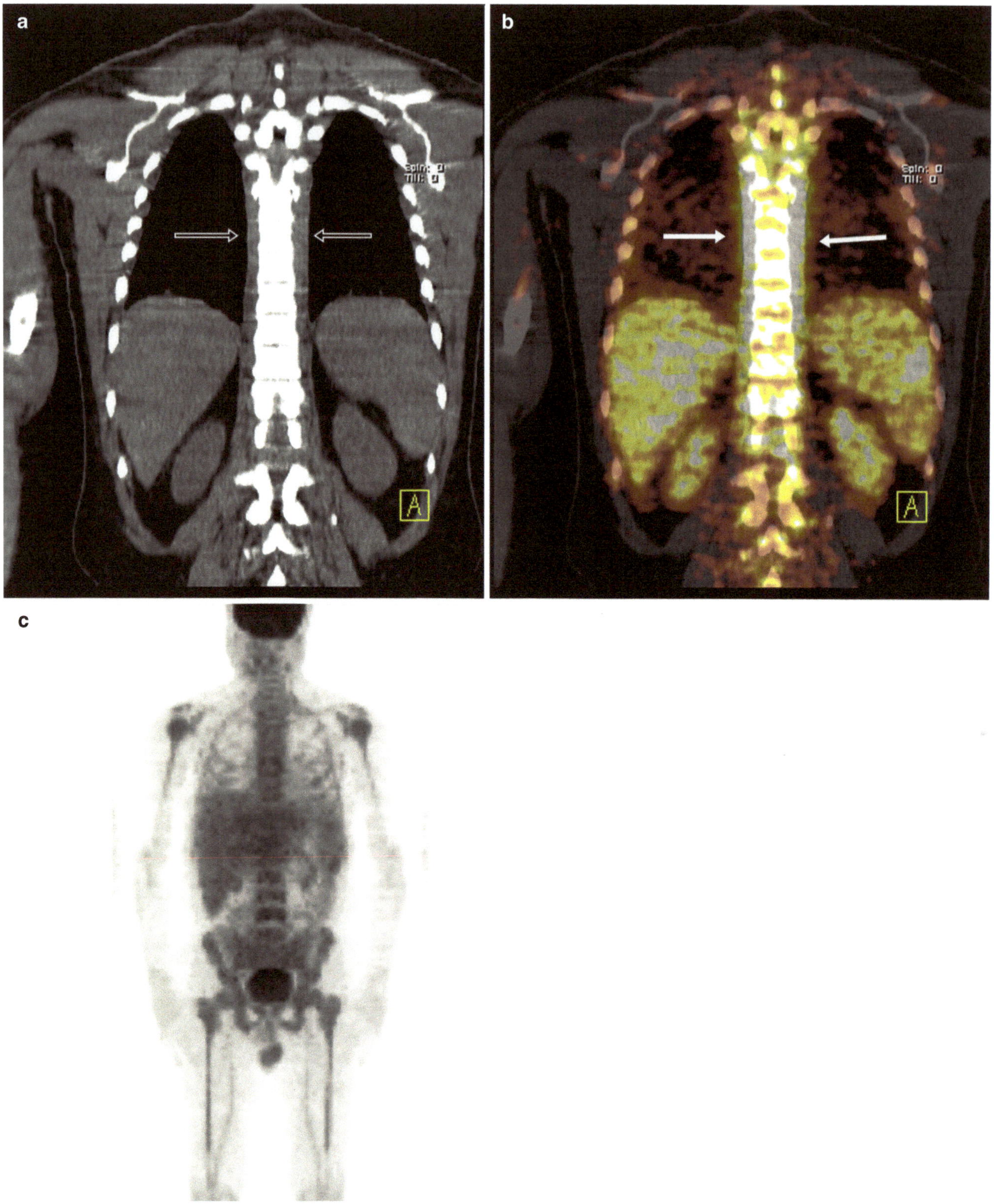

Fig. 2.155 A 36-year-old male patient who is being followed-up with the diagnosis of B-cell prolymphocytic leukemia underwent ^{18}F-FDG PET/CT scan. Coronal CT and fusion (**a**, **b**) and MIP (**c**) images of the patient show bilateral paraspinal soft tissue masses showing mild FDG uptake and extending along the vertebral column (*arrows*)

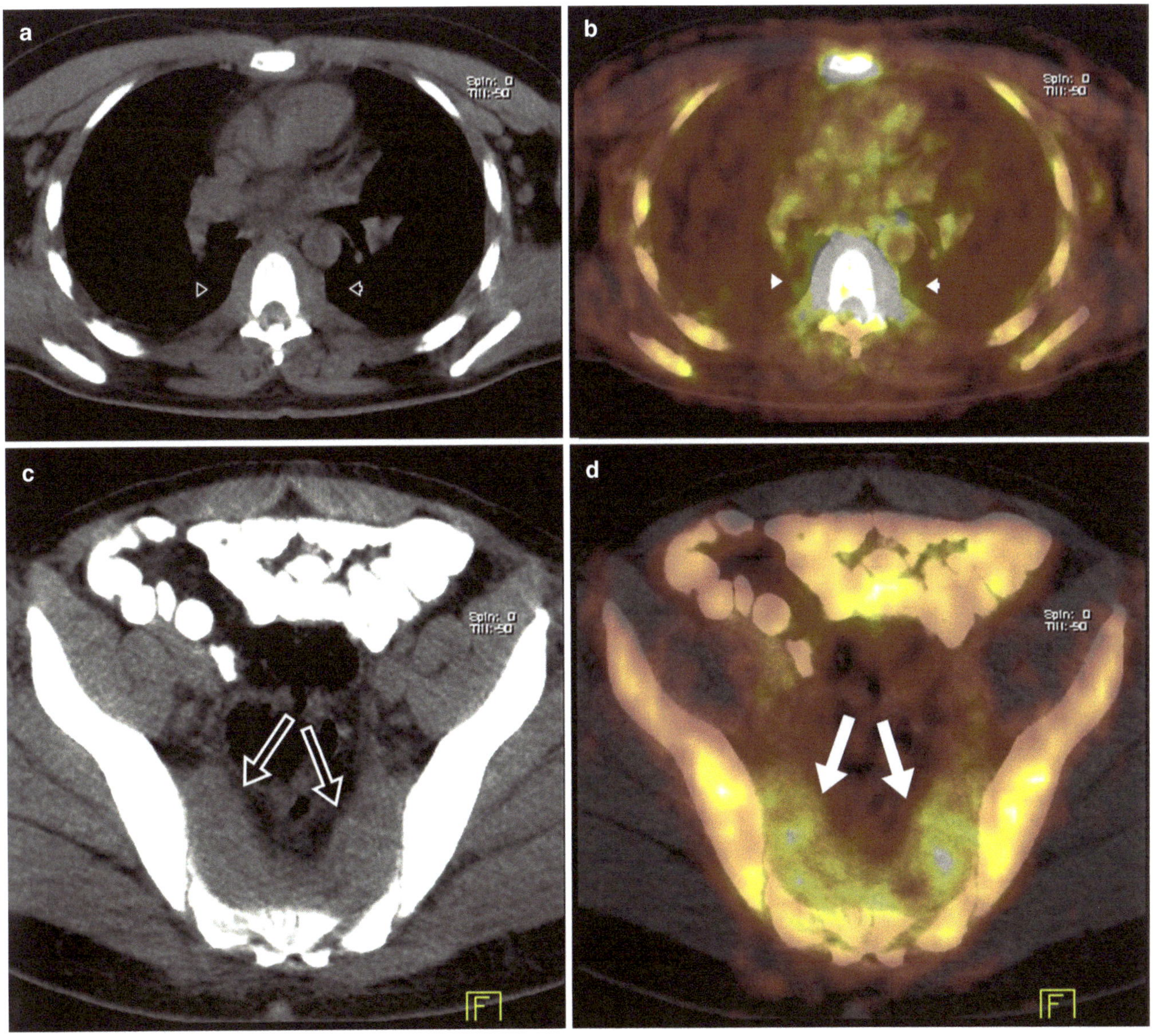

Fig. 2.156 Axial CT and fusion images from thorax (**a**, **b**) and pelvis (**c**, **d**) show mildly hypermetabolic soft tissue mass lesions at paravertebral and presacral areas (*arrows*). Extramedullary hematopoiesis (EMH) occurs in various disorders that goes with anemia like chronic myeloid leukemia, sickle cell anemia, and polycythemia vera. It occurs as a result of intramedullary erythroid destruction and peripheral hemolysis. It may cause paravertebral/intrathoracic, intraabdominal, or pelvic masses and often involves liver, spleen, and lymph nodes

Vasculitis

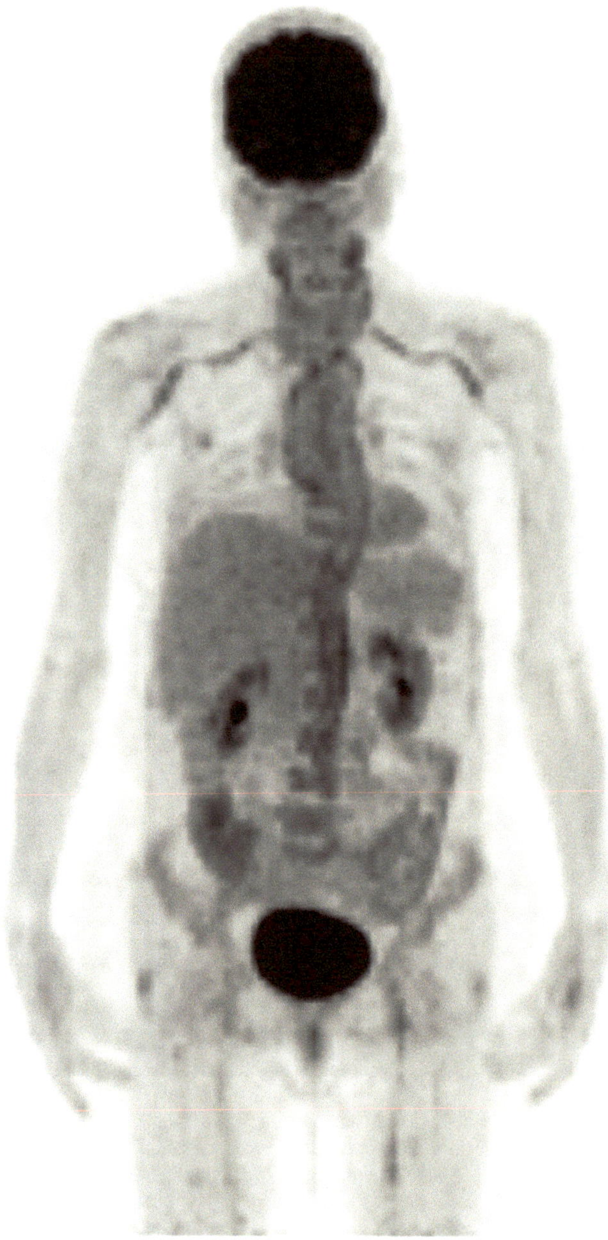

Fig. 2.157 A 60-year-old female who had an unexplained elevated ESR and weight loss history, underwent ^{18}F-FDG PET/CT scan for identification of any possible malignancy. MIP image demonstrates intense ^{18}F-FDG uptake in the aorta, bilateral subclavian, and brachiocephalic arteries consistent with giant cell arteritis. ^{18}F-FDG PET/CT can detect the extent and activity of large-vessel vasculitis in untreated patients and it may be useful in the assessment of therapy monitoring. The level of ^{18}F-FDG uptake may also give prognostic information in large-vessel vasculitis

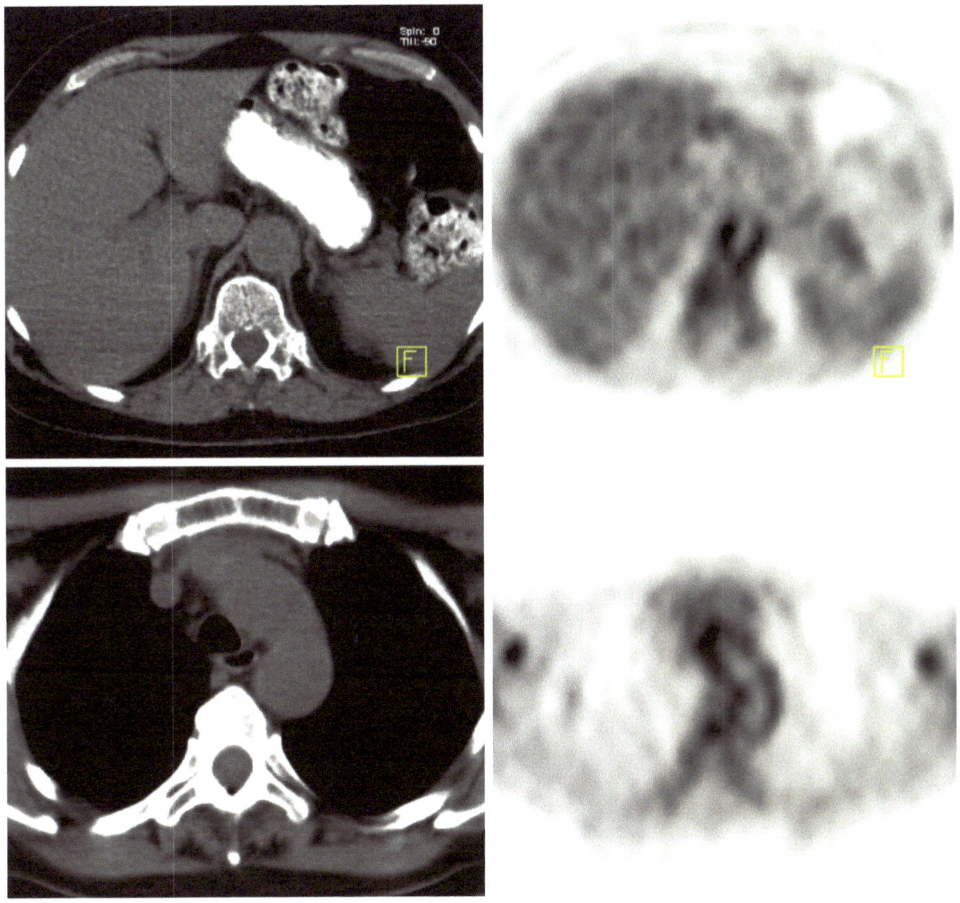

Fig. 2.158 Axial slices of CT and PET images

FDG Uptake at Atherosclerotic Blood Vessels

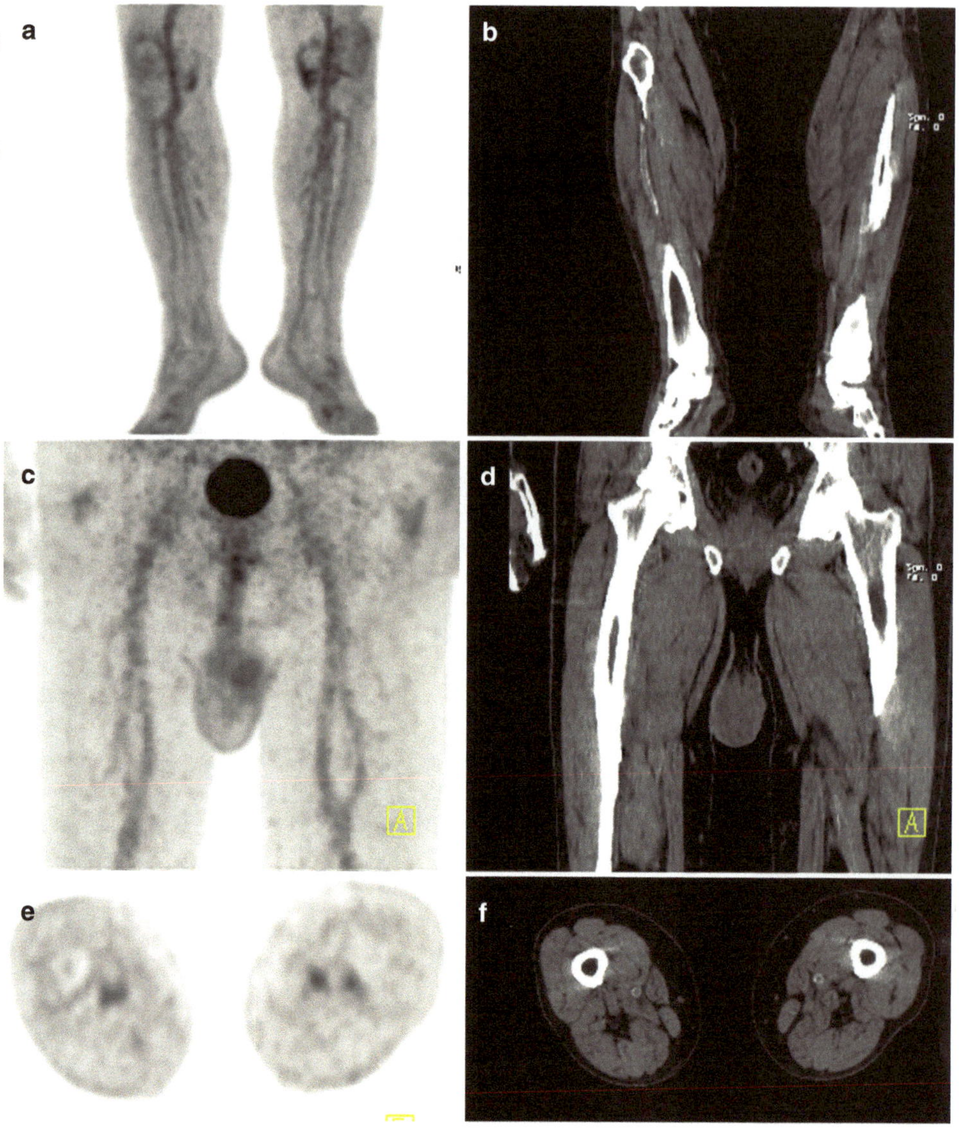

Fig. 2.159 MIP PET (**a**, **c**) and coronal CT (**b**, **d**) and axial PET and CT (**e**, **f**) images show increased FDG uptake at atherosclerotic vessels. In one study atherosclerosis imaging with ^{18}F-FDG PET is found useful for tracking inflammation within plaque and monitoring the response to drug therapy

Parathyroid Adenoma and Brown Tumor

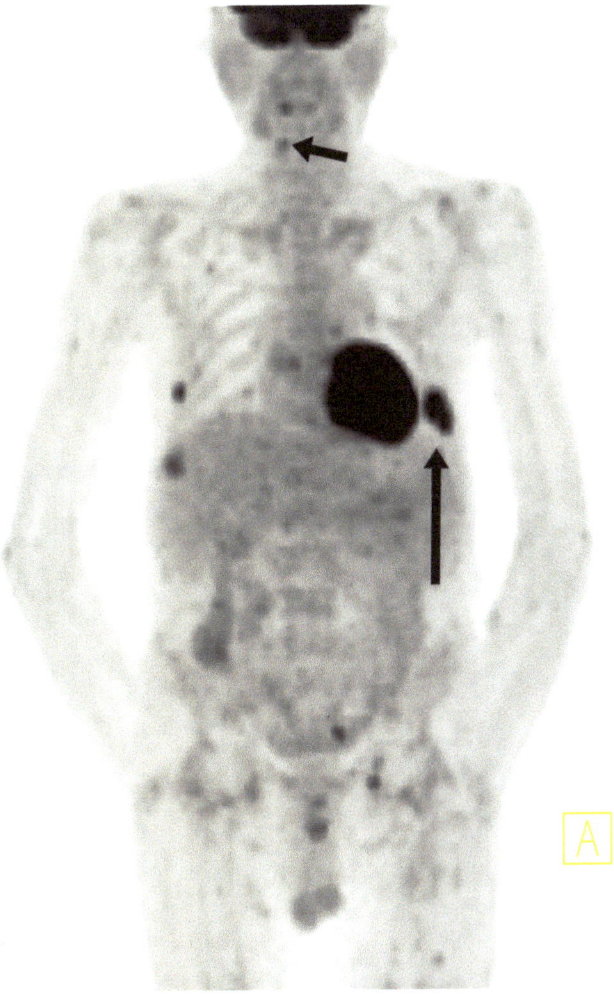

Fig. 2.160 MIP image show focal increased FDG uptake at left hemithorax consistent with brown tumor at rib (*long arrow*) and subtle FDG accumulation at neck region representing a parathyroid adenoma (*short arrow*)

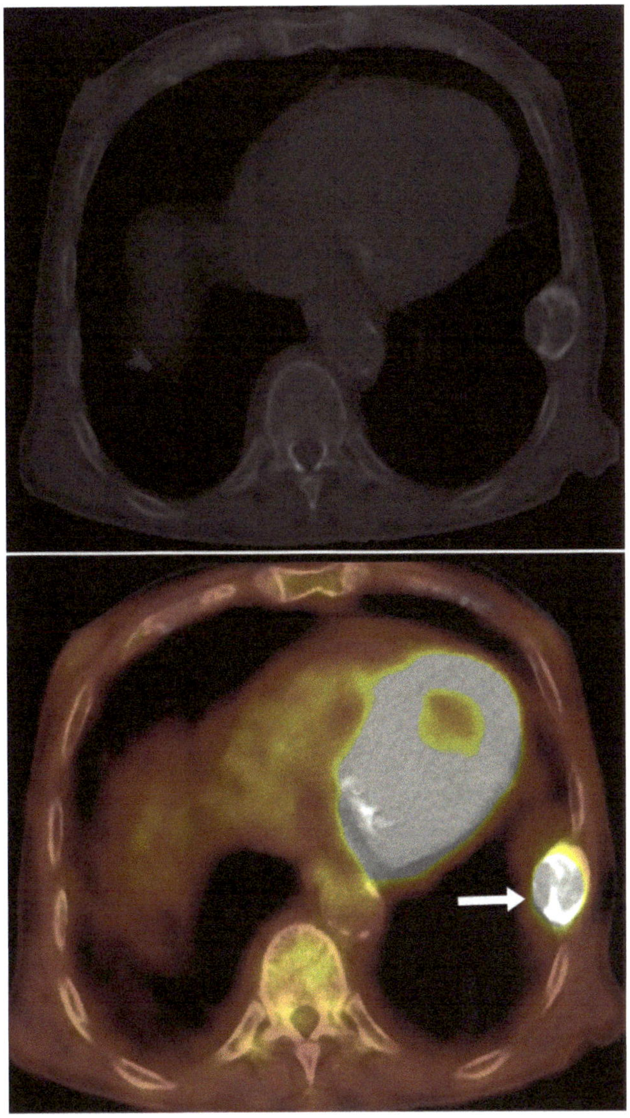

Fig. 2.161 Axial CT and fusion images display intensely increased FDG uptake at expansile lesion of rib representing a brown tumor (*arrow*)

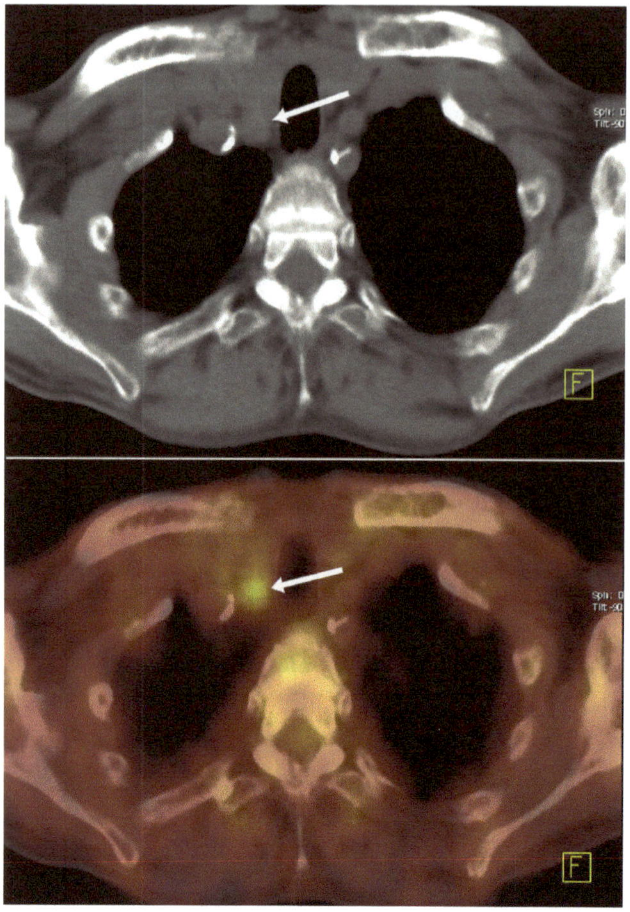

Fig. 2.162 Axial CT and fusion images show focal increased FDG accumulation right lower cervical region posterior to right lobe of thyroid gland. This lesion turned out to be parathyroid adenoma (*arrow*)

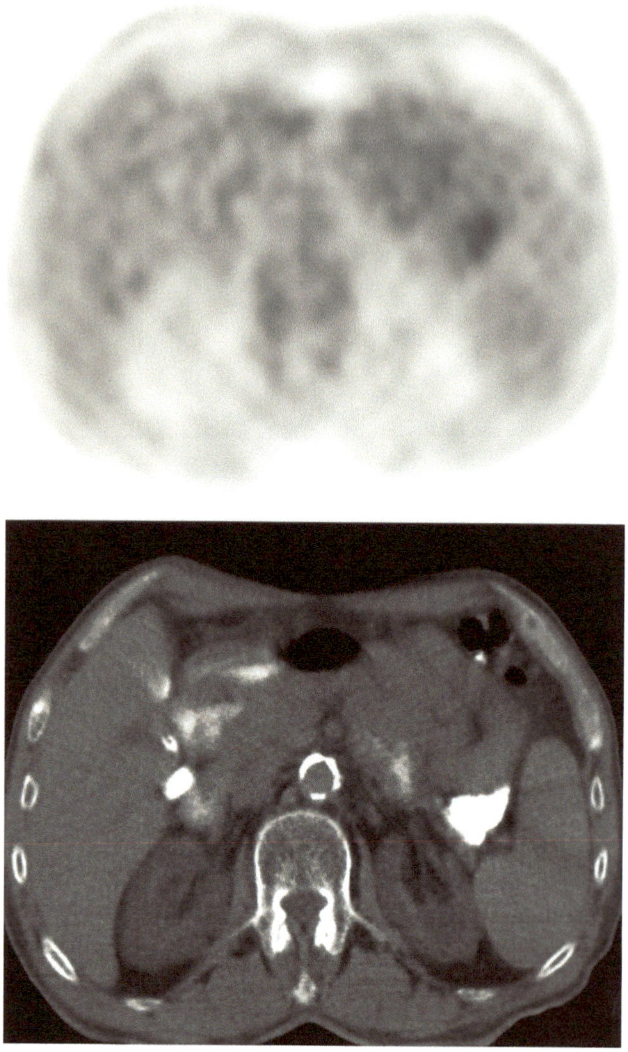

Fig. 2.163 Axial PET and CT images display no FDG uptake at both kidneys reflecting renal insufficiency which imply that the patient has secondary hyperparathyroidism

Granulomatous Foreign Body Reaction Due to Sunflower Oil Injection to Skin

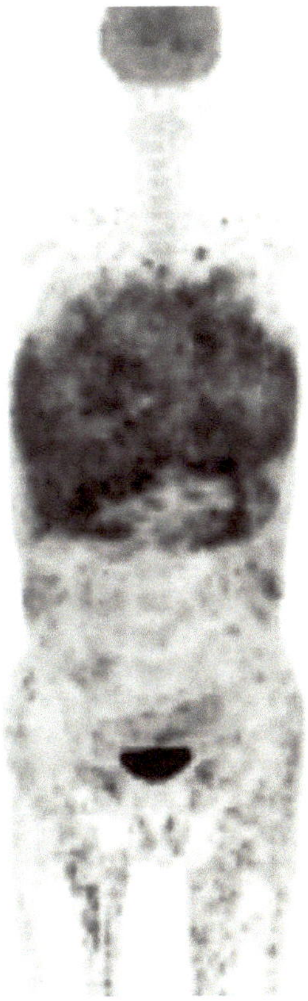

Fig. 2.164 MIP image of a patient showing intense heterogenous FDG uptake at thorax due to granulomatous foreign body reaction that occurred as a result of repeated intradermal self-injections of sunflower oil

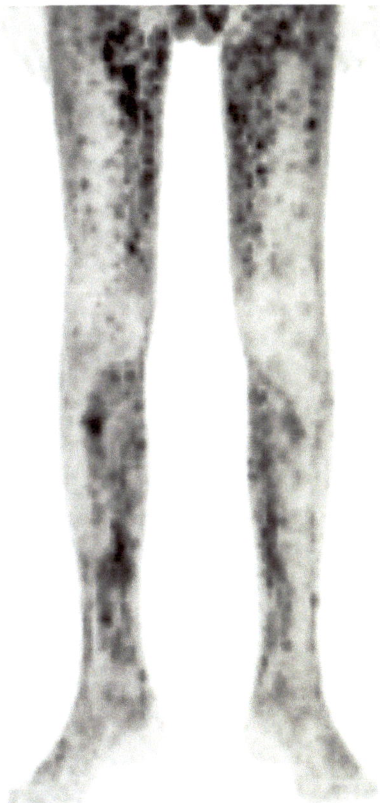

Fig. 2.165 MIP image of legs of the patient showing multiple focal increased FDG uptake at injection sites

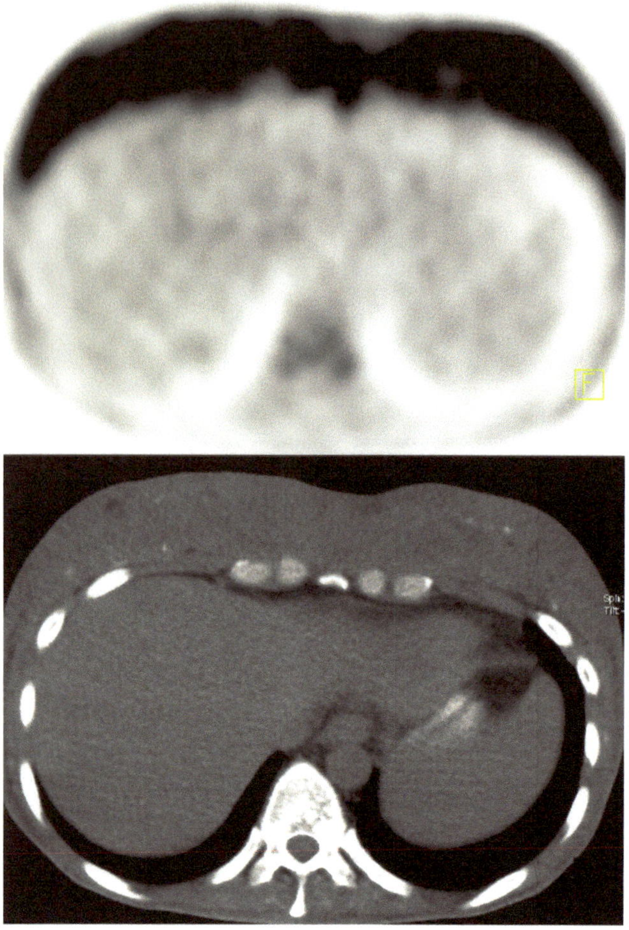

Fig. 2.166 Axial PET and CT image of thorax showing intense FDG uptake corresponding to thickening at anterior wall of thorax

Sarcoidosis

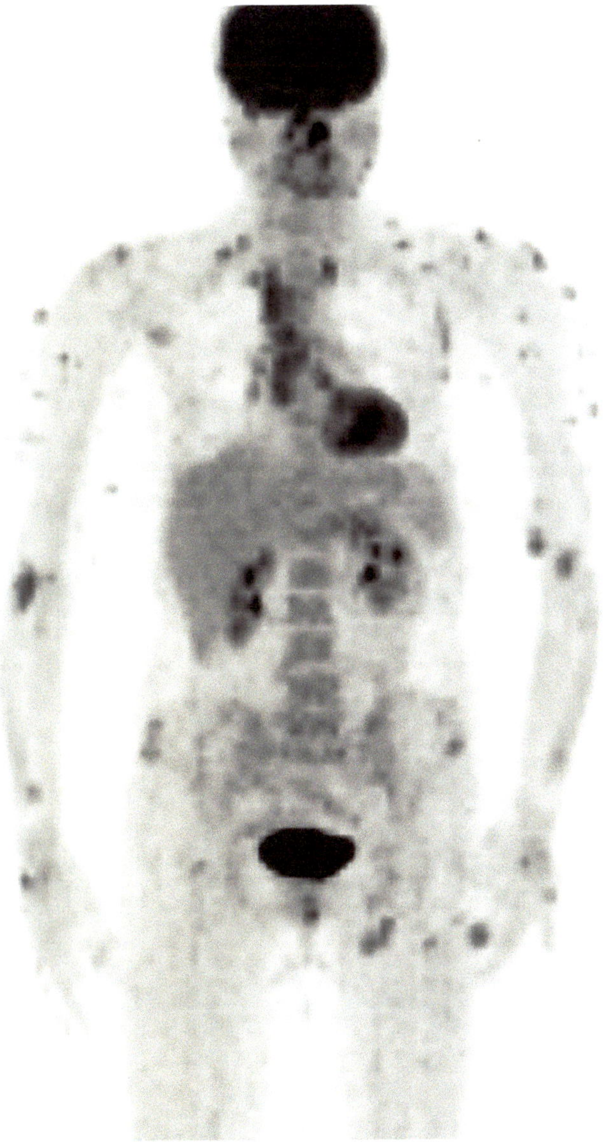

Fig. 2.167 A 60-year-old female with a known history of sarcoidosis underwent ^{18}F-FDG PET/CT for the evaluation of the disease. MIP image shows multiple hypermetabolic bone lesions at cranium, long bones of upper and lower extremities, phalanges of hand and foot, and pelvic bones (SUVmax 7.6). There are also multiple lymph nodes showing increased FDG uptake at mediastinum, both axillary fossa and both femoroinguinal regions (SUVmax 7.3). The prevalence of bone involvement in sarcoidosis has been estimated to be 3–5 %, mostly affecting the phalanges. The majority of these lesions could not be detected on CT. FDG PET scanning is effective in the detection of sarcoidosis with systemic distribution, including osseous lesions

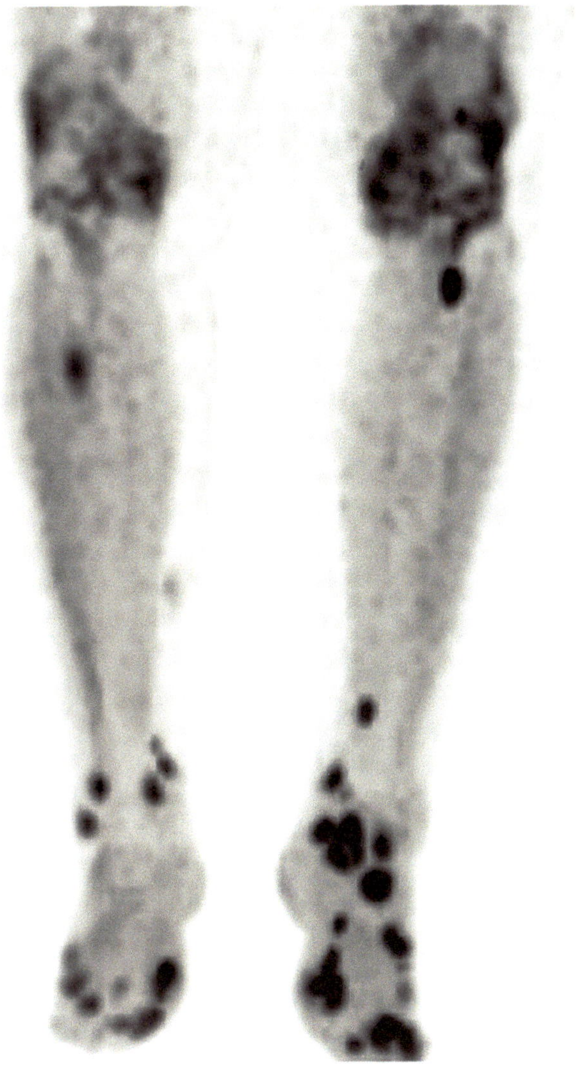

Fig. 2.168 MIP image of lower extremities show numerous hypermetabolic bone lesions

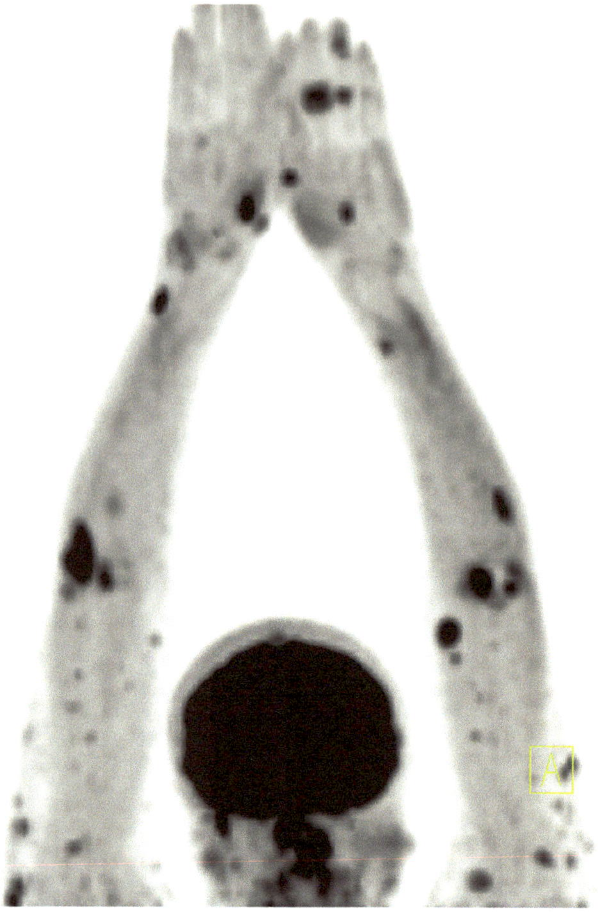

Fig. 2.169 MIP image of upper extremities shows hypermetabolic foci at bony structures as well as subcutaneous tissues

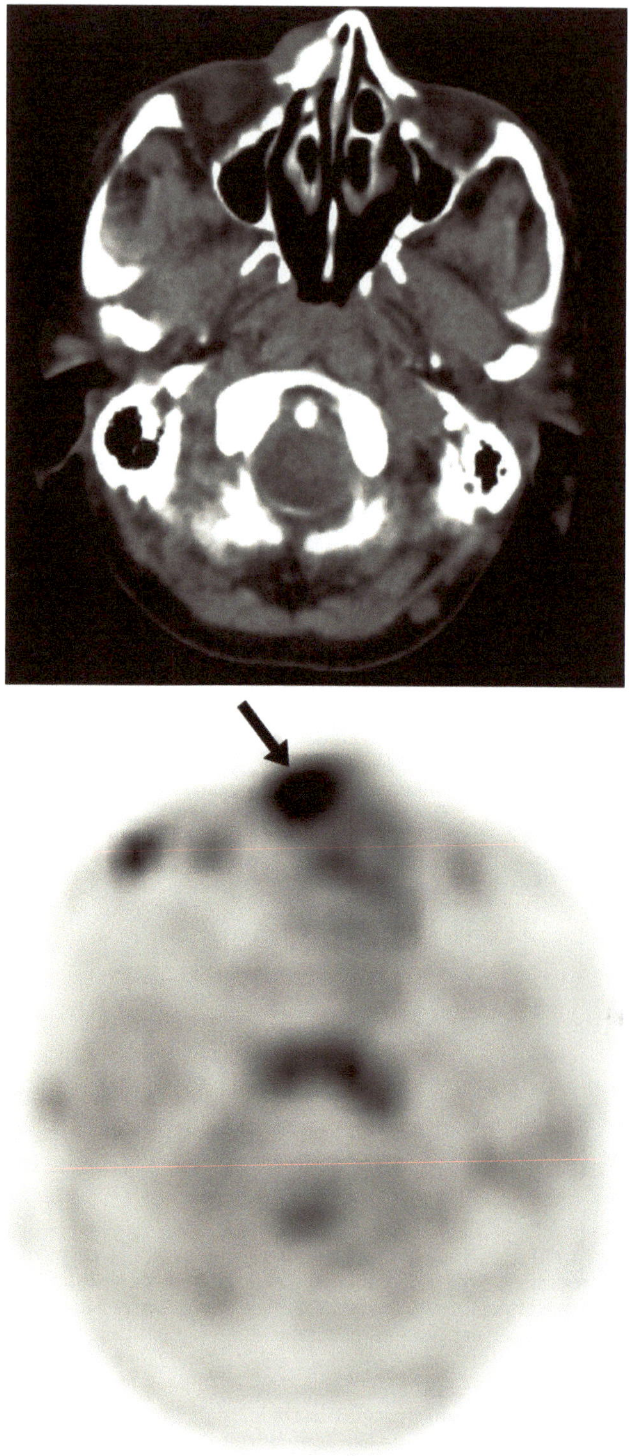

Fig. 2.170 Axial slices of CT and PET images of cranium show focal increased FDG uptake at right side of nasal bone (*arrow*)

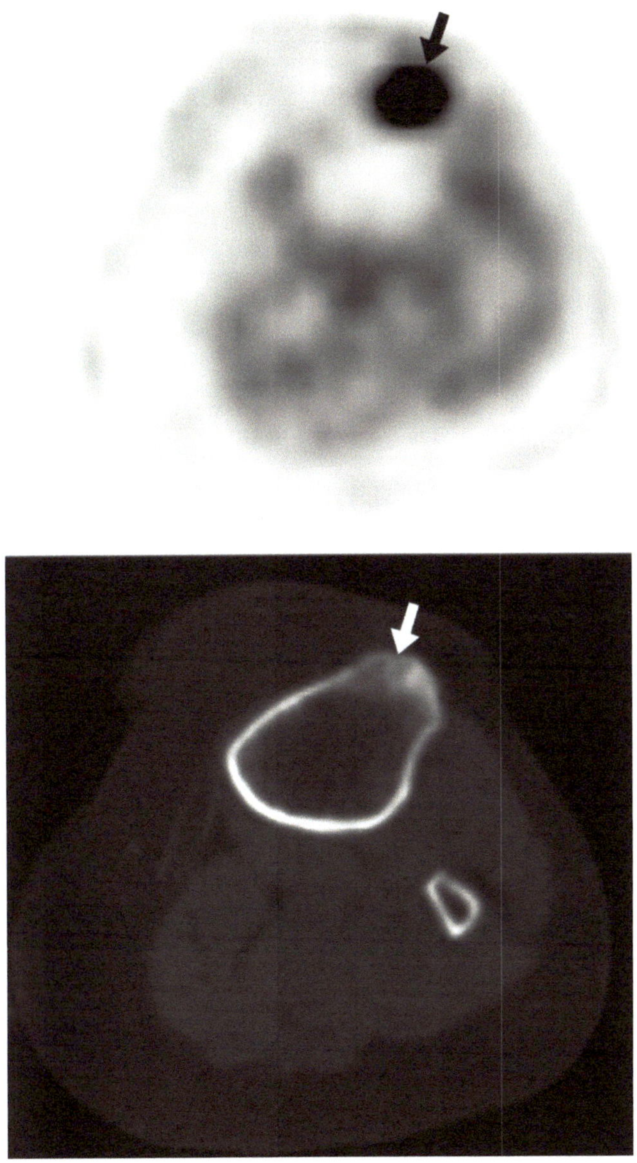

Fig. 2.171 Axial slices of PET and CT images show focal hypermetabolic lytic lesion at anterior cortex of tibia (*arrows*)

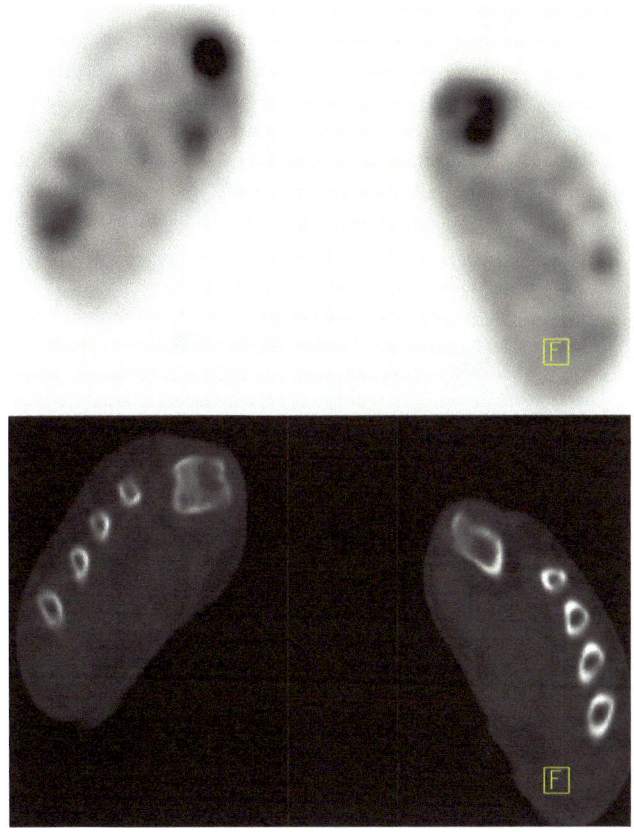

Fig. 2.172 Axial slices PET and CT images of both feet show hypermetabolic lytic lesions at distal phalanges of feet

Bibliography

1. Abele JT, Fung CI. Effect of hepatic steatosis on liver FDG uptake measured in mean standard uptake values. Radiology. 2010;254:917–24.
2. Bogsrud TV, Karantanis D, Nathan MA, Mullan BP, Wiseman GA, Collins DA, et al. The value of quantifying 18F-FDG uptake in thyroid nodules found incidentally on whole-body PET-CT. Nucl Med Commun. 2007;28:373–81.
3. Bredella MA, Essary B, Torriani M, Ouellette HA, Palmer WE. Use of FDG-PET in differentiating benign from malignant compression fractures. Skeletal Radiol. 2008;37:405–13.
4. Courtois A, Nusgens BV, Hustinx R, Namur G, Gomez P, Somja J, et al. 18F-FDG uptake assessed by PET/CT in abdominal aortic aneurysms is associated with cellular and molecular alterations prefacing wall deterioration and rupture. J Nucl Med. 2013;54:1740–7.
5. Ferdinand B, Gupta P, Kramer EL. Spectrum of thymic uptake at 18F-FDG PET. Radiographics. 2004;24:611–6.
6. Harisankar CN. Focal fat sparing of the liver: a nonmalignant cause of focal FDG uptake on FDG PET/CT. Clin Nucl Med. 2014;39:359–61.
7. Hollinger EF, Alibazoglu H, Ali A, Green A, Lamonica G. Hematopoietic cytokine-mediated FDG uptake simulates the appearance of diffuse metastatic disease on whole-body PET imaging. Clin Nucl Med. 1998;23:93–8.
8. Hoffmann M, Kletter K, Becherer A, Jäger U, Chott A, Raderer M. 18F-fluorodeoxyglucose positron emission tomography (18F-FDG-PET) for staging and follow-up of marginal zone B-cell lymphoma. Oncology. 2003;64:336–40.
9. Hoffmann M, Kletter K, Diemling M, Becherer A, Pfeffel F, Petkov V, et al. Positron emission tomography with fluorine-18-2-fluoro-2-deoxy-D-glucose (F18-FDG) does not visualize extranodal B-cell lymphoma of the mucosa-associated lymphoid tissue (MALT)-type. Ann Oncol. 1999;10:1185–9.
10. Jeong SY, Lee SW, Lee HJ, Kang S, Seo JH, Chun KA, et al. Incidental pituitary uptake on whole-body 18F-FDG PET/CT: a multicentre study. Eur J Nucl Med Mol Imaging. 2010;37:2334–43.
11. Karapolat I, Oncel G, Kumanlıoğlu K. Clinically occult pituitary adenoma can appear as a hypermetabolic lesion on whole body FDG PET imaging in a patient with lymphoma. Mol Imaging Radionucl Ther. 2013;22:18–20.
12. Kazama T, Swanston N, Podoloff DA, Macapinlac HA. Effect of colony-stimulating factor and conventional- or high-dose chemotherapy on FDG uptake in bone marrow. Eur J Nucl Med Mol Imaging. 2005;32:1406–11.
13. Klein JS, Braff S. Imaging evaluation of the solitary pulmonary nodule. Clin Chest Med. 2008;29:15–38.
14. Kwek BH, Aquino SL, Fischman AJ. Fluorodeoxyglucose positron emission tomography and CT after talc pleurodesis. Chest. 2004;125:2356–60.
15. Limet R, Sakalihassan N, Albert A. Determination of the expansion rate and incidence of rupture of abdominal aortic aneurysms. J Vasc Surg. 1991;14:540–8.
16. Lin CY, Lin WY, Lin CC, Shih CM, Jeng LB, Kao CH. The negative impact of fatty liver on maximum standard uptake value of liver on FDG PET. Clin Imaging. 2011;35:437–41.
17. Makis W, Ciarallo A, Hickeson M, Rush C, Derbekyan V, Novales-Diaz JA, et al. Spectrum of gastric malignancy on 18F-FDG PET/CT: a pictorial essay. Clin Imaging. 2012;36:432–46.
18. Matsuda M, Sakamoto H, Okamura T, Nakai Y, Ohashi Y, Kawabe J, et al. Positron emission tomographic imaging of pleomorphic adenoma in the parotid gland. Acta Otolaryngol Suppl. 1998;538:214–20.
19. Mehta A, Blodgett TM. Retroperitoneal fibrosis as a cause of positive FDG PET/CT. J Radiol Case Rep. 2011;5:35–41.
20. Mert M, Kocabay G, Ozülker T, Temizel M, Yanar H, Uygun O, et al. Liver abscess due to Yersinia bacteremia in a well-controlled type I diabetic patient. Endokrynol Pol. 2011;62:357–60.
21. Mostard RL, Prompers L, Weijers RE, van Kroonenburgh MJ, Wijnen PA, Geusens PP, et al. F-18 FDG PET/CT for detecting bone and bone marrow involvement in sarcoidosis patients. Clin Nucl Med. 2012;37:21–5. doi:10.1097/RLU.0b013e3182335f9b.
22. Ozülker T, Ozülker F, Mert M, Ozpaçaci T. Clearance of the high intestinal (18)F-FDG uptake associated with metformin after stopping the drug. Eur J Nucl Med Mol Imaging. 2010;37:1011–7. doi:10.1007/s00259-009-1330-7.
23. Özülker T, Özülker F, Özpaçacı T. Incidental finding of bladder diverticula on F-18 FDG PET/CT and whole body bone scintigraphy. Turk J Nucl Med. 2009;18:55–7.
24. Rudd JH, Myers KS, Bansilal S, Machac J, Pinto CA, Tong C, et al. Atherosclerosis inflammation imaging with 18F-FDG PET: carotid, iliac, and femoral uptake reproducibility, quantification methods, and recommendations. J Nucl Med. 2008;49:871–8. doi:10.2967/jnumed.107.050294.
25. Sakalihasan N, Limet R, Defawe OD. Abdominal aortic aneurysm. Lancet. 2005;365:1577–89.
26. Stubbs E, Kraas J, Morton KA, Clark PB. Brain abnormalities detected on whole-body 18F-FDG PET in cancer patients: spectrum of findings. AJR Am J Roentgenol. 2007;188:866–73.

Part II

PET/CT in Oncology

3 Head and Neck Cancer

3.1 Case 1: Adenoid Cystic Carcinoma of Lacrimal Gland

History A 42-year-old female had undergone surgery for a mass in her left eye causing orbital pain and paresthesia and the pathology turned out to be adenoid cystic carcinoma of lacrimal gland. Patient was lost to follow up during 10 years period and eventually a ^{18}F-FDG PET/CT study was performed.

Findings

Interpretation Widespread metastatic lesions of adenoid cystic carcinoma at both lungs.

Teaching Point Adenoid cystic carcinomas of the lacrimal gland are rare FDG avid malignant tumors. They are indolent tumors, which tend to spread to adjacent structures and occasionally metastasize via hematogenous spread to lungs, brain, and bone.

T. Özülker, F. Özülker, *Atlas of PET-CT Imaging in Oncology: A Case-Based Guide to Image Interpretation*,
DOI 10.1007/978-3-319-18994-9_3

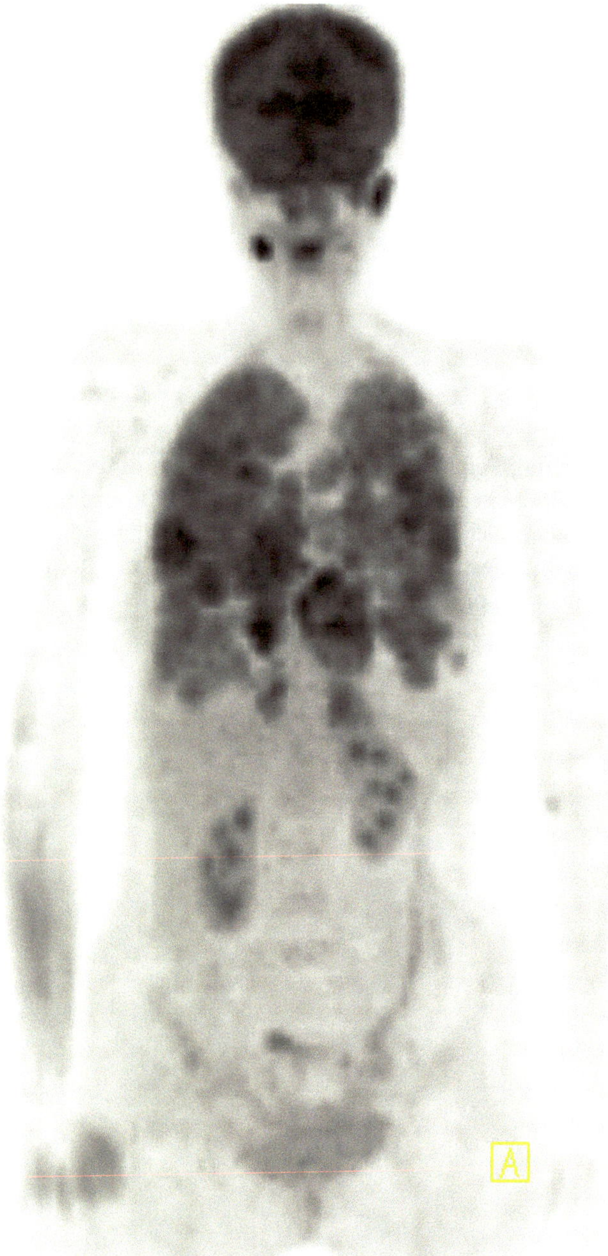

Fig. 3.1 MIP image shows intense and widespread FDG uptake at both lungs

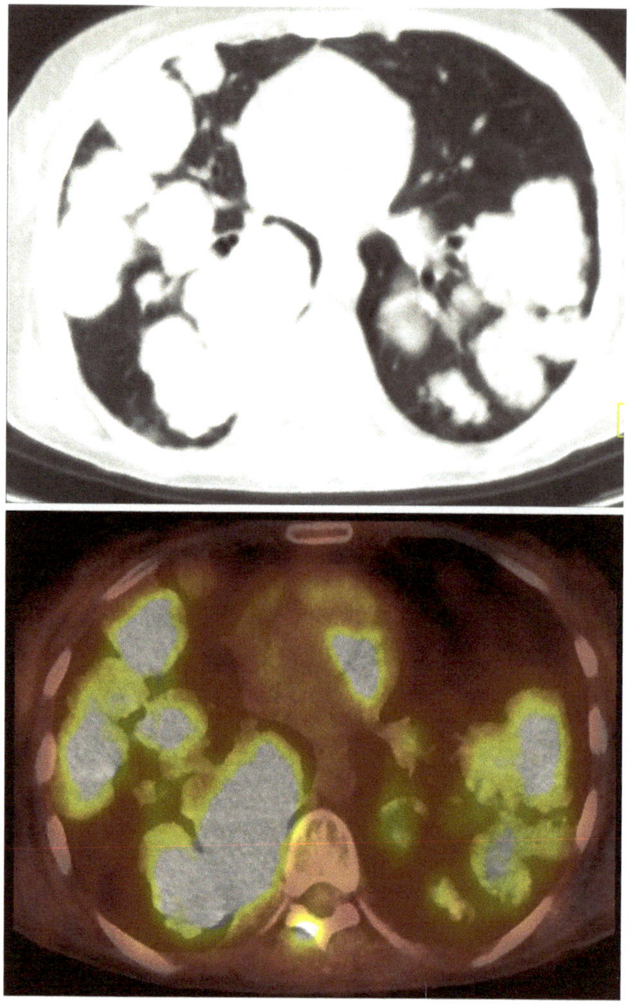

Fig. 3.2 Axial slices of CT and fusion images show mass lesions at both lungs with intense FDG uptake

3.2 Case 2: Basal Cell Adenocarcinoma of the Right Parotid Gland

History A 52-year-old male who was diagnosed with the basal cell adenocarcinoma of the right parotid gland underwent ^{18}F-FDG PET/CT before and after surgical resection of the tumor.

Findings

Interpretation ^{18}F-FDG PET/CT study showed the therapy response at right parotid gland tumor. The pathological uptake at the transverse process of Lomber 2 vertebra is due to simple fracture rather than being a metastasis.

Teaching Point

- Basal Cell Adenocarcinoma of parotid gland is a rare disease entity and it is FDG avid.
- Benign bone fractures should not be misinterpreted as metastasis while evaluating ^{18}F-FDG PET/CT studies.

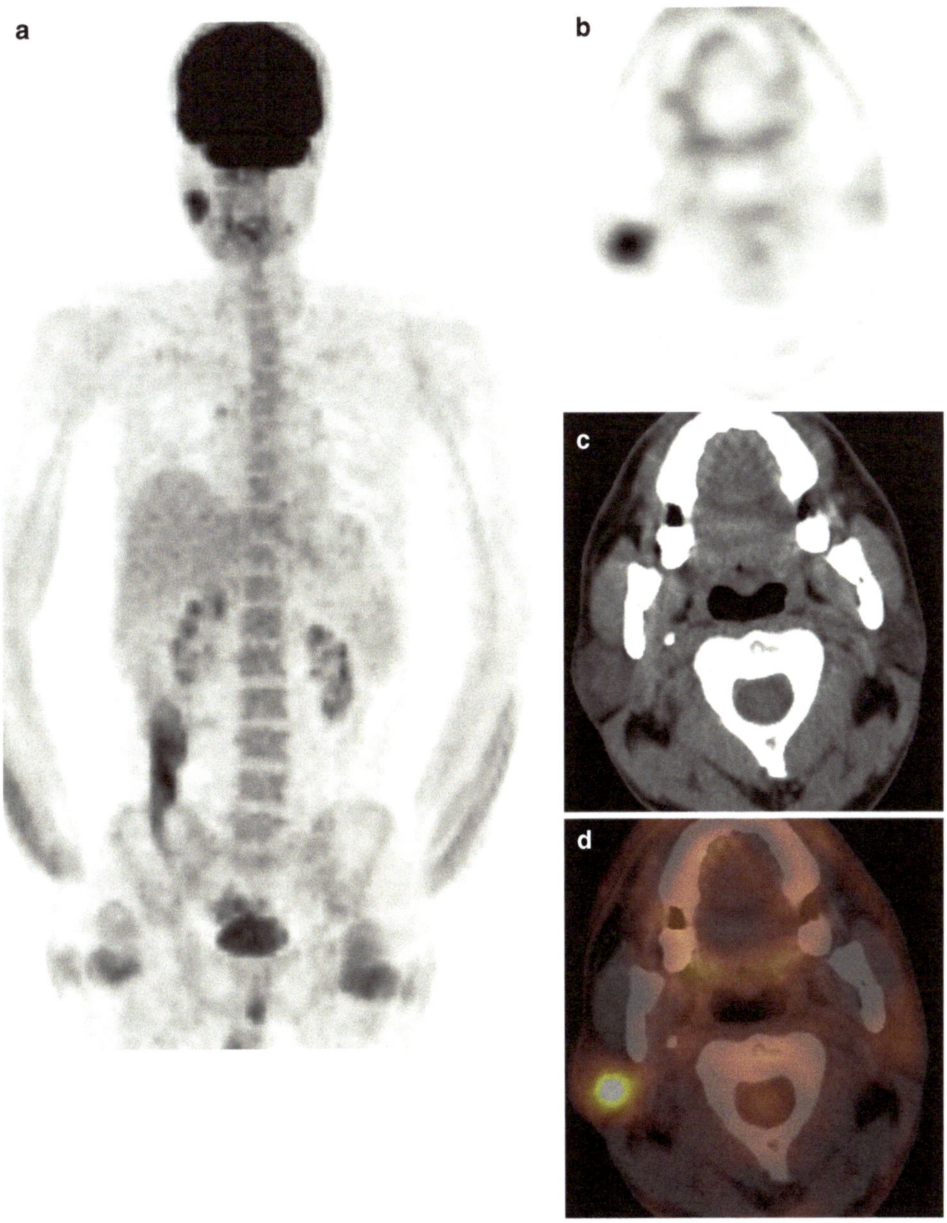

Fig. 3.3 MIP image (**a**), axial PET, CT, and fusion images show focal increased FDG uptake at right parotid gland (**b**–**d**)

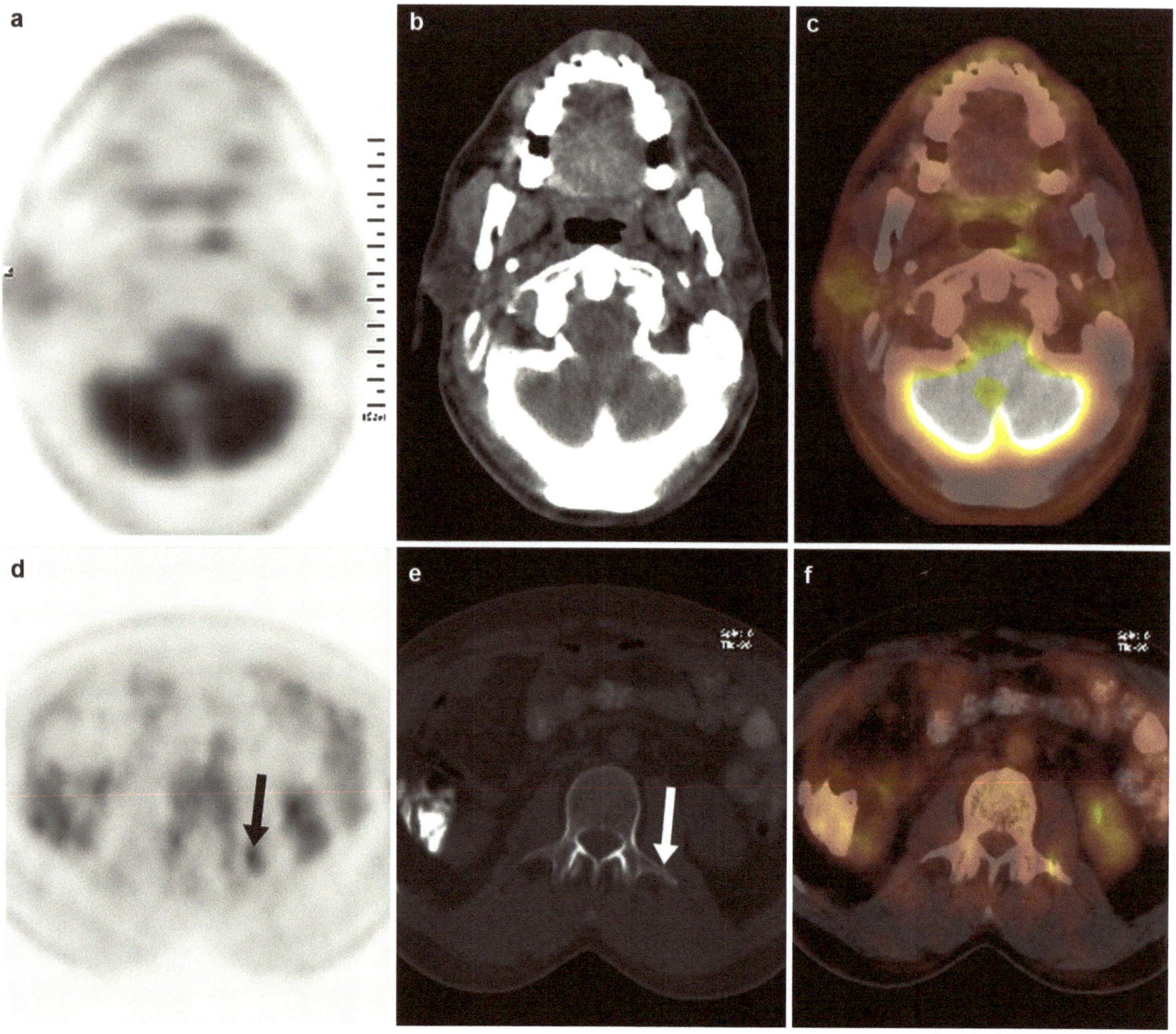

Fig. 3.4 ^{18}F-FDG PET/CT study performed while the patient is status post surgical resection of the lesion at right parotid gland shows the clearance of the pathological activity at right parotid gland (**a–c**), and FDG uptake at the left transverse process of Lomber 2 vertebra (*arrow*) corresponding to a fracture at this site (**d–f**)

3.3 Case 3: Oncocytic Carcinoma of Parotid Gland

History A 45-year-old female was diagnosed as oncocytic carcinoma of the right parotid gland and underwent ^{18}F-FDG PET/CT for staging.

Findings

Interpretation ^{18}F-FDG PET/CT study showed intensely increased FDG uptake at right parotid gland mass confirming the malignant nature of the lesion

Teaching Point Oncocytic carcinoma is an extremely rare malignancy in salivary glands, accounting only for 0.5 % of all epithelial salivary gland malignancies. Oncocytic carcinoma is an FDG avid malignancy but one must bear in mind that benign pathologies of salivary glands like oncocytoma, pleomorphic adenoma, and Warthin tumor are also FDG avid.

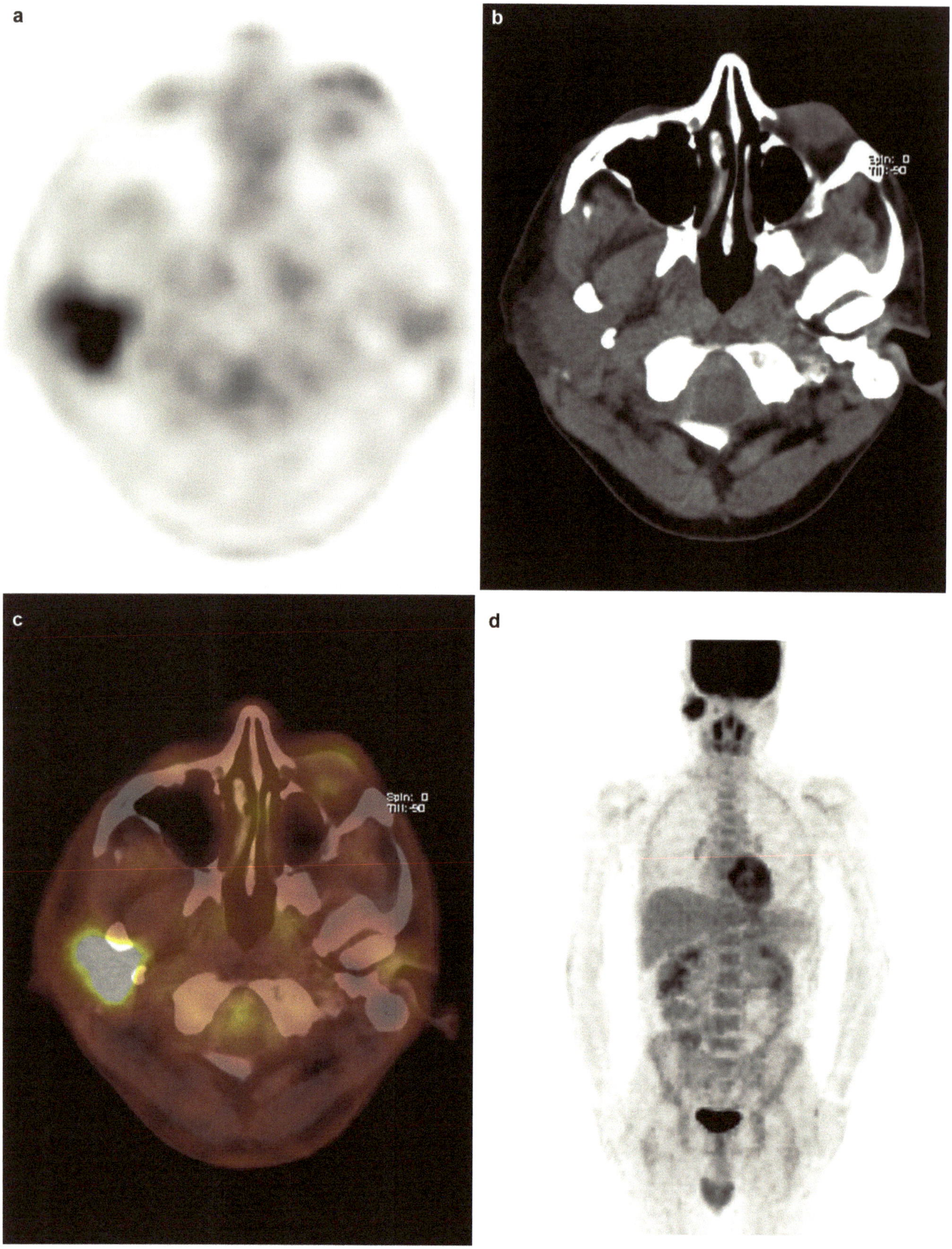

Fig. 3.5 Axial PET, CT, and fusion images (**a–c**) and MIP image (**d**) show intensely increased FDG uptake at right parotid gland

3.4 Case 4: Therapy Response in Nasopharyngeal Carcinoma

History A 34-year-old male with nasopharyngeal carcinoma was evaluated with PET/CT before and after having chemotherapy and radiotherapy.

Findings

Interpretation Intensely hypermetabolic mass lesion at nasopharynx consistent with nasopharyngeal carcinoma and right cervical metastatic lymph nodes. All of the pathological activities are cleared after treatment indicating complete metabolic response to therapy.

Teaching Point ^{18}F-FDG PET/CT can precisely assess response to therapy in nasopharyngeal carcinoma, which gives prognostic information for patients. The SUVmax corresponds well with response of tumor to treatment, with greater decreases in SUVmax correlating well with better survival.

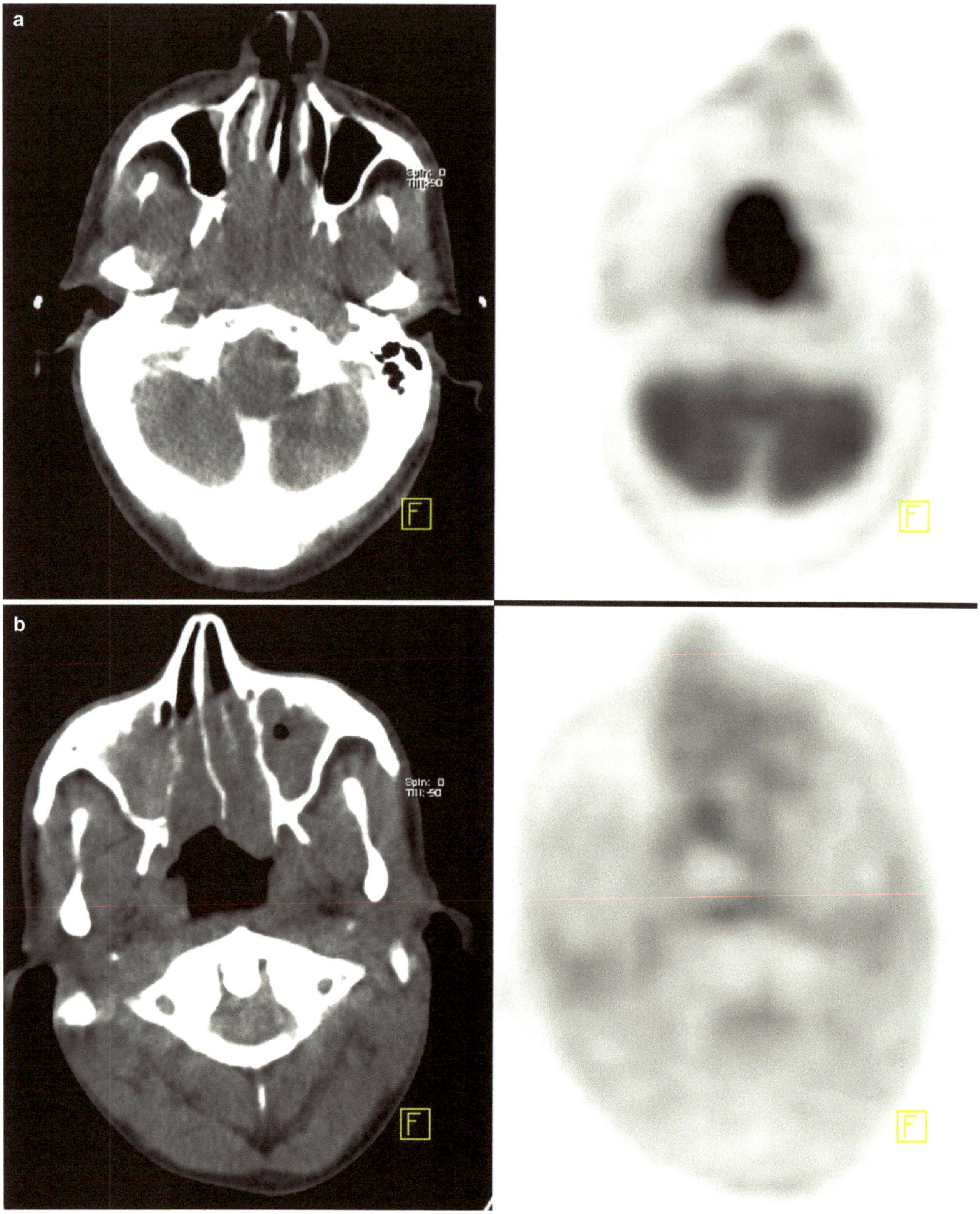

Fig. 3.6 Large mass with high FDG uptake (SUVmax 15) extending from right posterior nasal cavity to right posterolateral wall of nasopharynx (**a**). Axial slice of ^{18}F- FDG PET/CT study performed 10 months after initial staging study shows clearance of the pathological uptake after treatment (**b**)

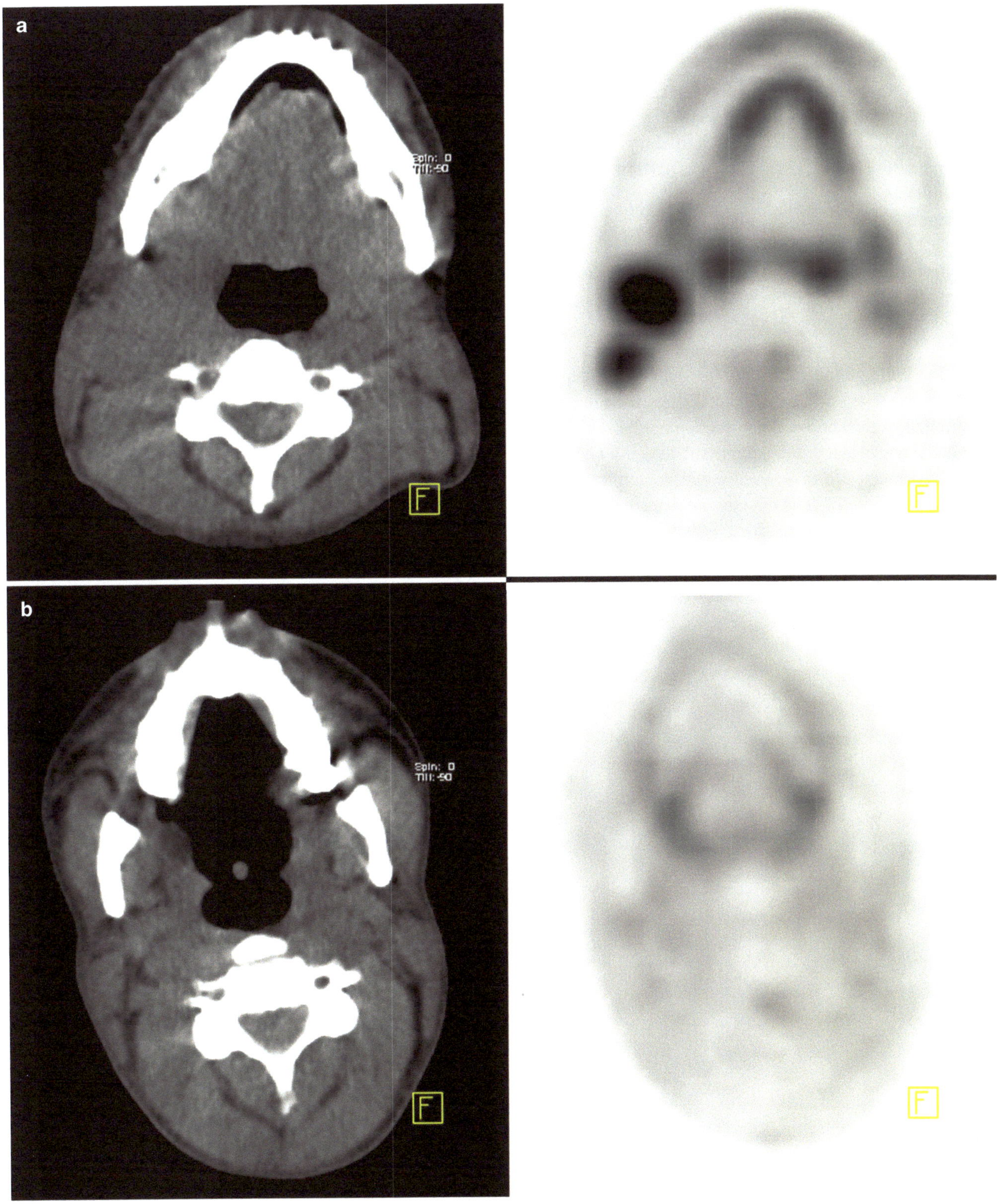

Fig. 3.7 Two intensely hypermetabolic foci (SUVmax 13) at the right level II lymph node station (**a**) Disappearance of the lesions after treatment (**b**)

3.5 Case 5: Detection of Recurrence in Tongue Carcinoma

History A 55-year-old male underwent resection of tongue for tongue carcinoma and after surgery had a flap reconstruction of the tongue. The patient was referred for restaging purpose and a ^{18}F-FDG PET/CT study was performed.

Findings

Interpretation Extensive FDG uptake at the posteromedial border of the flap compatible with recurrence of the primary malignant disease.

Teaching Point Recurrence of tumor may not be detectable clinically especially when the lesion is deep to the flap reconstruction. The thickening along the flap border due to postsurgical changes and granulation tissue may not be possible to be distinguished from recurrence with anatomical imaging methods. FDG PET/CT is effective in detecting the relapse of the tumor in such cases.

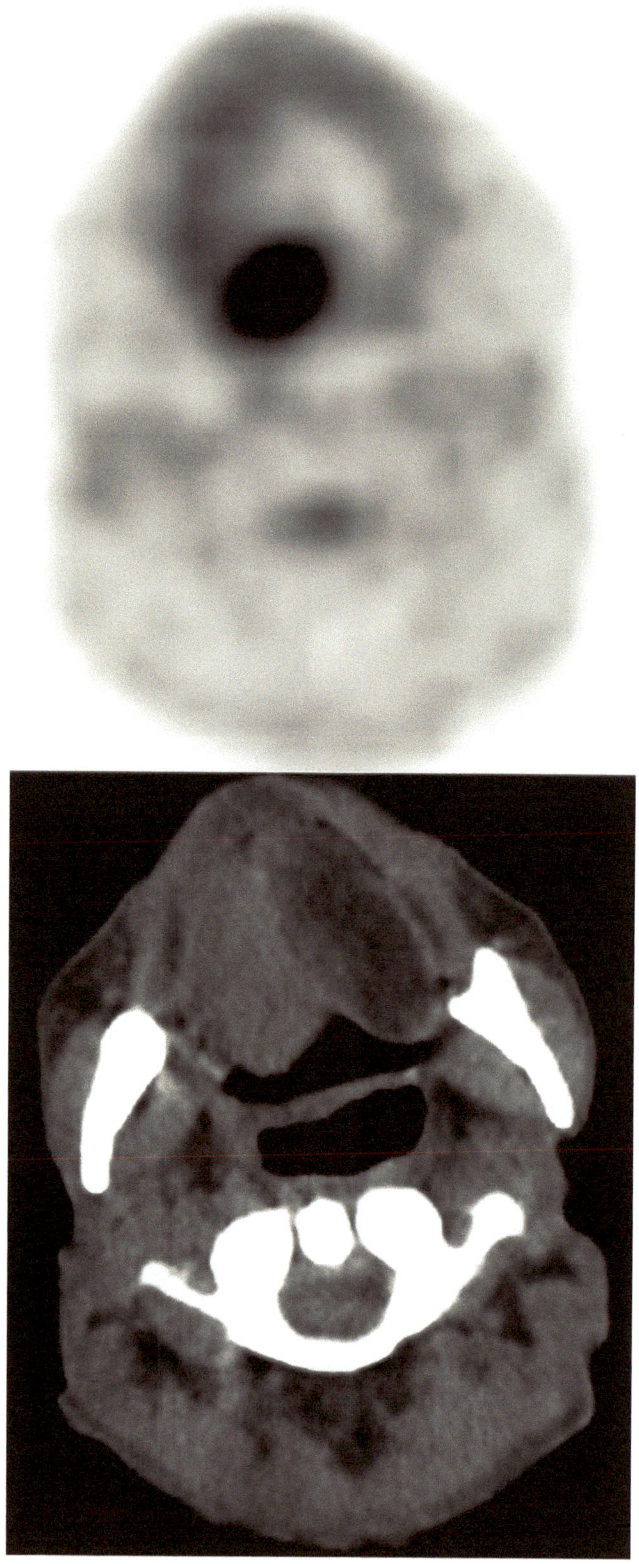

Fig. 3.8 Axial PET and CT images show intense focal FDG uptake at the posteromedial border of the flap

3.6 Case 6: Squamous Cell Carcinoma of the Epiglottis

History A 75-year-old female had the diagnosis of squamous cell carcinoma of the epiglottis after a biopsy and underwent ^{18}F-FDG PET/CT scan for pretreatment staging.

Findings

Interpretation Findings are consistent with primary malignancy at epiglottis without any lymph node involvement and distant metastasis.

Teaching Point Imaging of primary tumors of larynx is best done with CT and MRI. ^{18}F-FDG PET CT has limited applications in the evaluation of primary tumor. ^{18}F-FDG PET CT may establish a baseline from which to follow the patient posttreatment. PET may have a role in detection of metastatic disease and second primary tumors.

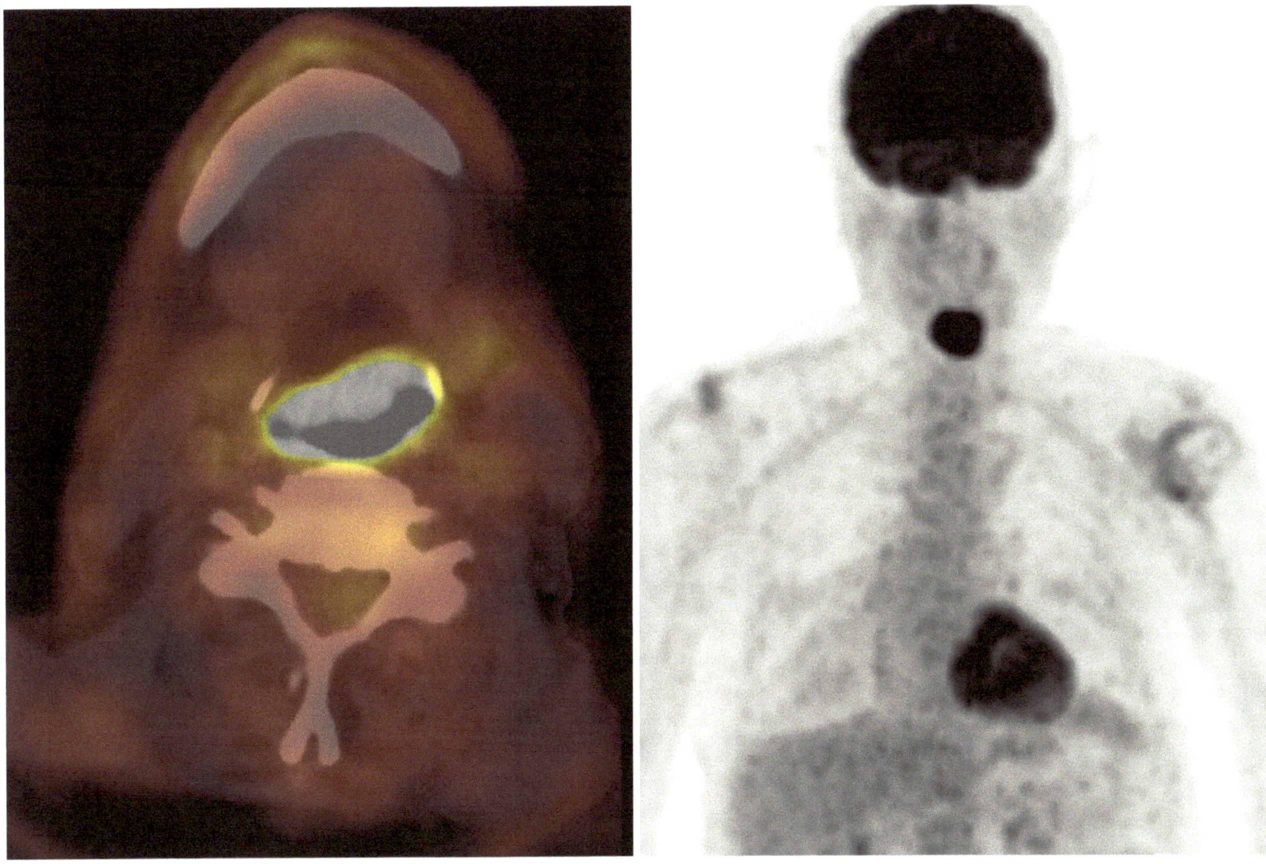

Fig. 3.9 Axial fusion and MIP images show intensely hypermetabolic lesion (SUVmax 12.9) at epiglottis. There is not any detectable cervical lymph node showing pathologically increased FDG uptake

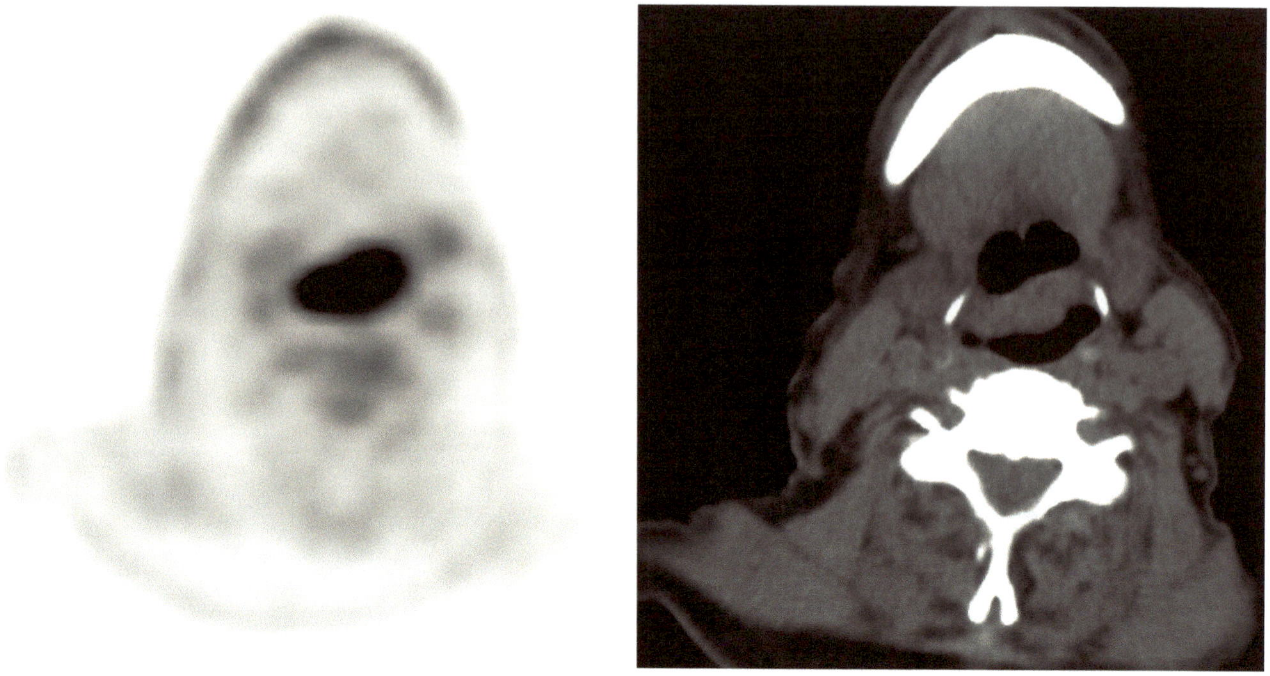

Fig. 3.10 Axial PET and CT images show intensely increased FDG uptake at epiglottis

3.7 Case 7: Staging of Larynx Malignant Mesenchymal Tumor

History A 41-year-old male was admitted to the hospital with the complaints of hoarseness and dyspnea. Excisional biopsy of the mass at larynx revealed malignant mesenchymal tumor. Evaluation with PET/CT for staging is requested.

Findings

Interpretation Primary malignant tumor at larynx showing high FDG uptake and metastatic left cervical lymph node.

Teaching Point

- Malignant mesenchymal tumors of the larynx constitutes 0.3–1 % of all laryngeal cancers and can be demonstrated with FDG PET studies.
- In the clinically N-0 neck, PET does not seem to be superior to conventional imaging, due to high false-negative rate. PET is more helpful in patients with T1 to T3 disease when the evaluation of neck metastases is concerned.
- Increased FDG uptake at tracheostomy site might be due to inflammation or attenuation correction artifact and should be distinguished from disease involvement.

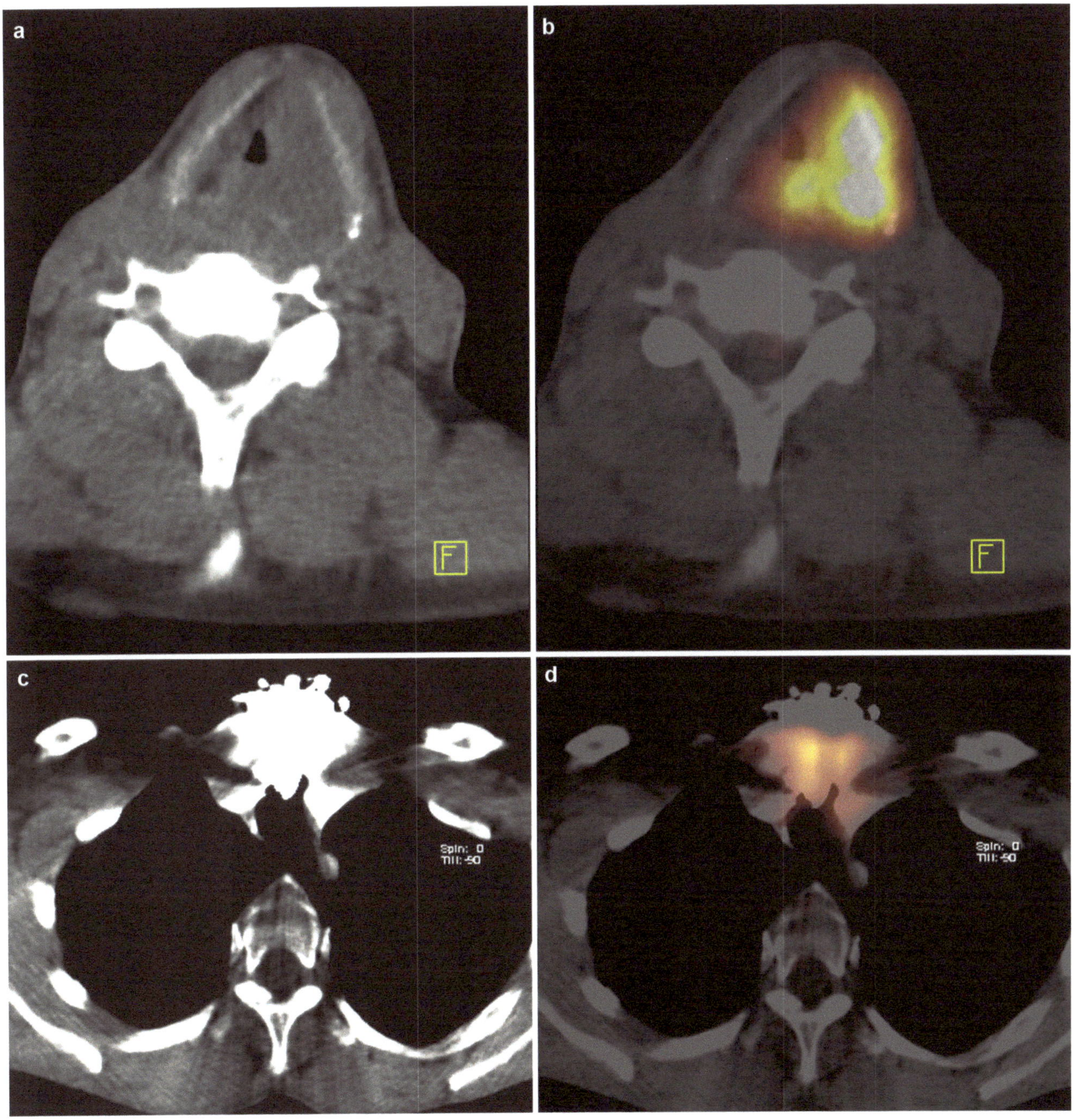

Fig. 3.11 Axial slices of CT and fusion images demonstrate transglottic tumor involving left aryepiglottic fold and showing high FDG uptake (**a**, **b**), mildly increased FDG uptake corresponding to tracheostomy of the patient (**c**, **d**)

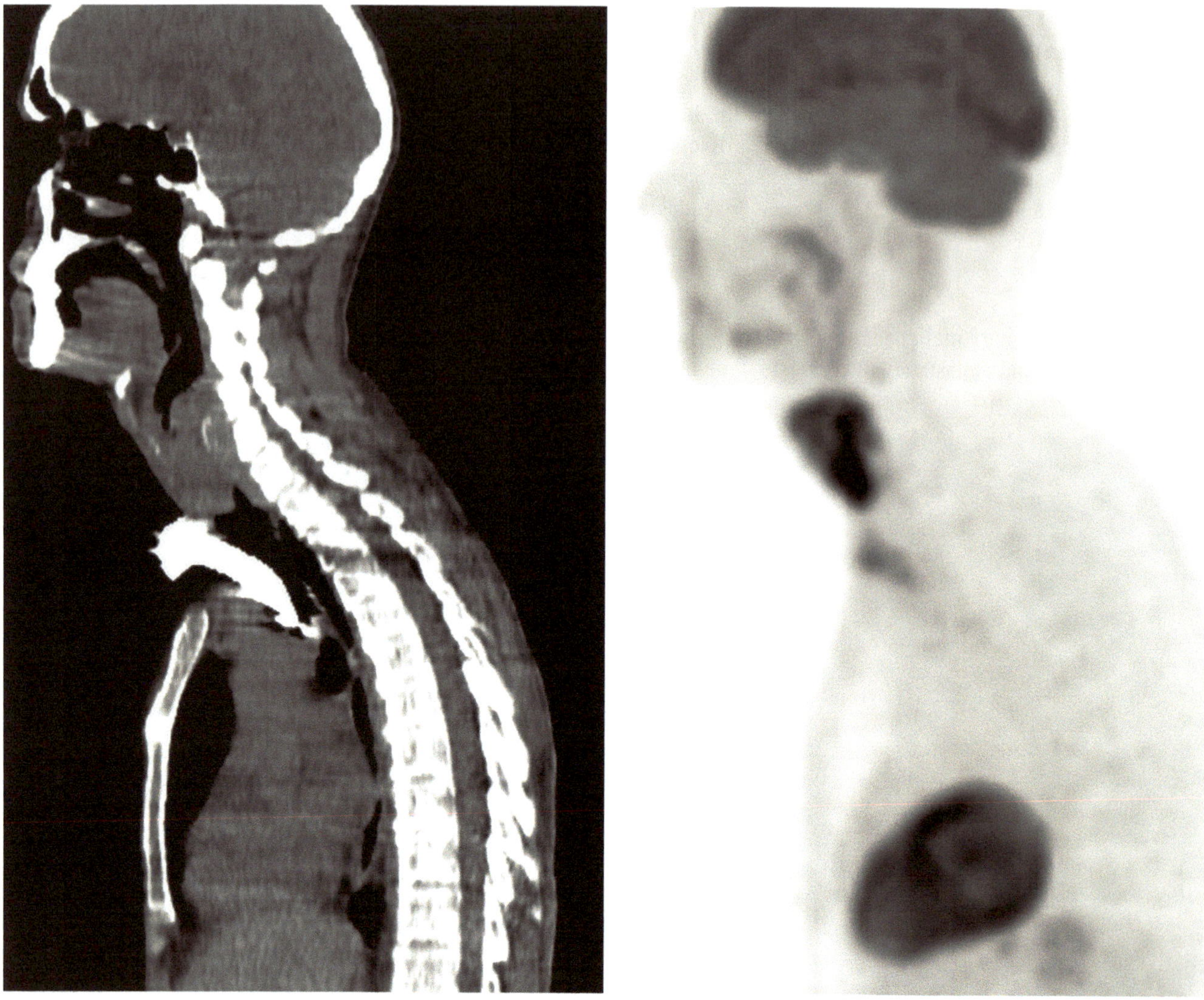

Fig. 3.12 Sagittal CT and PET images

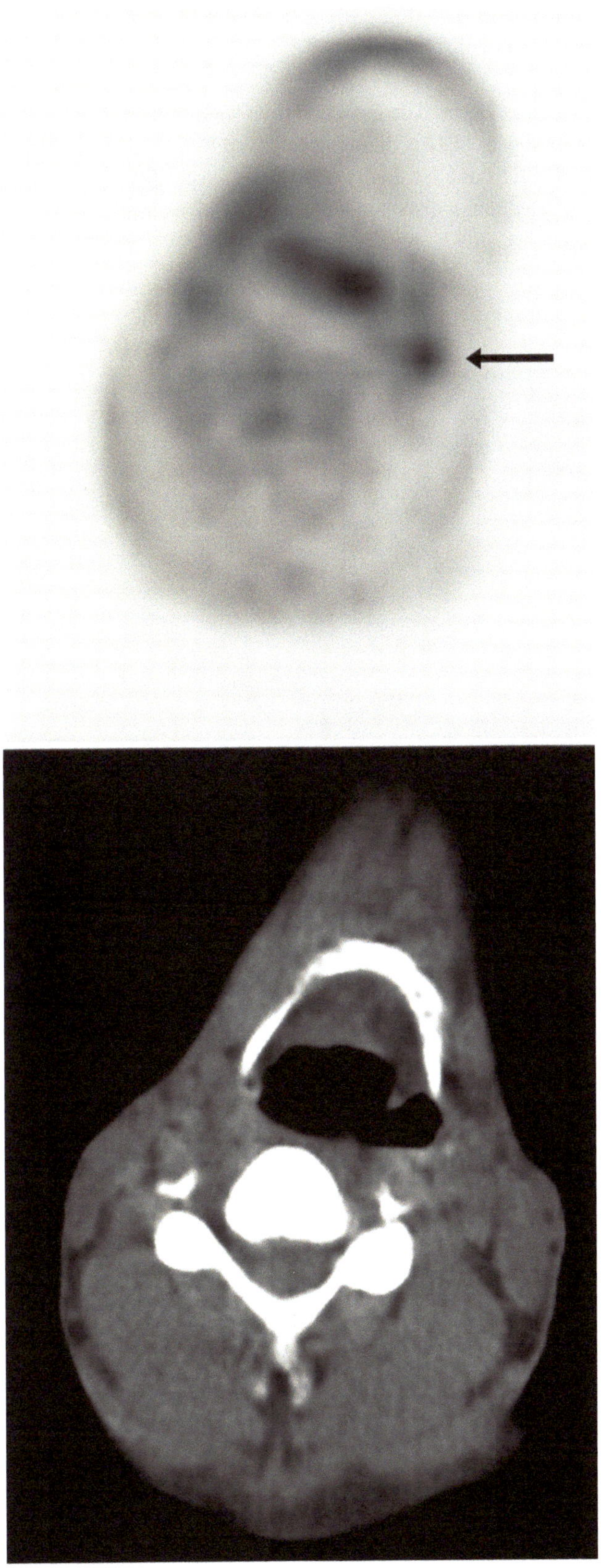

Fig. 3.13 Moderately increased focal FDG uptake at left level III lymph node station

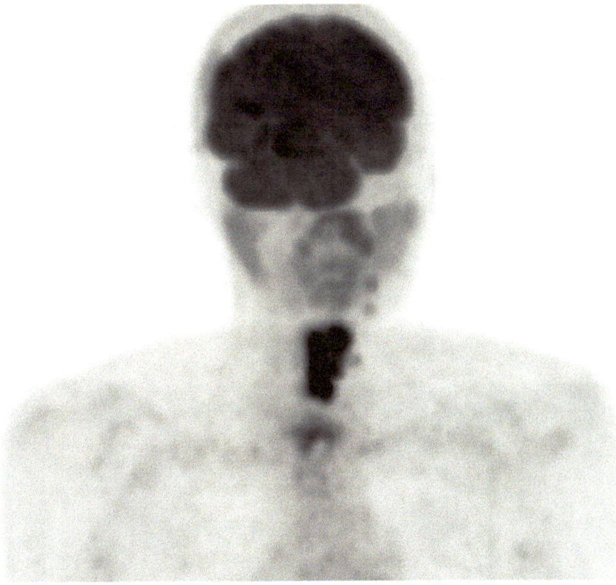

Fig. 3.14 MIP image

3.8 Case 8: Restaging of Larynx Carcinoma

History A 45-year-old male who has been operated for squamous cell carcinoma of the larynx is now being evaluated for the detection of any local or distant metastasis.

Findings

Interpretation Metastatic lesions at right lobe of liver and lower zone of right lung.

Teaching Point The most common site for distant metastases in laryngeal SCC is the lung, followed by bones and the liver. FDG PET has a sensitivity of 90 % and a specificity of 94 % for the detection of distant metastases of head and neck cancer.

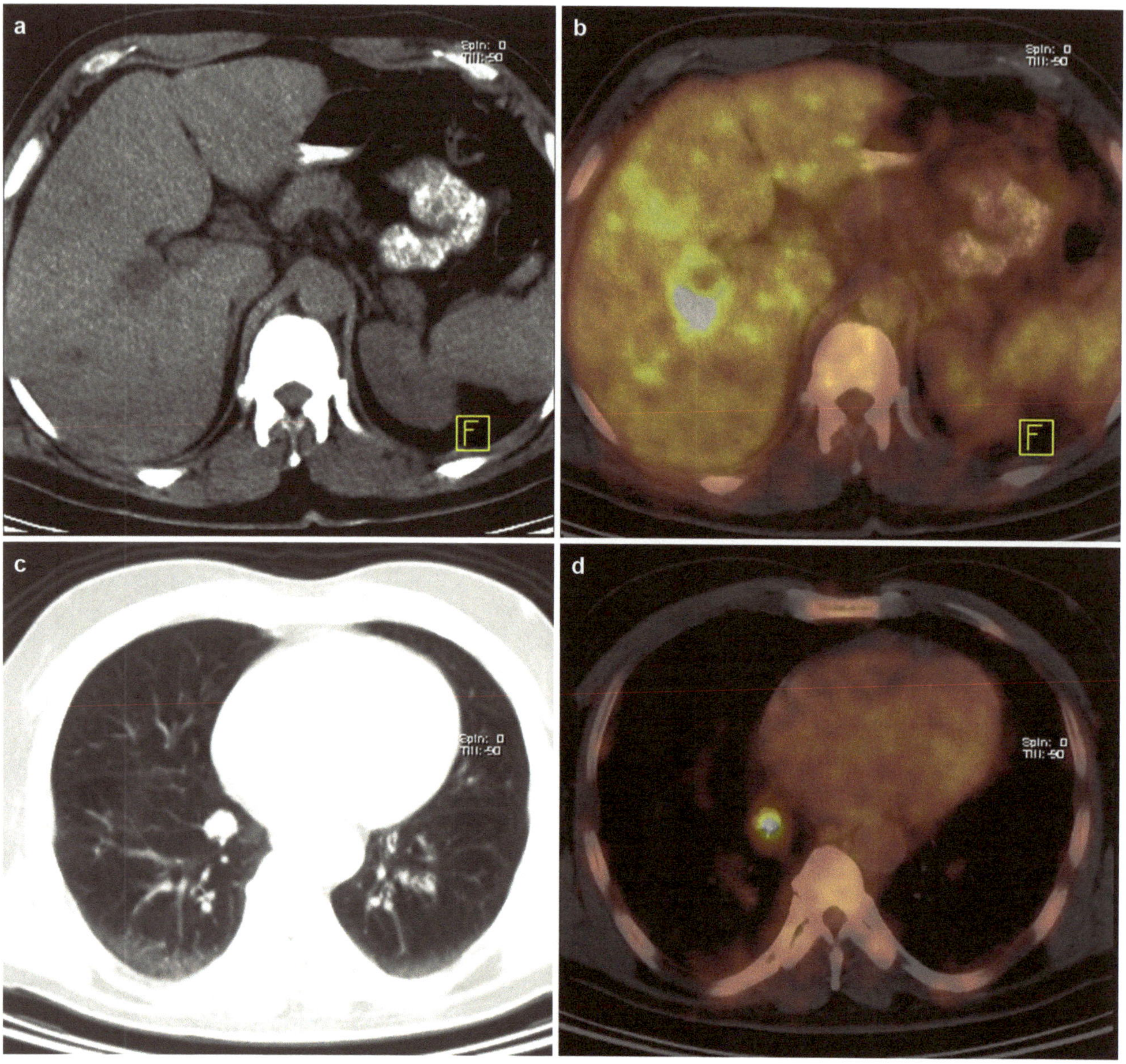

Fig. 3.15 Axial slices of CT and fusion images show hypermetabolic lesion at the right lobe of liver (**a, b**), lung nodule with increased metabolic activity at the medial basal segment of the lower lobe of right lung (**c, d**)

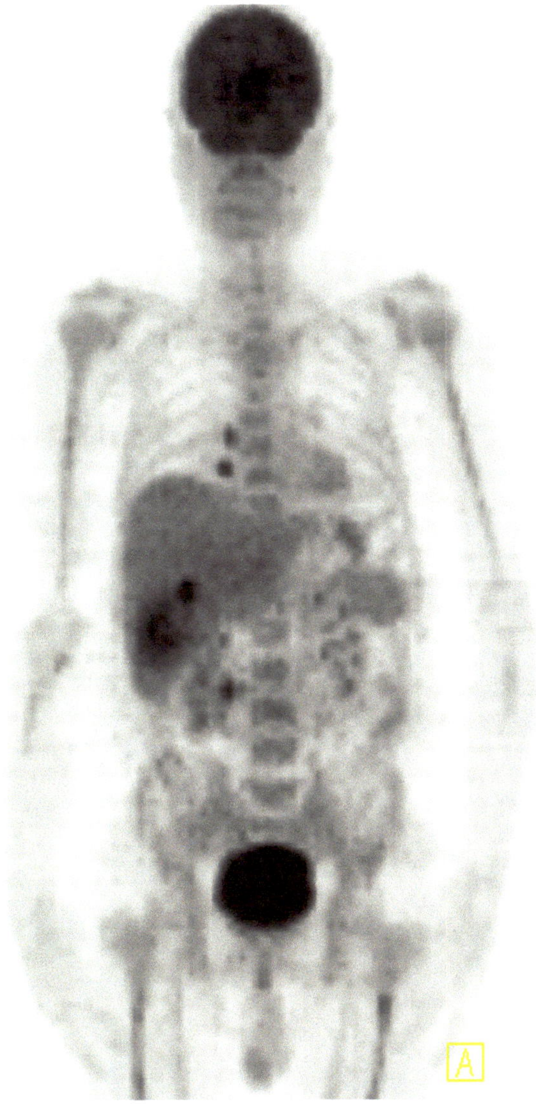

Fig. 3.16 The MIP image showing hypermetabolic lesion at right lobe of liver and two hypermetabolic lesions at lower zone of right lung

3.9 Case 9: Identification of Metastatic Neck Lymph Nodes in Larynx Carcinoma

History A 52-year-old male status post laryngectomy for supraglottic larynx cancer is currently being evaluated for restaging.

Findings

Interpretation Multiple metastatic lymph nodes at bilateral cervical juguler lymphatic chain.

Teaching Point Supraglottic larynx cancers have a propensity for bilateral nodal metastases and PET is more accurate than CT or magnetic resonance imaging (MRI) in nodal staging.

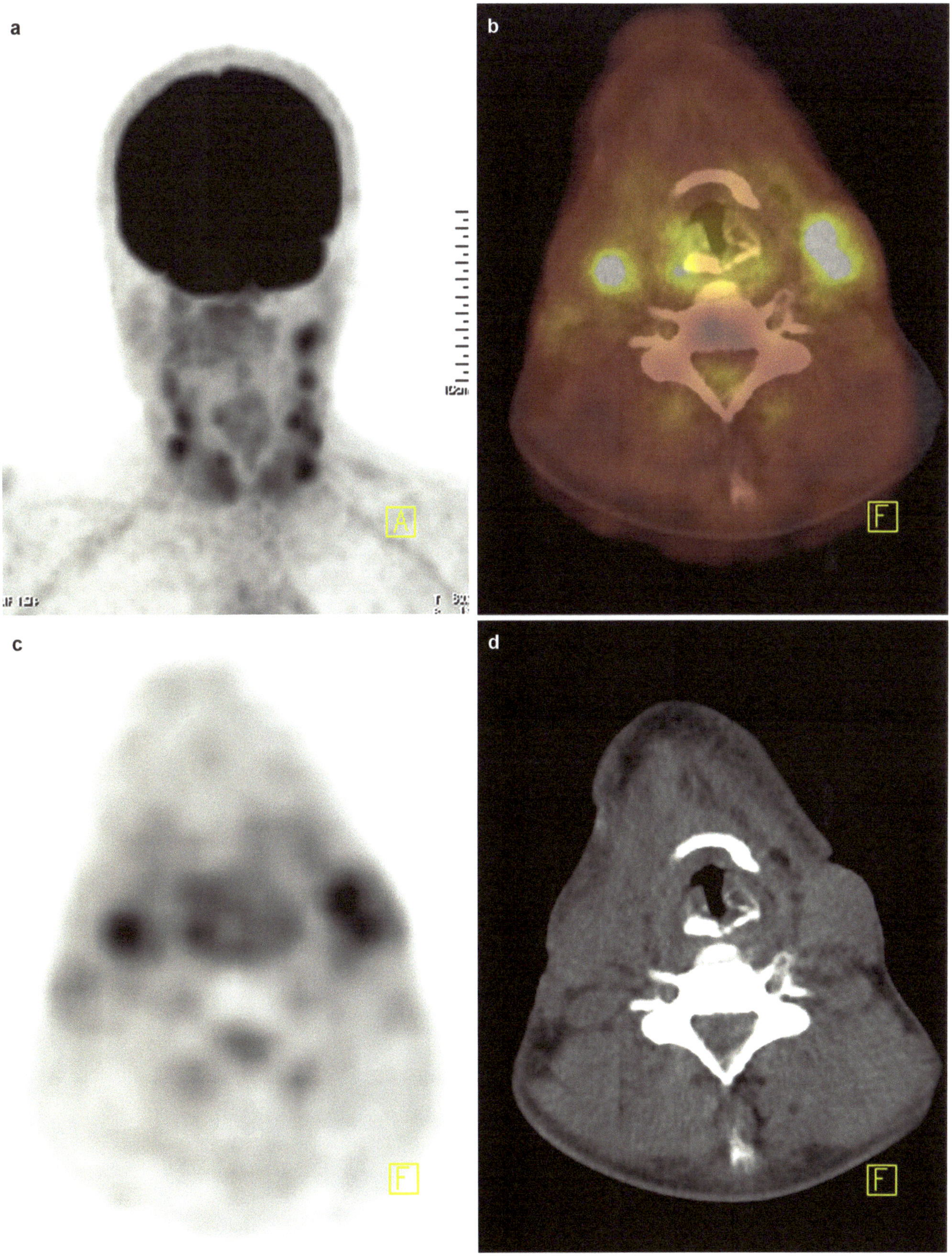

Fig. 3.17 MIP image (**a**), axial fusion, PET, and CT images show multiple foci of increased FDG uptake at bilateral cervical juguler lymphatic chain (**b**–**d**)

3.10 Case 10: Occult Primary Head and Neck Carcinoma

History A 50-year-old male was diagnosed with squamous cell carcinoma of the left neck without identifiable primary lesion. Patient underwent ^{18}F-FDG PET/CT study for the detection of occult primary lesion. Chemoradiotherapy was given to patient and ^{18}F-FDG PET/CT study was repeated 3 months after the completion of the therapy.

Findings

Interpretation Intense FDG uptake at left base of the tongue consistent with the primary malignant lesion and hypermetabolic lesions at left upper cervical juguler area representing lymph nodes with metastatic involvement.

Teaching Point Conventional diagnostic evaluation for an occult primary tumor consists of a meticulous clinical examination including fiberoptic endoscopy of all the mucosa of the superior aerodigestive tract, CT and/or MRI followed by panendoscopy with directed biopsies and tonsillectomy. Metastatic carcinoma in cervical lymph nodes of unknown primary origin accounts for 3–5 % of all head and neck tumors. Identification of occult primary lesion in head and neck tumors vary in the literature from 5 to 73 %, with a mean detection rate of 24.5 %.

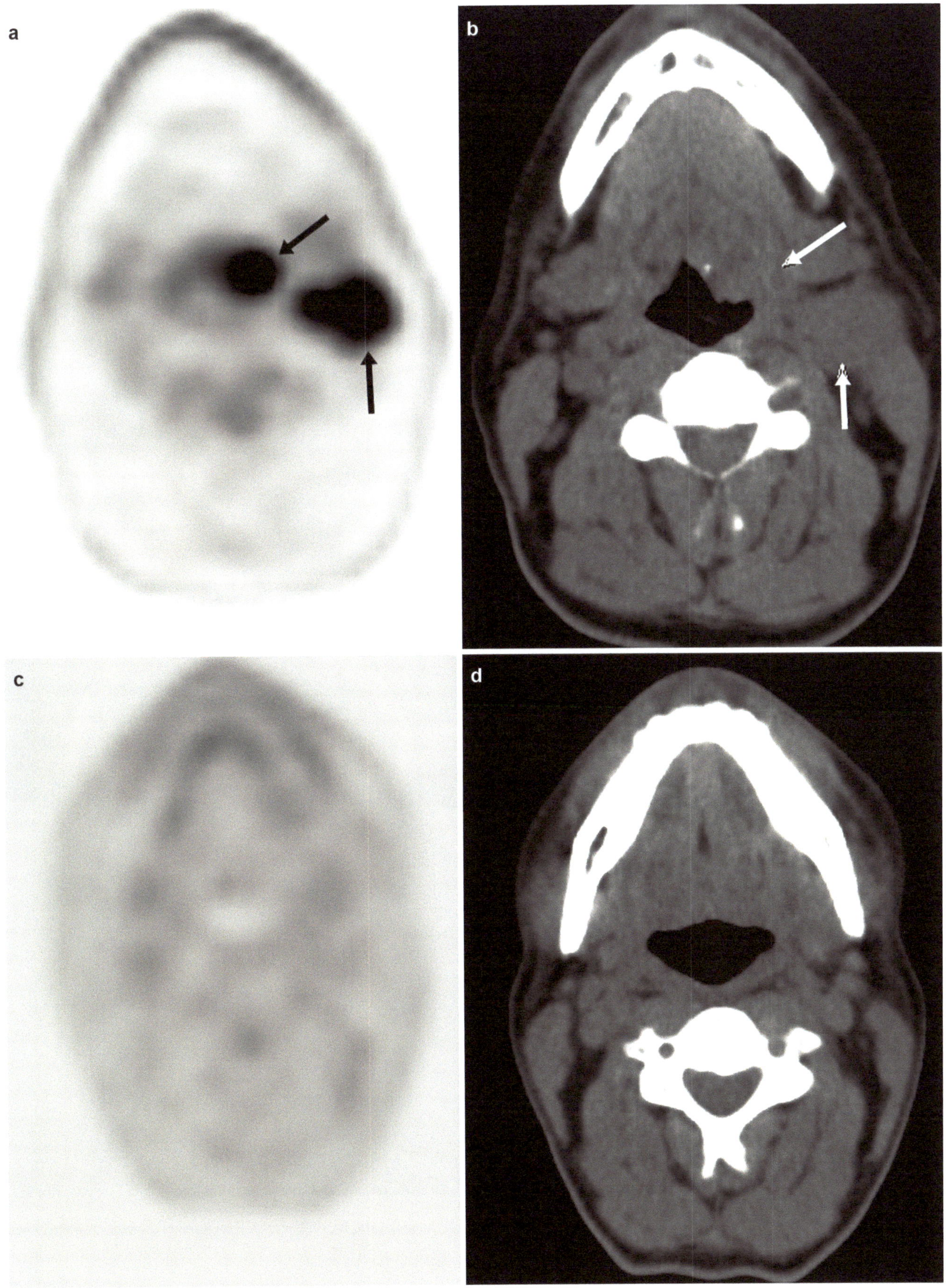

Fig. 3.18 Axial PET and CT images show intense FDG uptake at left upper cervical juguler area (SUVmax 15) and a focal accumulation of activity at the left side base of the tongue (SUVmax 16) (**a**, **b**), clearance of the pathological activities after therapy (**c**, **d**) (*arrows*)

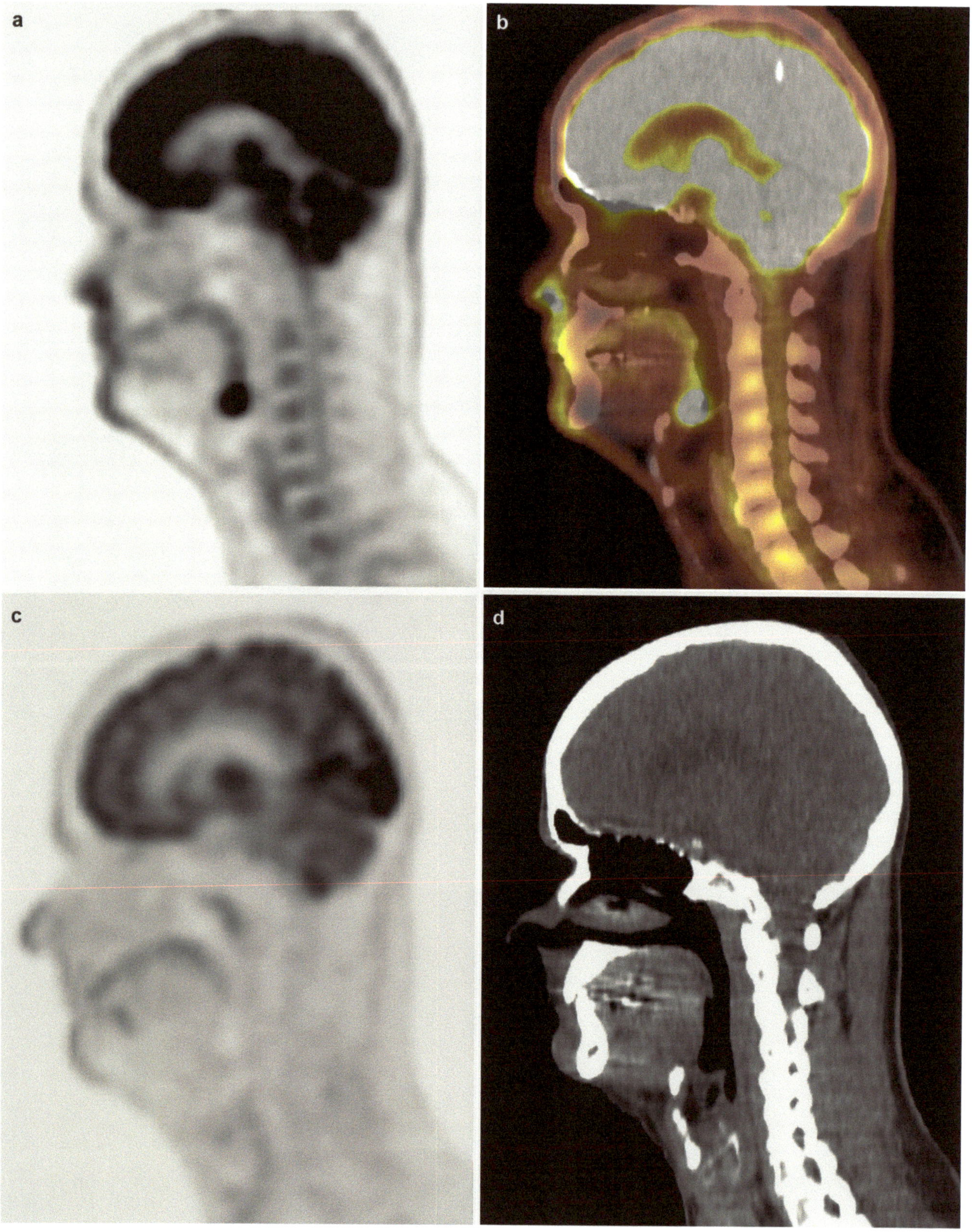

Fig. 3.19 Sagittal PET and fusion images show intense FDG uptake at base of the tongue (**a**, **b**), PET, and CT images after therapy show clearance of the pathological activity (**c**, **d**)

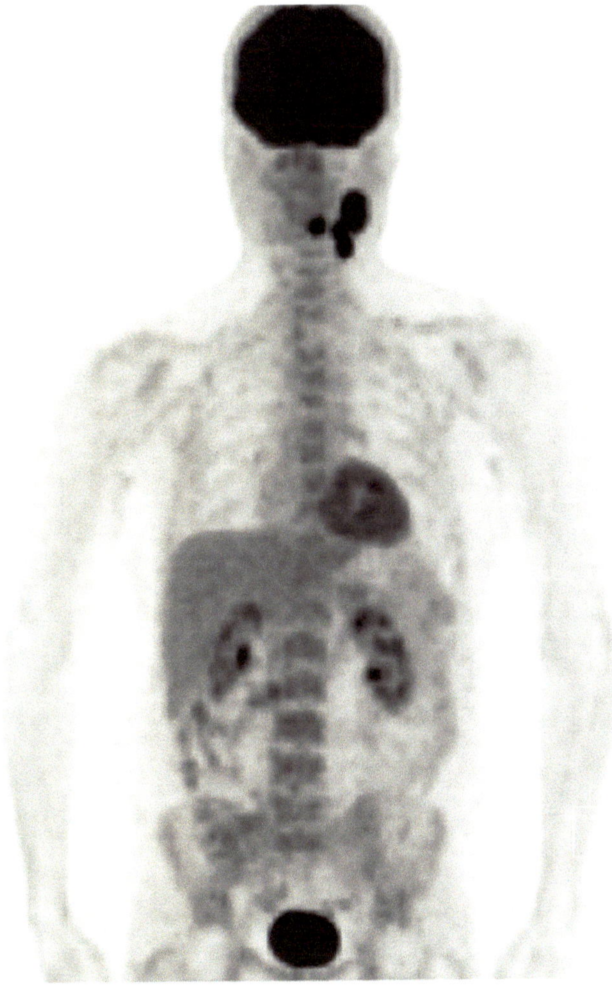

Fig. 3.20 MIP image before therapy

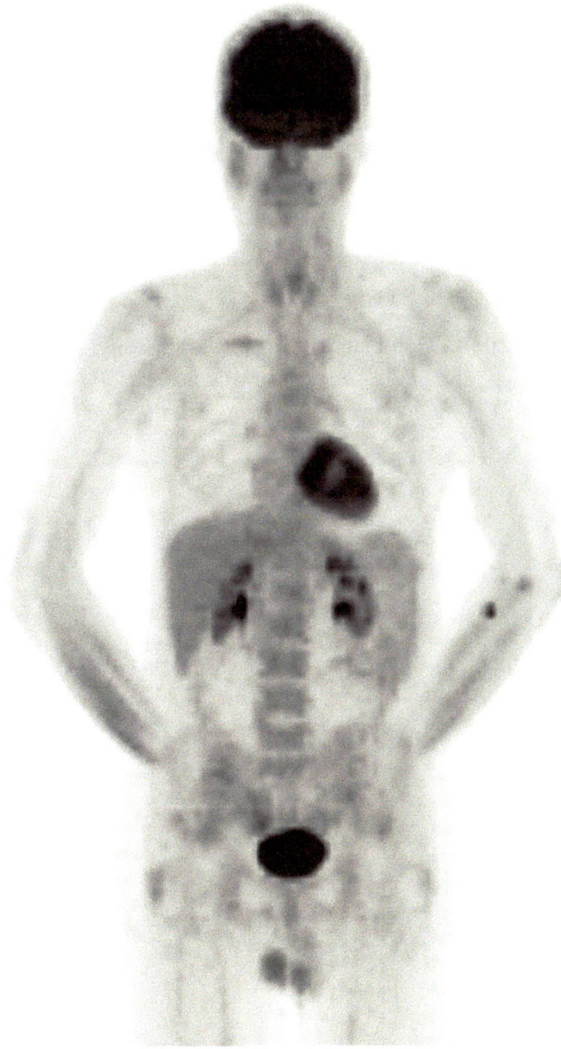

Fig. 3.21 MIP image after therapy

3.11 Case 11: Squamous Cell Carcinoma of Lip and Second Primary Lung Cancer

History A 64-year-old male diagnosed with squamous cell carcinoma of the lower lip underwent ^{18}F-FDG PET/CT for staging.

Findings

Interpretation Malignant hypermetabolic lesion at lower lip and hypermetabolic mass lesion at lower lobe of right lung representing either metastasis or second primary tumor of lung.

Result Histopathological examination of the lesion at right lung revealed nonsmall cell carcinoma of lung.

Teaching Point Incidence of coincidental second primary tumors of the aerodigestive tract in patients with head and neck tumors is between 6 and 36 %.

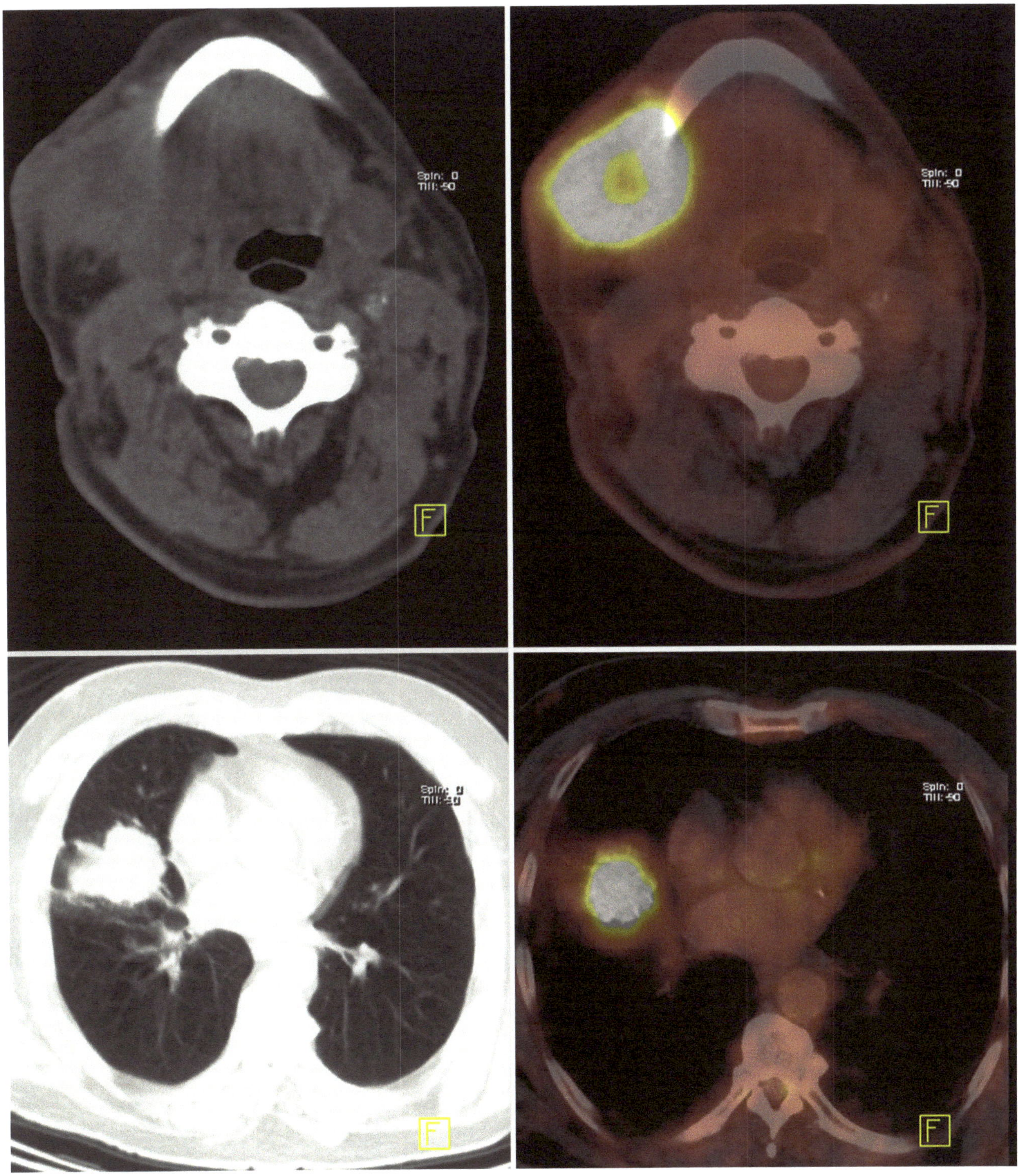

Fig. 3.22 Axial CT and fusion images show increased FDG uptake with a hypometabolic necrotic center at the malignant lesion located at lower lip (*upper row*) and mass lesion at lower lobe of right lung showing intense FDG uptake (*lower row*)

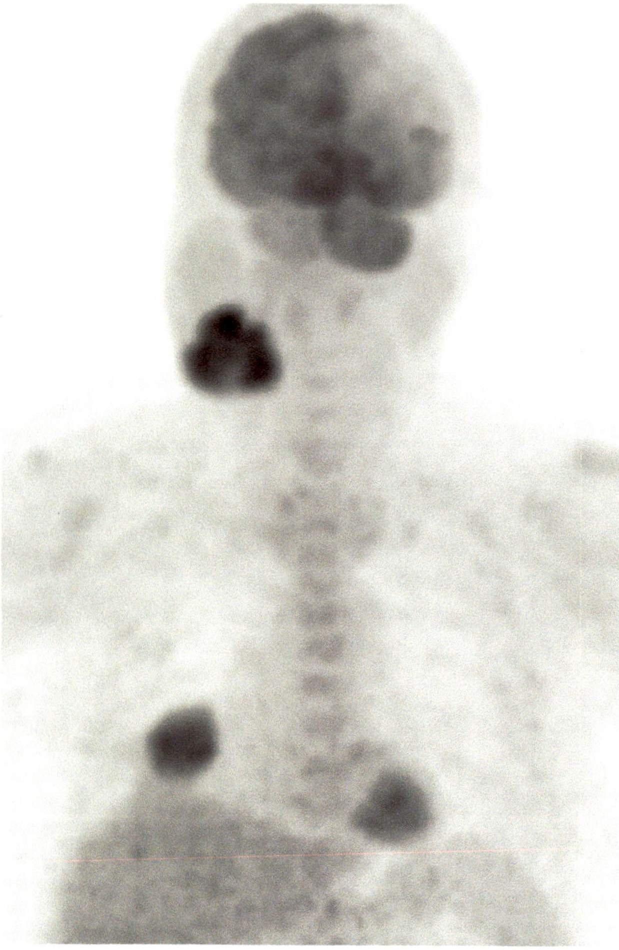

Fig. 3.23 MIP image

Bibliography

1. Berge JK, Kapadia SB, Myers EN. Osteosarcoma of the larynx. Arch Otolaryngol Head Neck Surg. 1998;124:207–10.
2. Dammann F, Horger M, Mueller-Berg M, Schlemmer H, Claussen CD, Hoffman J, et al. Rational diagnosis of squamous cell carcinoma of the head and neck region: comparative evaluation of CT, MRI, and 18F-FDG PET. AJR Am J Roentgenol. 2005;184: 1326–31.
3. Ellis GL, Auclair PL, Gnepp DR, Goode RK. Other malignant epithelial neoplasms. In: Surgical pathology of the salivary glands. Philadelphia: Saunders; 1991. p. 455–88.
4. Hagino K, Tsunoda A, Ishihara A, Kishimoto S, Suzuki T, Hara A. Oncocytoma in the parotid gland presenting a remarkable increase in fluorodeoxyglucose uptake on positron emission tomography. Otolaryngol Head Neck Surg. 2006;134:708–9.
5. Ilknur AK, Stokkel MP, Pauwels EK. Positron emission tomography with 2-[18F] fluoro-2-deoxy-D-glucose in oncology: Part II: the clinical value in detecting and staging primary tumours. J Cancer Res Clin Oncol. 2000;126:560–74.
6. Joshi VM, Wadhwa V, Mukherji SK. Imaging in laryngeal cancers. Indian J Radiol Imaging. 2012;22:209–26.
7. Kapoor V, Fukui MB, McCook BM. Role of 18F FDG PET/CT in the treatment of head and neck cancers: principles, technique, normal distribution, and initial staging. AJR Am J Roentgenol. 2005;184:579–87.
8. Khan AJ, DiGiovanna MP, Ross DA, Sasaki CT, Carter D, Son YH. Adenoid cystic carcinoma: a retrospective clinical review. Int J Cancer. 2001;96:149–58.
9. Lin Q, Yang R, Sun L, Chen S, Wu H. Biological response of nasopharyngeal carcinoma to radiation therapy: a pilot study using serial 18F-FDG PET/CT scans. Cancer Invest. 2012;30:528–36.
10. Mahoney EJ, Spiegel JH. Evaluation and management of malignant cervical lymphadenopathy with an unknown primary tumor. Otolaryngol Clin N Am. 2005;38:87–97.
11. McGuirt WF, Greven K, Williams D, Keyes Jr JW, Watson N, Cappellari JO, et al. PET scanning in head and neck oncology. Head Neck. 1998;20:208–15.
12. Miller FR, Hussey D, Beeram M, Eng T, McGuff HS, Otto RA. Positron emission tomography in the management of unknown primary head and neck carcinoma. Arch Otolaryngol Head Neck Surg. 2005;131:626–9.
13. Mohandas A, Marcus C, Kang H, Truong MT, Subramaniam RM. FDG PET/CT in the management of nasopharyngeal carcinoma. Am J Roentgenol. 2014;203:146–57.
14. Pereira G, Silva JC, Monteiro E. Positron emission tomography in the detection of occult primary head and neck carcinoma: a retrospective study. Head Neck Oncol. 2012;18;4:34.
15. Rusthoven KE, Koshy M, Paulino AC. The role of fluorodeoxyglucose positron emission tomography in cervical lymph node metastases from an unknown primary tumor. Cancer. 2004;101: 2641–9.
16. Shah VN, Branstetter BF. Oncocytoma of the parotid gland: a potential false-positive finding on 18F-FDG PET. AJR Am J Roentgenol. 2007;189:212–4.
17. Spiro RH, Huvos AG. Stage means more than grade in adenoidcystic carcinoma. Am J Surg. 1992;164:623–8.
18. Wilson TC, Robinson RA. Basal cell adenocarcinoma and basal cell adenoma of the salivary glands: a clinicopathological review of seventy tumors with comparison of morphologic features and growth control indices. Head Neck Pathol. 21 Aug 2014 (Epub ahead of print).
19. Xie P, Yue JB, Fu Z, Feng R, Yu JM. Prognostic value of 18F-FDG PET/CT before and after radiotherapy for locally advanced nasopharyngeal carcinoma. Ann Oncol. 2010;21:1078–82.
20. Yen RF, Chen TH, Ting LL, Tzen KY, Pan MH, Hong RL. Early restaging whole-body (18)F-FDG PET during induction chemotherapy predicts clinical outcome in patients with locoregionally advanced nasopharyngeal carcinoma. Eur J Nucl Med Mol Imaging. 2005;32:1152–9.

4 Thyroid Cancer

4.1 Case 1: Thyroid Incidentaloma Identified by ^{18}F-FDG PET/CT

History A 42-year-old man had the surveillance FDG PET/CT scan because of history of a malignant melanoma.

Findings

Interpretation Hypermetabolism at the right thyroid lobe is suspicious for malignancy.

Outcome FNA of the hypermetabolic nodule at right thyroid lobe revealed papillary thyroid carcinoma.

Teaching Point The prevalence of focal thyroid lesions on FDG PET/CT is 1.2–4.0 %. Of the thyroid incidentalomas that underwent FNA and surgery, 14–47 % were found to be malignant.

T. Özülker, F. Özülker, *Atlas of PET-CT Imaging in Oncology: A Case-Based Guide to Image Interpretation*,
DOI 10.1007/978-3-319-18994-9_4

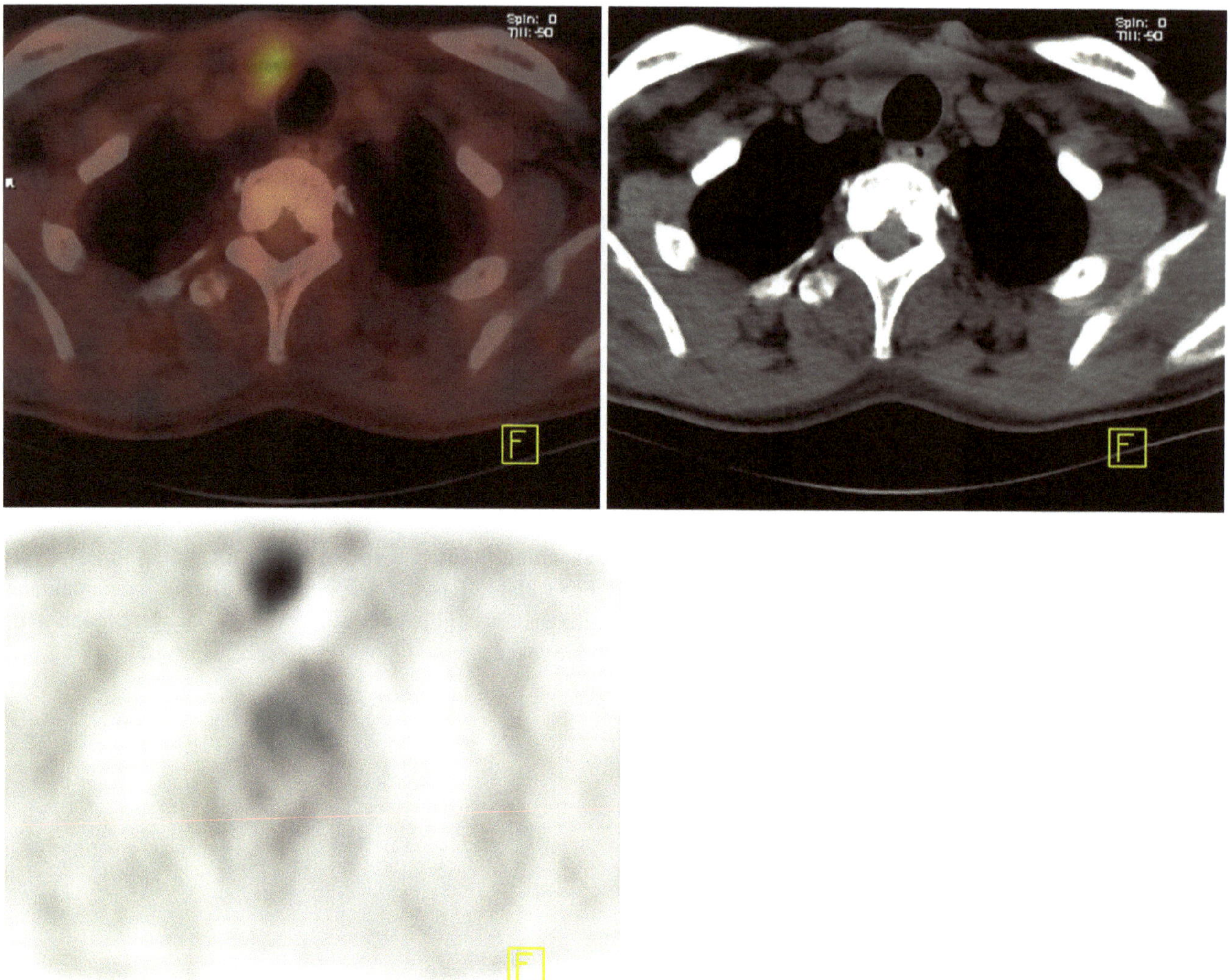

Fig. 4.1 Hypermetabolic thyroid nodule at right lobe of thyroid gland with an SUVmax 7

4.2 Case 2: ^{18}F-FDG PET CT Performed for Evaluation of Thyroid Nodule

History A 38-year-old female was found to have a rapidly growing single nodule on USG measuring 1.5 × 1.9 × 1.3 cm and having microcalcifications in it. The nodule was hypoactive on thyroid scintigraphy and the thyroid function tests of the patient was normal. After an indeterminate fine needle aspiration biopsy, the patient underwent ^{18}F-FDG PET CT scan for determination of the malignant nature of the nodule.

Findings

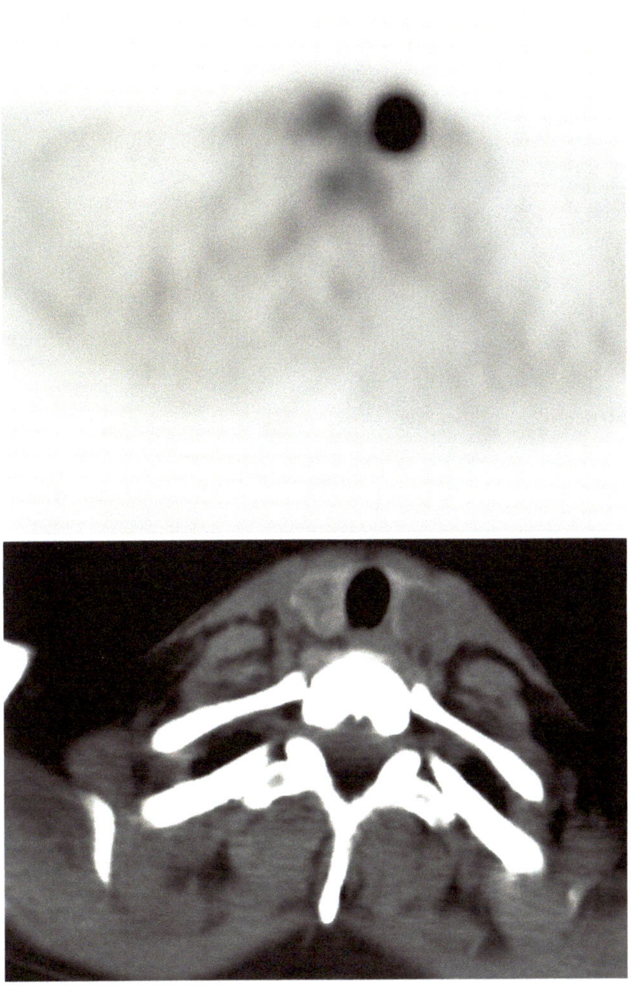

Fig. 4.2 Axial PET and CT images show intensely hypermetabolic thyroid nodule at left lobe of thyroid gland (SUVmax 33)

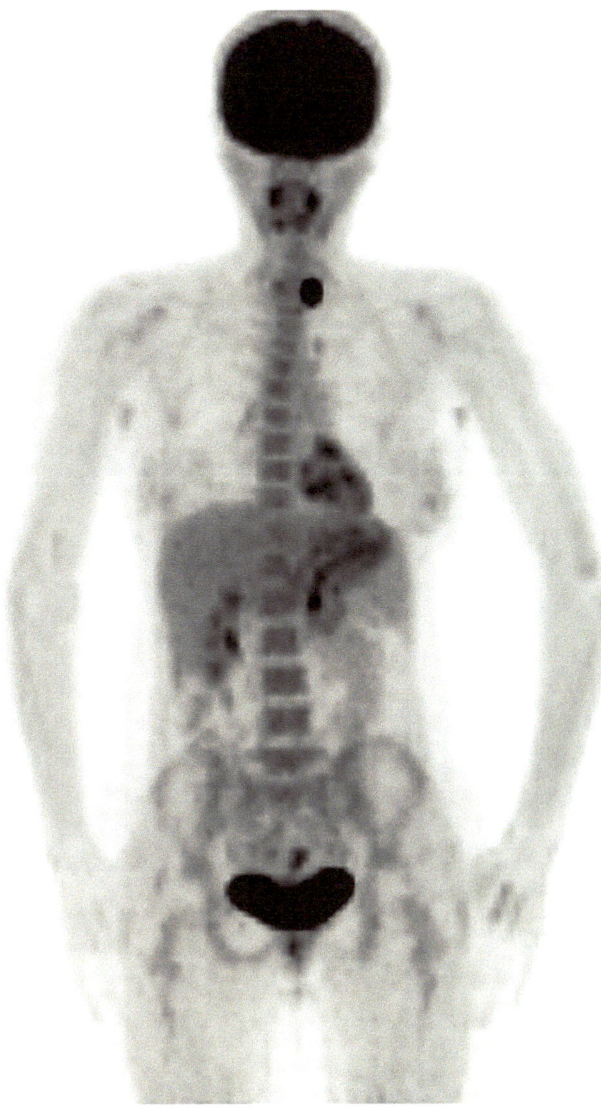

Fig. 4.3 MIP image

Interpretation The nodule showing high FDG uptake at the left thyroid lobe is suspicious for malignancy.

Result The patient underwent left lobectomy and isthmectomy and histopathology turned out to be papillary thyroid cancer.

Teaching Point ^{18}F-FDG PET CT showed a high sensitivity in detecting malignancy in patients with indeterminate FNAB results. In a meta-analysis, ^{18}F-FDG PET or PET/CT correctly detected malignant lesions, with a very high pooled sensitivity of 89.0 %. The malignant nodules with a dimension >1–1.5 cm rarely become negative on FDG PET.

4.3 Case 3: Staging of Insular Thyroid Carcinoma

History A 88-year-old female who was diagnosed with poorly differentiated thyroid carcinoma underwent ^{18}F-FDG PET/CT study.

Findings

Interpretation FDG avid primary malignancy at thyroid gland and multiple metastases at lung parenchyme and bony structures

Teaching Point

- Well differentiated thyroid carcinoma shows poor FDG uptake and high I-131 uptake, whereas more malignant types (PDTC) appear to retain FDG more avidly while their I-131 uptake is low. This flip-flop phenomenon is attributed to the characterization of progressive dedifferentiation of thyroid tumors by upregulation of glucose transporters (GLUT1) and reduction of expression of sodium-iodide symporter (NIS).
- ^{18}F-FDG PET/CT is currently used for initial staging and follow-up of high-risk patients with poorly differentiated thyroid cancers. It is also used as a prognostic tool in patients with metastases, for the evaluation of posttreatment response, and as selection tool in patients not eligible to radioiodine therapy.

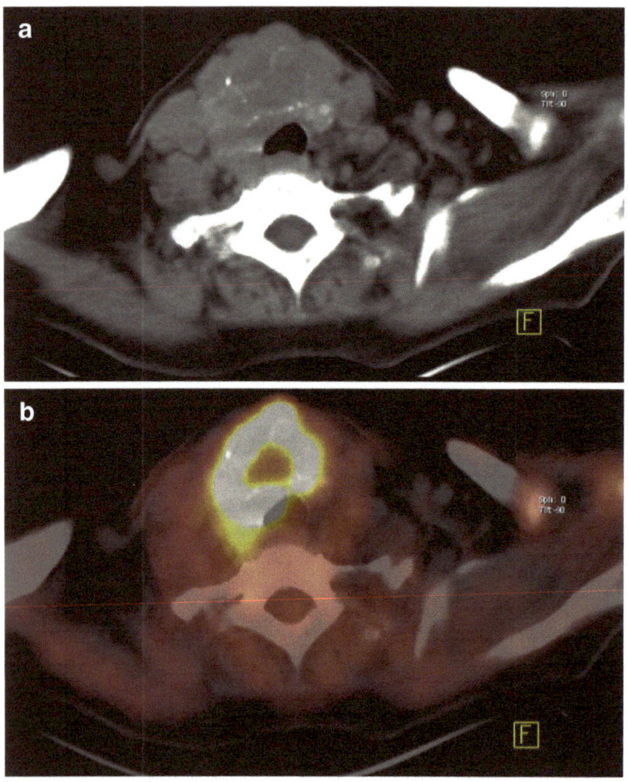

Fig. 4.4 Axial CT and fusion images of PET/CT show intensely hypermetabolic lesion with irregular borders and hypometabolic necrotic center at thyroid gland (**a**, **b**)

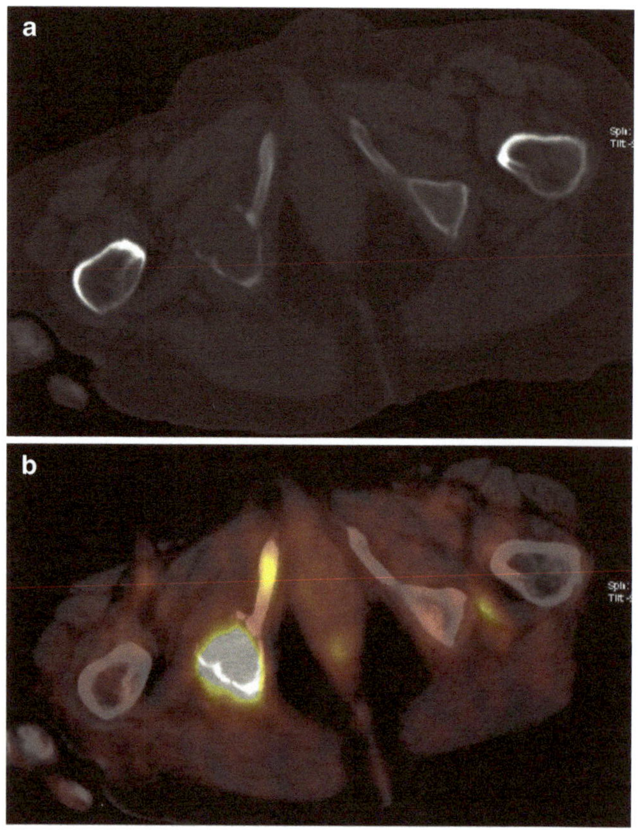

Fig. 4.5 Axial CT and fusion images show intensely hypermetabolic lytic lesion at right ischium (**a**, **b**)

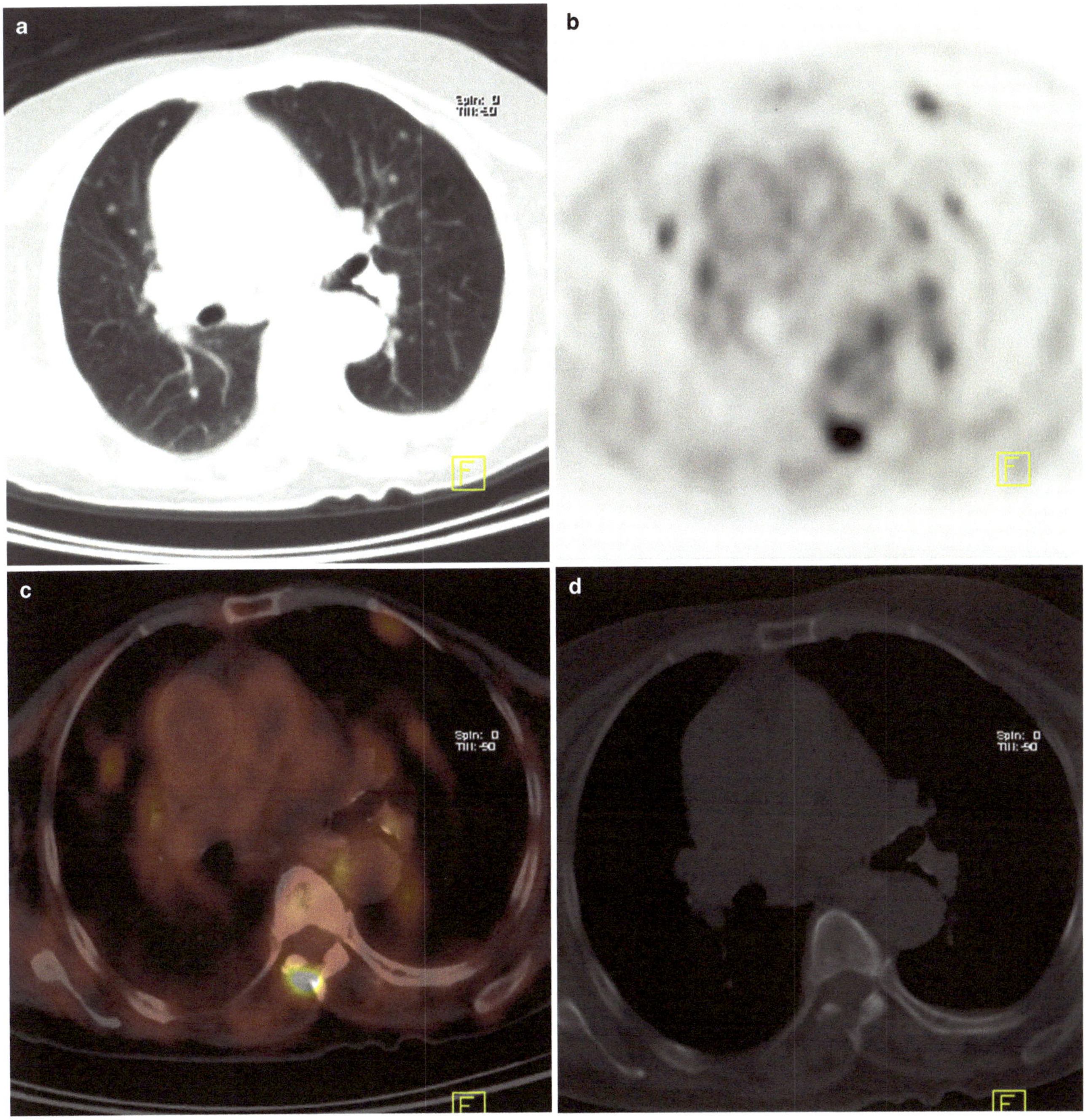

Fig. 4.6 Axial images show multiple lung nodules showing increased FDG uptake and hypermetabolic activity at the lytic lesion at right posterior elements of D6 vertebra (**a**–**d**)

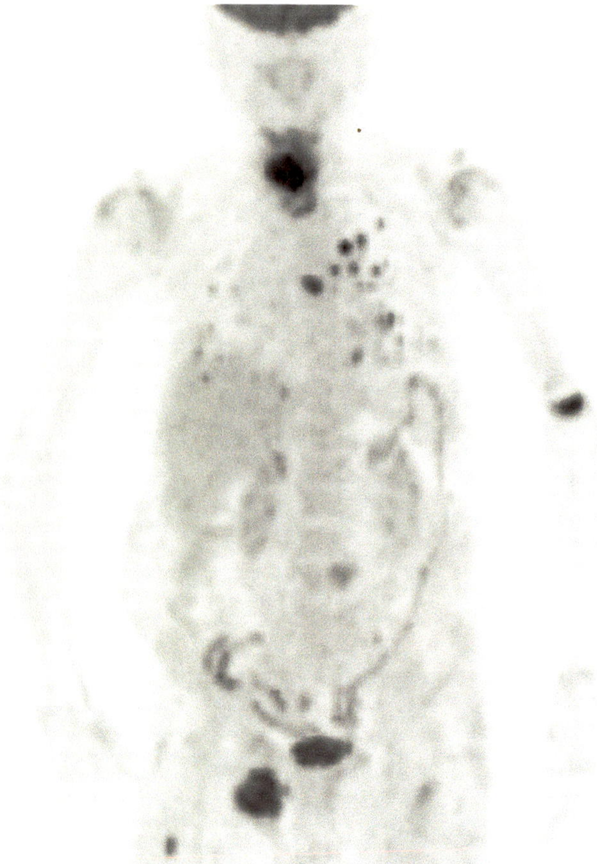

Fig. 4.7 MIP image shows additional pathologically increased FDG uptake sites at distal diaphysis of left humerus, left side of corpus of L4 vertebra, and proximal right femur diaphysis

4.4 Case 4: Restaging of Insular Thyroid Carcinoma

History A 71-year-old female who has a history of insular thyroid carcinoma. The patient is status postthyroidectomy and I-131 ablation. He is now being evaluated for high thyroglobulin levels (500 ng/ml). The patient is referred to ^{18}F-FDG PET/CT scan after a diagnostic whole body I-131 scan gave negative result.

Findings

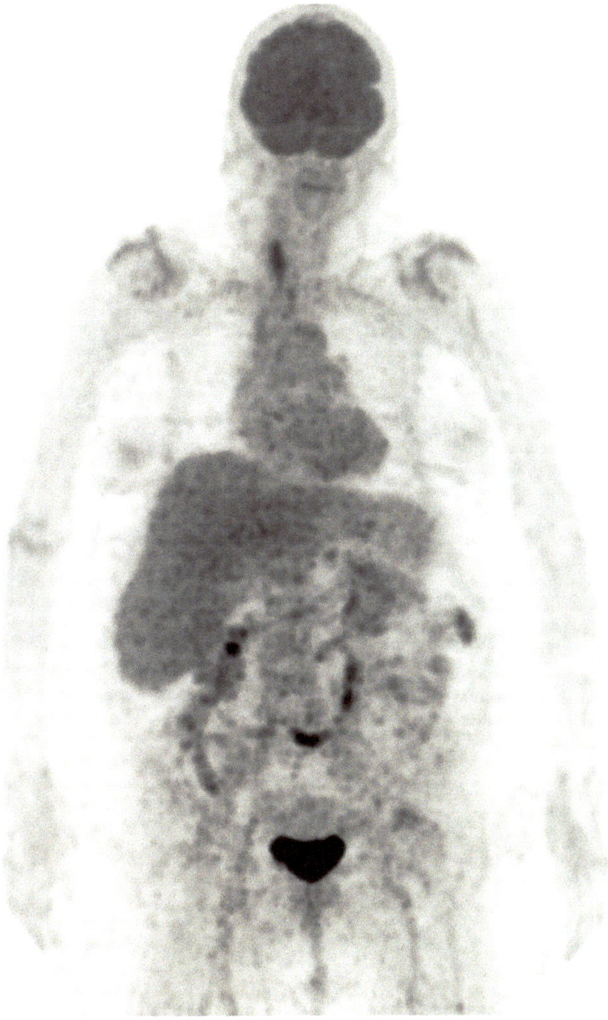

Fig. 4.8 MIP image shows pathologically increased FDG uptake at right side of the neck

Interpretation Local recurrence of primary thyroid malignancy.

Outcome The patient underwent operation for the mass lesion suspicious for recurrence and histopathology turned out to be metastasis of thyroid malignancy.

Teaching Point ^{18}F-FDG PET CT scan is effective in the evaluation of recurrence of poorly differentiated thyroid malignancies when Tg levels are high but I-131 DxWBS is negative.

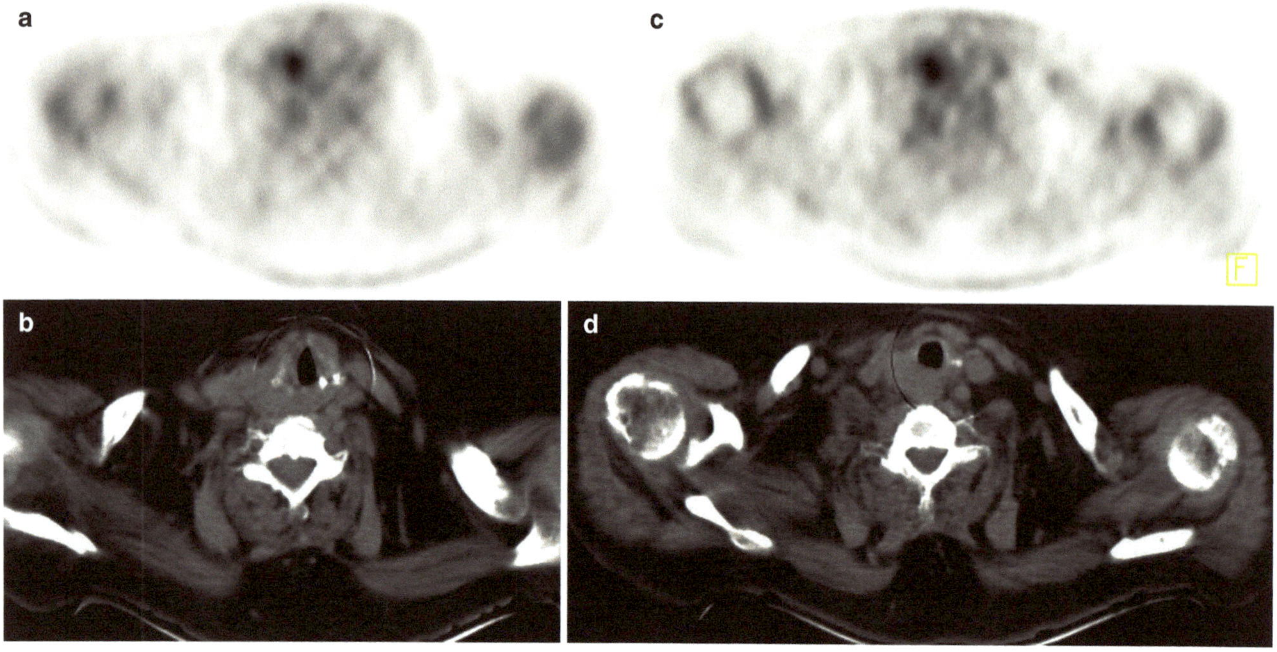

Fig. 4.9 Axial PET and CT images show moderately hypermetabolic lesion in soft tissue density at right posterolateral aspect of thyroid cartilage (SUVmax 7.1) (**a–d**)

4.5 Case 5: Restaging of Hurthle Cell Carcinoma

History A 88-year-old male who has a history of Hurthle cell carcinoma of thyroid gland. The patient is status post-thyroidectomy and I-131 ablation. He is now being evaluated for a mass lesion on USG at left side of the neck at the thyroid bed, negative on I-131 scan but suggestive of a recurrence. Patient underwent FDG PET/CT study with the purpose of restaging.

Findings

Interpretation Recurrent malignant lesion at left neck and metastatic lung nodules.

Teaching Point

- FDG PET/CT is useful in initial staging and restaging of Hurthle cell carcinoma.
- FDG PET/CT is efficient in revealing the malignant nature of the suspicious lesions especially when I-131 scan is negative.

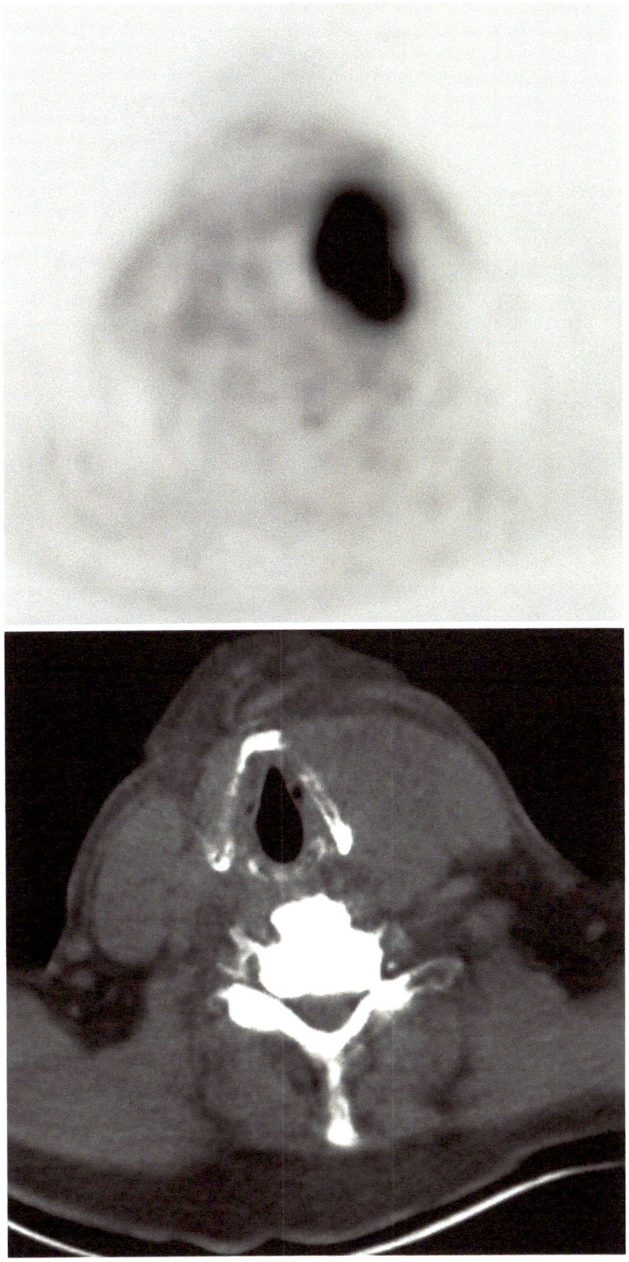

Fig. 4.10 Axial PET and CT images show intensely increased FDG uptake at the mass lesion near to the left side of thyroid cartilage

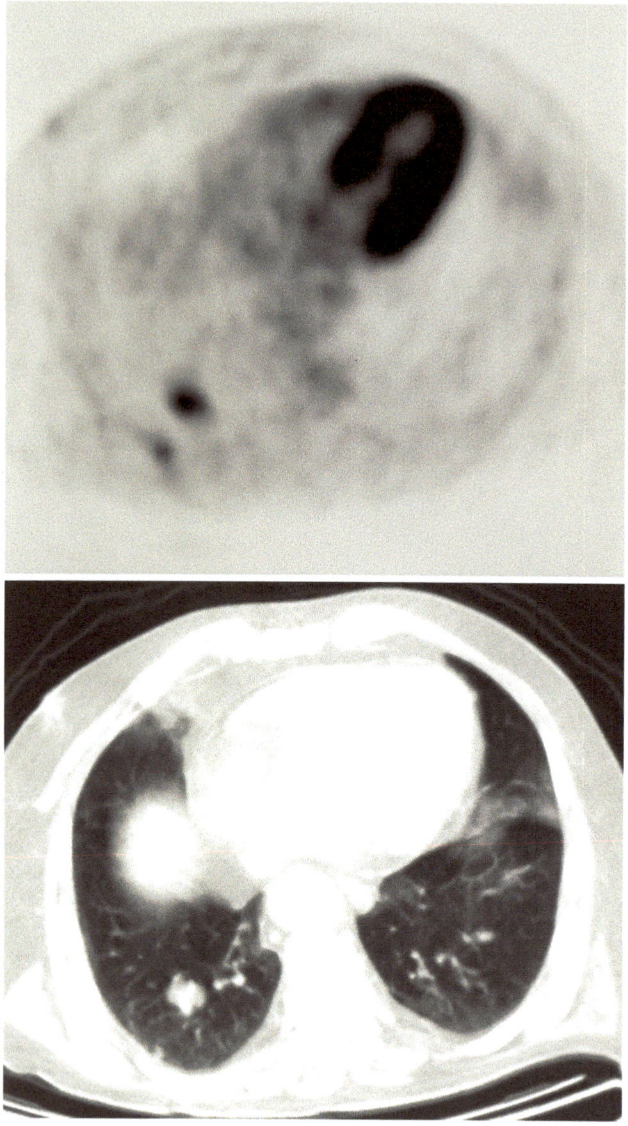

Fig. 4.11 Axial PET and CT images show two hypermetabolic lung nodules at lower lobe of right lung

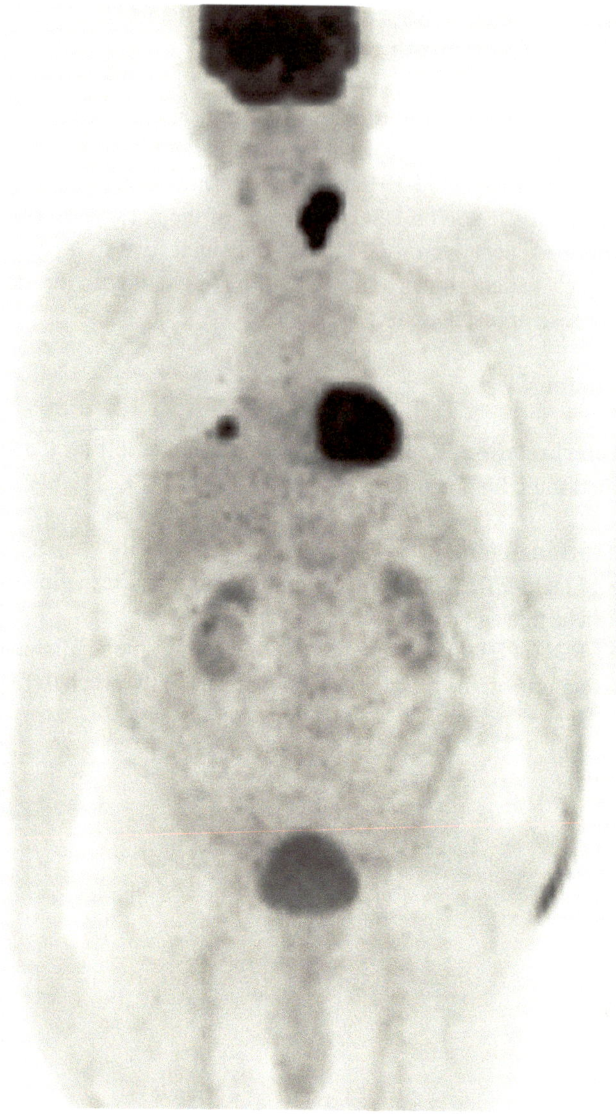

Fig. 4.12 MIP image

4.6 Case 6: Staging of Anaplastic Carcinoma

History A 54-year-old female who was diagnosed as anaplastic carcinoma of thyroid gland (ATC) underwent ^{18}F-FDG PET/CT study with the purpose of staging.

Findings

Interpretation Hypermetabolic mass lesion at left thyroid lobe consistent with primary malignancy, metastatic cervical and mediastinal lymph nodes, and metastatic lung nodules.

Teaching Point ^{18}F-FDG PET/CT is an efficient imaging modality for ATC at initial staging and also seems to be effective in the early evaluation of treatment response and follow up.

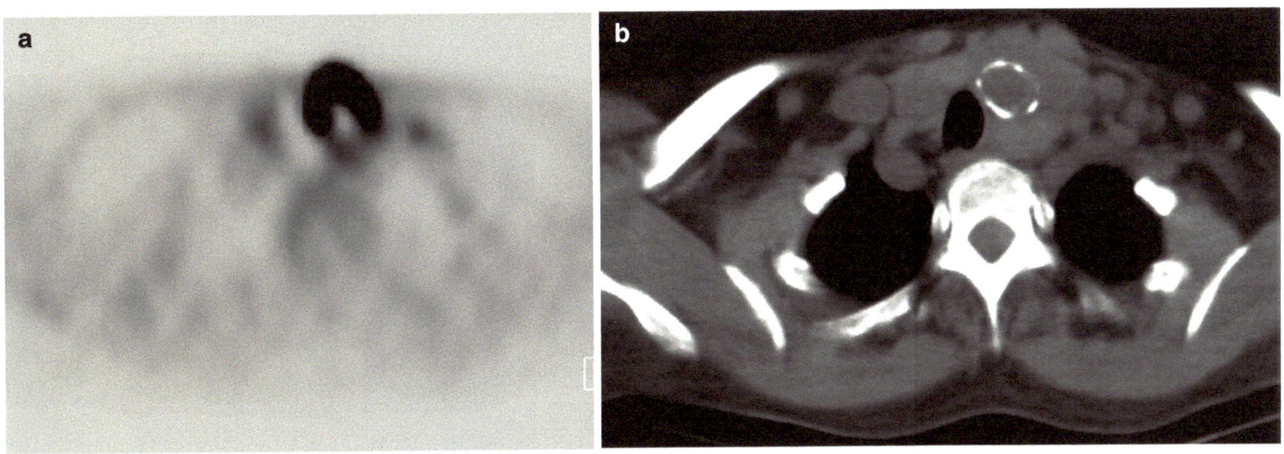

Fig. 4.13 Axial PET and CT images show intensely increased FDG uptake at the left thyroid lobe (**a**, **b**)

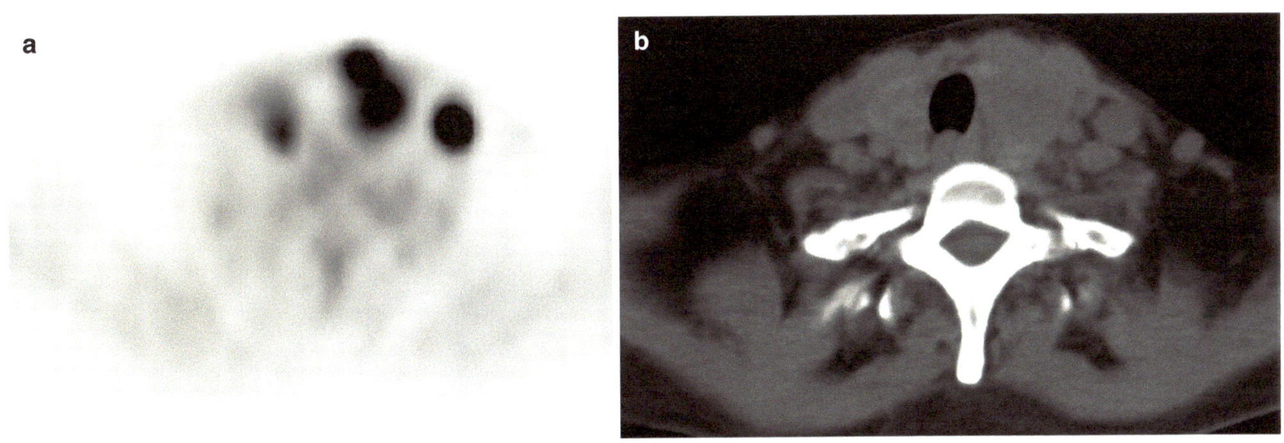

Fig. 4.14 Bilateral hypermetabolic cervical lymph nodes (**a**, **b**)

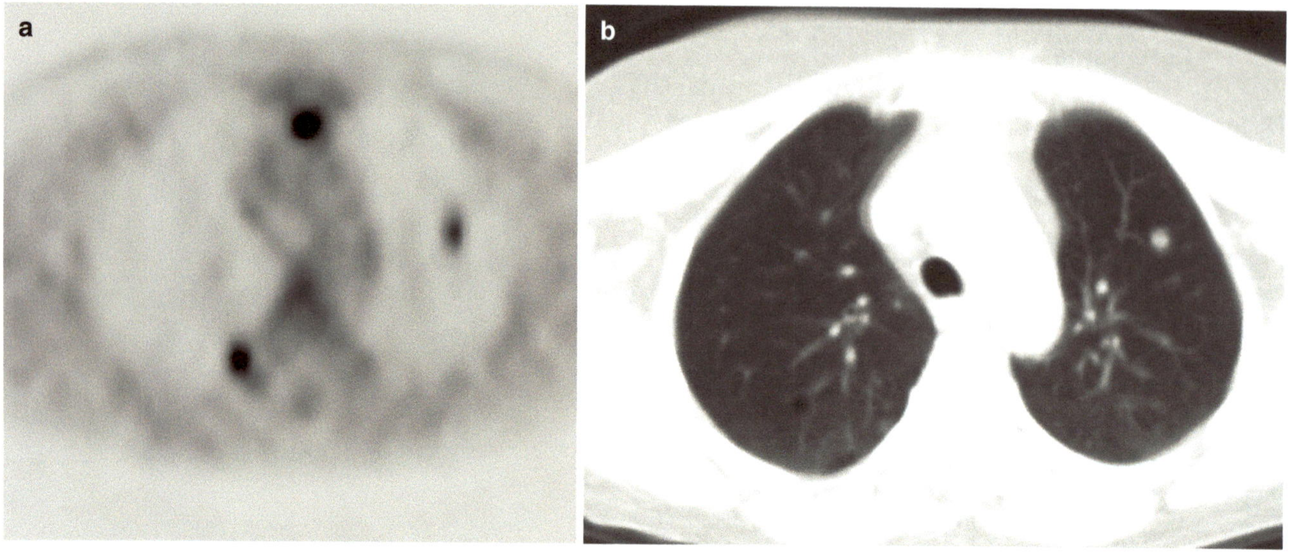

Fig. 4.15 Hypermetabolic lung nodules at parenchyme of both lungs (**a**, **b**)

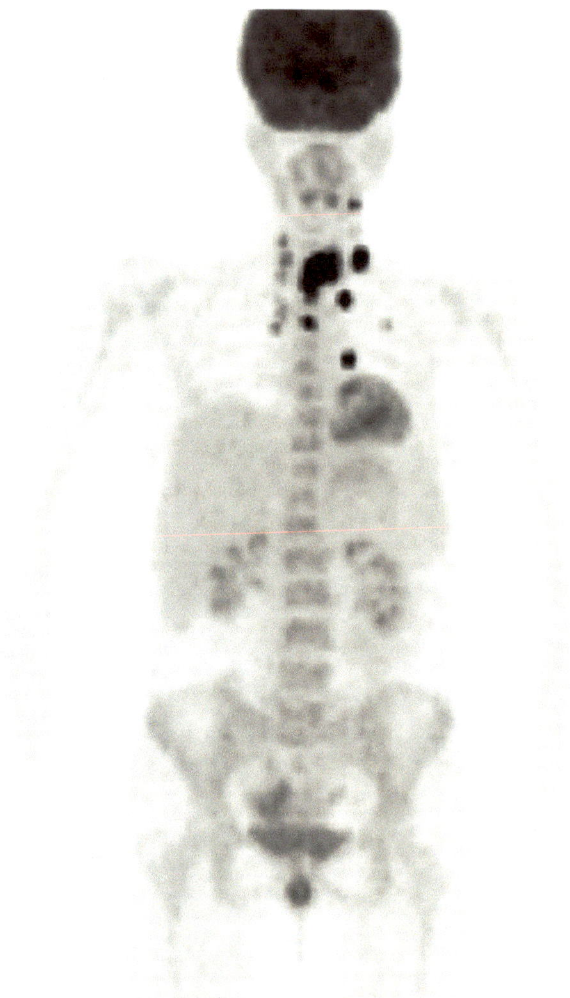

Fig. 4.16 MIP image

4.7 Case 7: Staging of Medullary Thyroid Cancer

History A 60-year-old female whose FNA from thyroid nodule was suspicious for medullary thyroid cancer (MTC) underwent ^{18}F-FDG PET/CT scan before operation.

Findings

Interpretation Hypermetabolism at the right thyroid lobe nodule is suggestive of malignancy.

Teaching Point FDG PET/CT imaging is not recommended for routine initial screening for MTC metastases in patients when an FNA is diagnostic or suspicious for MTC. Sensitivity of FDG PET/CT imaging in the detection of recurrent disease varies between 47.4–80 %. FDG PET/CT imaging can be used as complementary to conventional imaging modalities in situations where they are inconclusive while calcitonin and carcinoembryonic antigen (CEA) are elevated.

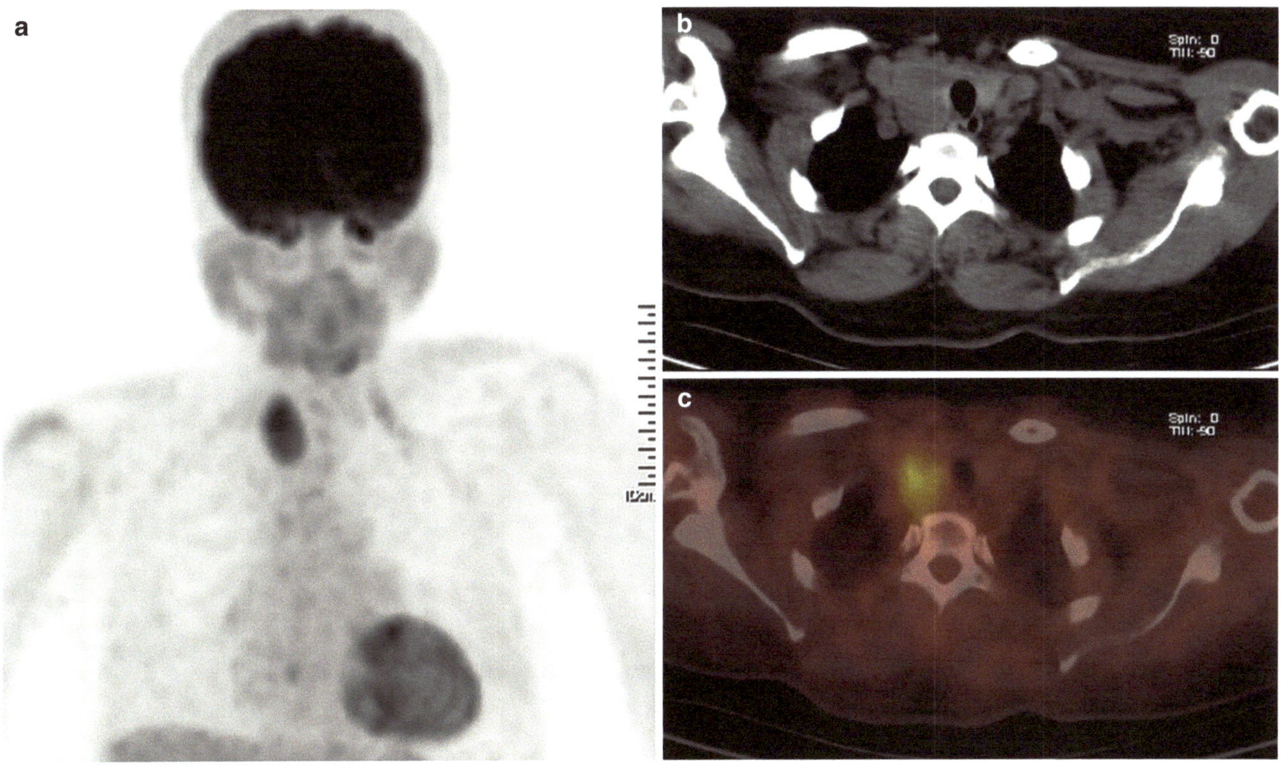

Fig. 4.17 MIP (**a**), axial CT, and fusion images (**b**), (**c**) show moderately increased FDG uptake (SUVmax 9.2) at the thyroid nodule at right thyroid lobe. There was no additional FDG avid pathological lesion in the rest of the body

Bibliography

1. Bockisch A, Brandt-Mainz K, Görges R, Müller S, Stattaus J, Antoch G. Diagnosis in medullary thyroid cancer with [18F]FDG PET and improvement using a combined PET-CT scanner. Acta Med Austriaca. 2003;30:22–5.
2. Bogsrud TV, Karantanis D, Nathan MA, Mullan BP, Wiseman GA, Kasperbauer JL. 18F-FDG PET in the management of patients with anaplastic thyroid carcinoma. Thyroid. 2008;18:713–9.
3. Chen YK, Ding HJ, Chen KT, Chen YL, Liao AC, Shen YY, et al. Prevalence and risk of cancer of focal thyroid incidentaloma identified by 18F-fluorodeoxyglucose positron emission tomography for cancer screening in healthy subjects. Anticancer Res. 2005;25: 1421–6.
4. Cohen MS, Arslan N, Dehdashti F, Doherty GM, Lairmore TC, Brunt LM, et al. Risk of malignancy in thyroid incidentalomas identified by fluorodeoxyglucose-positron emission tomography. Surgery. 2001;130:941–6.
5. Kang KW, Kim SK, Kang HS, Lee ES, Sim JS, Lee IG, et al. Prevalence and risk of cancer of focal thyroid incidentaloma identified by 18F-fluorodeoxyglucose positron emission tomography for metastasis evaluation and cancer screening in healthy subjects. J Clin Endocrinol Metab. 2003;88:4100–4.
6. Kloos RT, Eng C, Evans DB, Francis GL, Gagel RF, Gharib H. Medullary thyroid cancer: management guidelines of the American Thyroid Association. Thyroid. 2009;19:565–612. doi:10.1089/thy.2008.0403.
7. Nanni C, Rubello D, Fanti S, Farsad M, Ambrosini V, Rampin L, et al. Role of 18FFDG-PET and PET-CT imaging in thyroid cancer. Biomed Pharmacother. 2006;60:409–13.
8. Patel KN, Shaha AR. Poorly differentiated and anaplastic thyroid cancer. Cancer Control. 2006;13:119–28.
9. Poisson T, Deandreis D, Leboulleux S, Bidault F, Bonniaud G, Baillot S, et al. 18F-fluorodeoxyglucose positron emission tomography and computed tomography in anaplastic thyroid cancer. Eur J Nucl Med Mol Imaging. 2010;37:2277–85.
10. Skoura E, Rondogianni P, Alevizaki M, Tzanela M, Tsagarakis S, Piaditis G, et al. Role of [(18)F]FDG-PET-CT in the detection of occult recurrent medullary thyroid cancer. Nucl Med Commun. 2010;31:567–75.
11. Treglia G, Annunziata S, Muoio B, Salvatori M, Ceriani L, Giovanella L. The role of fluorine-18-fluorodeoxyglucose positron emission tomography in aggressive histological subtypes of thyroid cancer: an overview. Int J Endocrinol. doi:10.1155/2013/856189.
12. Wang N, Zhai H, Lu Y. Is fluorine-18 fluorodeoxyglucose positron emission tomography useful for the thyroid nodules with indeterminate fine needle aspiration biopsy? A meta-analysis of the literature. J Otolaryngol Head Neck Surg. 2013;42:38. doi:10.1186/1916-0216-42-38.
13. Yi JG, Marom EM, Munden RF, Truong MT, Macapinlac HA, Gladish GW, et al. Focal uptake of fluorodeoxyglucose by the thyroid in patients undergoing initial disease staging with combined PET/CT for non-small cell lung cancer. Radiology. 2005;236:271–5.

5 Lung Cancer

5.1 Case 1: Staging of Lung Carcinoma

History A 58-year-old male underwent ^{18}F-FDG PET/CT scan after he was diagnosed to have nonsmall cell lung carcinoma (NSCLC) with a bronchoscopic biopsy.

Findings

Interpretation Increased uptake at the known primary lesions at right lung and metastatic lesion at left surrenal gland.

Teaching Point PET detects unsuspected distant metastases in 10 % of patients. Adrenal metastasis, at the initial diagnosis of nonsmall cell lung cancer, occurs in less than 10 % of lung cancer patients. Sensitivity and specificity of PET/CT for adrenal metastasis is 94 % and 85 %, respectively.

T. Özülker, F. Özülker, *Atlas of PET-CT Imaging in Oncology: A Case-Based Guide to Image Interpretation*,
DOI 10.1007/978-3-319-18994-9_5

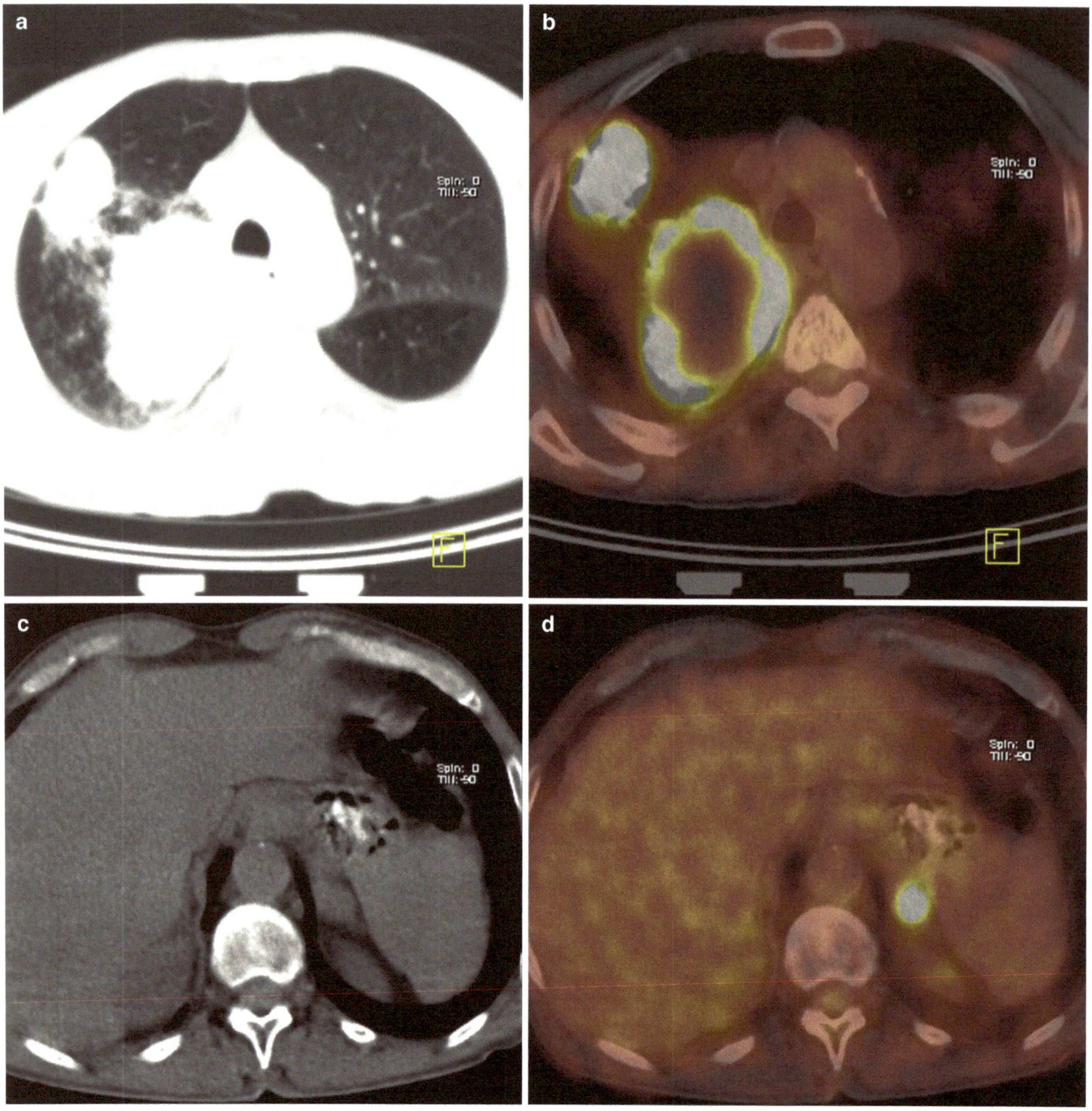

Fig. 5.1 Axial CT and fusion images show intensely hypermetabolic mass lesion (SUVmax 12.9) at right upper lobe adjacent to mediastinum with a hypometabolic necrotic center and another solid lesion located anteriorly with increased FDG uptake (SUVmax 13.9) (**a**, **b**), hypermetabolism at the nodular lesion at left surrenal gland (SUVmax8.9) (**c**, **d**)

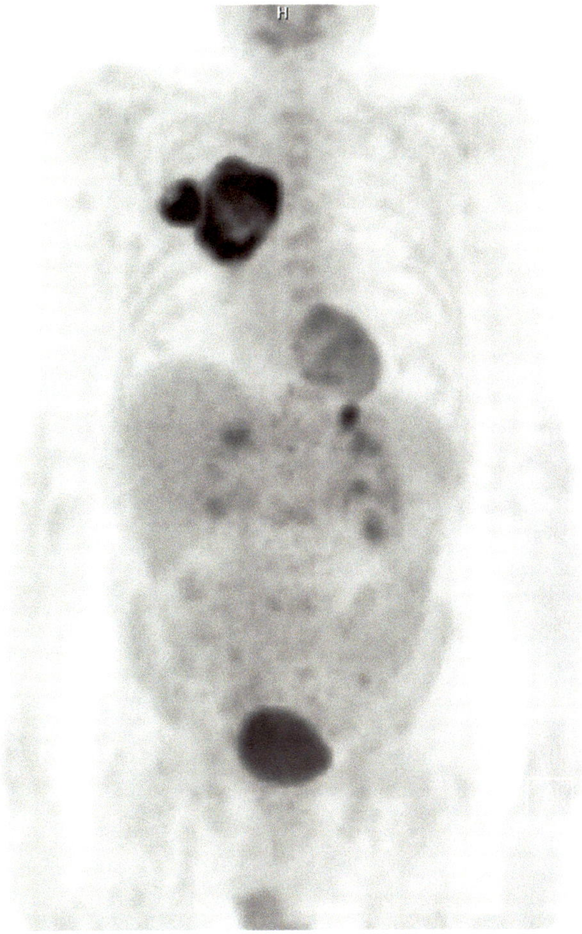

Fig. 5.2 MIP image

5.2 Case 2: Staging of Lung Carcinoma

History A 55-year-old male with known NSCLC at right lung. The current ^{18}F-FDG PET/CT imaging is being done to evaluate the extent of disease.

Findings

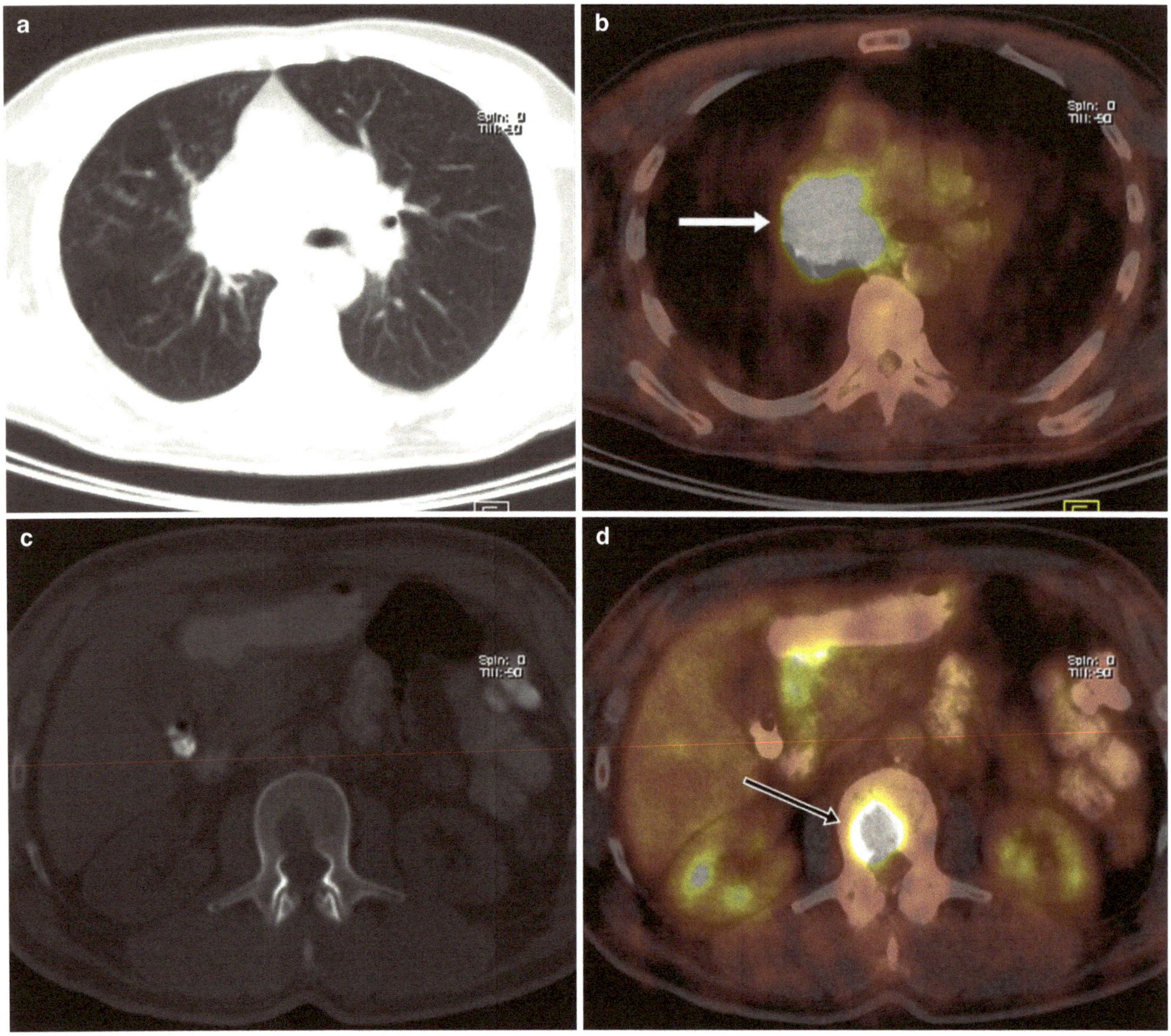

Fig. 5.3 Axial CT and fusion images show intensely hypermetabolic solid lesion (SUVmax 13.6) at right hilus adjacent to the right main bronchus (*arrow*). There is not any hypermetabolic mediastinal lymph node suspicious for metastatic invasion (**a**, **b**). Intensely increased FDG uptake is seen in the lytic lesion at L2 vertebra (*arrow*) (SUVmax 14) (**c**, **d**)

Interpretation Increased uptake at the primary malignant lesion at right lung and metastatic lesion at L2 vertebra.

Teaching Point ^{18}F-FDG PET/CT is useful in detecting any possible distant metastasis in Stage II, III, and IV.

5.3 Case 3: Staging of Lung Carcinoma

History A 55-year-old male who was admitted with the complaint of cough was found to have a cavitary lesion at lower lobe of left lung on CT. Bronchoscopic biopsy revealed squamous cell carcinoma of lung (SLC). The current ^{18}F-FDG PET/CT imaging is being done to stage the disease.

Findings

Interpretation Primary malignant lesion at lower lobe of left lung and metastatic involvement of left lower paratracheal lymph node.

Result Patient is regarded as Stage IIIA and underwent neoadjuvant chemotherapy before operation.

Teaching Point

- If the ^{18}F-FDG PET/CT scan is positive in mediastinum, the lymph node status needs pathological confirmation and mediastinoscopy is done for this purpose.
- Cavitating lesions are frequently seen in patients with SLC and these lesions might mimic infectious processes. They are characterized with increased chemoresistance and worse prognosis.

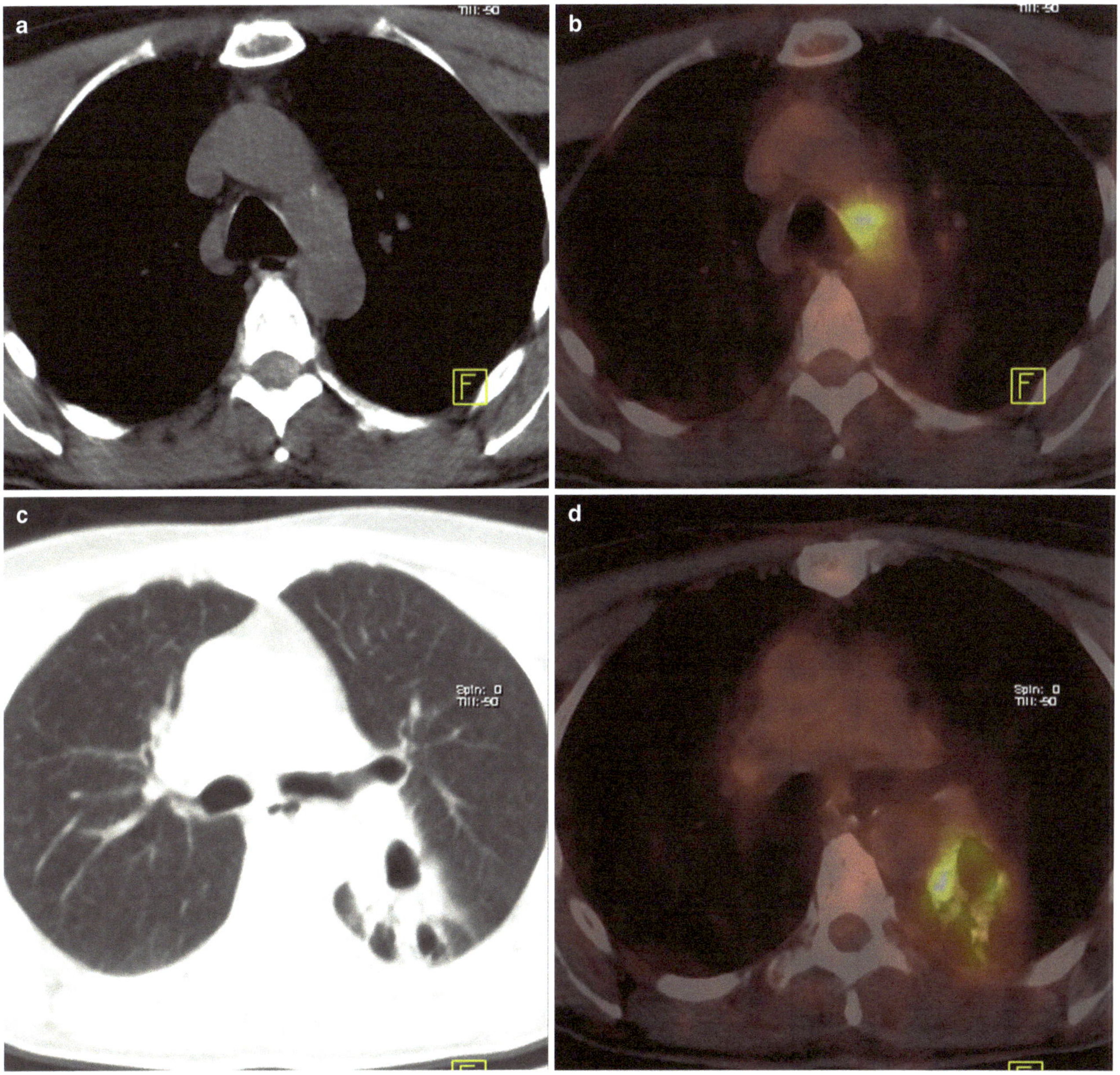

Fig. 5.4 Axial CT and fusion images show hypermetabolic lesion at left lower paratracheal area (SUVmax 10.8) (**a**, **b**) and cavitary lesion at left lower lobe with moderately increased FDG uptake (SUVmax 10.6) (**c**, **d**)

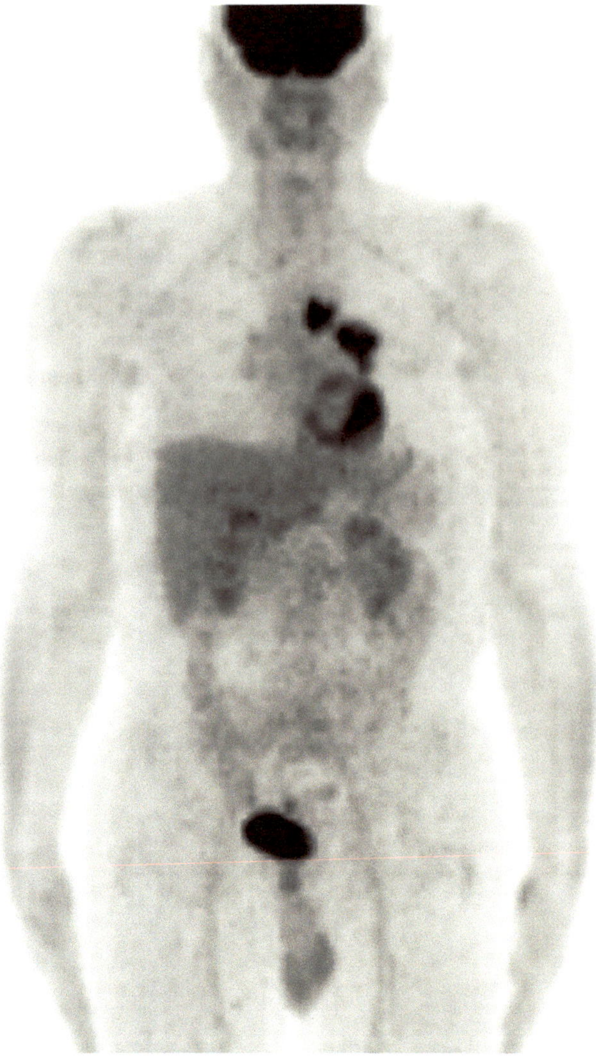

Fig. 5.5 MIP image

5.4 Case 4: Restaging of Lung Carcinoma

History A 54-year-old female status post left pneumonectomy for adenocarcinoma of lung underwent ^{18}F-FDG PET/CT imaging for evaluation of the extent of the disease.

Findings

Interpretation Recurrent metastatic lesion at left frontal lobe of brain.

Teaching Point F-18 FDG PET/CT studies can be done as whole-body imaging; from the top of the head through the feet or torso imaging; base of the skull to mid-thigh. Although torso imaging is usually preferred because of high physiological FDG uptake at brain that can mask metastatic hypermetabolic foci, this case shows the importance of obtaining whole-body imaging when likelihood for metastasis to brain is high.

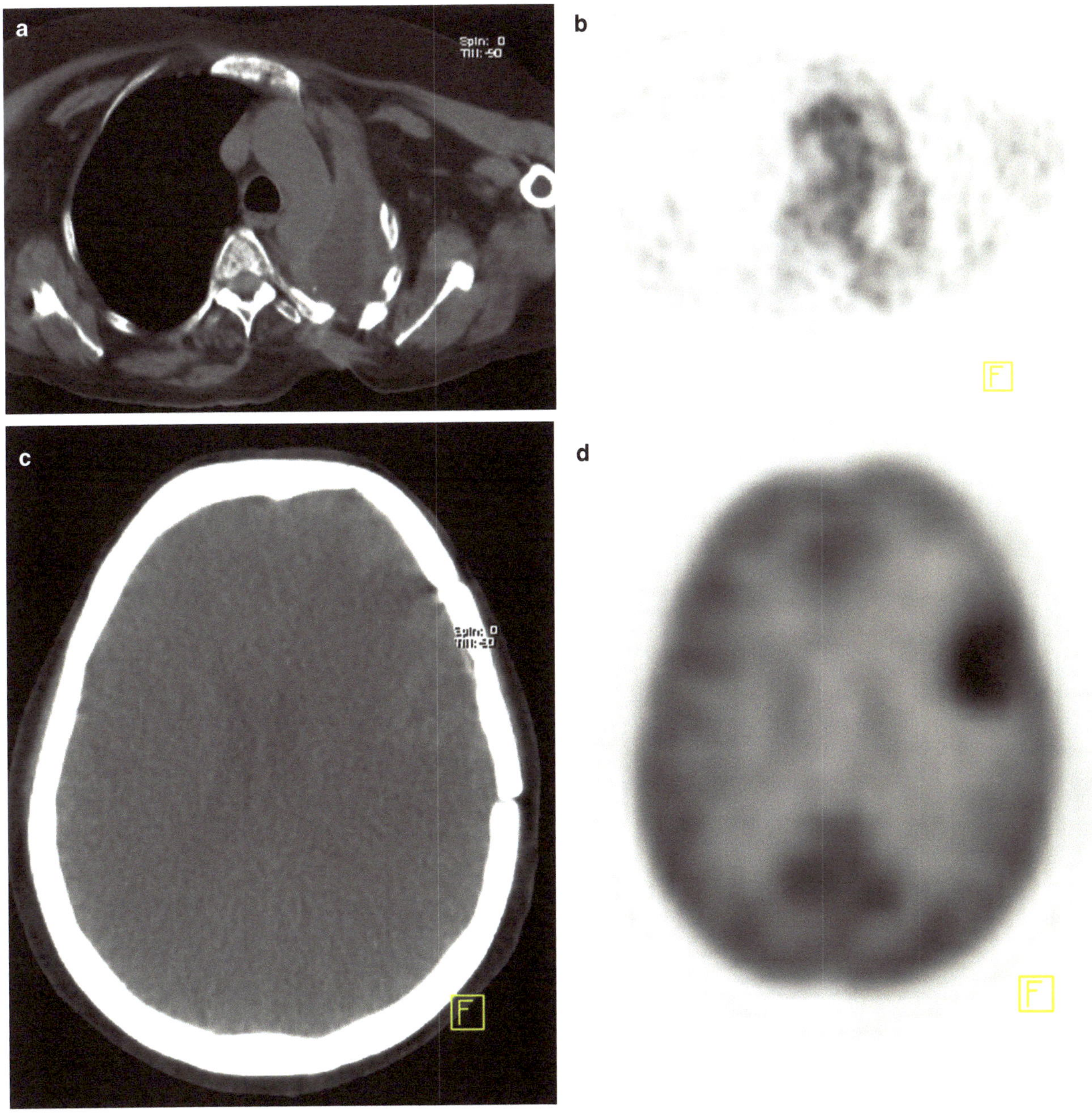

Fig. 5.6 Axial CT and PET images show collapse of left lung due to pneumonectomy and no pathological FDG uptake in favor of local recurrence (**a**, **b**) and increased focal FDG uptake at left frontal lobe of brain (SUVmax 10.4) (**c**, **d**)

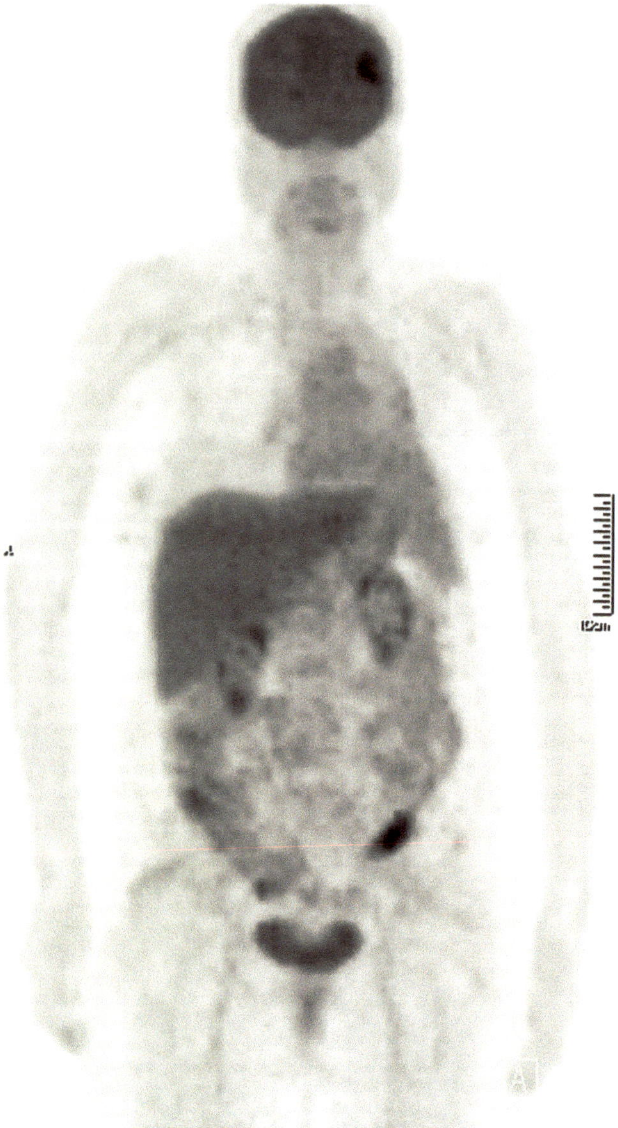

Fig. 5.7 MIP image

5.5 Case 5: Detection of Bone Metastasis in Lung Carcinoma

History A 55-year-old male with NSCLC underwent ^{18}F-FDG PET/CT imaging while being followed-up after having chemotherapy and radiotherapy.

Findings

Interpretation Metastatic sclerotic lesions at corpus of dorsal vertebras.

Teaching Point ^{18}F-FDG PET/CT is less sensitive in detecting sclerotic metastases since they are relatively hypocellular and consequently contain lower volumes of viable tumor tissue causing low degree of uptake of FDG. FDG nonavid osteoblastic lesions can be detected as sclerotic lesions on CT part of the PET/CT studies.

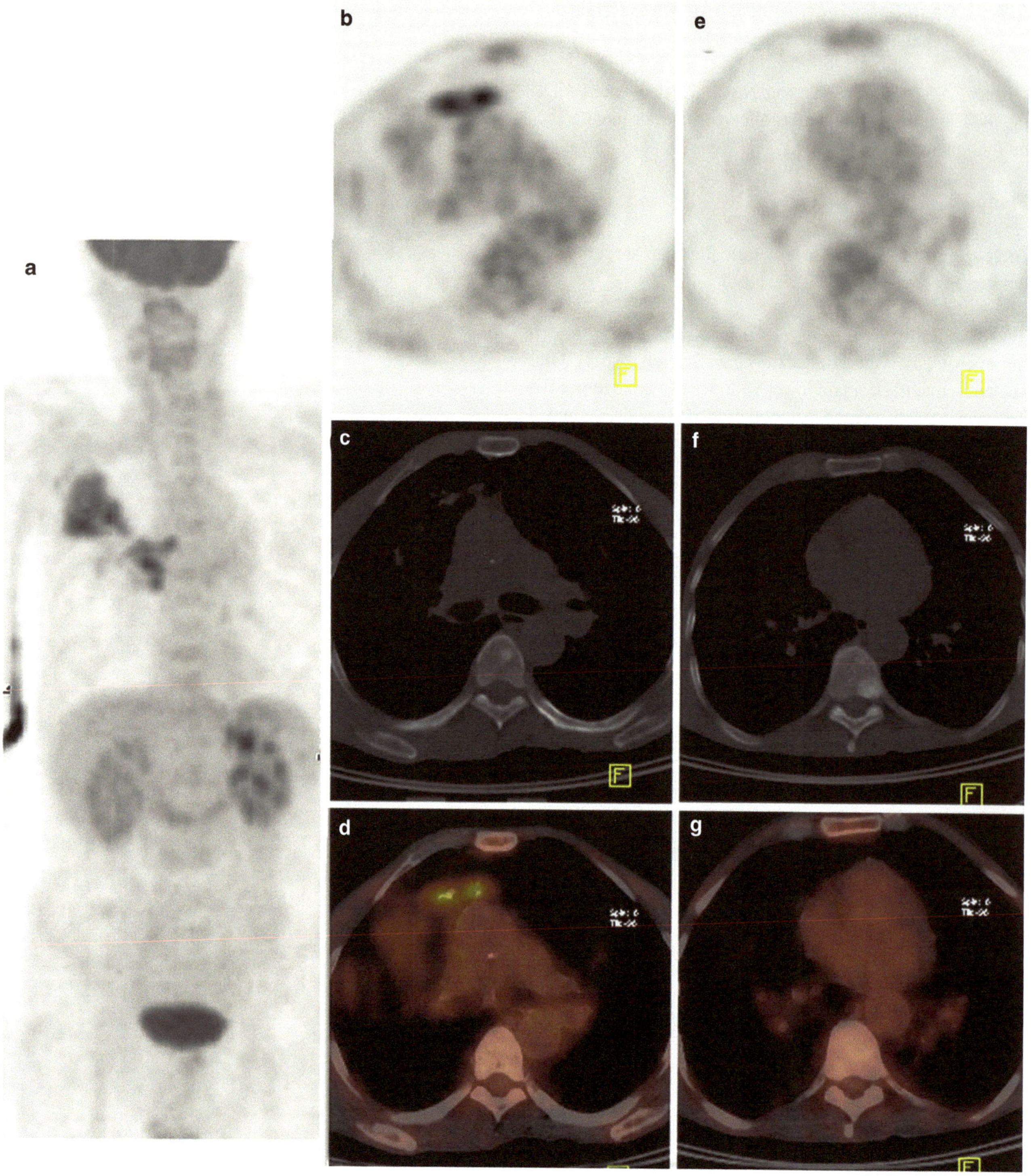

Fig. 5.8 MIP image (**a**), axial PET, CT, and fusion images showing focal hyperdense lesion at dorsal vertebras without corresponding FDG uptake (**b**, **c**, **d**) and (**e**, **f**, **g**). Diffuse FDG uptake at upper lobe of right lung represents inflammatory process following radiotherapy

5.6 Case 6: Differentiation of Lung Carcinoma from Atelectasis

History A 75-year-old female with known right-sided adenocarcinoma. Patient underwent ^{18}F-FDG PET/CT imaging to evaluate the extent of disease.

Findings

Interpretation Compression of the bronchus by the tumor caused atelectasis.

Teaching Point Atelectasis caused by the compression of the bronchus sometimes may not be differentiated from tumor itself on CT. PET might be helpful in that respect, since there is little or no FDG uptake at area with atelectasis.

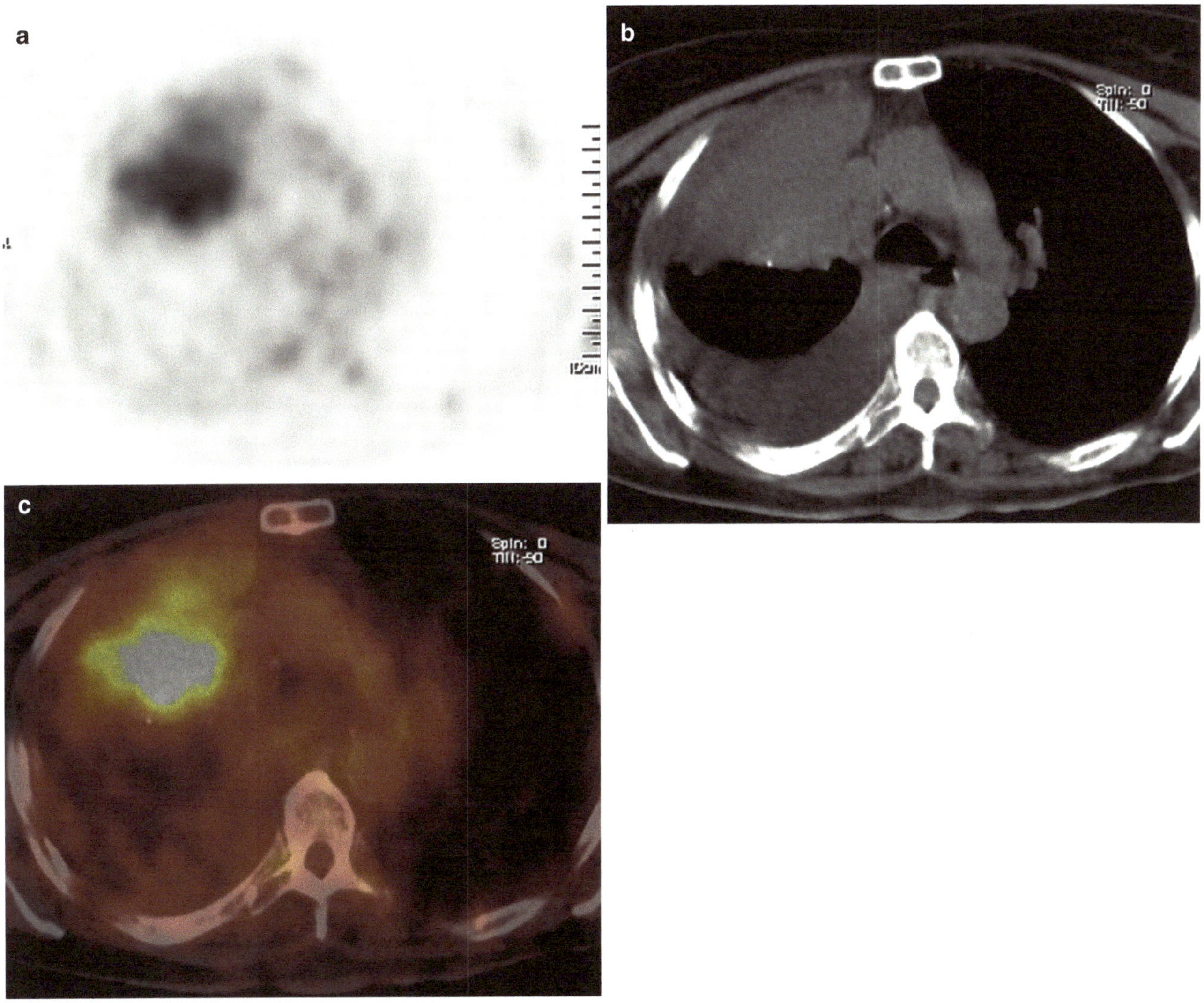

Fig. 5.9 Axial PET, CT, and fusion images show increased FDG uptake in the mass lesion at anterior segment of upper lobe of right lung. Anterior to the mass lesion, soft tissue density which exhibits minimally increased FDG uptake on PET image is seen (**a**–**c**). Pleural effusion without FDG uptake is also noted at right lung

5.7 Case 7: Tumor Thrombus in Superior Vena Cava from Lung Carcinoma

History A 70-year-old man presented to the hospital with a history of progressive edema of the head, neck, arms, and upper chest, followed by dyspnea and distention of the jugular and chest veins. The patient underwent ^{18}F-FDG PET/CT imaging.

Findings

Interpretation Malignant thrombosis of superior vena cava.

Teaching Point

- NSCLC is the most common cause of superior vena cava syndrome, as a result of either compression of the SVC by an adjacent tumor or compression by mediastinal lymph nodes. But since the speed of blood flow in the SVC is too fast for thrombus formation in blood, the development of SVC thrombosis alone is not frequently seen·
- ^{18}F-FDG-PET/CT is helpful in discriminating between benign and malignant thrombus but interpretation should be made carefully since the benign lesions like inflammatory and infectious venous processes might complicate the cases by showing F-18 FDG uptake.

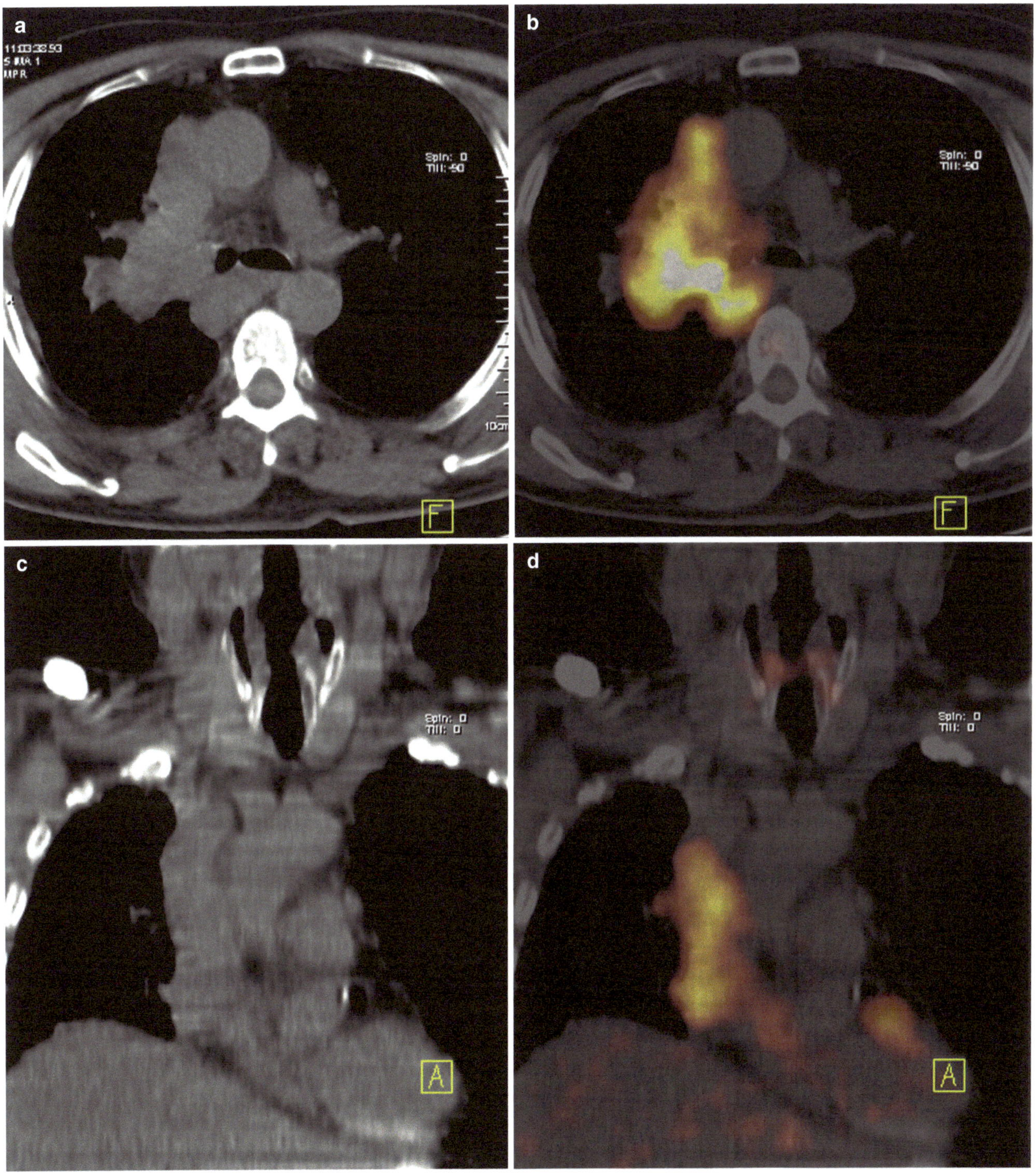

Fig. 5.10 Axial (**a**, **b**) and coronal (**c**, **d**) CT and fusion images show an intensely hypermetabolic mass at hilus of right lung with a SUVmax 13.6. There is also increased FDG uptake extending from the primary tumor into the mediastinum and ending just above the right atrium

5.8 Case 8: Tumor Thrombus in Left Atrium and Right Pulmonary Vein from Lung Carcinoma

History A 64-year-old man who was diagnosed to have NSCLC 2 months ago underwent ^{18}F-FDG PET CT scan.

Findings

Interpretation Malignant thrombosis of left atrium and right pulmonary vein. There is also hypermetabolic N3 lymph node consistent with metastatic invasion.

Teaching Point Surgical treatment with pneumonectomy combined with left atrium resection of T4 lung cancer invading the left atrium or the base of the pulmonary vein is possible, particularly in N0 and N1 patients. In our case N3 lymph node is positive for metastatic invasion making this therapeutic approach invalid.

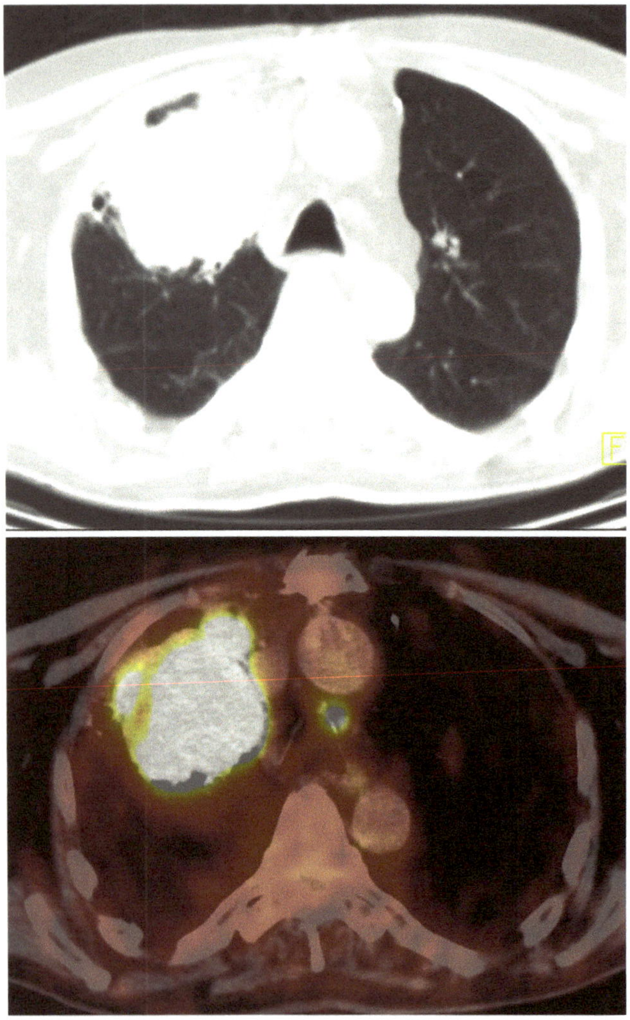

Fig. 5.11 Axial CT and fusion images show an extensively hypermetabolic mass (SUVmax 23.2) at anterior segment of upper lobe of right lung abutting the mediastinal and pleural surface. Hypermetabolic lymph node at left lower paratracheal area is also noted

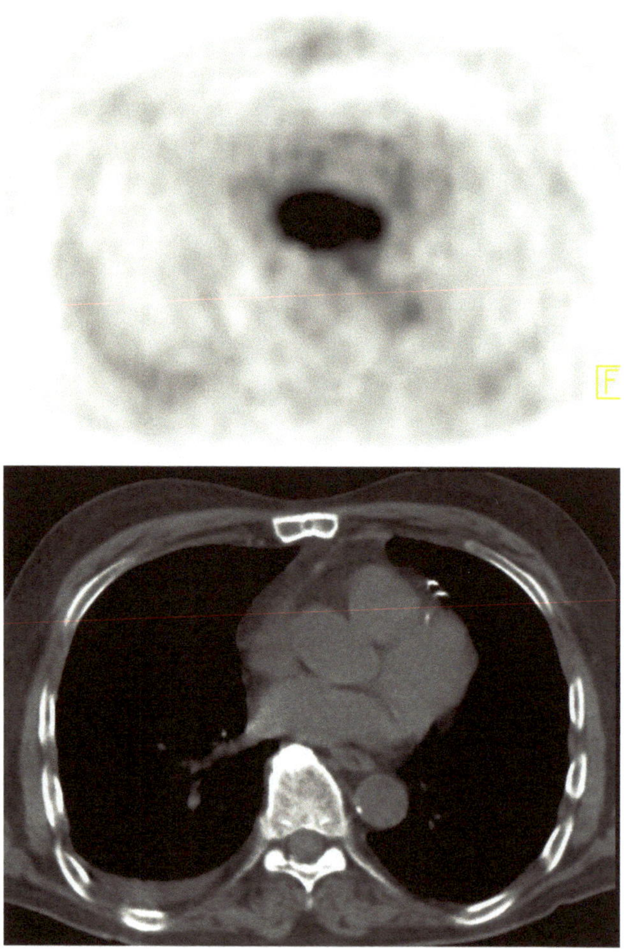

Fig. 5.12 Axial PET and CT images. Intensely increased FDG uptake at left atrium is detected (SUVmax 19.3)

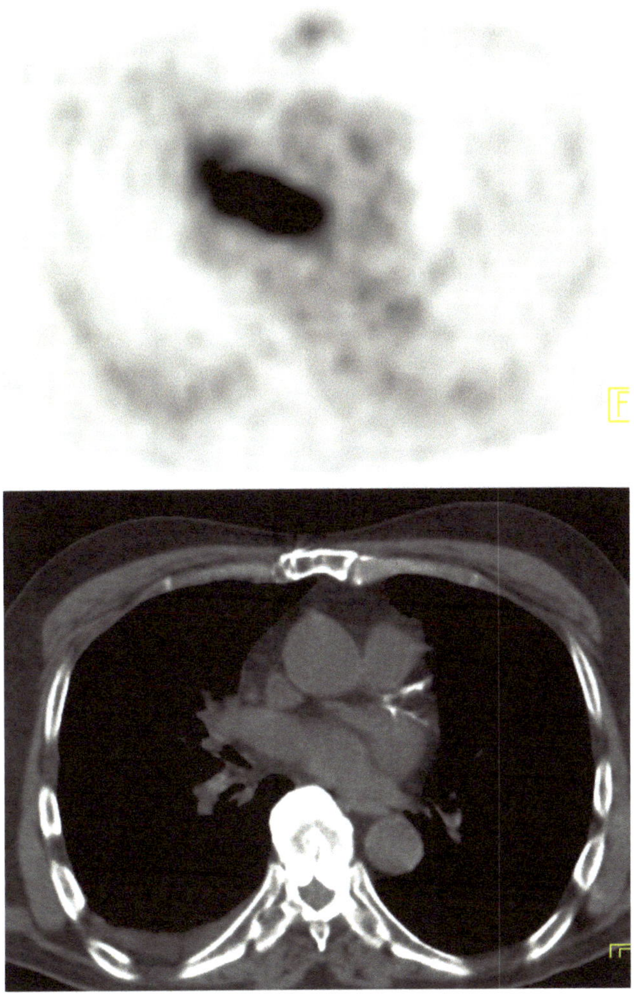

Fig. 5.13 Axial PET and CT images. Intensely increased FDG uptake at right pulmonary vein is detected

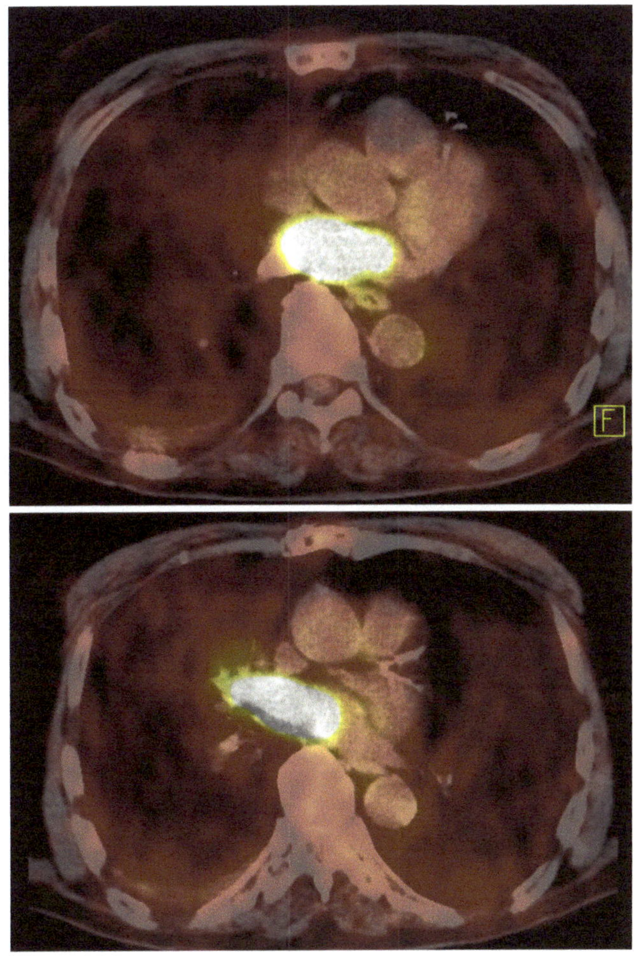

Fig. 5.14 Axial fusion images show hypermetabolism at left atrium and right pulmonary vein

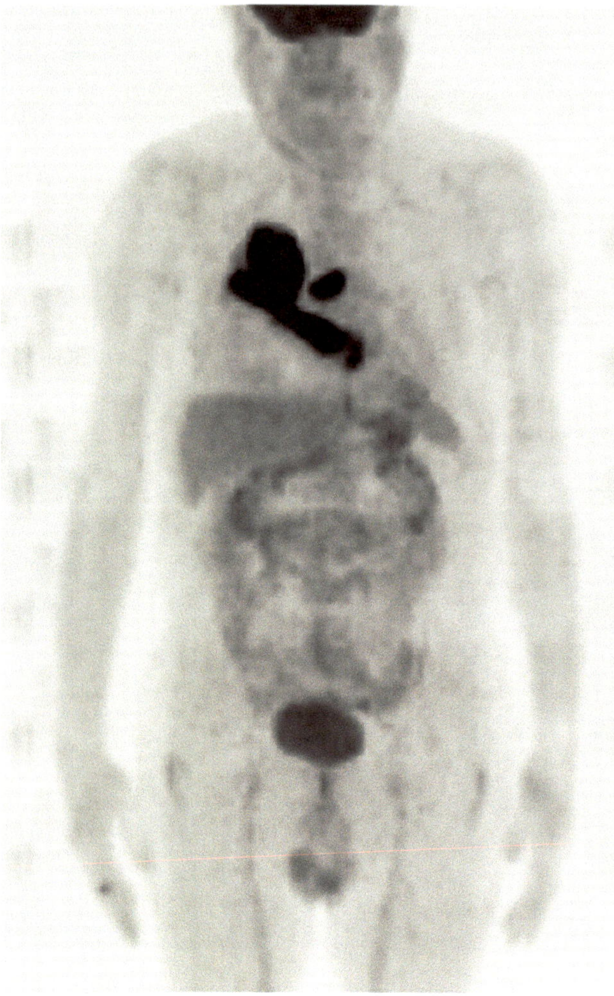

Fig. 5.15 MIP image

5.9 Case 9: Metastatic Supraclavicular Lymph Node Changes the Stage

History A 65-year-old male who was diagnosed as NSCLC underwent ^{18}F-FDG PET/CT imaging to for staging.

Findings

Interpretation Known malignant lesion at right hilus together with metastatically involved lymph nodes at right paratracheal and supraclavicular lymph node stations.

Teaching Point Metastasis at supraclavicular lymph node makes the case inoperable by upstaging to stage IIIB, which is otherwise could be operated after neoadjuvant chemotherapy.

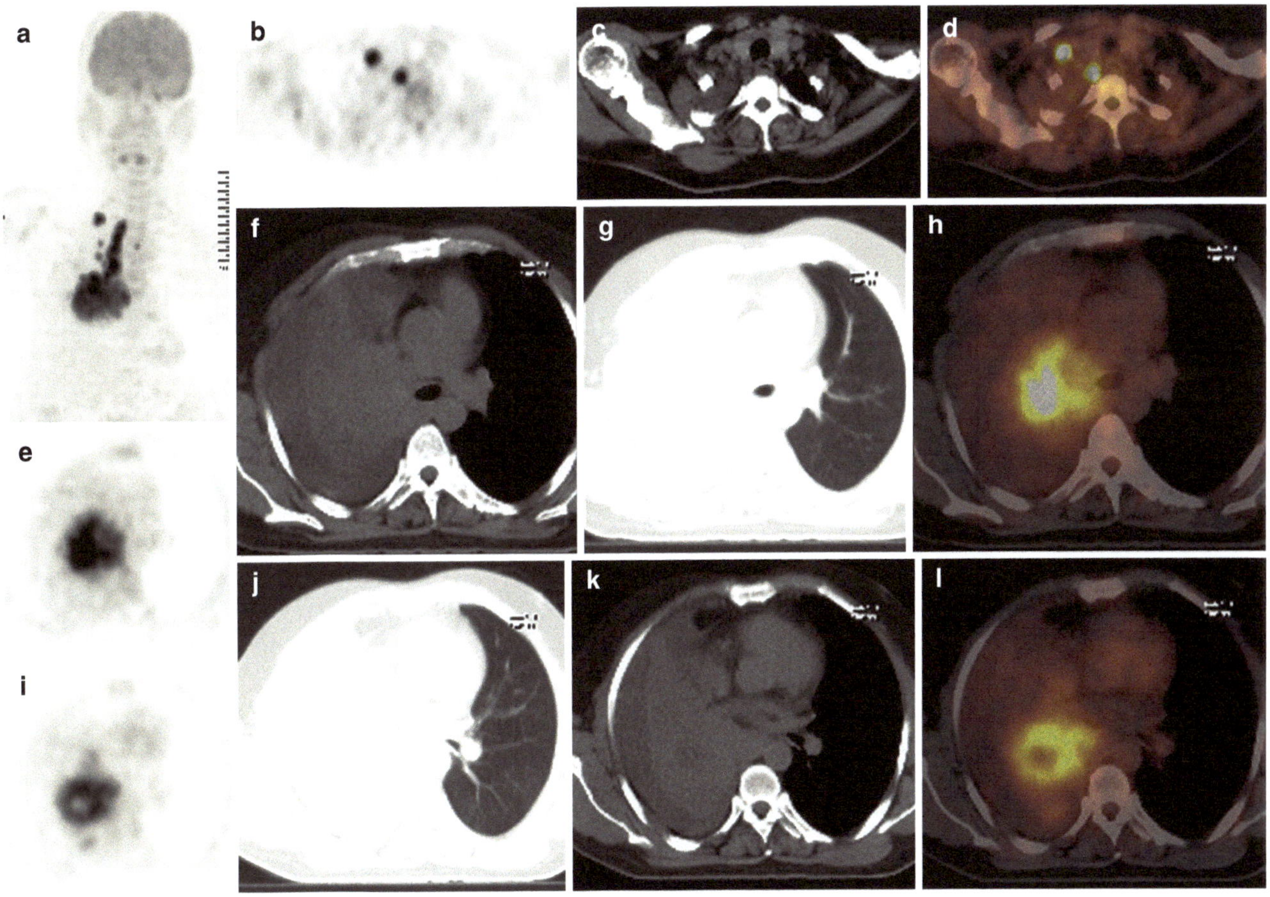

Fig. 5.16 At *upper row* MIP and axial slices of PET, CT, and fusion images show focal hypermetabolism at right supraclavicular area and hypermetabolic lymph nodes at lower and upper paratracheal area. At *middle* and *lower row* right hilar mass lesion showing intense FDG uptake is detected. Anterior to the mass lesion atelectasis due to compression of bronchus is also noted (**a–l**)

5.10 Case 10: Staging of Mesothelioma

History A 63-year-old male underwent ^{18}F-FDG PET/CT after having diagnosed as malignant mesothelioma following a biopsy from a mass lesion located at left parasternal region.

Findings

Interpretation Increased FDG uptake at left pleural thickening areas are consistent with primary malignant disease of pleura and a hypermetabolic retrocrural focus representing a lymph node with metastatic deposit. Hypermetabolic foci at iliac bone and ischium are compatible with metastases.

Teaching Point Although ^{18}F-FDG PET/CT does not identify the local extent of tumor or mediastinal nodal metastases reliably, it detects extrathoracic metastases, thereby obviating inappropriate thoracotomy. Detection of metastatically involved lymph nodes is crucial because patients with negative regional lymph nodes on multimodality imaging had a significantly better survival than patients with positive nodes.

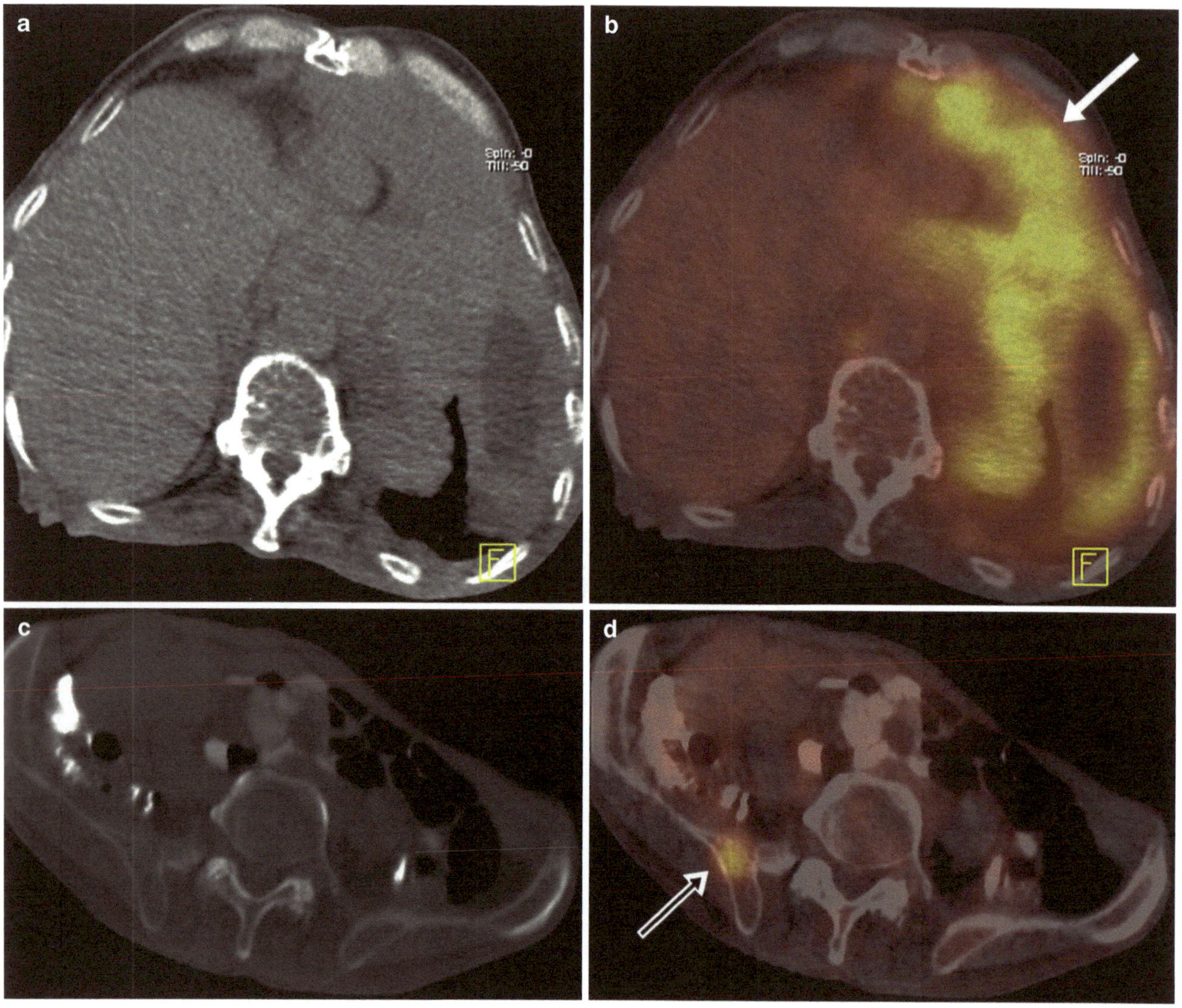

Fig. 5.17 Axial CT and fusion images shows diffuse and intensely increased FDG uptake corresponding the pleural thickening at left lung (*arrow*) which invades left costosternal junction and extends to subcutaneous fatty tissues (SUVmax 11), mildly hypermetabolic lymph node at right retrocrural area (**a**, **b**), and increased FDG uptake at right iliac bone (*arrow*) (**c**, **d**)

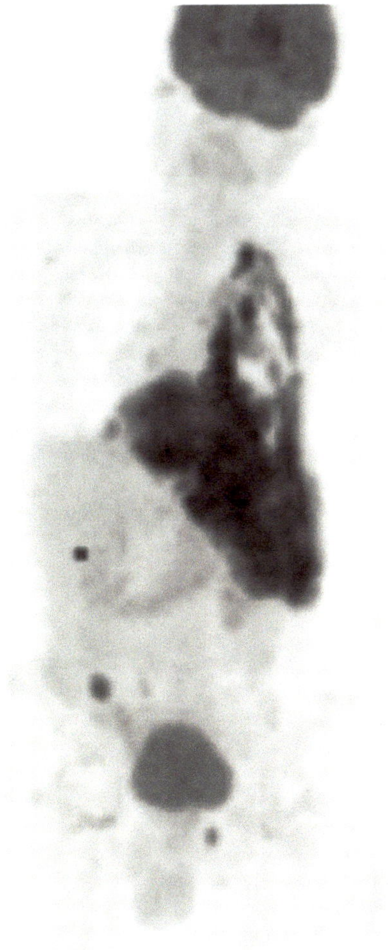

Fig. 5.18 MIP image showed intensely increased FDG uptake at left pleura, right iliac bone, and left ischium

5.11 Case 11: Pleural Mesothelioma with Synchronous Peritoneal Mesothelioma

History A 49-year-old female underwent ^{18}F-FDG PET/CT following a biopsy from umbilicus which revealed mesothelioma.

Findings

Interpretation Mesothelioma involving pleura and peritoneum synchronously.

Teaching Point Synchronous pleural malignant mesothelioma and peritoneal mesothelioma is a very rare finding.

a

b

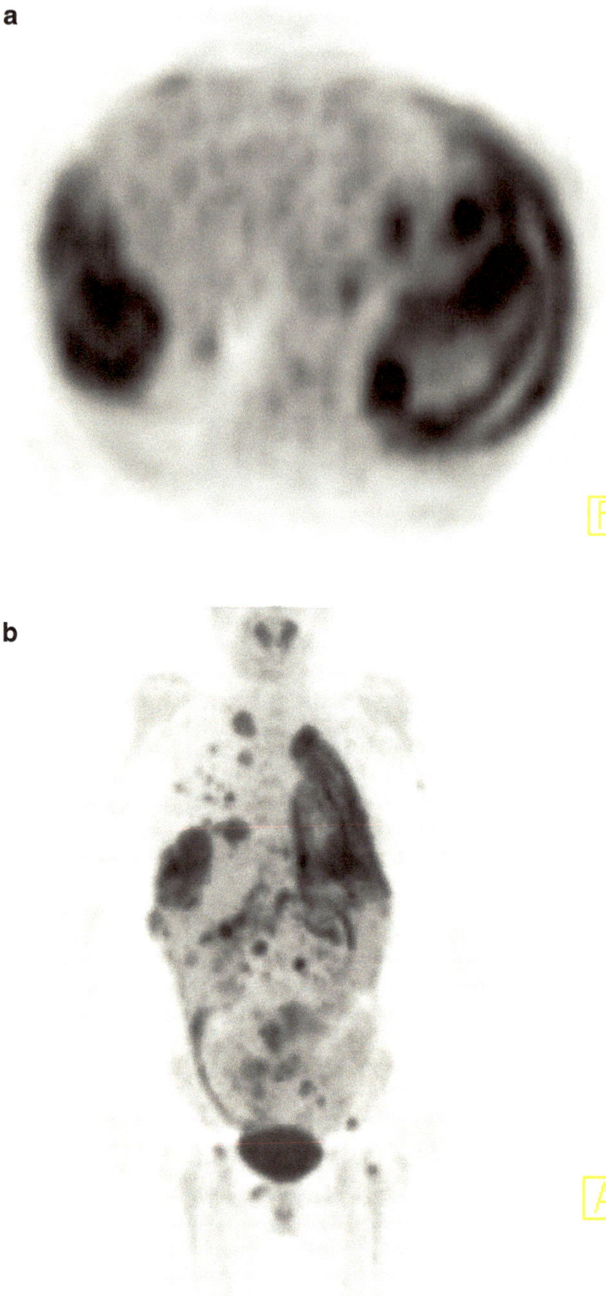

Fig. 5.19 Axial PET and MIP images show diffuse and intensely increased FDG uptake corresponding the pleural thickening at left lung (SUVmax 11.8), pleural involvement at right costophrenic sulcus, hypermetabolic nodules at right lung parenchyme, and increased FDG uptake at peritoneum (**a**, **b**)

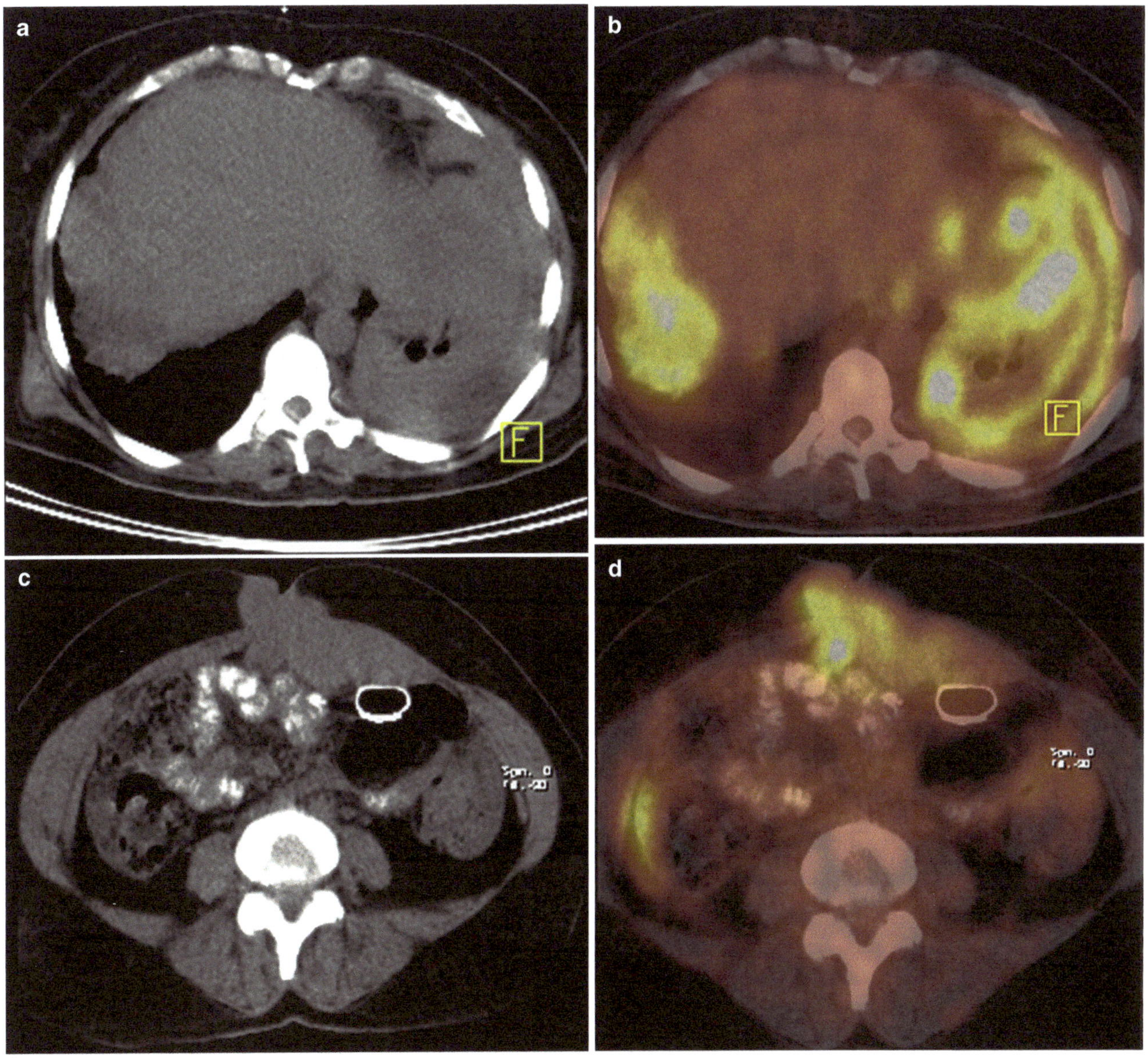

Fig. 5.20 Axial CT and fusion images show hypermetabolism at left pleural thickening and right costophrenic sulcus with possible invasion of liver (**a**, **b**) and intensely increased FDG uptake at peritoneal thickening invading anterior wall of abdomen (SUVmax 13) (**c**, **d**)

5.12 Case 12: Response to Therapy and Restaging in Mesothelioma

History A 36-year-old male underwent ^{18}F-FDG PET/CT after having diagnosed as malignant mesothelioma after a biopsy. Six months after the completion of chemotherapy he underwent second ^{18}F-FDG PET/CT imaging for evaluating therapy response and 10 months after this study, ^{18}F-FDG PET/CT scan was repeated for restaging purpose.

Findings

Interpretation Increased FDG uptake at left pleural thickening areas are compatible with primary malignant disease of pleura and there are metastatic nodules at right lung parenchyme. After therapy we observe disappearance of the right lung nodules and the decrease of the FDG uptake at left lung pleural thickening representing partial but not complete metabolic response. Last ^{18}F-FDG PET/CT shows progression of the disease.

Teaching Point FDG PET/CT showed 100 % sensitivity, 94.8 % in identifying malignant disease, which was confirmed by histopathologic examination in the diagnosis of pleural diseases. Reduction in FDG uptake in comparison with pretreatment values suggested response to chemotherapy.

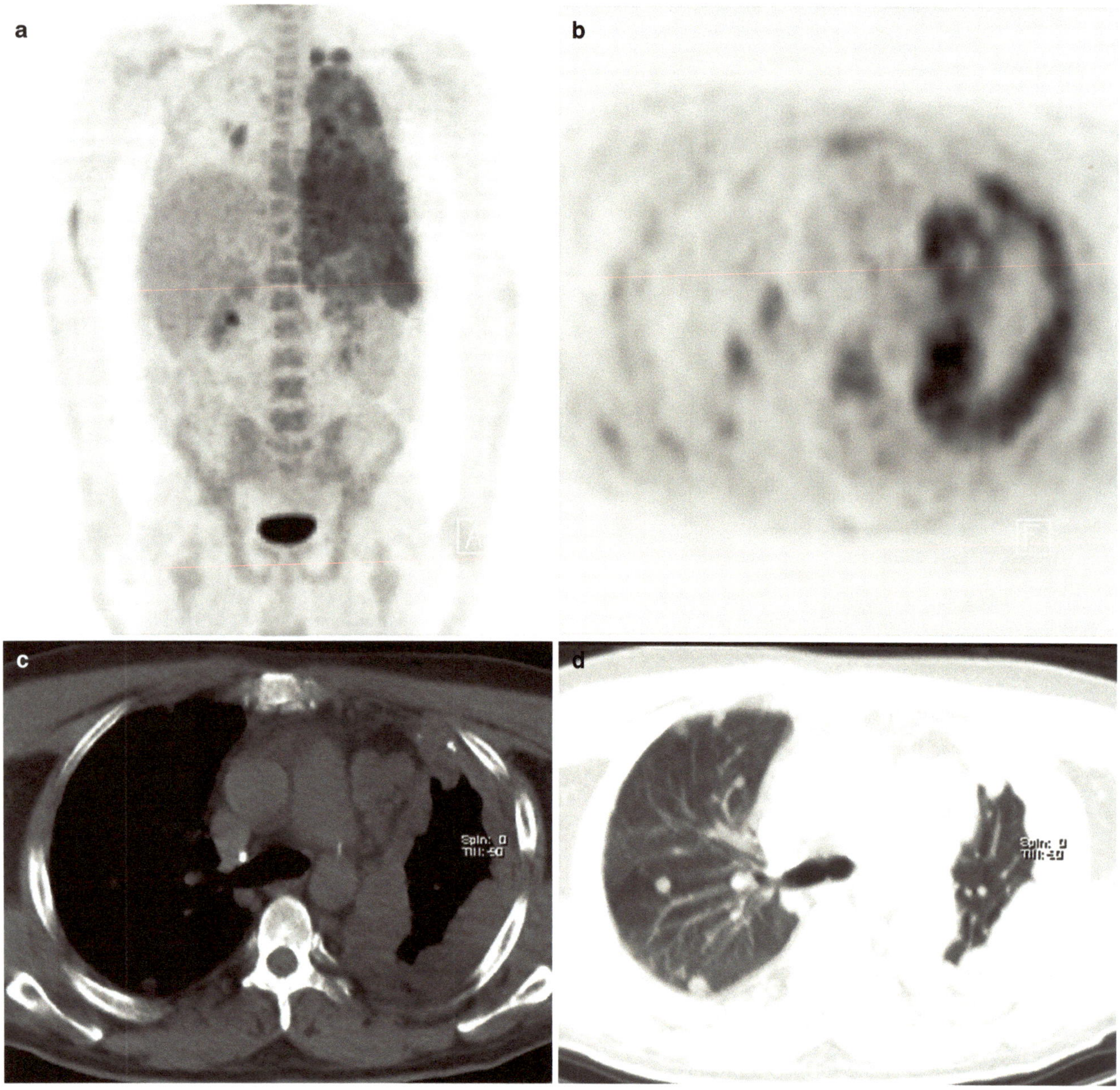

Fig. 5.21 Baseline ^{18}F-FDG PET/CT scan. MIP (**a**), axial PET (**b**), and CT (**c, d**) images show intensely increased FDG uptake at circumferential pleural thickening at left lung (SUVmax 6.6) and slightly hypermetabolic pulmonary nodules at right lung

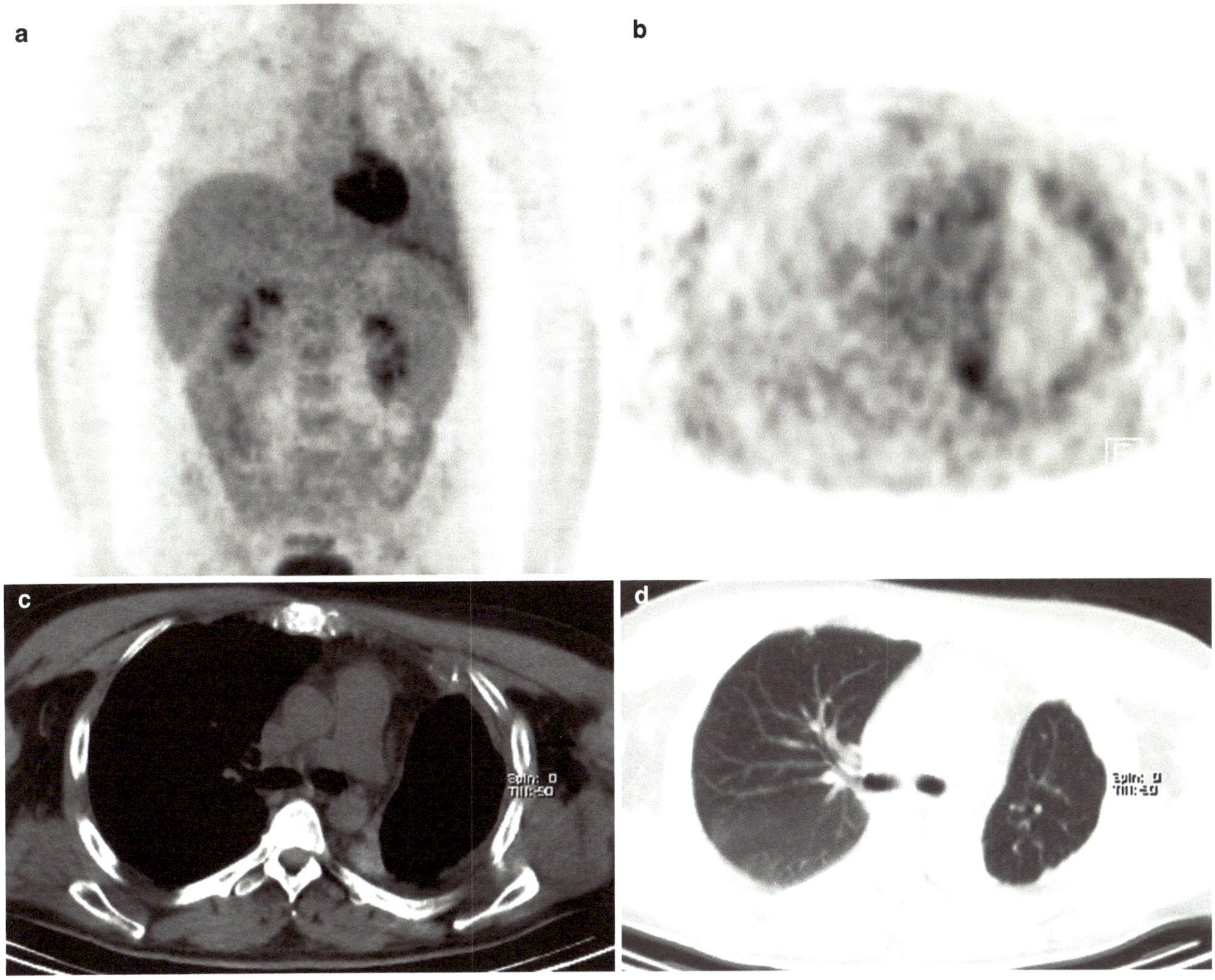

Fig. 5.22 ^{18}F-FDG PET/CT scan performed 6 months after chemotherapy. MIP (**a**), axial PET (**b**), and CT (**c**, **d**) images shows mildly increased FDG uptake at mediastinal and costal pleura of left lung (SUVmax 3.6) and clearance of hypermetabolic pulmonary nodules at right lung that were seen at previous study

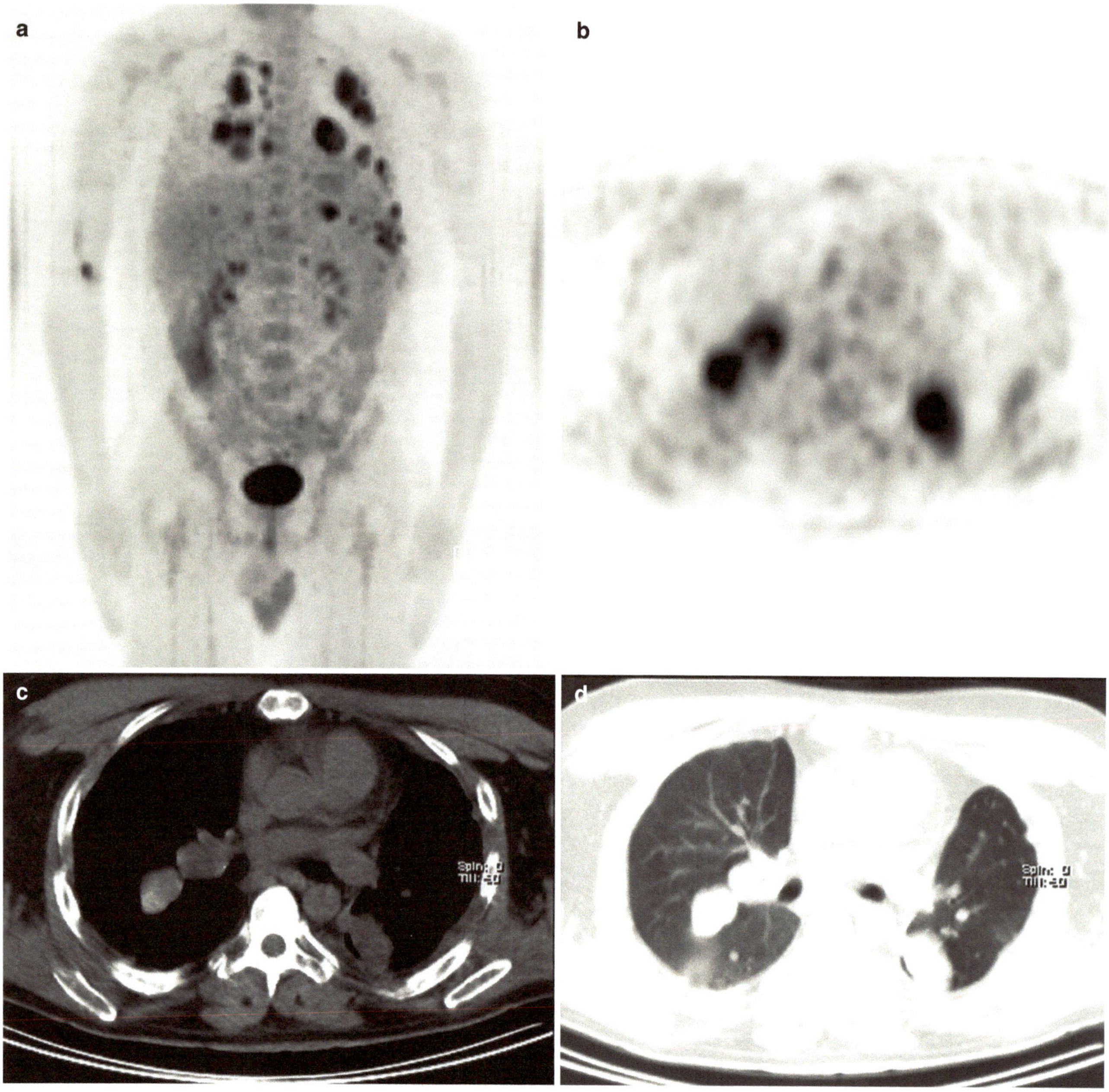

Fig. 5.23 ^{18}F-FDG PET/CT scan 10 months after second study. MIP (**a**), axial PET (**b**), and CT (**c**, **d**) images shows intensely increased FDG uptake (SUVmax 12) at newly developed multiple pulmonary nodules in the parenchyme of both lungs

Bibliography

1. Allard P, Yankaskas BC, Fletcher RH, Parker LA, Halvorsen RA. Sensitivity and specificity of computed tomography for the detection of adrenal metastatic lesions among 91 autopsied lung cancer patients. Cancer. 1990;66:457–62.
2. Carretta A, Landoni C, Melloni G, Ceresoli GL, Compierchio A, Fazio F, et al. 18-FDG positron emission tomography in the evaluation of malignant pleural diseases: a pilot study. Eur J Cardiothorac Surg. 2000;17:377–83.
3. Del Gobbo A, Fiori S, Gaudioso G, Bonaparte E, Tabano S, Palleschi A, et al. Synchronous pleural and peritoneal malignant mesothelioma: a case report and review of literature. Int J Clin Exp Pathol. 2014;7:2484–9.
4. Detterbeck FC, Falen S, Rivera MP, Halle JS, Socinski MA. Seeking a home for a PET, part 2: defining the appropriate place for positron emission tomography imaging in the staging of patients with suspected lung cancer. Chest. 2004;125:2300–8.
5. Flores RM, Akhurst T, Gonen M, Larson SM, Rusch VW. Positron emission tomography defines metastatic disease but not locoregional disease in patients with malignant pleural mesothelioma. J Thorac Cardiovasc Surg. 2003;126:11–6.
6. Orki A, Akin O, Tasci AE, Ciftci H, Urek S, Falay O, et al. The role of positron emission tomography/computed tomography. Thorac Cardiovasc Surg. 2009;57:217–21.
7. Özülker T, Özülker F, Eker Ö, Aydın T, Özpaçacı T. Tumor thrombus in inferior vena cava from renal cell carcinoma showing F-18 FDG uptake on positron emission tomography. Turk J Nucl Med. 2009;18:19–22.
8. Pieterman RM, van Putten JW, Meuzelaar JJ, Mooyaart EL, Vaalburg W, Koëter GH, et al. Preoperative staging of non-small-cell lung cancer with positron-emission tomography. N Engl J Med. 2000;343:254–61.
9. Silvestri GA, Gonzalez AV, Jantz MA, Margolis ML, Gould MK, Tanoue LT, et al. Methods for staging non-small cell lung cancer: diagnosis and management of lung cancer, 3rd ed: American College of Chest Physicians evidence-based clinical practice guidelines. Chest. 2013;143 Suppl 5:211–50. doi:10.1378/chest.12-2355.
10. Stone WZ, Wymer DC, Canales BK. Fluorodeoxyglucose-positron-emission tomography/computed tomography imaging for adrenal masses in patients with lung cancer: review and diagnostic algorithm. J Endourol. 2014;28:104–11. doi:10.1089/end.2013.0380.
11. Sugarbaker DJ, Strauss GM, Lynch TJ, Richards W, Mentzer SJ, Lee TH, et al. Node status has prognostic significance in the multimodality therapy of diffuse, malignant mesothelioma. J Clin Oncol. 1993;11:1172–8.
12. Wu L, Xu Z, Zhao X, Li J, Zhong L, Pang T, et al. Surgical treatment of lung cancer invading the left atrium or base of the pulmonary vein. World J Surg. 2009;33:492–6. doi:10.1007/s00268-008-9873-5.
13. Zarogoulidis P, Terzi E, Kouliatsis G, Zervas V, Kontakiotis T, Mitrakas A, et al. Subclavian thrombosis in a patient with advanced lung cancer: a case report. J Med Case Rep. 2011;5:173. doi:10.1186/1752-1947-5-173.

6 Breast Cancer

6.1 Case 1: Initial Evaluation of Breast Mass with ^{18}F-FDG PET/CT

History A 48-year-old female underwent ^{18}F-FDG PET/CT after suspicious mass lesion at left breast was detected on thorax CT and USG.

Findings

Interpretation Intense FDG uptake at left breast mass lesions is indicative of malignant disease of breast and hypermetabolic foci at left axilla and retroclavicular region reflect metastatically involved lymph nodes.

Result Biopsy of the mass lesion at left breast turned out to be invasive ductal carcinoma.

Teaching Point ^{18}F-FDG PET/CT has high specificity in the detection of metastatic axillary lymph nodes, but sensitivity is not satisfactory especially in lymph nodes with low tumor burden. So ^{18}F-FDG PET/CT may preclude axillary dissection with sentinel lymph node mapping when FDG positive lymph nodes are detected.

T. Özülker, F. Özülker, *Atlas of PET-CT Imaging in Oncology: A Case-Based Guide to Image Interpretation*,
DOI 10.1007/978-3-319-18994-9_6

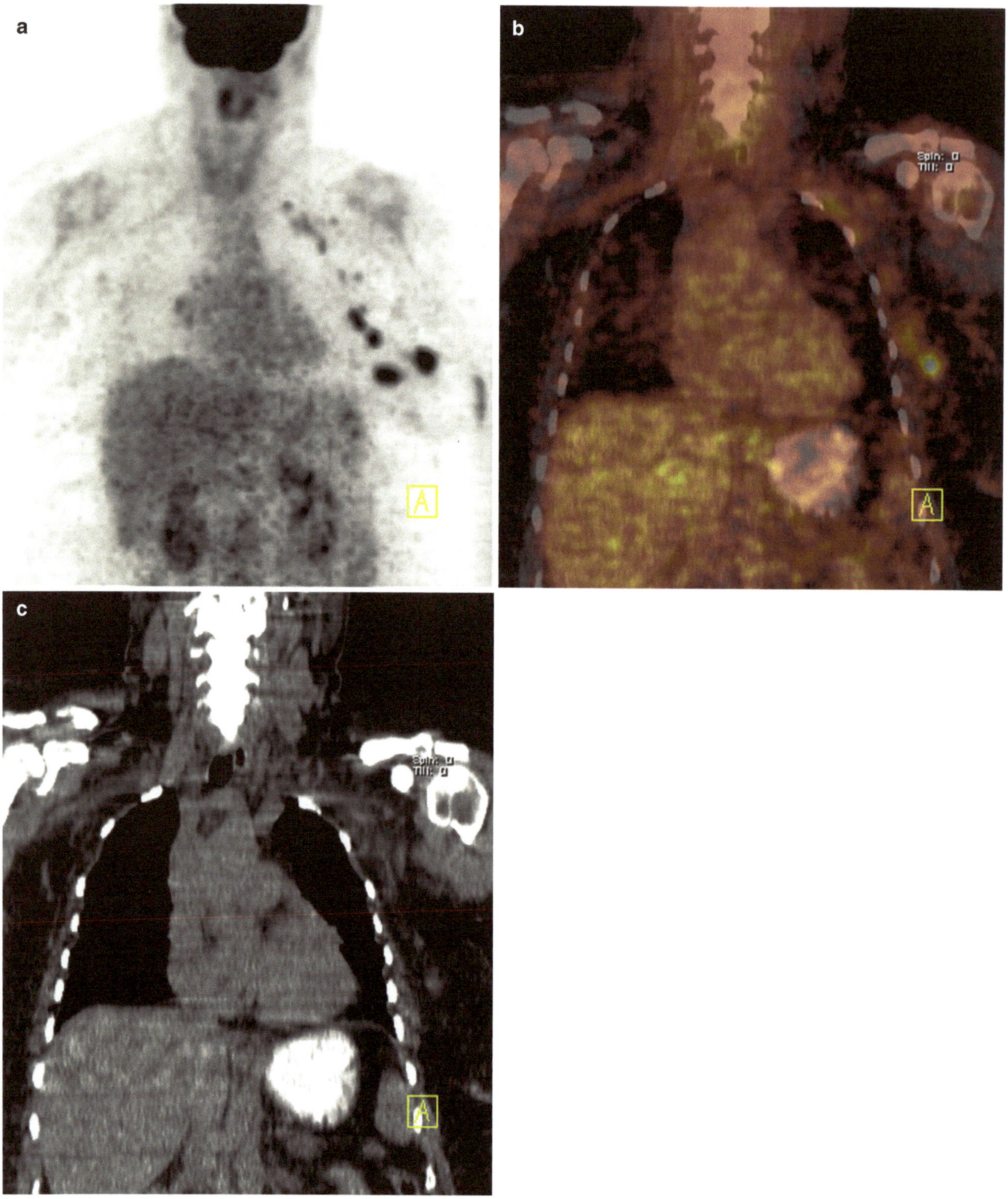

Fig. 6.1 MIP image (**a**), coronal fusion, and CT images (**b**, **c**) show two intensely hypermetabolic foci at lateral aspect of left breast corresponding to mass lesions on CT (SUVmax 9.7). There are also lymph nodes at left axillary fossa and left retroclavicular region showing significant FDG uptake (SUVmax 7.9)

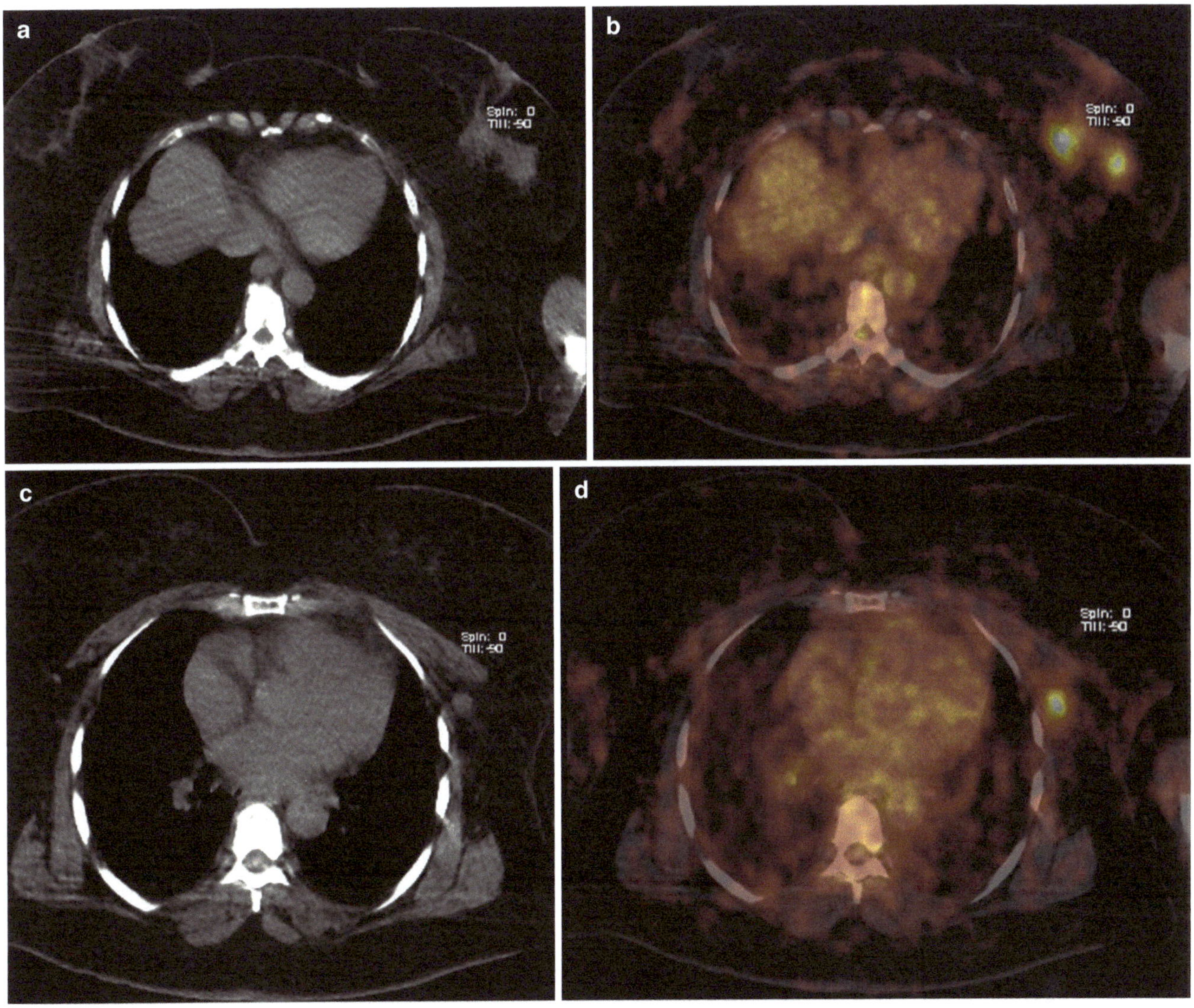

Fig. 6.2 Axial slices of CT and fusion images (**a–d**) show mass lesions at left breast and lymph nodes at left axillary fossa which show increased FDG uptake

6.2 Case 2: Invasive Ductal Carcinoma and Fibroadenoma

History A 26-year-old female status post biopsy proven to be invasive ductal carcinoma at right breast and fibroadenoma at left breast underwent ^{18}F-FDG PET/CT for pretreatment staging.

Findings

Interpretation Intense FDG uptake at right breast mass lesion is indicative of a malignant disease, whereas mild uptake at left breast mass lesion is suggestive for a benign lesion but malignancy cannot be ruled out.

Result Histopathology revealed invasive ductal carcinoma at right breast and fibroadenoma at left breast.

Teaching Point ^{18}F-FDG PET/CT has good sensitivity in detecting invasive ductal carcinomas. Benign neoplasms like ductal adenoma, fibrous dysplasia, and fibroadenomas may give false positive results and should be taken into account while evaluating breast lesions. Low levels of SUVmax at benign lesions might help to discriminate them from malignancies.

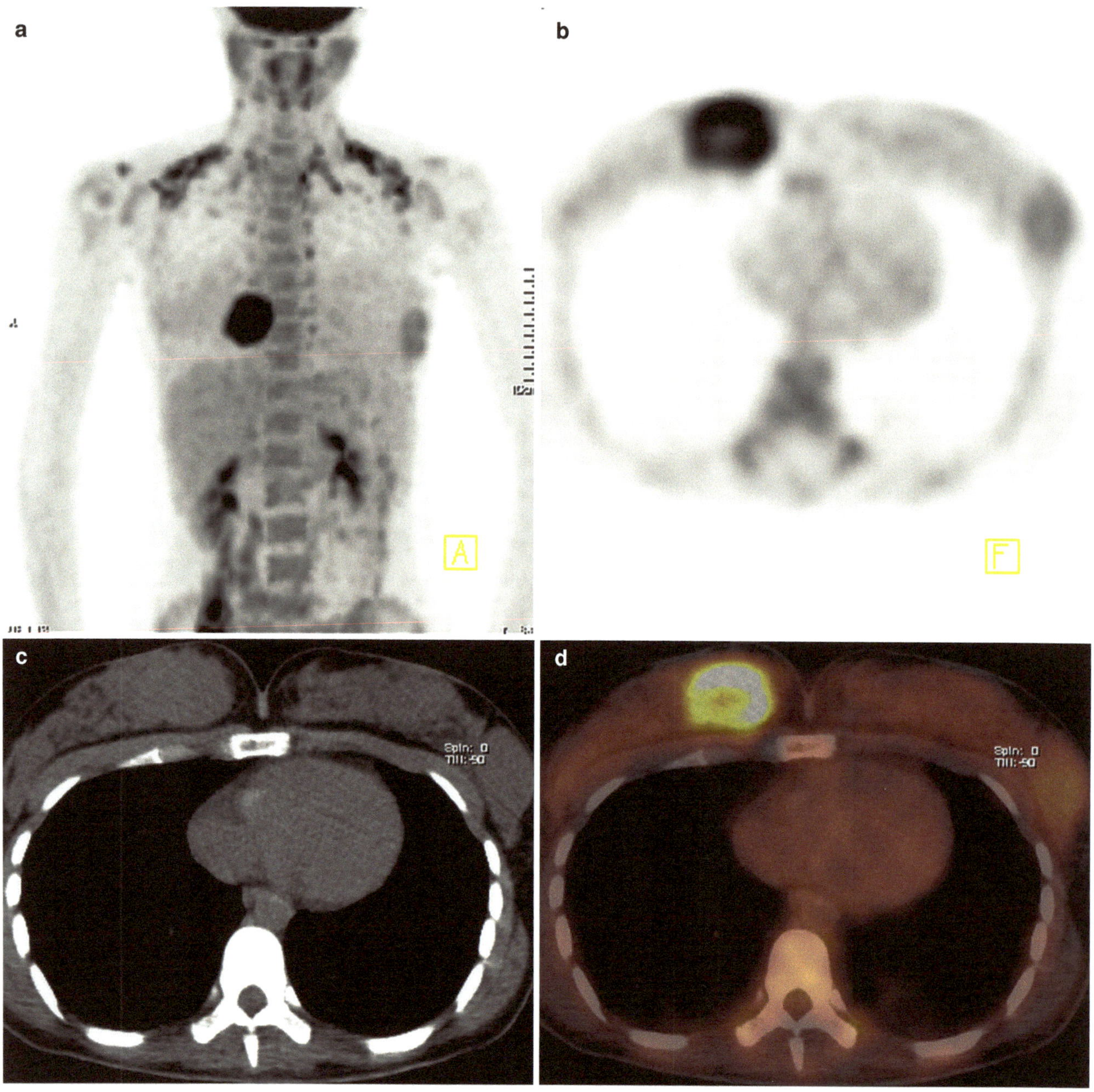

Fig. 6.3 MIP image (**a**), axial slices of PET, CT, and fusion images (**b**, **c**, **d**) show intensely hypermetabolic round mass lesion at right breast measuring 5.7×5 cm and having hypometabolic necrotic center (SUVmax 10). There is also another mass lesion located laterally at left breast measuring 4×4 cm and showing mild FDG uptake (SUVmax 3). Increased FDG uptake at supraclavicular and paravertebral areas representing uptake at brown adipose tissue (BAT) is also noted

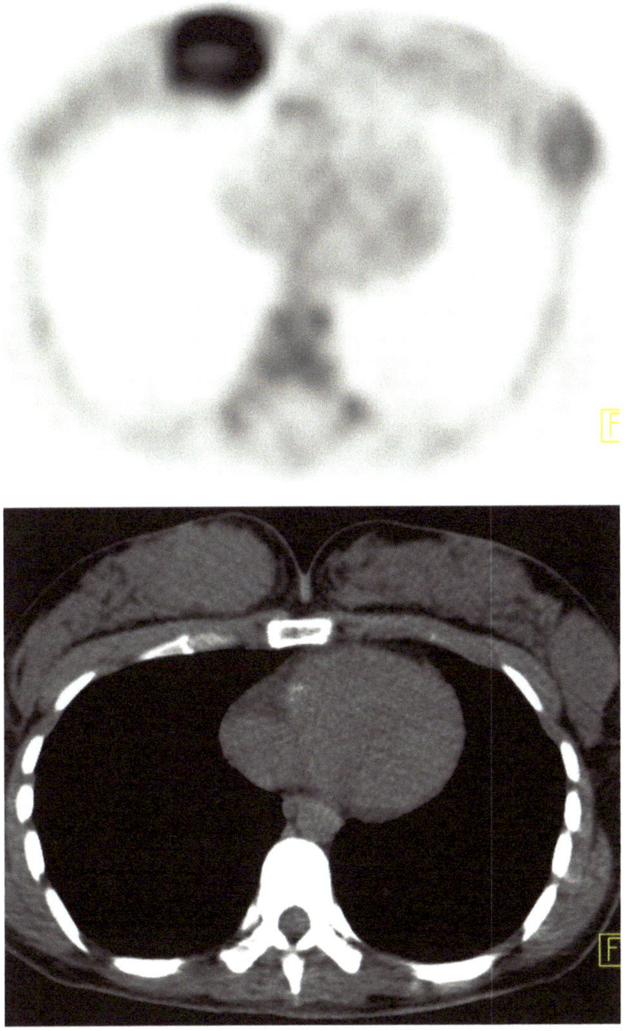

Fig. 6.4 Axial PET and CT images

6.3 Case 3: Pretreatment Staging in Locally Advanced Breast Cancer

History A 52-year-old female with right sided locally advanced breast cancer (LABC) (invasive ductal carcinoma) underwent ^{18}F-FDG PET/CT for pretreatment staging.

Findings

Interpretation Hypermetabolic mass lesion at right breast is consistent with primary malignant disease of breast. There is metastatic involvement of right axillary lymph nodes, metastatic deposits at liver, pelvic bones, and both femurs.

Teaching Point According to NCCN guideline, ^{18}F-FDG PET CT is most helpful in situations where standard staging studies are equivocal or suspicious and it may also be helpful in identifying unsuspected regional nodal disease and/or distant metastases in LABC when used in addition to standard staging studies. However, there are studies claiming that ^{18}F-FDG PET CT should be a substitute rather than an additional imaging procedure in staging of LABC, depending on the fact that it can change the clinical stage in approximately half of the patients.

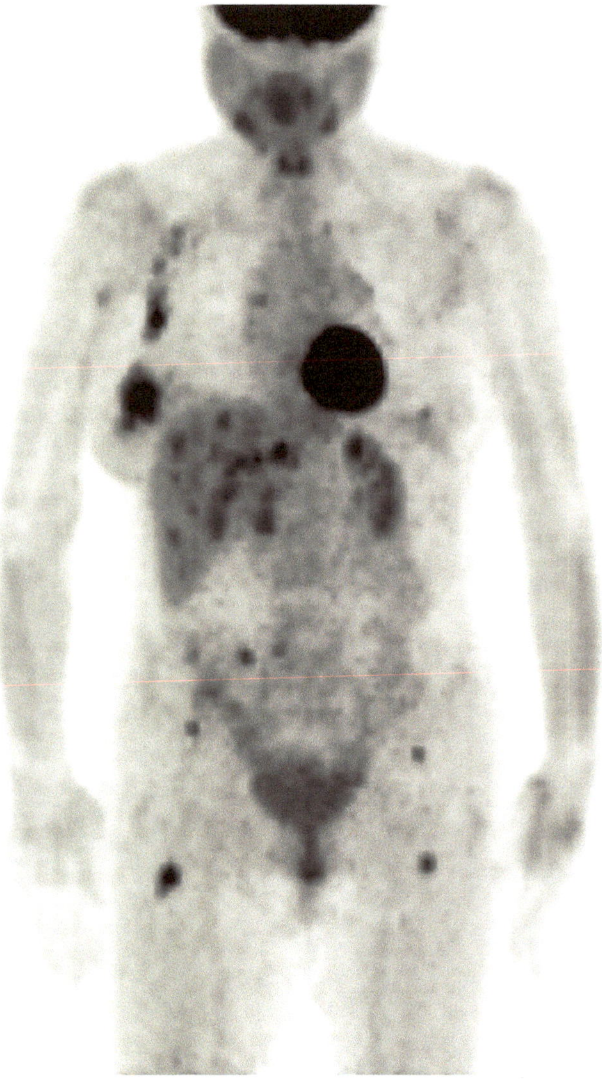

Fig. 6.5 MIP image shows intensely hypermetabolic lesion at right breast, hypermetabolic right axillary lymph nodes, multiple hypermetabolic foci at liver, hypermetabolic lesions at pelvic bones and both proximal femurs

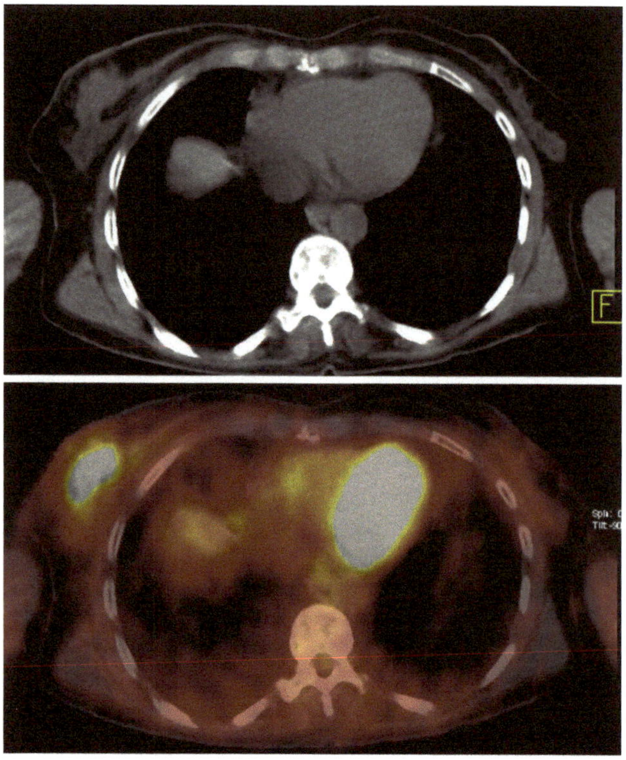

Fig. 6.6 Axial slices of CT and fusion images show pathologically increased FDG uptake at right sided breast lesion

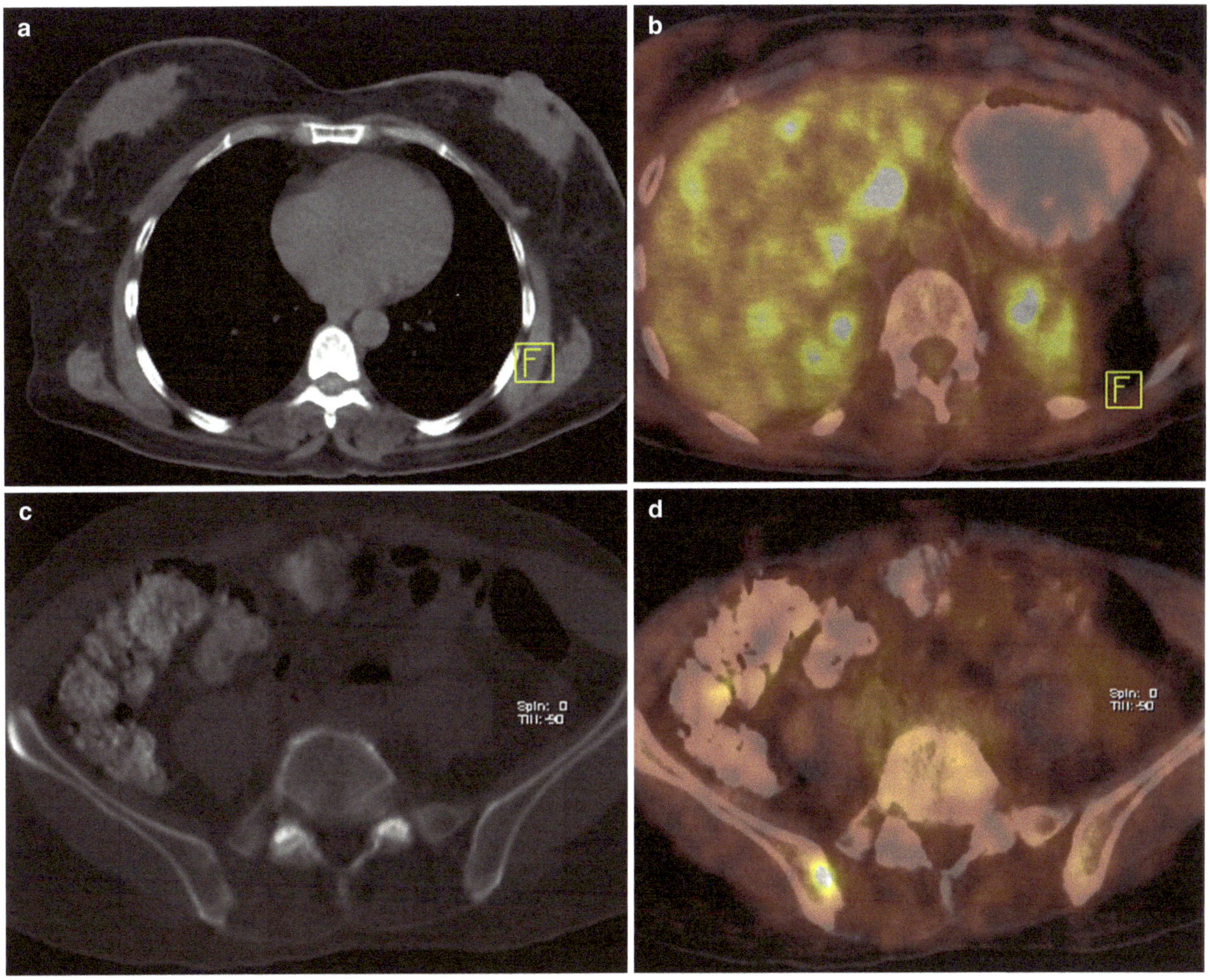

Fig. 6.7 Axial slices of CT and fusion (**a**–**d**) images demonstrate multiple hypermetabolic foci at both lobes of liver and hypermetabolic focus located at right posterior iliac bone

6.4 Case 4: Monitoring Response to Therapy in Breast Cancer

History A 60-year-old female status post biopsy proven to be invasive ductal carcinoma at left and right breast underwent ^{18}F-FDG PET/CT for pretreatment staging. Six months after the completion of chemotherapy PET/CT study was repeated for the evaluation of chemotherapy response.

Findings

Interpretation Hypermetabolic lesions at both breasts are compatible with primary malignant disease and increased FDG uptake at axillary lymph nodes and bony structures represent metastatic lesions. Clearance of all pathological FDG accumulations in the second study reflects complete response to therapy.

Teaching Point ^{18}F-FDG PET/CT is effective in assessment of therapy response during induction therapy for advanced disease and neoadjuvant chemotherapy. ^{18}F-FDG PET/CT also differentiates responders from nonresponders early in the course of therapy. After the first course, all responders can be correctly identified with a sensitivity of 100 % and a specificity of 85 % by a standardized uptake value decrease below 55 % of the baseline scan.

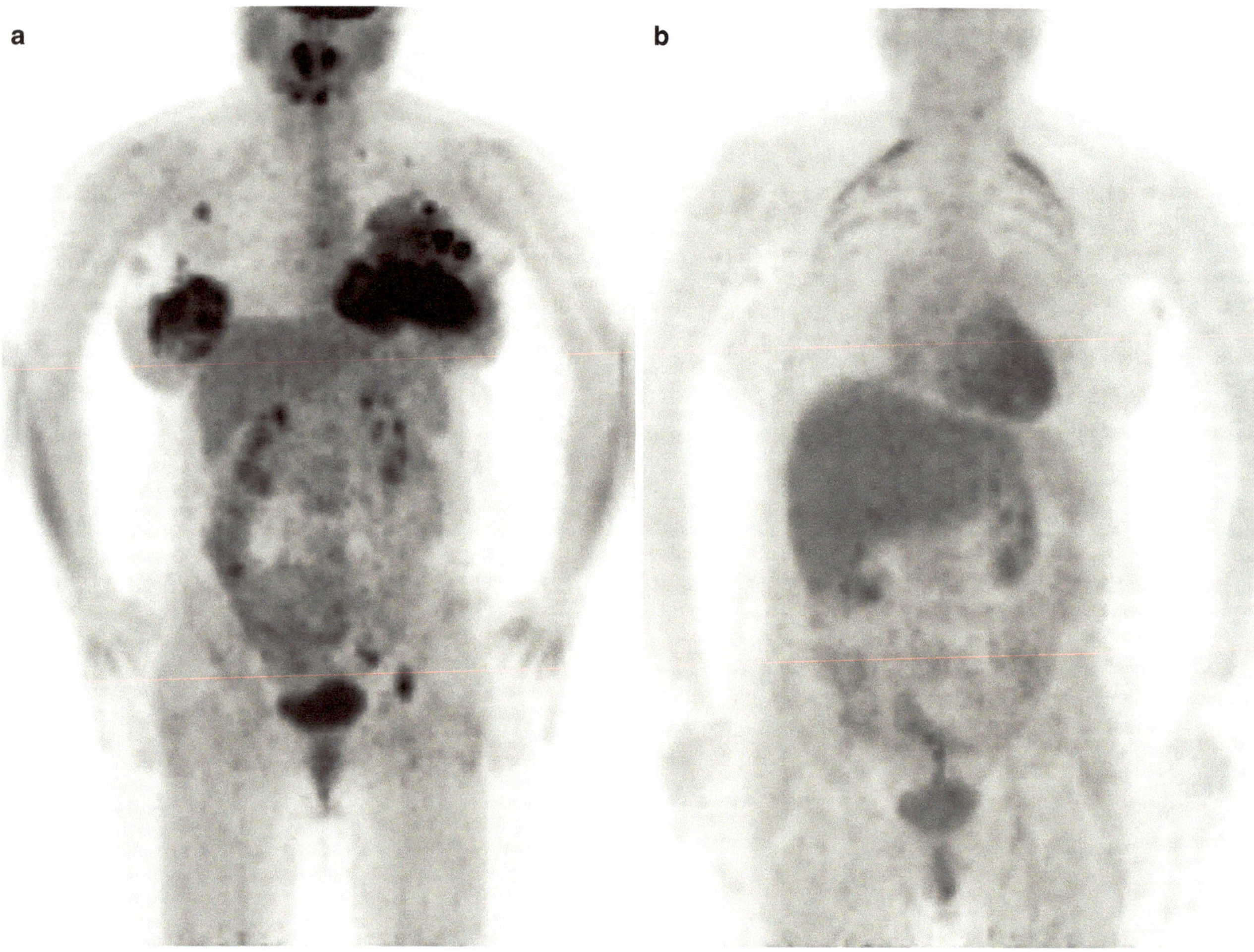

Fig. 6.8 MIP images before (**a**), and after (**b**) chemotherapy. First study shows intensely hypermetabolic lesions at right (SUVmax 7.4) and left (SUVmax 13.8) breasts being more prominent at left. There are also pathologically increased FDG uptake sites at sternum, left 7th rib, and left acetabulum. Hypermetabolic lymph nodes at both axillary fossa is seen. There is no pathologically increased FDG uptake at second study

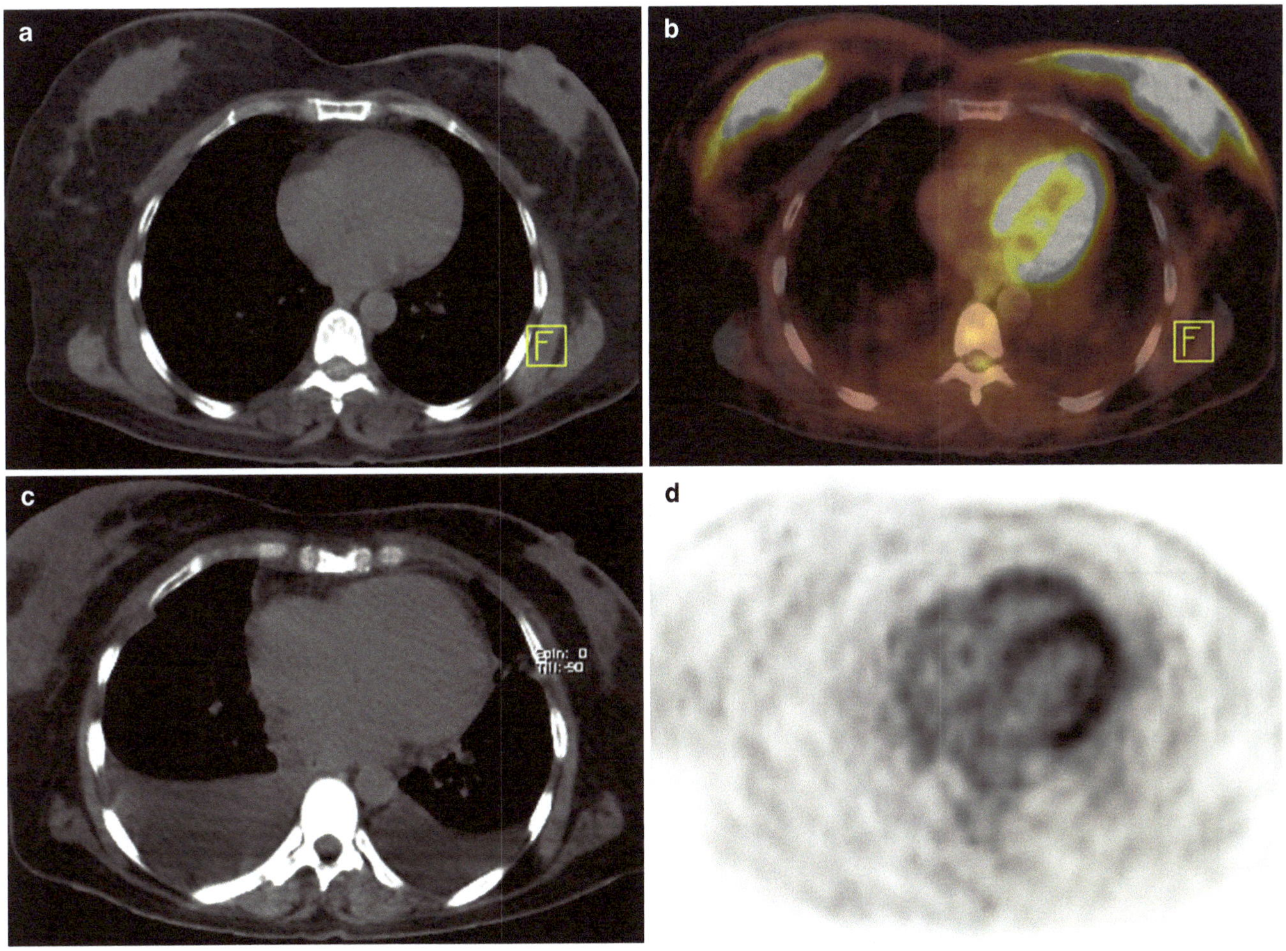

Fig. 6.9 Axial slices of CT and fusion (**a**, **b**), CT and PET (**c**, **d**) images show pathologically increased FDG uptake at both breasts and resolution of the activities after chemotherapy

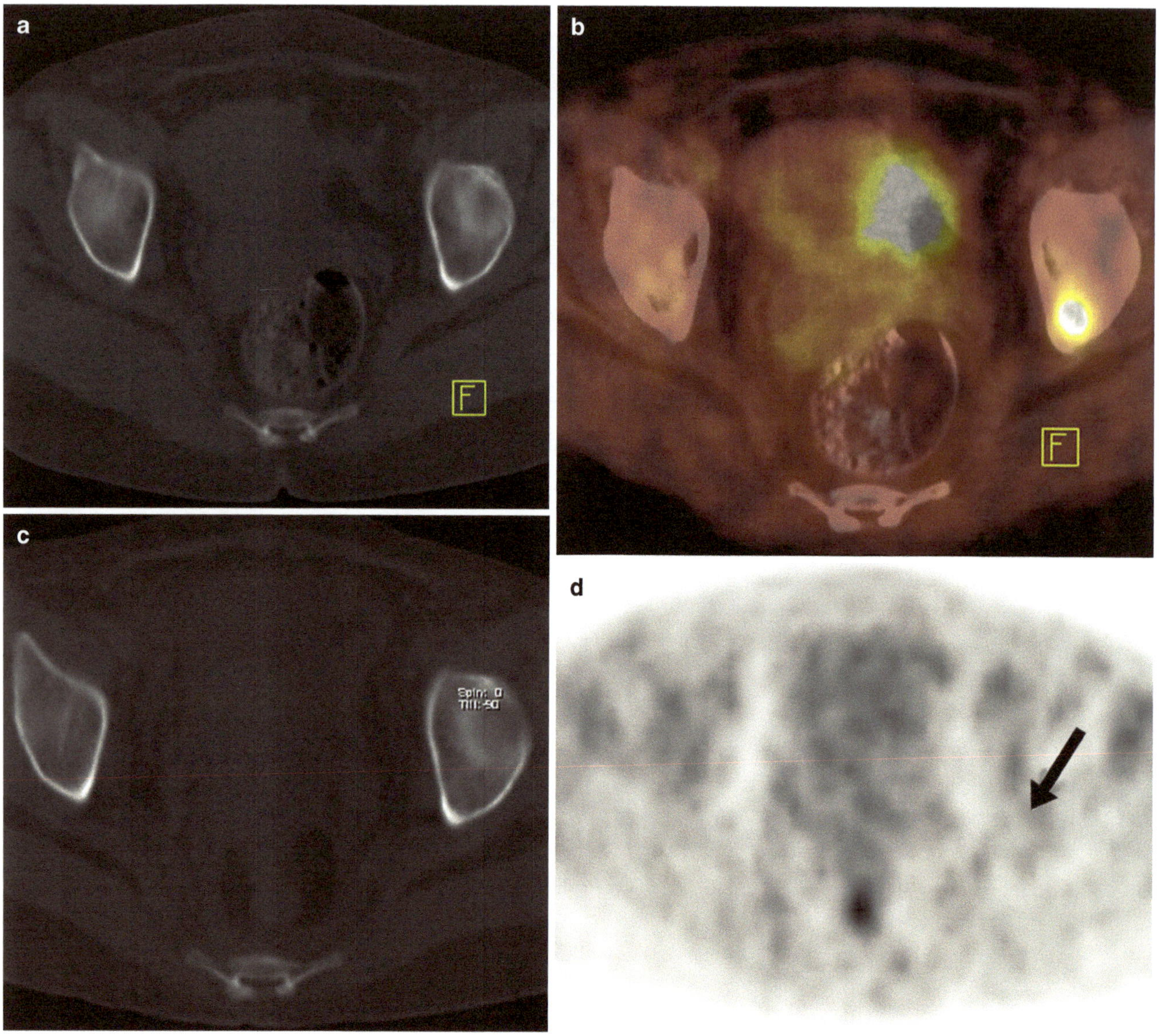

Fig. 6.10 Axial slices of CT and fusion (**a**, **b**), CT and PET (**c**, **d**) images show hypermetabolic focus at left acetabulum and clearance of the activity after therapy (*arrow*)

6.5 Case 5: Male Breast Cancer

History A 47-year-old male patient who has been followed up with the diagnosis of male breast cancer (invasive carcinoma) for 3 years underwent ^{18}F-FDG PET/CT for restaging.

Findings

Interpretation Hypermetabolic lesions at bony structures are compatible with widespread metastases.

Teaching Point Breast cancer in men is a rare disease. Less than 1 % of all breast cancers occur in men. Most tumors are detected at more advanced stages than in women. FDG PET/CT is a powerful imaging method to perform staging, restaging, and treatment response assessment in male patients with breast cancer. Sensitivity and specificity of FDG PET/CT to detect distant metastases are 100 % and 67 %.

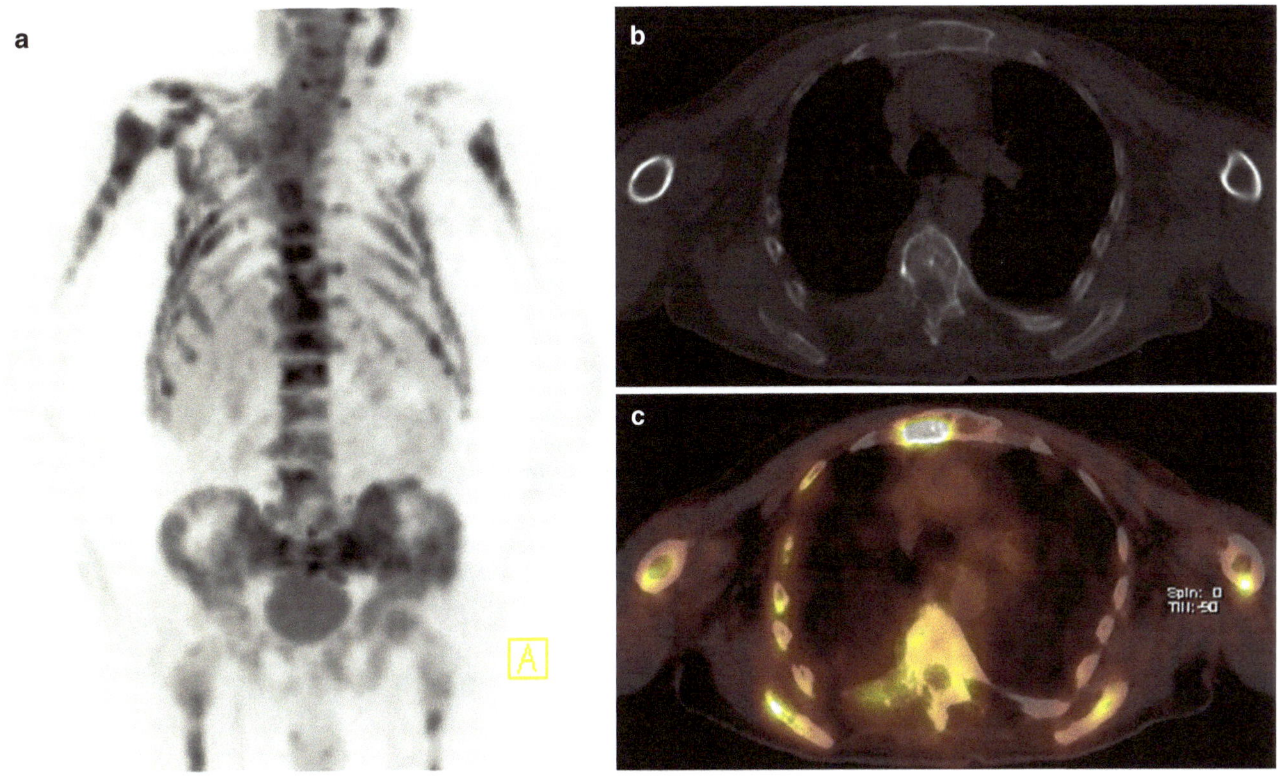

Fig. 6.11 MIP (**a**), axial slices of CT and fusion (**b**, **c**) images show heterogenously increased FDG uptake at axial and appendicular skeleton

6.6 Case 6: Bilateral Ovarian Metastases From Breast Cancer

History A 39-year-old female patient who has been followed up with the diagnosis of breast cancer (invasive ductal carcinoma) for 6 years underwent ^{18}F-FDG PET/CT for restaging.

Findings

Interpretation Hypermetabolic lesions at both ovaries may represent primary ovarian malignancy or metastatic lesions.

Result The patient underwent surgical resection of lesions at both ovaries and the histopathology revealed metastasis from breast cancer.

Teaching Point Breast cancers may be associated with ovarian metastases and surgical resection may increase survival. While interpreting PET studies it must be kept in mind that bilateral physiological ovarian FDG uptake may simulate malignancy.

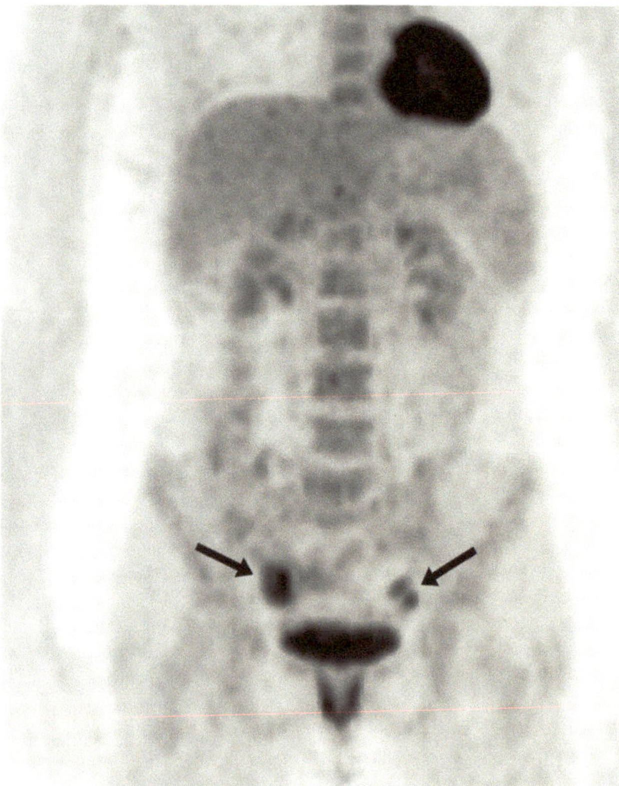

Fig. 6.12 MIP image shows bilateral increased FDG uptake at both adnexa (*arrows*)

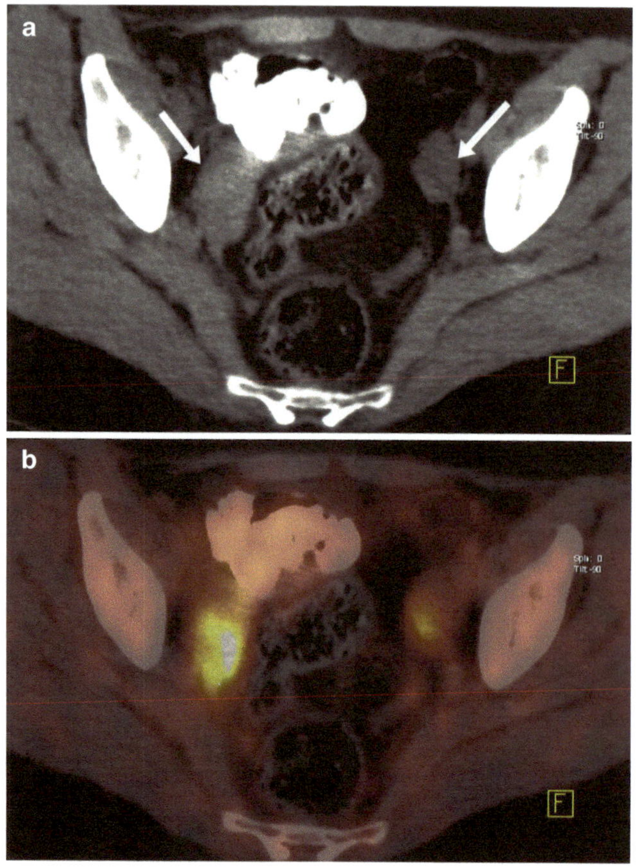

Fig. 6.13 Axial slices of CT and fusion (**a**, **b**) images show significantly increased FDG uptake at both ovaries being more prominent at right (*arrows*)

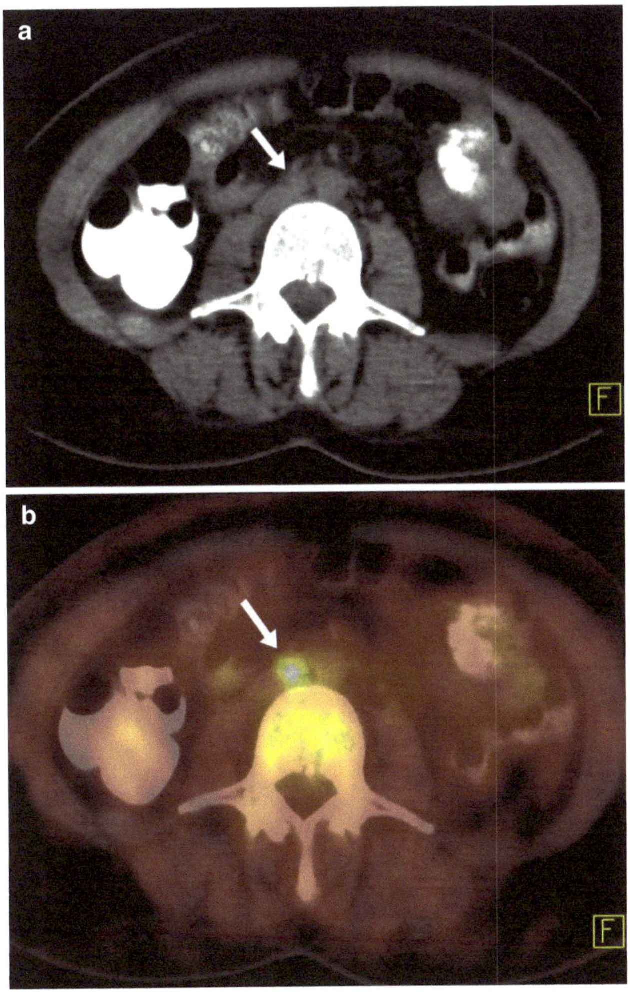

Fig. 6.14 Axial slices of CT and fusion (**a**, **b**) images show hypermetabolic focus at interaortocaval area (*arrow*)

Bibliography

1. Avril N, Rosé CA, Schelling M, Dose J, Kuhn W, Bense S, et al. Breast imaging with positron emission tomography and fluorine-18 fluorodeoxyglucose: use and limitations. Clin Oncol. 2000;18: 3495–502.
2. Bigorie V, Morice P, Duvillard P, Antoine M, Cortez A, Flejou JF, et al. Ovarian metastases from breast cancer: report of 29 cases. Cancer. 2010;116:799–804. doi:10.1002/cncr.24807.
3. Groheux D, Giacchetti S, Delord M, Hindié E, Vercellino L, Cuvier C, et al. ^{18}F-FDG PET/CT in staging patients with locally advanced or inflammatory breast cancer: comparison to conventional staging. Nucl Med. 2013;54:5–11. doi:10.2967/jnumed.112.106864.
4. Groheux D, Hindié E, Marty M, Espié M, Rubello D, Vercellino L, et al. ^{18}F-FDG-PET/CT in staging, restaging, and treatment response assessment of male breast cancer. Eur J Radiol. 2014;83:1925–33. doi:10.1016/j.ejrad.2014.05.037.
5. NCCN Clinical Practice Guidelines in Oncology (NCCN Guidelines): breastcancer—version 3.2012. National Comprehensive Cancer Network Web site. http://www.nccn.org/professionals/physician_gls/pdf/breast.pdf. Accessed 15 Nov 2012.
6. Schelling M, Avril N, Nährig J, Kuhn W, Römer W, Sattler DJ, et al. Positron emission tomography using [(18)F]Fluorodeoxyglucose for monitoring primary chemotherapy in breast cancer. Clin Oncol. 2000;18:1689–95.

7 Lymphoma

7.1 Case 1: Staging of Anaplastic Large Cell Lymphoma

History A 49-year-old male underwent ^{18}F-FDG PET/CT after having diagnosed as anaplastic lymphoma kinase (ALK) negative anaplastic large cell lymphoma (ALCL) following a biopsy from a lesion located at left inguinal area.

Findings

Interpretation Hypermetabolism at lymph nodes, liver, spleen, vertebral colon, and pelvic bones is compatible with multiple metastases.

Teaching Point ALCL is a rare type of non-Hodgkin lymphoma (NHL). It is divided into two entities according to the expression of ALK. It is an FDG avid malignancy and ALK expression is related to higher FDG uptake. ALK-positive patients tend to have better progression free survival than ALK-negative patients.

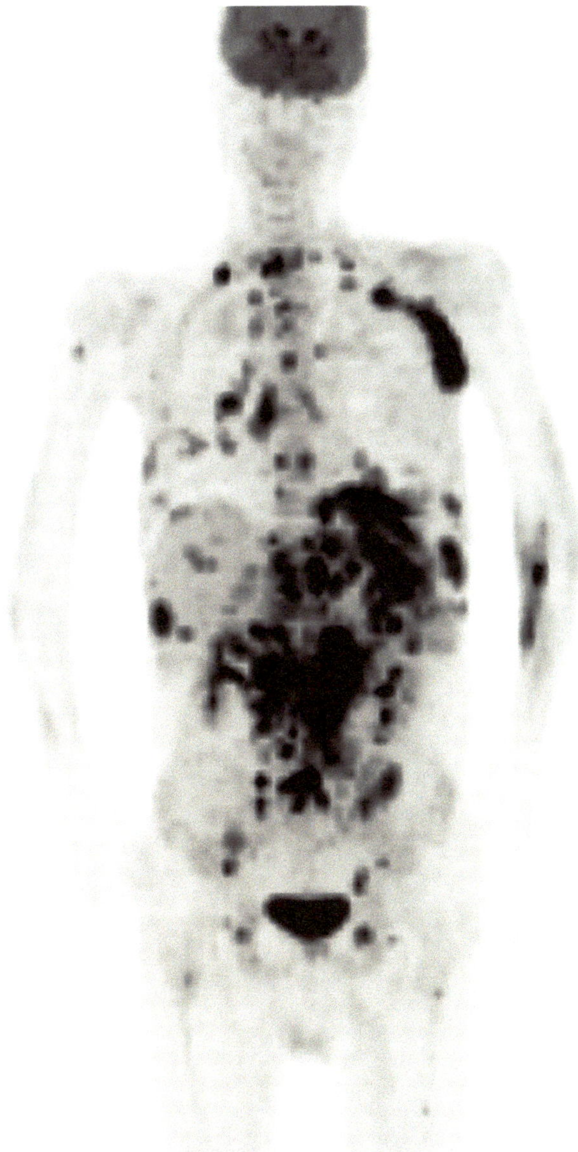

Fig. 7.1 MIP image shows intensely increased FDG uptake at cervical jugular, mediastinal, and intraabdominal lymph nodes (SUVmax 10); hypermetabolic foci at liver and spleen (SUVmax 9); multiple hypermetabolic foci at vertebral colon and pelvic bones

T. Özülker, F. Özülker, *Atlas of PET-CT Imaging in Oncology: A Case-Based Guide to Image Interpretation*,
DOI 10.1007/978-3-319-18994-9_7

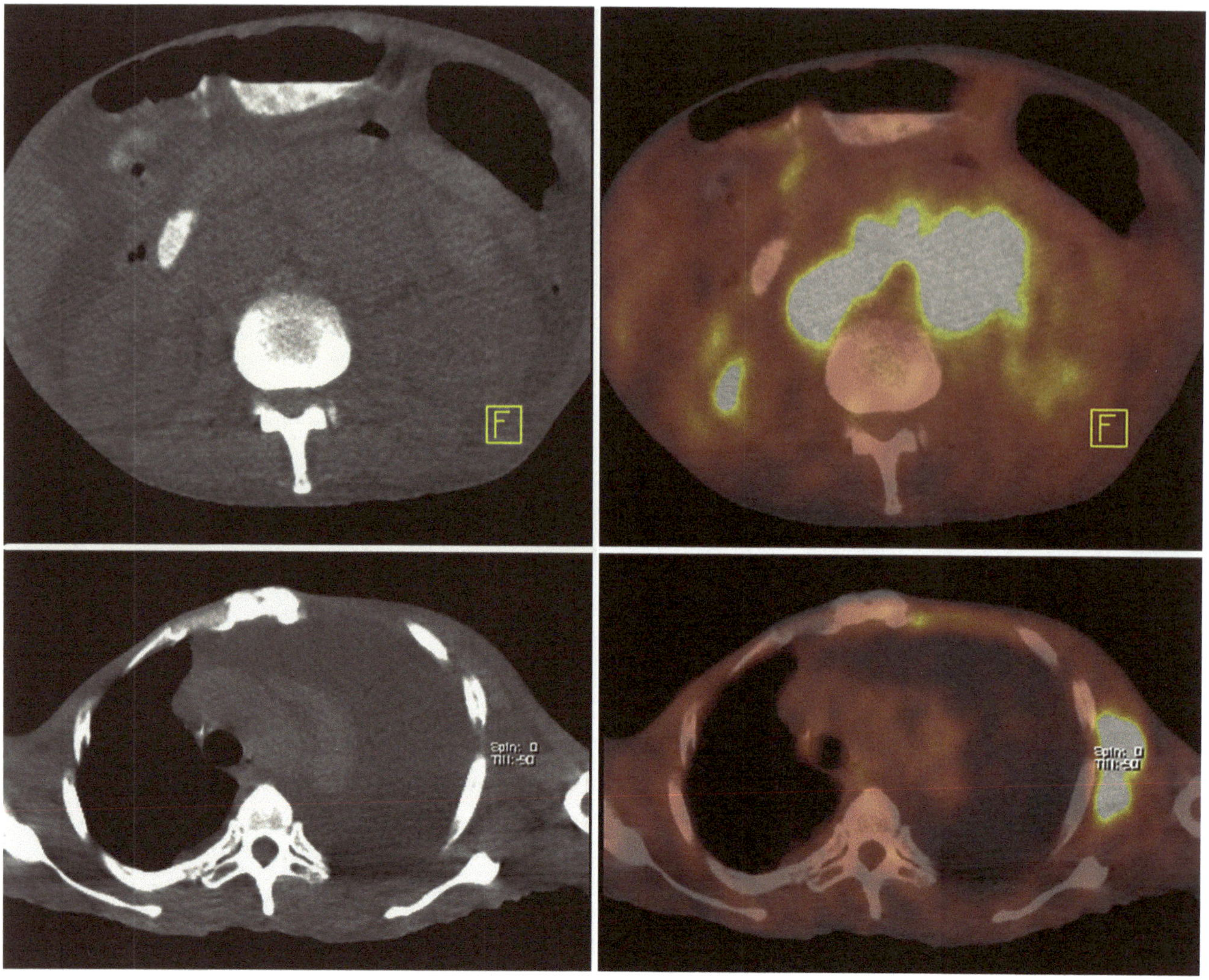

Fig. 7.2 Axial CT and fusion images show intensely hypermetabolic lymph nodes at paraaortic, interaortocaval, and left axillary fossa lymph node stations

7.2 Case 2: Staging of non-Hodgkin Lymphoma

History A 72-year-old male underwent ^{18}F-FDG PET/CT for pretreatment staging after having diagnosed as NHL with small lymphocytic lymphoma subtype.

Findings

Interpretation Splenomegaly together with increased FDG uptake is consistent with metastatic involvement of spleen. Although FDG uptake is not intense, hypermetabolism at lymph nodes is also suggestive of metastasis.

Teaching Point ^{18}F-FDG PET/CT is an effective method in the evaluation of metastatically involved lymph nodes which are reported as normal on CT depending on the size criterion. It is also superior to CT in the evaluation of diffusely infiltrated sites, such as the spleen or bone marrow. Sensitivity and specificity of PET/CT were higher than those of the other diagnostic modalities alone when the initial staging of splenic lymphomatous involvement is concerned.

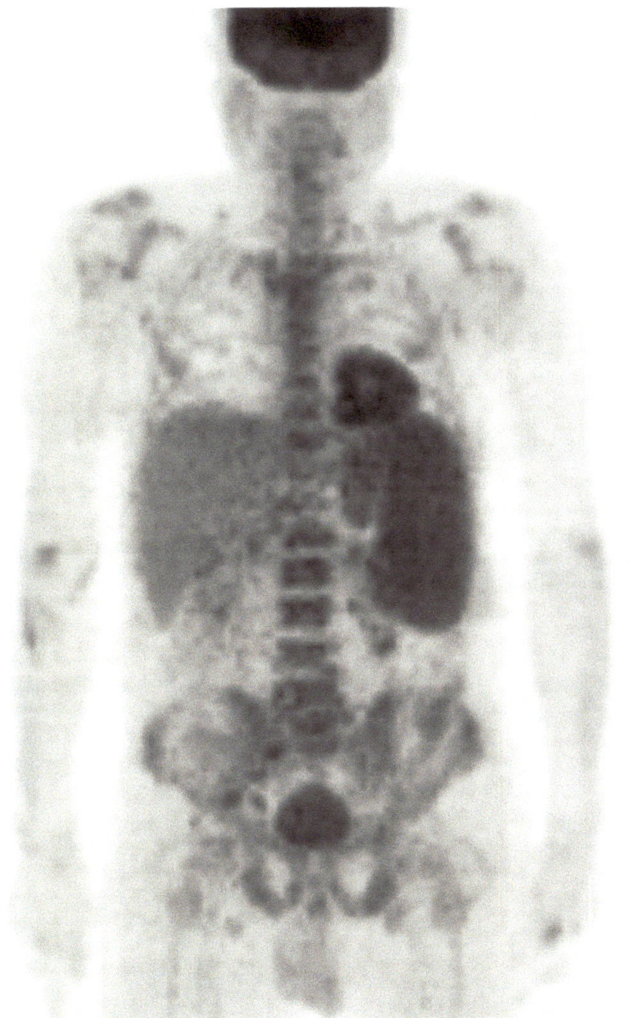

Fig. 7.3 MIP image shows enlargement and diffuse increased FDG uptake (SUVmax 5.2) at spleen. There are also mildly hypermetabolic lymph nodes barely visualized at perigastric, peripancreatic, and bilateral inguinal areas. The spleen/liver SUVmax ratio is 5.2/3

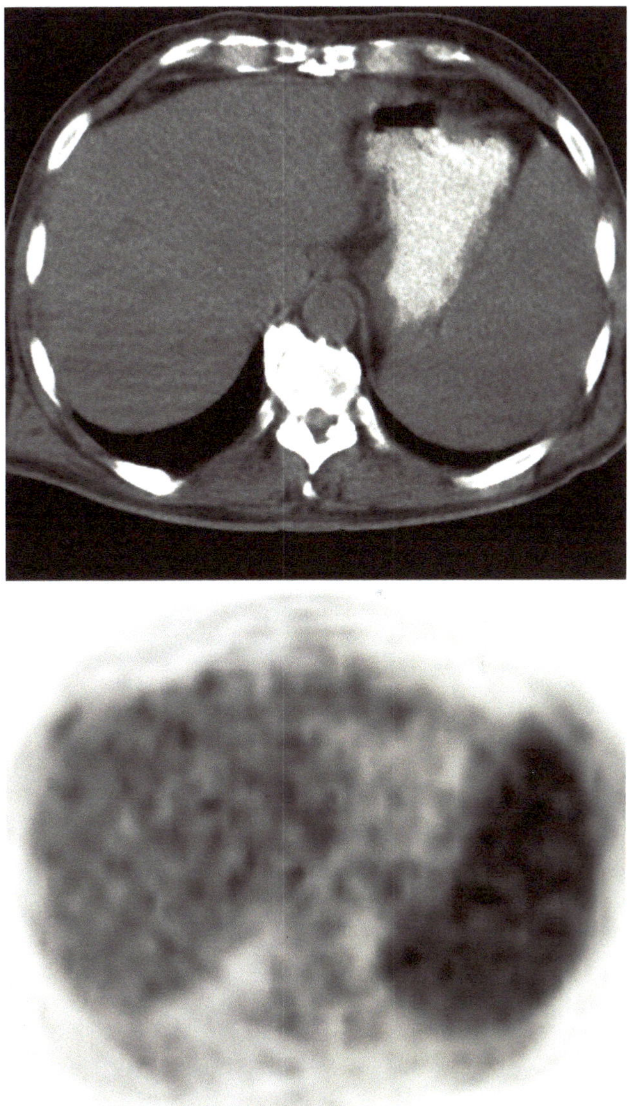

Fig. 7.4 Axial CT and PET images show diffuse hypermetabolism at spleen

7.3 Case 3: Diffuse Large B-Cell Lymphoma

History A 72-year-old male, status post left axillary lymph node excisional biopsy proven to be Diffuse Large B-Cell Lymphoma (DLBCL) underwent ^{18}F-FDG PET/CT for pretreatment staging.

Findings

Interpretation Increased FDG uptake sites at infra- and supraabdominal lymph node stations, liver, spleen, and bony structures are compatible with metastatic involvement of lymphoma. Diffuse increased bone marrow uptake at proximal humeri and both femurs is due to hematopoietic activation.

Teaching Point FDG uptake pattern in spleen is heterogenous and multifocal in metastatic infiltration, whereas diffuse and mild in bone marrow activation.

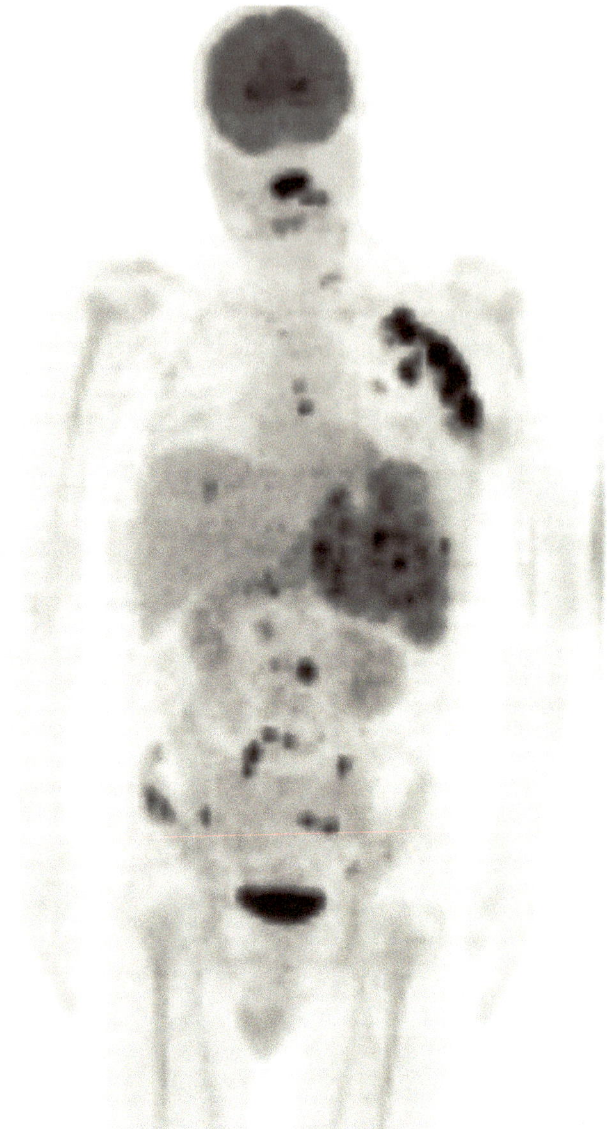

Fig. 7.5 MIP image shows hypermetabolic lymph nodes at left axillary fossa; intraabdominal lymph stations; focal hypermetabolic lesion at liver; increased FDG uptake sites at vertebral colon and pelvic bones. Spleen shows enlargement with intense heterogeneous FDG uptake with hypermetabolic foci dispersed through the organ. There is also minimal diffuse hypermetabolism at proximal humeri and both femurs

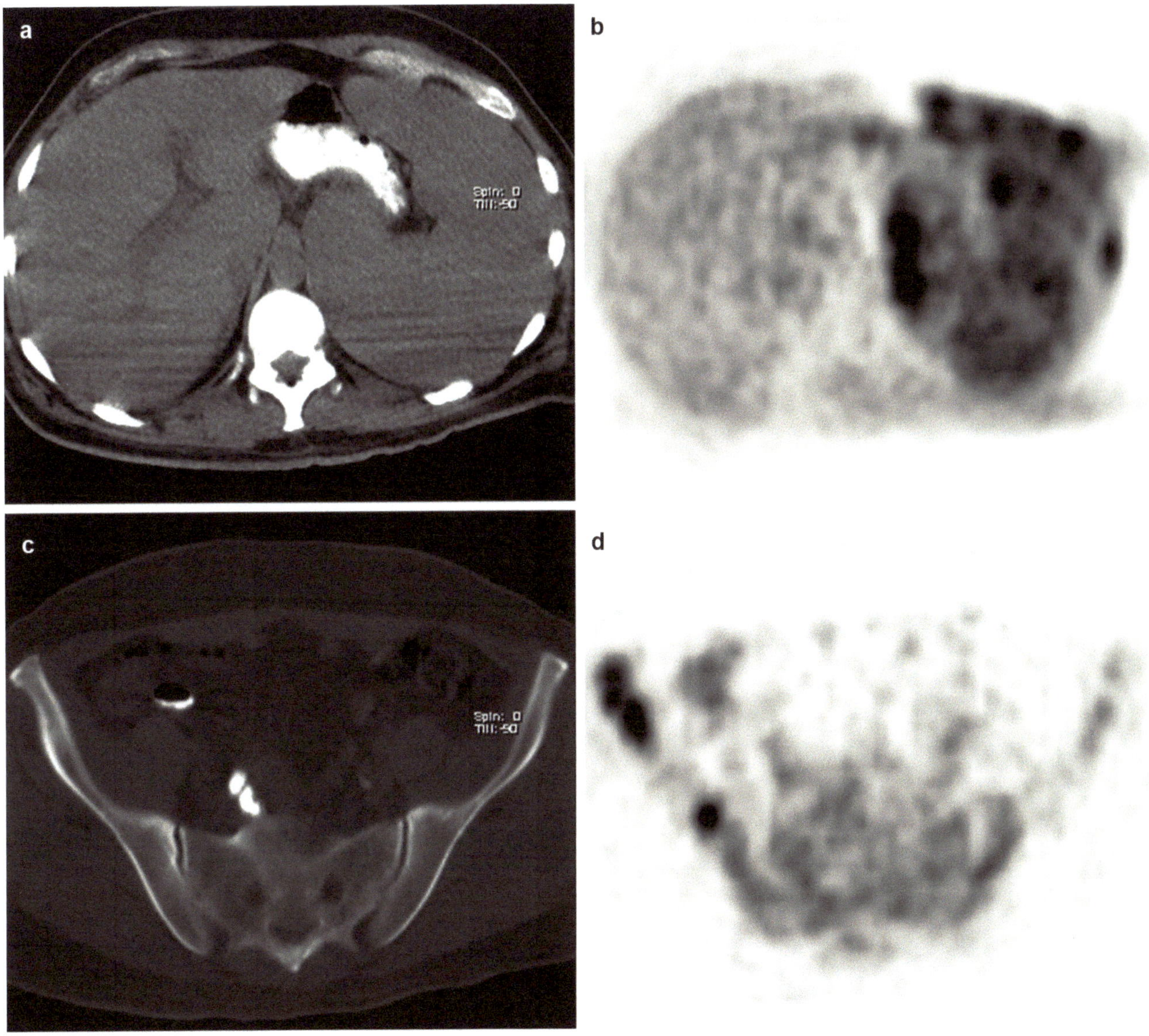

Fig. 7.6 Axial CT and PET images shows hypermetabolic foci disseminated throughout enlarged spleen (**a**, **b**) and right iliac wing (**c**, **d**)

7.4 Case 4: Testicular Lymphoma

History A 49-year-old male, status post left orchiectomy proven to be DLBCL, underwent ^{18}F-FDG PET/CT scan for pretreatment staging.

Findings

Interpretation Hypermetabolic retroperitoneal lymph node masses at left iliac lymphatic chain is compatible with metastatic involvement of lymphoma. The lesions showed complete remission after chemoradiotherapy.

Teaching Point Primary testicular lymphoma (PTL) comprises around 1–2 % of all NHL. It primarily affects men, with a median age of 67 years. The most common histological subtype is DLBCL, accounting for 80–90 % of PTLs. ^{18}F-FDG PET/CT is currently the standard procedure for assessment of the posttreatment response for most lymphoma subtypes.

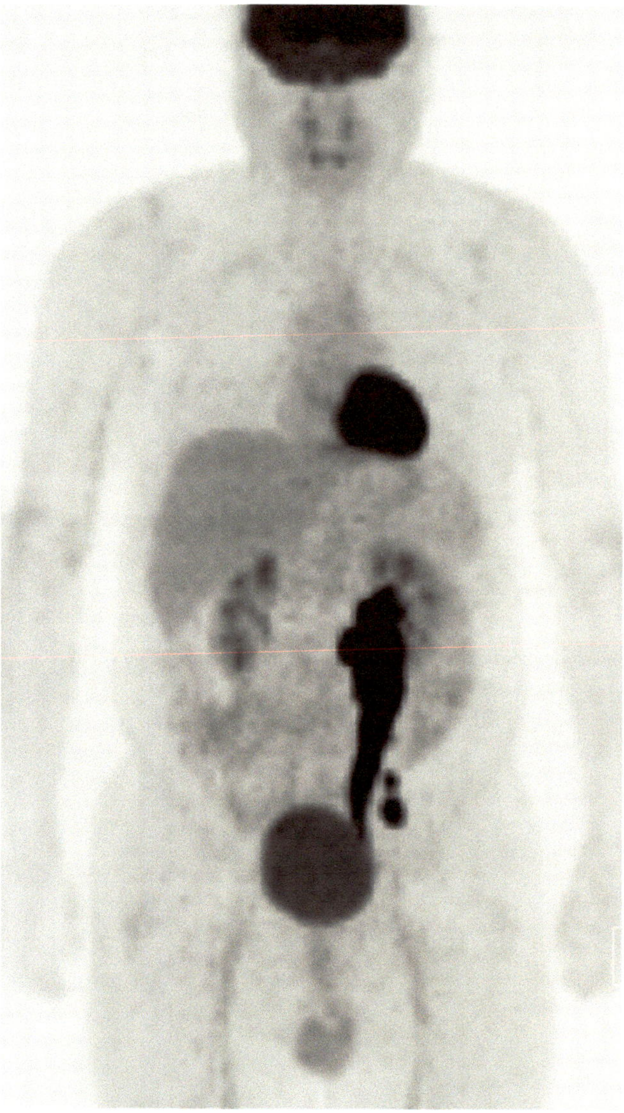

Fig. 7.7 MIP image shows intensely hypermetabolic conglomerate of retroperitoneal lymph nodes at left iliac lymphatic chain (SUVmax 15)

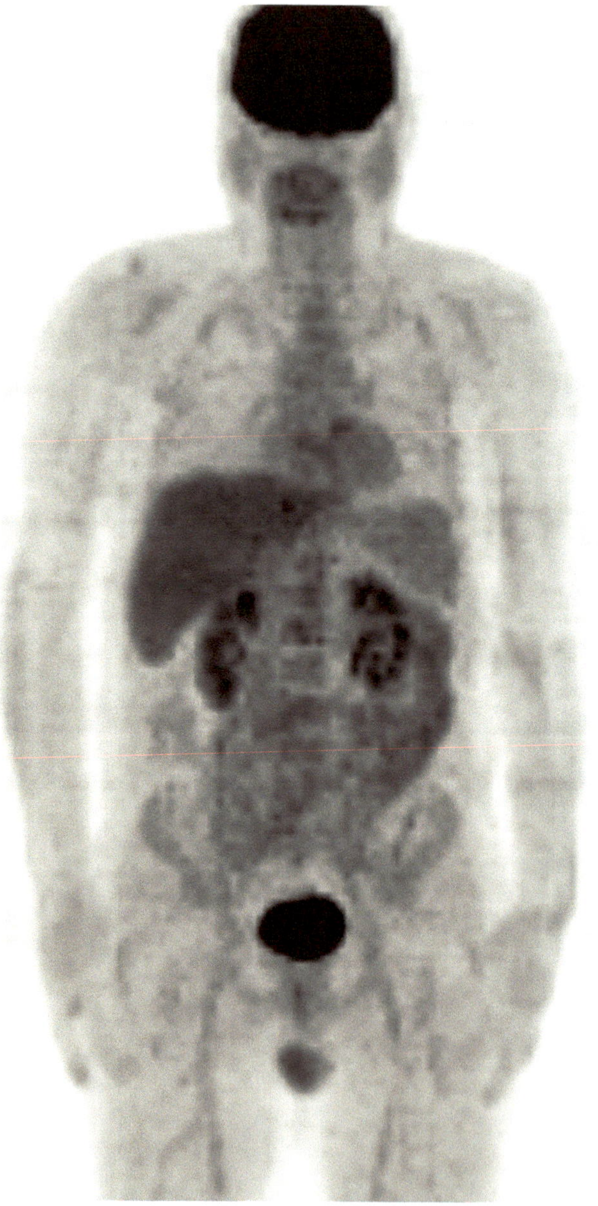

Fig. 7.8 MIP image of study performed 6 months after the patient received chemotherapy and radiotherapy. Lymph nodes with pathological FDG uptake disappeared

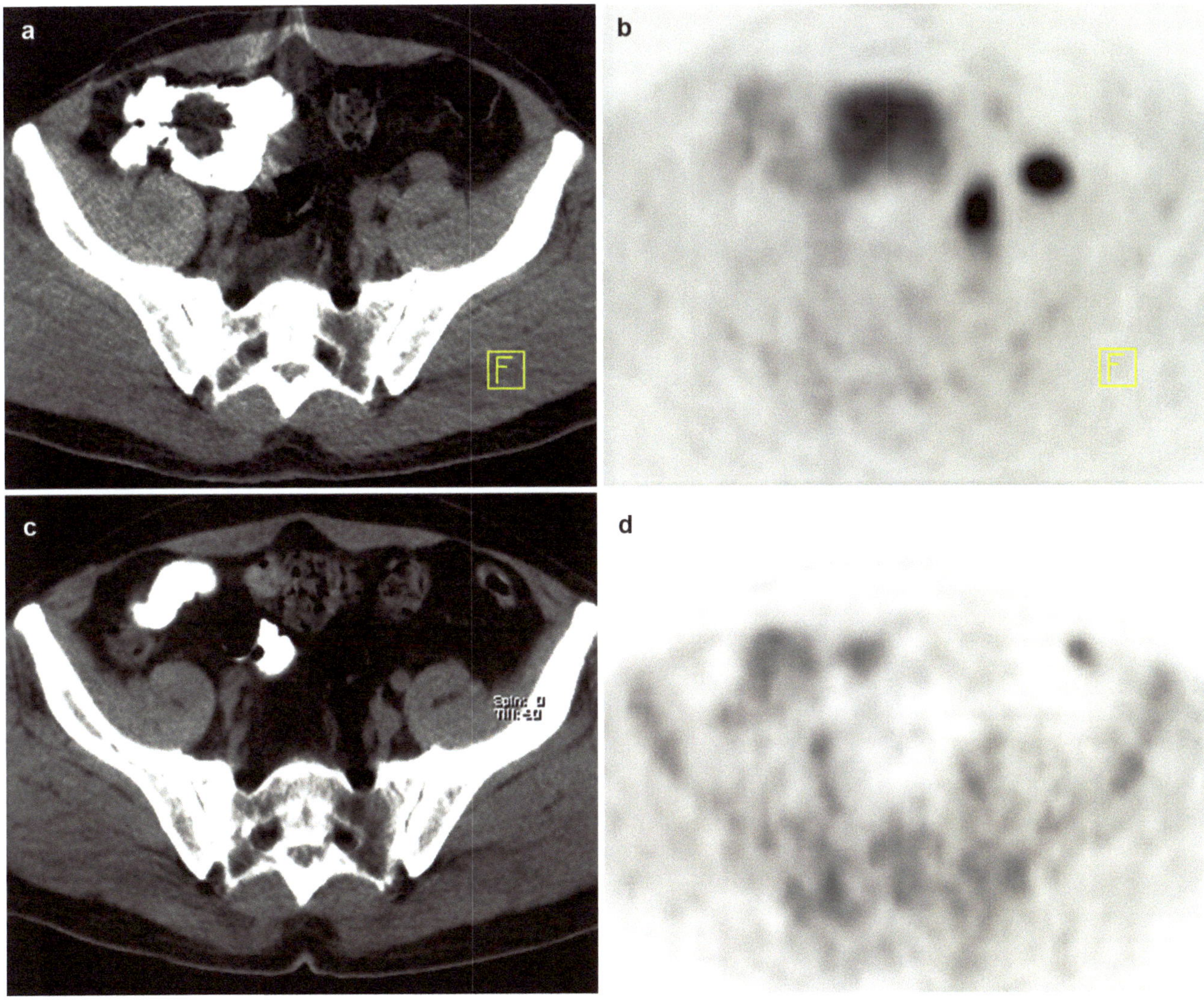

Fig. 7.9 Axial CT and PET images shows hypermetabolic foci at left external iliac region (**a**, **b**); resolution of metabolic activity at lymph nodes at PET/CT scan obtained 6 months after the first one (**c**, **d**)

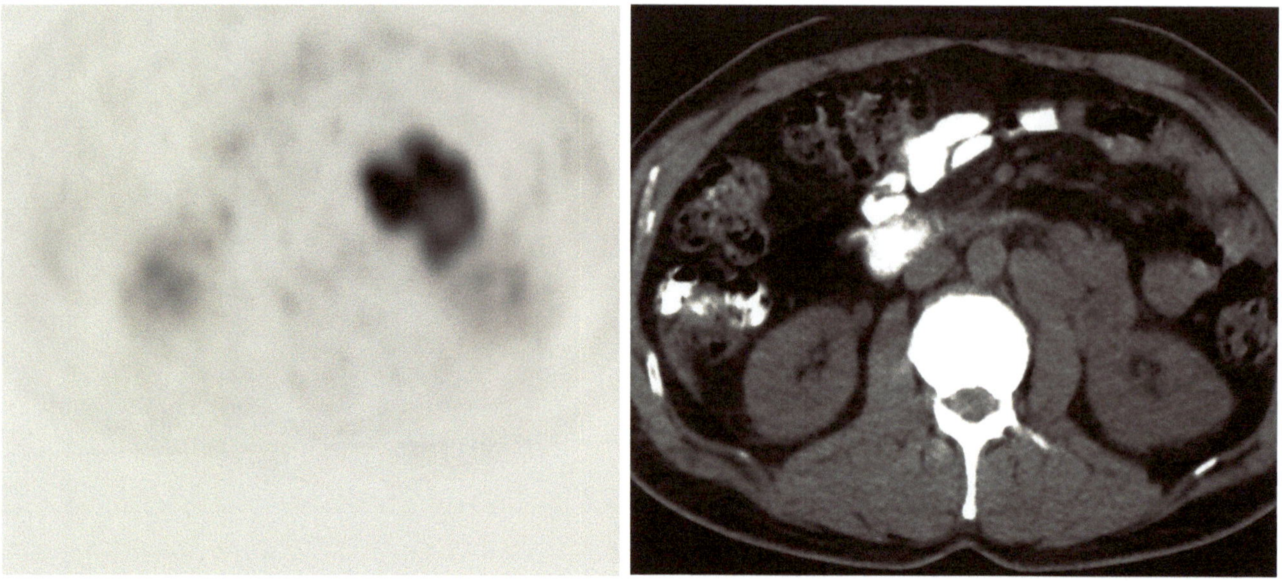

Fig. 7.10 Axial PET and CT images show hypermetabolic foci at left paraaortic region

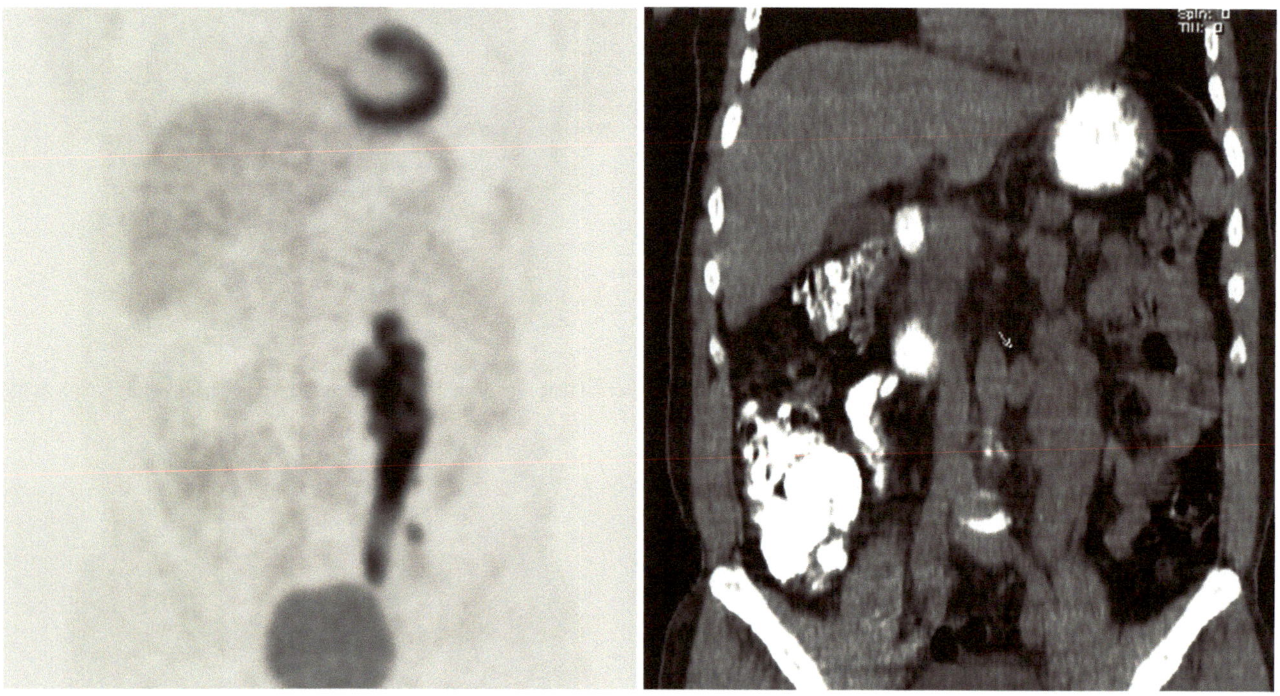

Fig. 7.11 Coronal PET and CT images show hypermetabolic conglomerate retroperitoneal lymph node masses at left iliac lymphatic chain

7.5 Case 5: Diffuse Large B-Cell Lymphoma Involving Duodenum

History A 72-year-old male, status post duodenum biopsy proven to be DLBCL, underwent ^{18}F-FDG PET/CT for pre-treatment staging.

Findings

Interpretation Hypermetabolism involving the duodenum compatible with extranodal lymphoma.

Teaching Point Although the GI tract is the predominant site of extranodal lymphomas (ENL), primary lymphomas of the GI tract are rare. 50–60 % of all primary GI lymphomas are NHL. Many of these tumors are of the B-cell type. The duodenum is the most infrequent site of these lesions. ^{18}F-FDG PET-CT has a significant advantage for the diagnosis of diffusely infiltrating organ involvements and is superior to contrast enhanced CT.

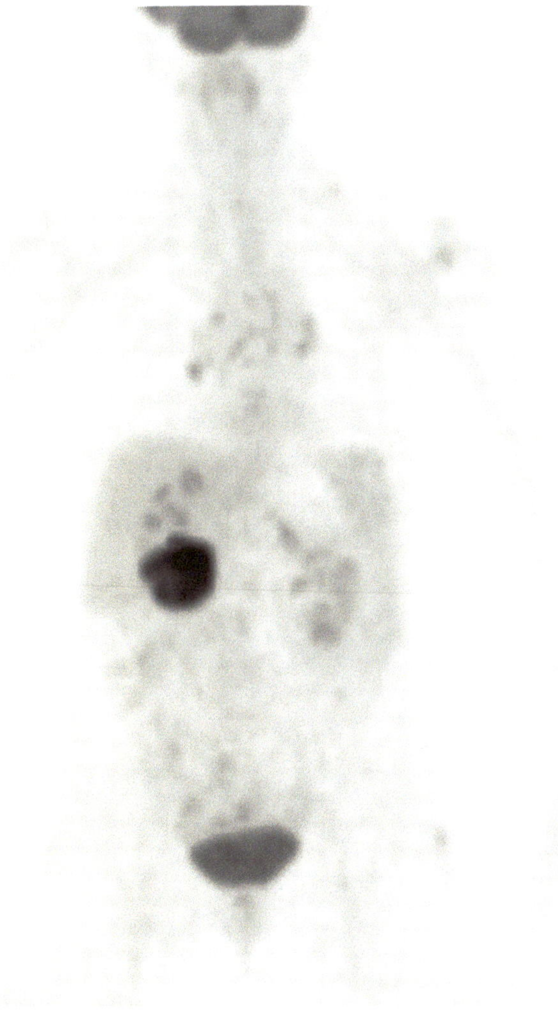

Fig. 7.12 MIP image

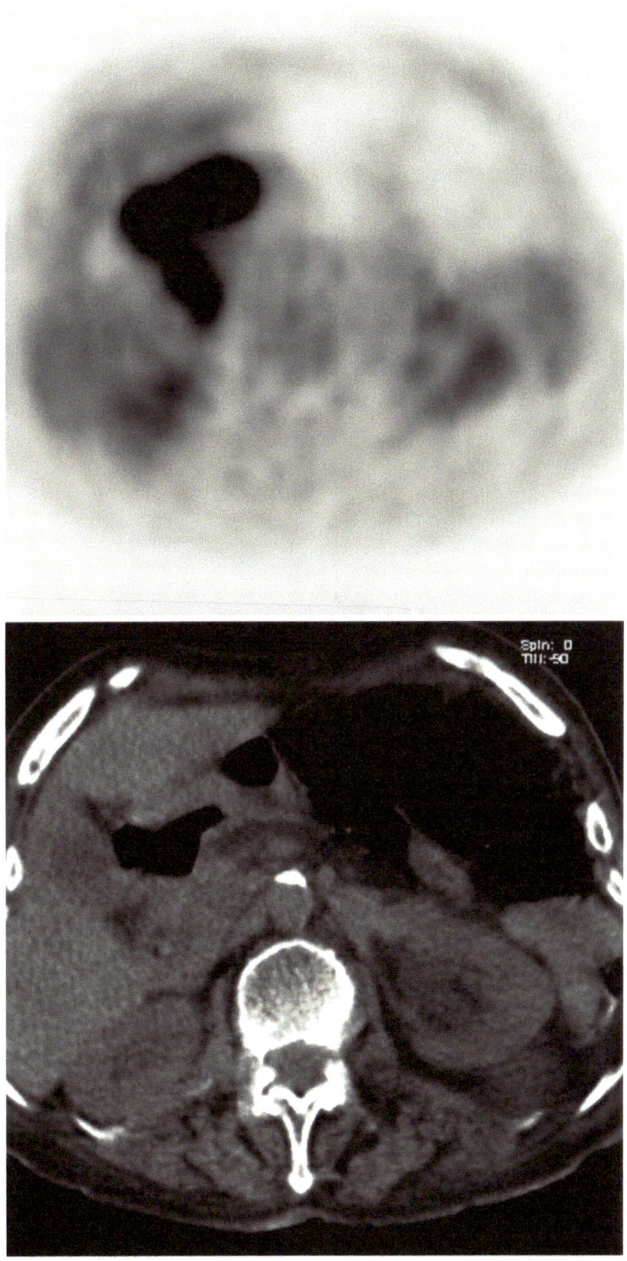

Fig. 7.13 Axial PET and CT images showed intensely increased FDG uptake (SUVmax 25) at duodenum

7.6 Case 6: Gastric Lymphoma and Virchow's node

History A 39-year-old male underwent ^{18}F-FDG PET/CT after having diagnosed as gastric NHL following a biopsy from stomach. PET/CT study was repeated 4.5 months after the patient received chemotherapy and radiotherapy.

Findings

Interpretation Diffuse and intensely increased FDG uptake at gastric wall represents primary malignant disease and hypermetabolic intraabdominal and supraclavicular (Virchow's node) lymph nodes reflect involvement with primary malignancy. Resolution of all lesions at second study indicates complete remission as a result of chemoradiotherapy.

Teaching Point Defining FDG avidity and PET/CT patterns in aggressive NHL before treatment may be important for further monitoring therapy response. The left supraclavicular lymph node (Virchow's node) may be involved by metastatic malignancies, including those of abdominal or pelvic origin, sometimes being the first manifestation of the disease.

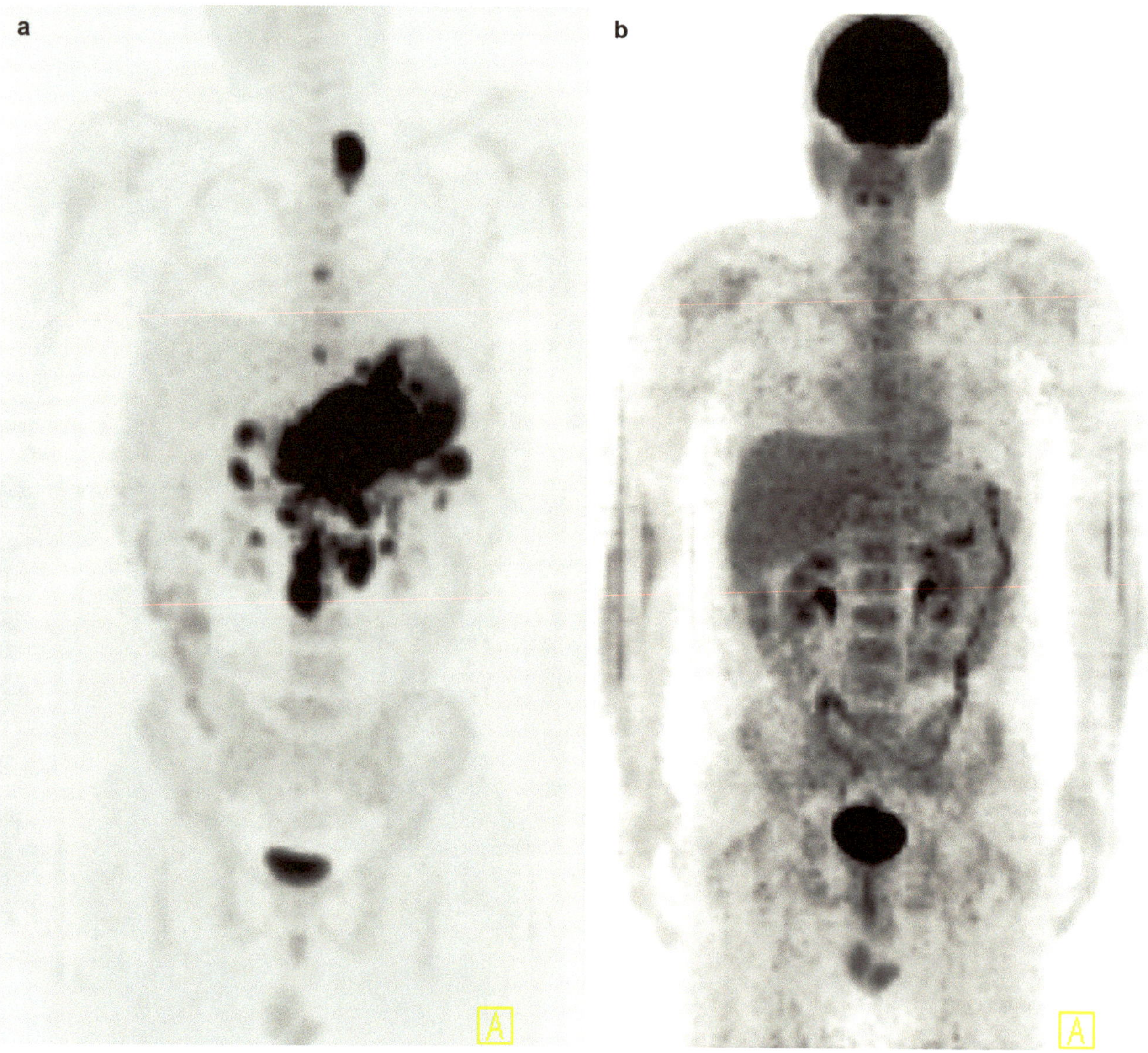

Fig. 7.14 MIP images shows intensely increased FDG uptake at gastric wall (SUVmax 45), numerous hypermetabolic intraabdominal lymph nodes (SUVmax 56) and hypermetabolic lymph node at left supraclavicular area (**a**), disappearance of all lesions with pathological FDG uptake at study performed 4.5 months after the patient received chemotherapy and radiotherapy (**b**)

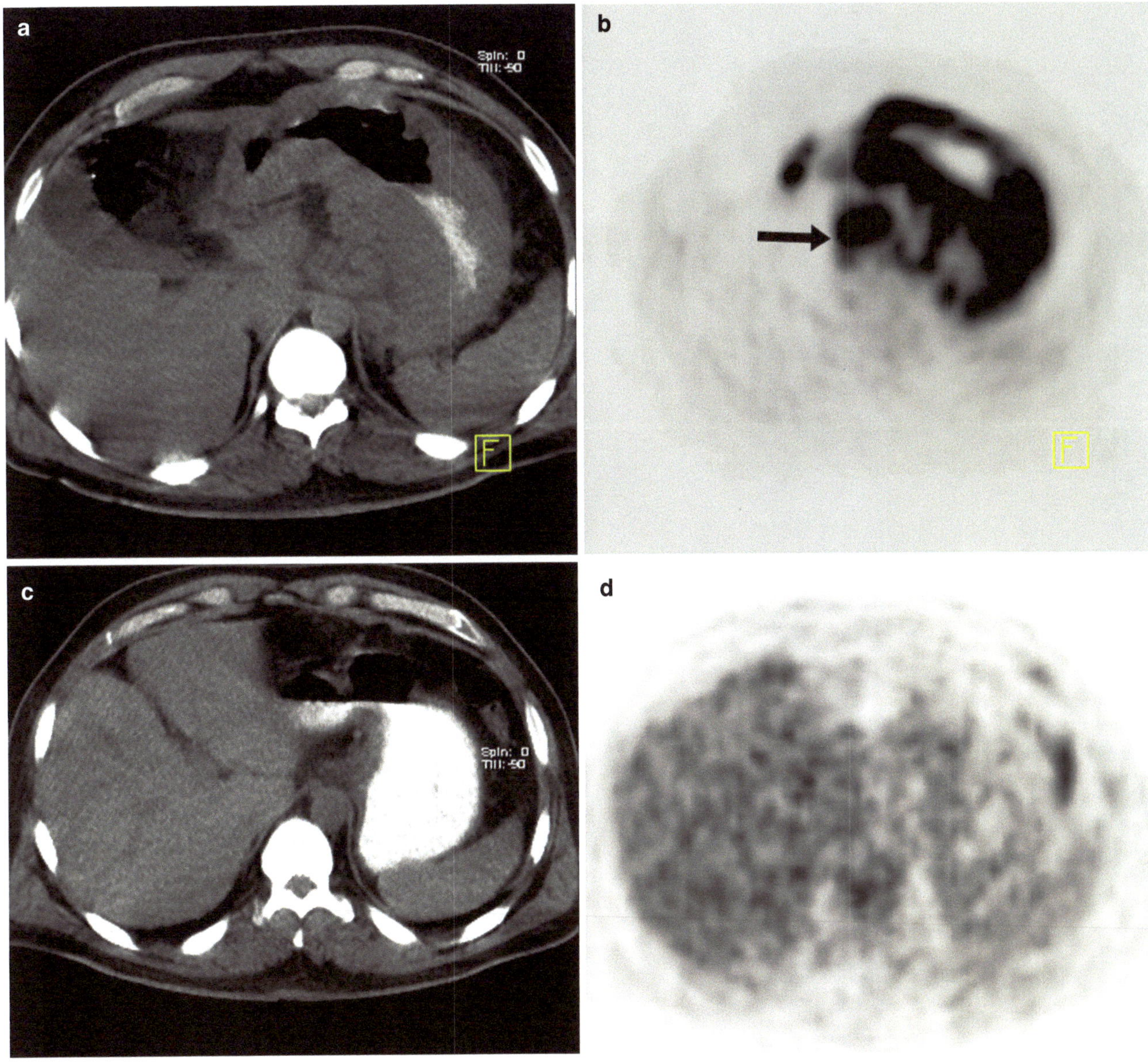

Fig. 7.15 Axial CT and PET images shows highly increased FDG uptake with corresponding abnormal gastric wall thickening and a few perigastric hypermetabolic lymph nodes (*arrow*) (**a**, **b**), resolution of metabolic activity at gastric wall and lymph nodes at ^{18}F-FDG PET CT scan obtained 4.5 months after the first one (**c**, **d**)

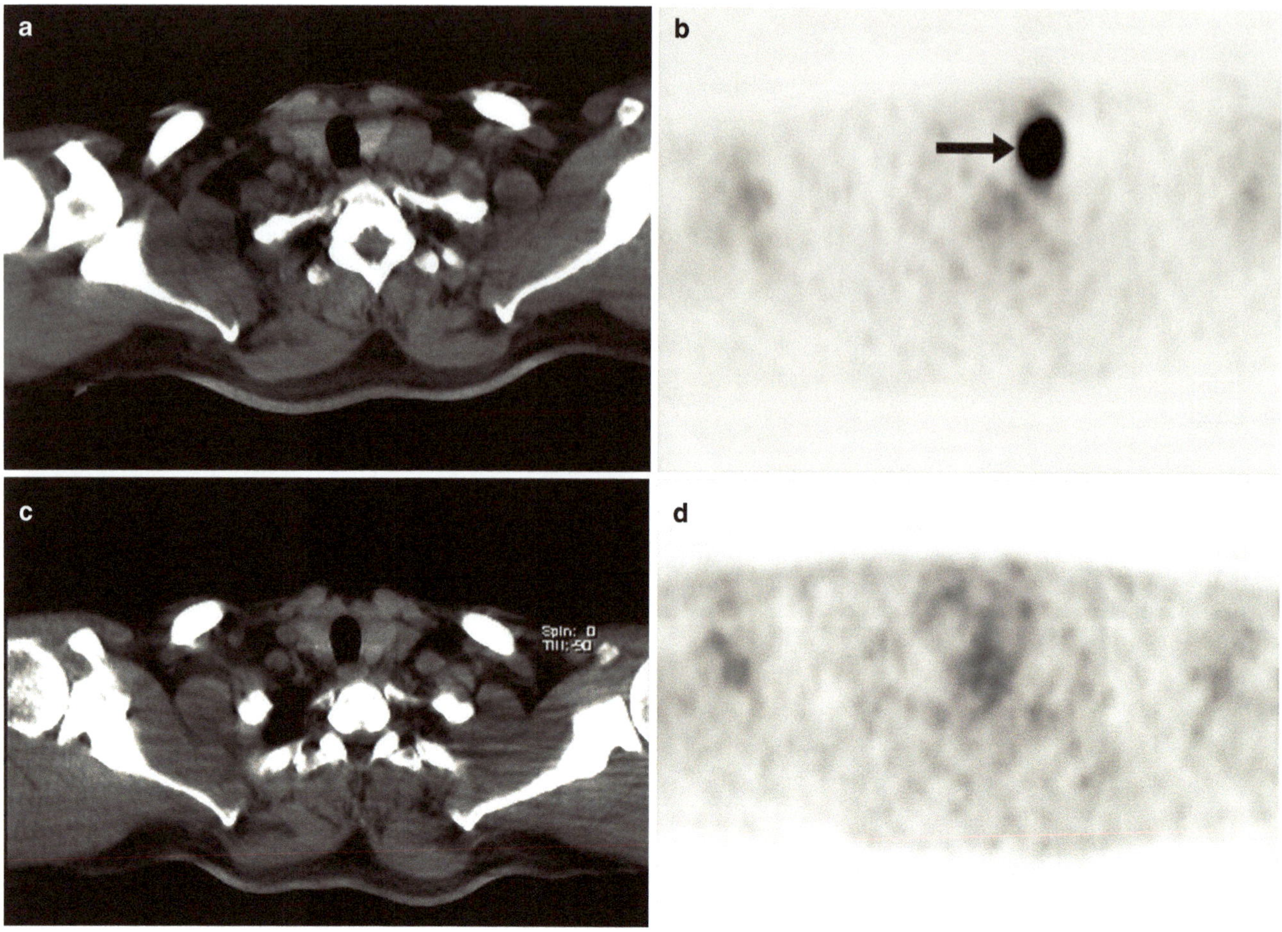

Fig. 7.16 Axial CT and PET images shows intensely hypermetabolic lymph node at supraclavicular region (*arrow*) (**a**, **b**), resolution of the lesion at the second study (**c**, **d**)

7.7 Case 7: Extranodal Non-Hodgkin Lymphoma

History A 26-year-old female patient underwent laminectomy from 4th, 5th, and 6th thoracic vertebras and histopathology revealed DLBCL. Two months later ^{18}F-FDG PET/CT scan was obtained.

Findings

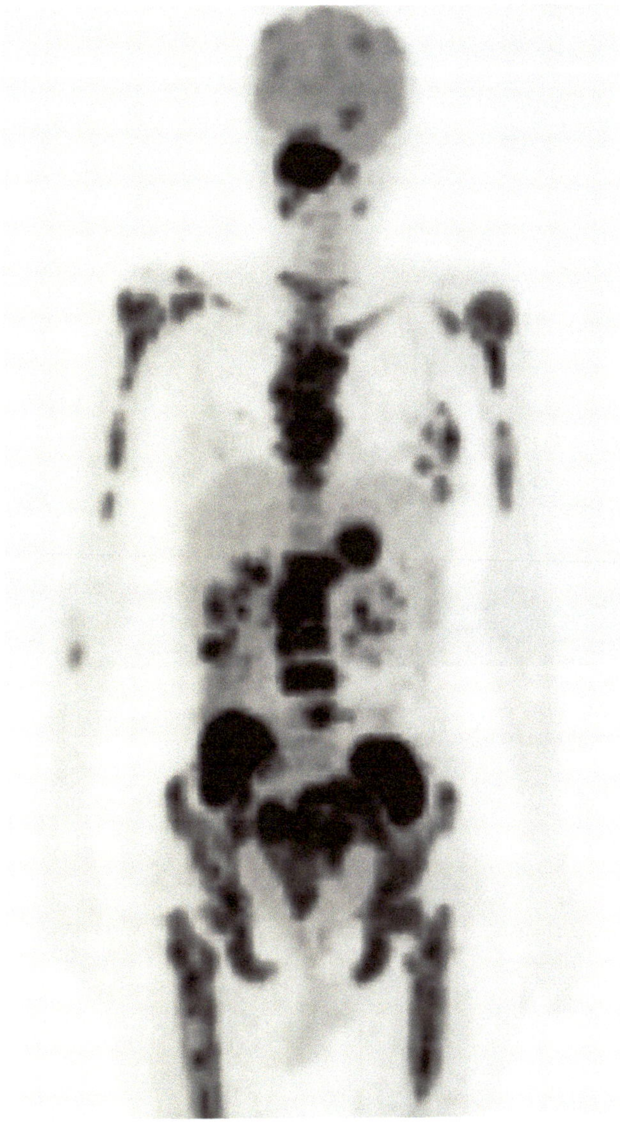

Fig. 7.17 MIP image shows intense FDG uptake at skeletal system, bone marrow, nasopharynx, pancreas, both kidneys, and ovaries

Interpretation This is a case of extranodal NHL with multiple and rare sites of organ involvement.

Teaching Point Malignant lymphoma (ML), especially NHL, may occur outside the lymph nodes and ENL occurs in about 40 % of ML patients. It is important to determine the number and location of extranodal lesions, because the existence of extranodal disease is a key factor in the prognosis of patients. Several studies have specifically addressed the superiority of PET/CT over CT for assessment of extranodal involvement.

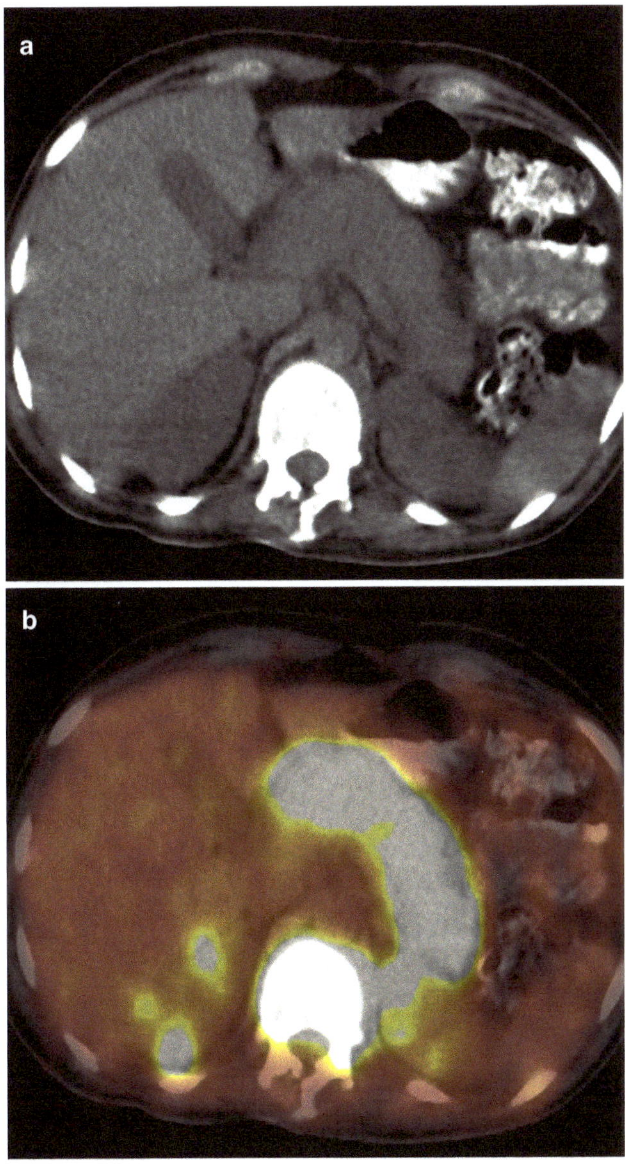

Fig. 7.18 Diffuse FDG uptake of pancreas due to NHL involvement is seen at axial CT and fusion images (**a**, **b**)

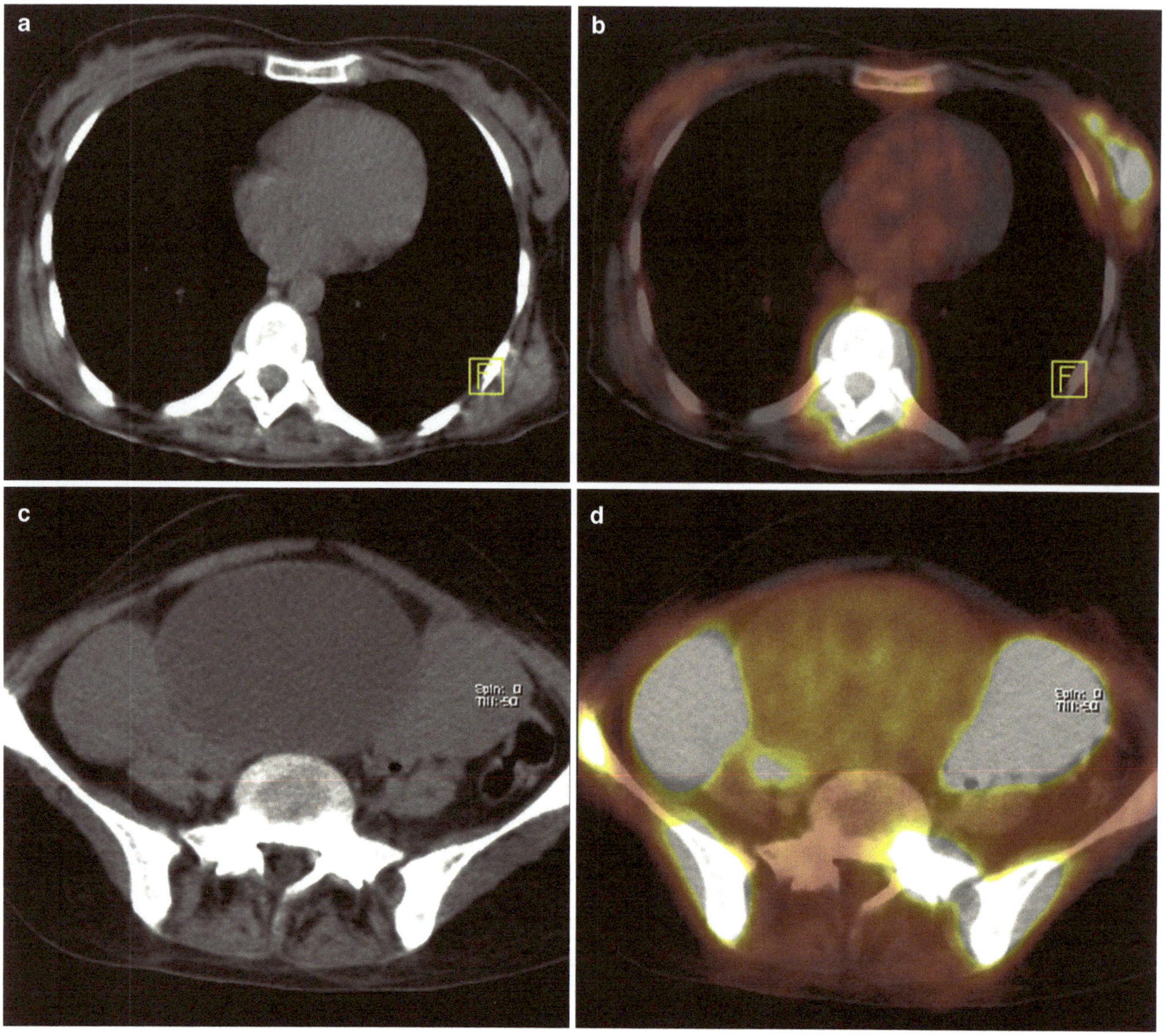

Fig. 7.19 Axial CT and fusion images demonstrates pathologically increased FDG uptake at vertebral body and left pectoralis major muscle (**a**, **b**), enlargement of both ovaries with intense FDG uptake due to involvement with NHL (**c**, **d**)

7.8 Case 8: Marginal Zone Splenic Lymphoma

History A 63-year-old male underwent ^{18}F-FDG PET/CT after having diagnosed as marginal zone splenic lymphoma (SMZL) after a biopsy from spleen.

Findings

Interpretation Diffuse and moderately increased FDG uptake at spleen which is higher than the metabolic activity of liver (SUVmax 3) is compatible with primary malignant lymphoma involvement. There are also hypermetabolic metastatic intraabdominal lymph nodes. Increased bone marrow uptake might be due to hematopoietic activation as well as metastatic infiltration.

Teaching Point SMZL is generally an indolent lymphoma that involves the spleen, bone marrow, and other organs. It comprises about less than 2 % of all cases of NHL. People with SMZL often respond very well when they undergo splenectomy. Diagnostic splenectomy is frequently performed in patients with suspected or known lymphoma. Preoperative ^{18}F-FDG PET/CT may correlate with splenic pathology. Low activity might be associated with benign findings or mantle cell lymphoma, intermediate activity with marginal zone lymphoma and high activity with DLBCL.

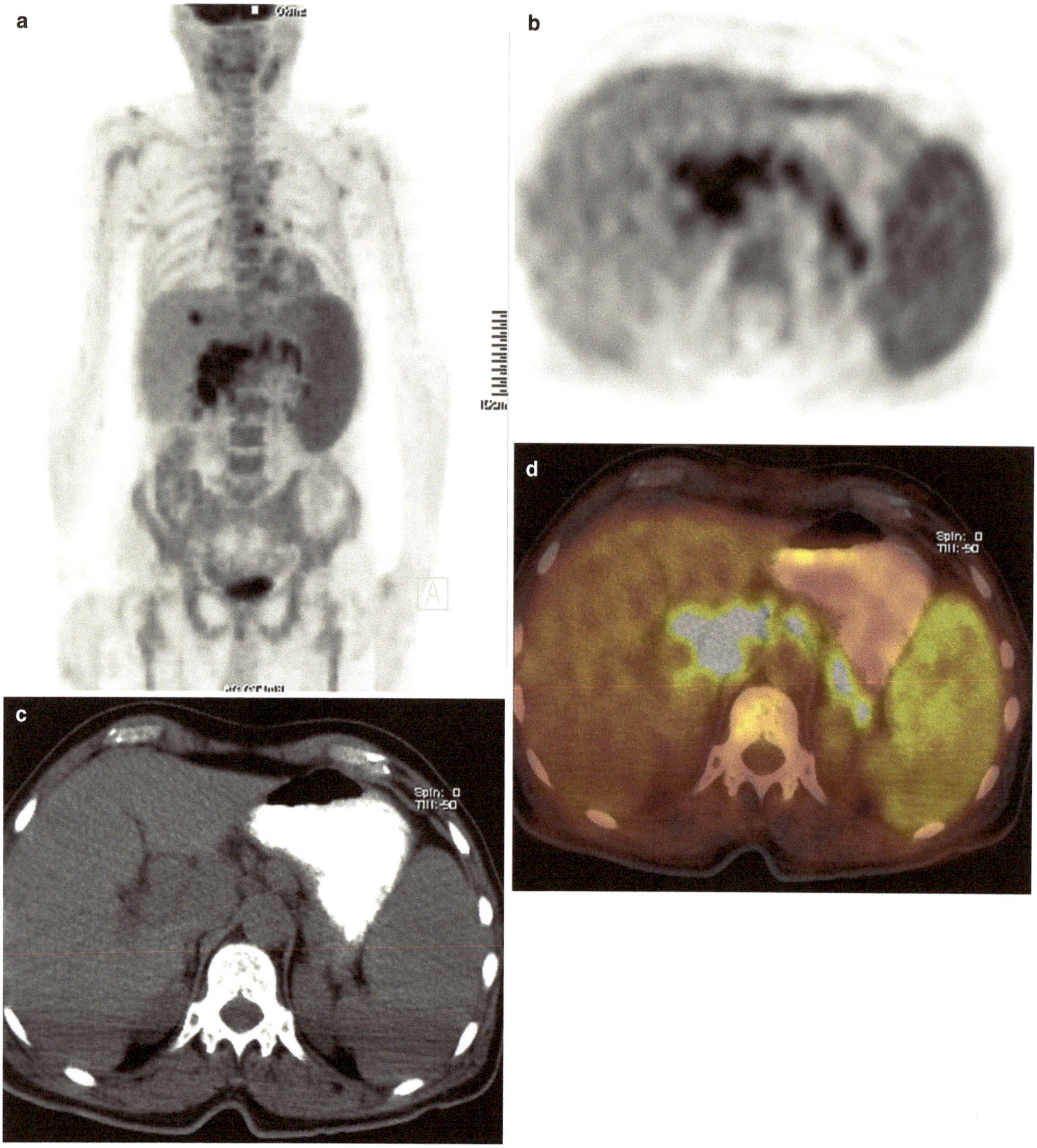

Fig. 7.20 MIP image (**a**) and axial PET, CT, and fusion images (**b–d**) shows moderately increased diffuse FDG uptake at spleen (SUVmax 5.3). There are intensely hypermetabolic intraabdominal lymph nodes at portal hilus, peripancreatic, and paraceliac areas (SUVmax 10). There is remarkably increased FDG uptake at bone marrow at axial and appendicular skeleton

7.9 Case 9: Mantle Cell Lymphoma

History A 70-year-old male, status post left axillary biopsy proven to be mantle cell lymphoma (MCL), underwent ^{18}F-FDG PET/CT for pretreatment staging.

Findings

Interpretation Intraabdominal lymph nodes without any metabolic activity represent metastatic involvement with lymphoma of low FDG affinity. The linear activity at sternum reflects inflammatory reaction secondary to bypass operation

Teaching Point MCL is a rare but aggressive NHL subtype with a poor prognosis. In our case, the lymph nodes are not FDG avid but generally PET imaging is superior to anatomic imaging techniques and has a high sensitivity in detecting both nodal and extranodal involvement in patients who have MCL. However, evaluation of the disease, especially when therapy response is concerned, is only possible in patients with highly FDG-avid MCL.

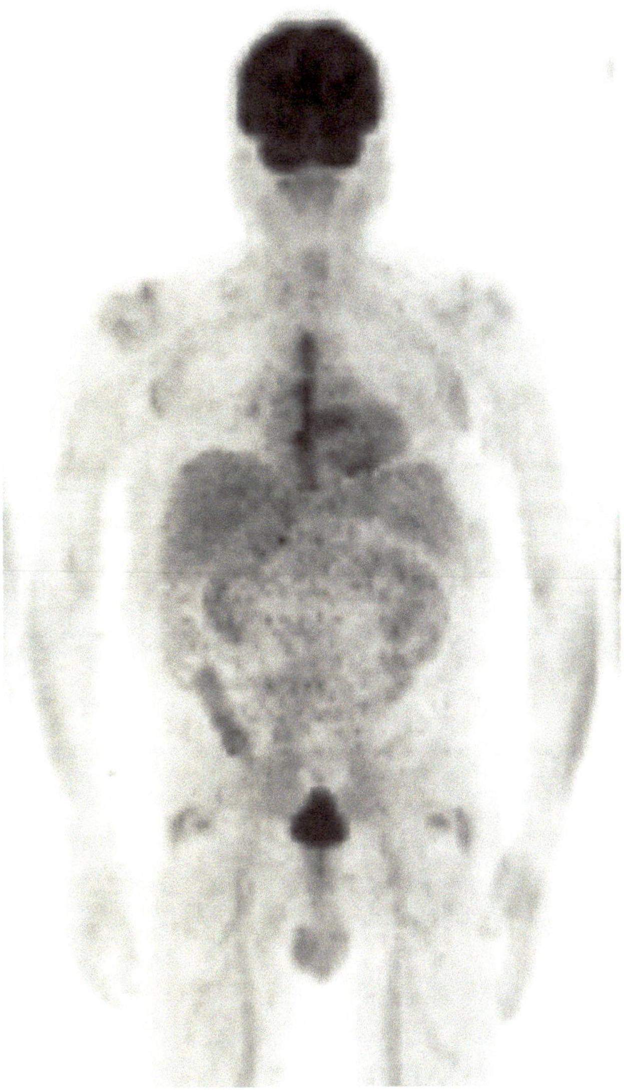

Fig. 7.21 MIP image shows linear activity at sternum and there is not any remarkable pathological metabolic activity other than this

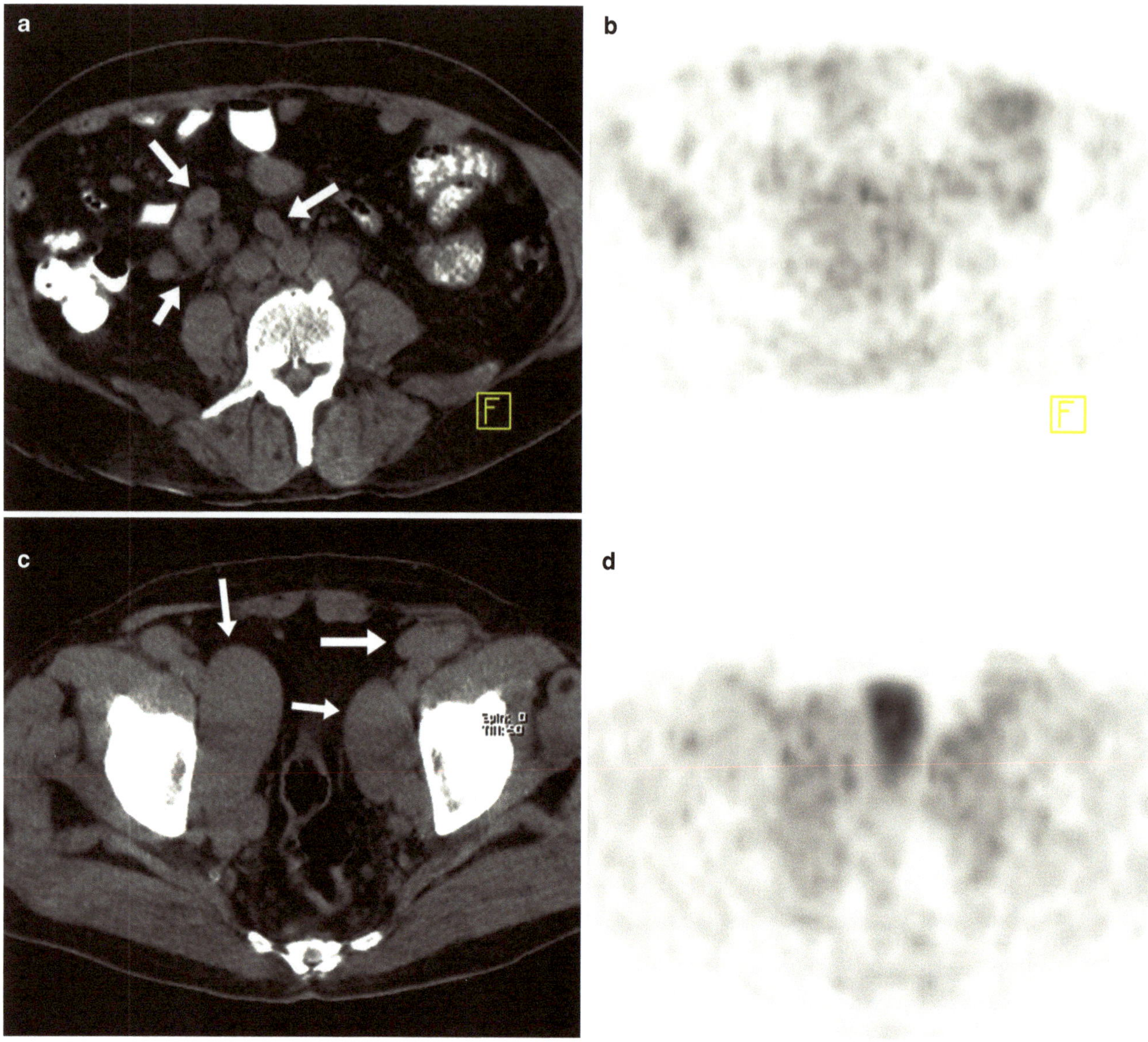

Fig. 7.22 Axial CT and PET images show paraortic, interaortocaval, mesenteric (**a**, **b**), and external iliac (**c**, **d**) lymph nodes (*arrows*) without any significant corresponding metabolic activity at PET study

7.10 Case 10: Bone Marrow Infiltration of non-Hodgkin's Lymphoma

History A 60-year-old male underwent ^{18}F-FDG PET/CT for restaging of NHL.

Findings

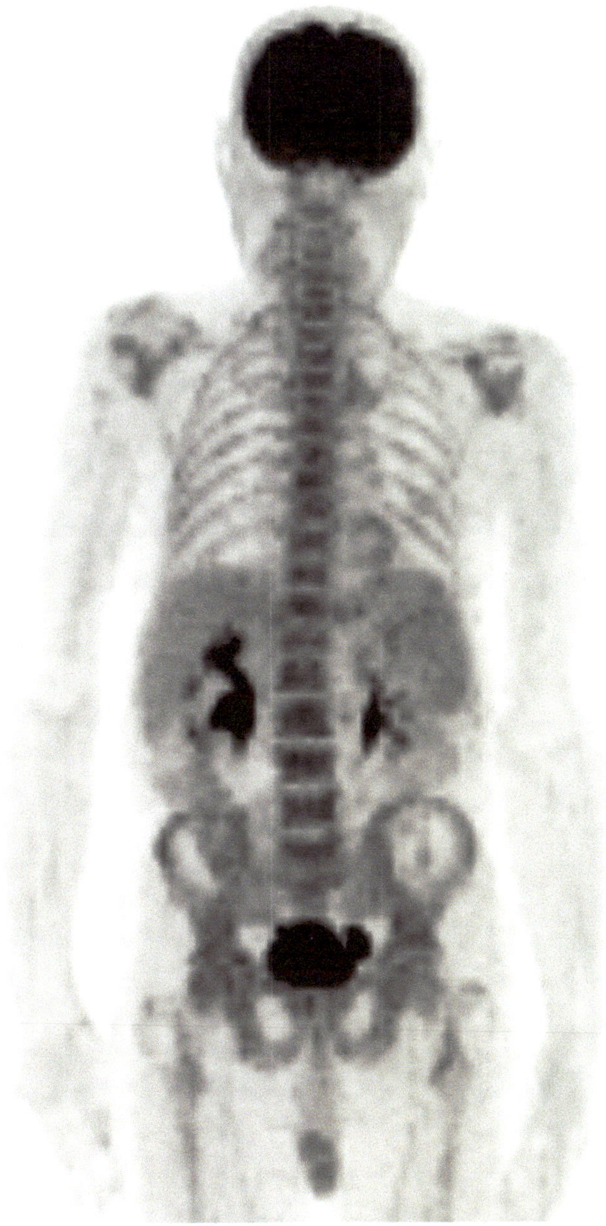

Fig. 7.23 MIP image shows heterogenous hypermetabolism at bone marrow of vertebral colon and pelvic bones

Interpretation Heterogenous FDG uptake at bone marrow is consistent with infiltration of bone marrow with primary malignancy.

Result Patient underwent bone marrow biopsy which revealed metastatic involvement with primary malignancy.

Teaching Point Heterogenous FDG uptake at bone marrow with relatively hypermetabolic foci is compatible with metastatic infiltration and should be distinguished from hematopoietic activation. ^{18}F-FDG PET has overall good diagnostic performance for detecting bone marrow involvement, but this may depend also on the type of lymphoma. ^{18}F-FDG PET may complement biopsy in the staging of primary or recurrent lymphoma. Sensitivity of ^{18}F-FDG PET/CT in detecting bone marrow involvement is 51 % and it is effective especially in HD and high-grade lymphoma.

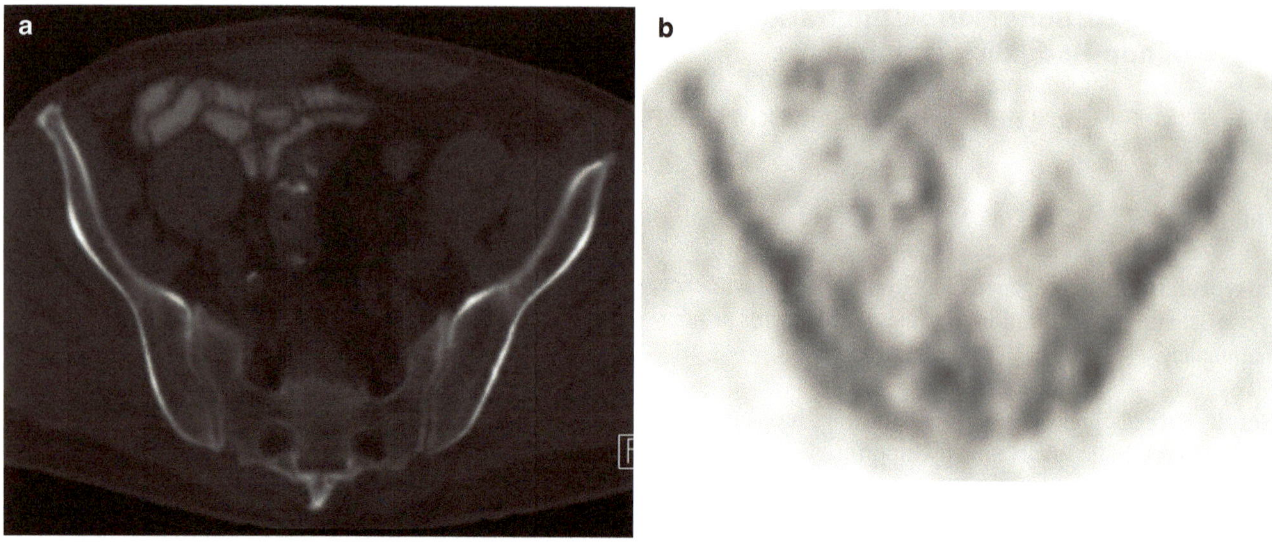

Fig. 7.24 Axial CT and PET images (**a**, **b**) show heterogenous FDG uptake at bone marrow without any corresponding bone lesion

7.11 Case 11: Nodular Sclerosis Hodgkin's Lymphoma

History A 20-year-old male underwent ^{18}F-FDG PET/CT scan after having diagnosed as nodular sclerosis Hodgkin's lymphoma (HL) following a biopsy from intraabdominal lymph nodes. PET/CT study was repeated after the patient received chemotherapy.

Findings

Interpretation First PET/CT study shows metastatic involvement of lymph nodes and pelvic bones; the second study displays complete resolution of all lesions reflecting therapy response.

Teaching Point FDG PET/CT is effective in assessing response to therapy in HL.

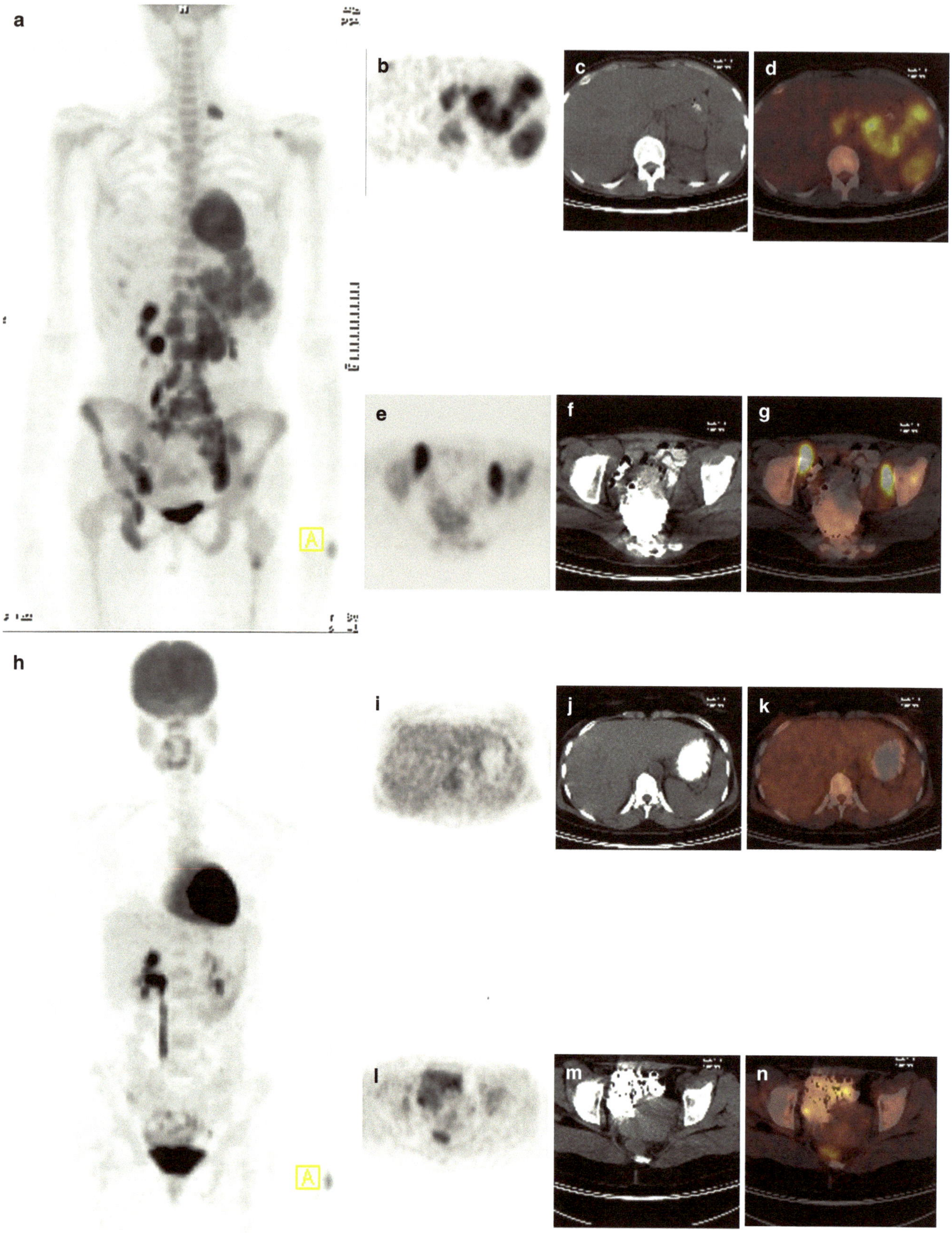

Fig. 7.25 MIP image (**a**), axial PET, CT, and fusion images (**b–g**) show hypermetabolic lymph nodes at left supraclavicular and intraabdominal lymph stations (SUVmax 8.6); increased FDG uptake at pelvic bones (SUVmax 10). MIP image (**h**), axial PET, CT, and fusion images (**i–n**) of PET/CT study performed 7 months after the first one do not show any pathologically increased FDG uptake site

7.12 Case 12: Therapy Response Evaluation in Hodgkin Lymphoma

History A 45-year-old male who was diagnosed to have mixed type HL underwent ^{18}F-FDG PET/CT before therapy and 3 months after chemotherapy.

Findings

Interpretation Diminished pathological FDG uptake at left cervical lymph nodes reflects complete response to therapy.

Teaching Point ^{18}F-FDG PET/CT is effective in assessing response to therapy in HL. Second study for evaluation of therapy response should be performed at least 3 months after the completion of the chemotherapy, in order to avoid misinterpretations.

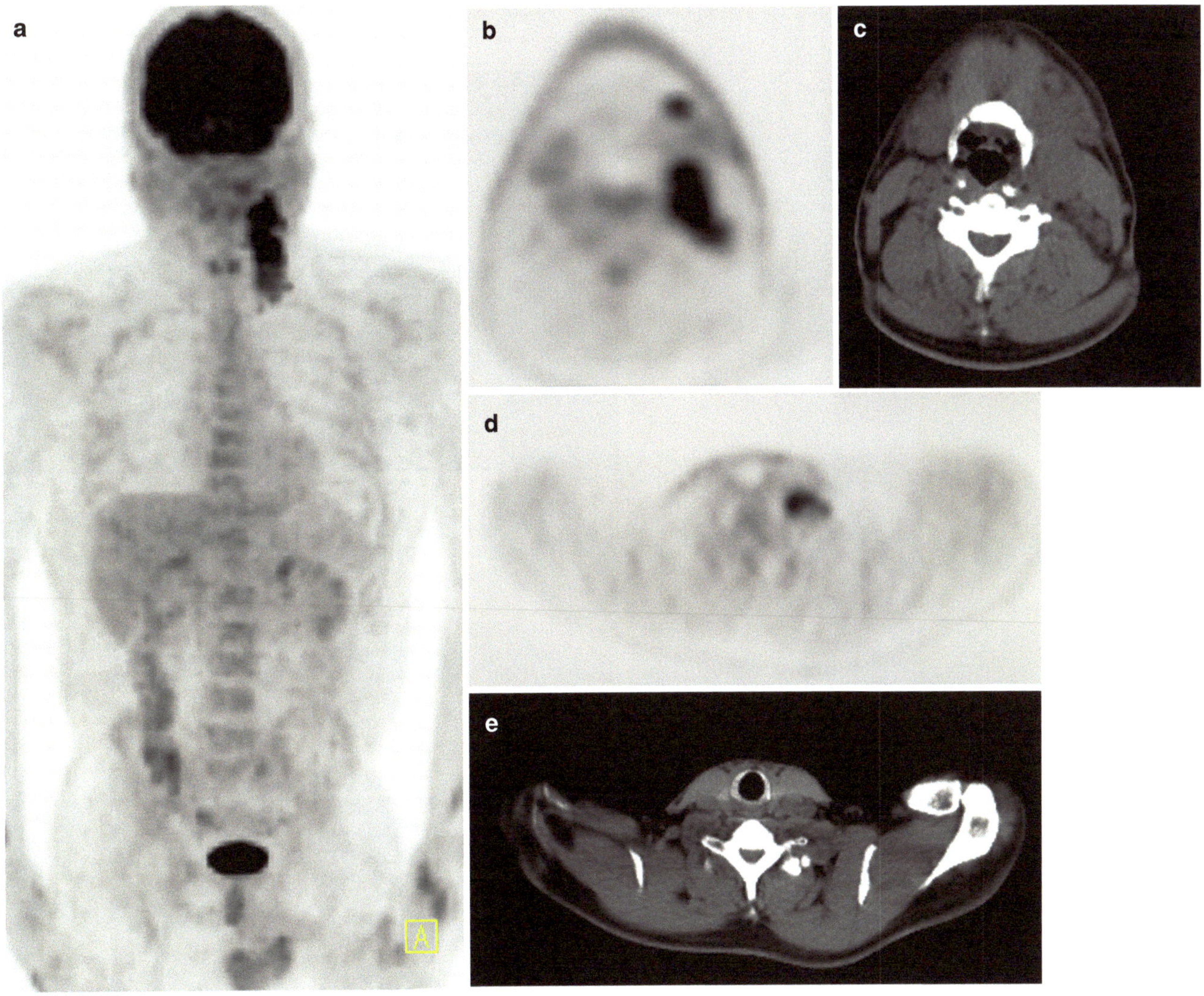

Fig. 7.26 MIP image (**a**) and axial PET and CT images (**b–e**) of ^{18}F-FDG PET/CT study before therapy show intensely increased FDG uptake at left cervical lymph nodes

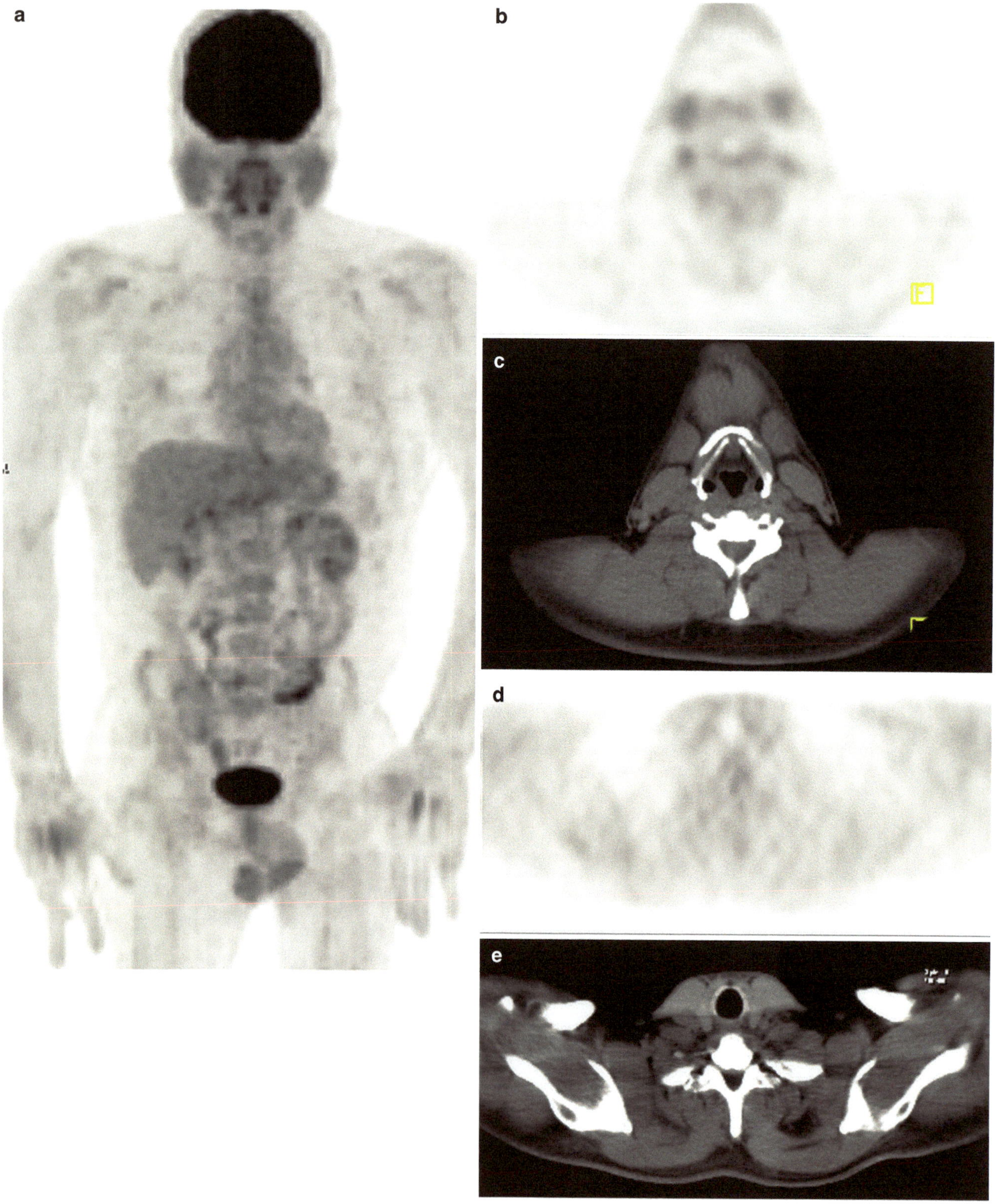

Fig. 7.27 MIP image (**a**) and axial PET and CT slices (**b–e**) of the study performed 3 months after the end of therapy show resolution of the pathological uptake at left cervical lymph nodes

7.13 Case 13: Hematopoietic Activation Due to Neupogen in Hodgkin's Lymphoma

History 25-year-old male, underwent ^{18}F-FDG PET/CT study for staging of HL. PET/CT study was repeated 3 weeks after the patient received chemotherapy and while he was on neupogen therapy.

Findings

Interpretation First PET/CT study shows metastatic involvement of lymph nodes; the second study show complete resolution of all lesions reflecting therapy response. Diffuse homogeneous bone marrow FDG uptake represents hematopoietic activation secondary to colony-stimulating factor (neupogen) administration.

Teaching Point ^{18}F-FDG PET/CT is effective in assessing response to therapy in Hodgkin's lymphoma but bone marrow FDG uptake due to hematopoietic activation should not be confused with metastatic infiltration.

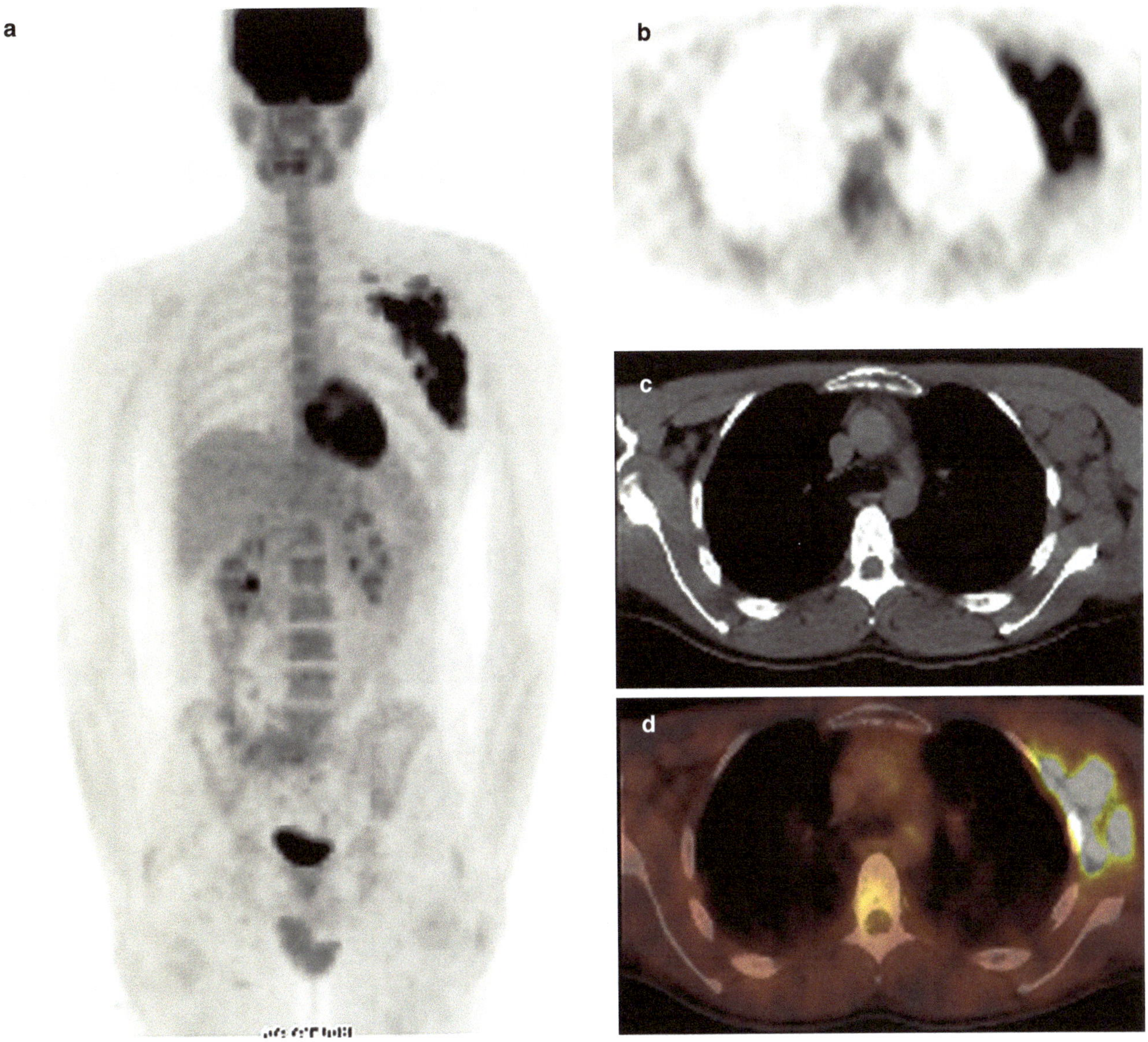

Fig. 7.28 MIP image (**a**), axial PET, CT, and fusion images (**b–d**) show hypermetabolic lymph nodes at left axillary fossa. MIP image (**e**), axial PET, CT, and fusion images (**f–h**) of the second study show clearance of pathologically increased metabolic activity at lymph nodes but newly appeared diffuse hypermetabolism at bone marrow of axial skeleton

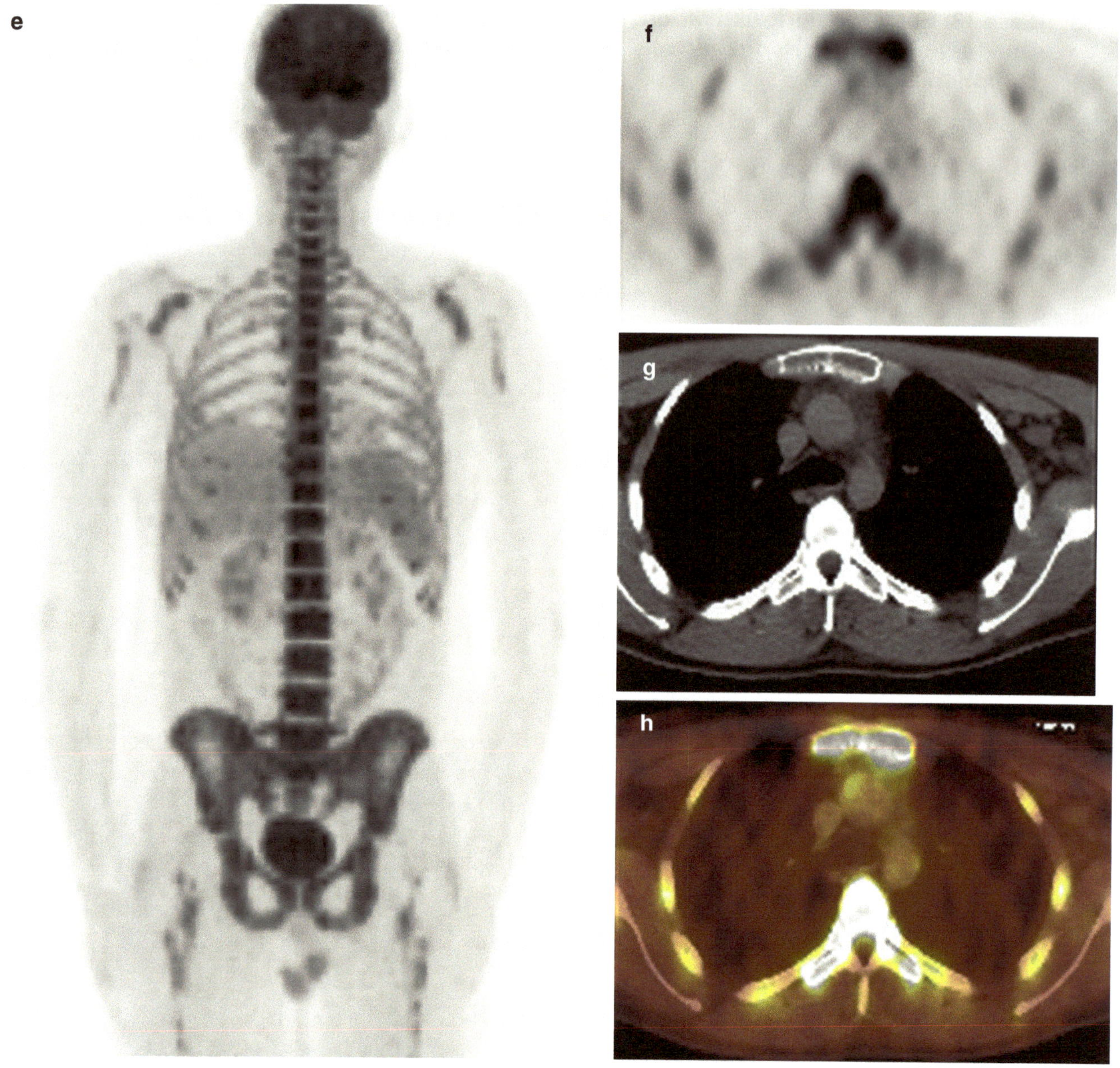

Fig. 7.28 (continued)

7.14 Case 14: Metastatic Involvement of Pulmonary Artery in Hodgkin's Lymphoma

History A 47-year-old male who was diagnosed to have HL 10 years ago was lost to follow up. The patient underwent ^{18}F-FDG PET/CT for restaging, and 6 months later PET/CT study was repeated to assess response to chemotherapy.

Findings

Interpretation Intensely increased FDG uptake at right pulmonary artery and hypermetabolic mass lesion at right paramediastinal area are consistent with metastatic involvement with primary malignancy.

Teaching Point Vascular invasion of lymphoma is a rare finding. FDG PET/CT detects the lesion at vascular structures effectively and it is helpful in evaluation of response to therapy.

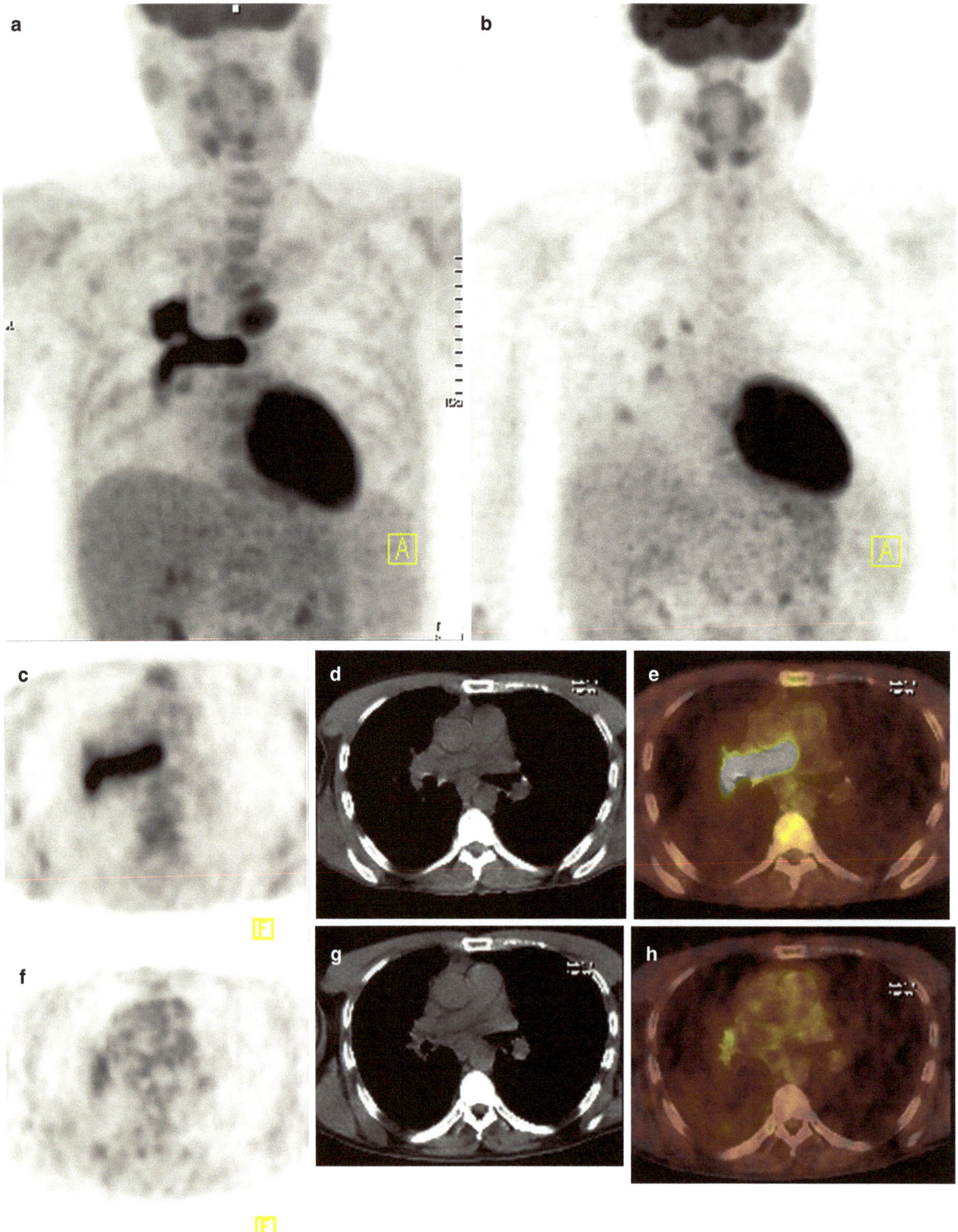

Fig. 7.29 The first MIP image (**a**) shows intensely increased FDG uptake at right pulmonary artery (SUVmax 11.6), hypermetabolic mass lesion at right paramediastinal area (SUVmax 11.2), a few hypermetabolic mediastinal lymph nodes. The second MIP image (**b**) reflects resolution of hypermetabolism at pulmonary artery and paramediastinal mass lesion. There are few residual mildly hypermetabolic mediastinal lymph nodes. Axial PET, CT, and fusion images (**c–e**) show increased FDG uptake at right pulmonary artery, and images after therapy (**f–h**) show resolution of metabolic activity at pulmonary artery

7.15 Case 15: Pulmonary Infection After Treatment of non-Hodgkin Lymphoma

History A 60-year-old male who was diagnosed to have NHL underwent ^{18}F-FDG PET/CT for pretreatment staging. Patient received chemotherapy and ^{18}F-FDG PET/CT was repeated 4 months after the first study.

Findings

Interpretation The second PET/CT scan showed complete remission of disease after chemotherapy. Hypermetabolism at infiltration area at right lung represents infectious process.

Teaching Point Any hypermetabolic lesion at lung appearing after complete remission of NHL is strongly suspicious for pulmonary infection, especially in immunecompromised patients.

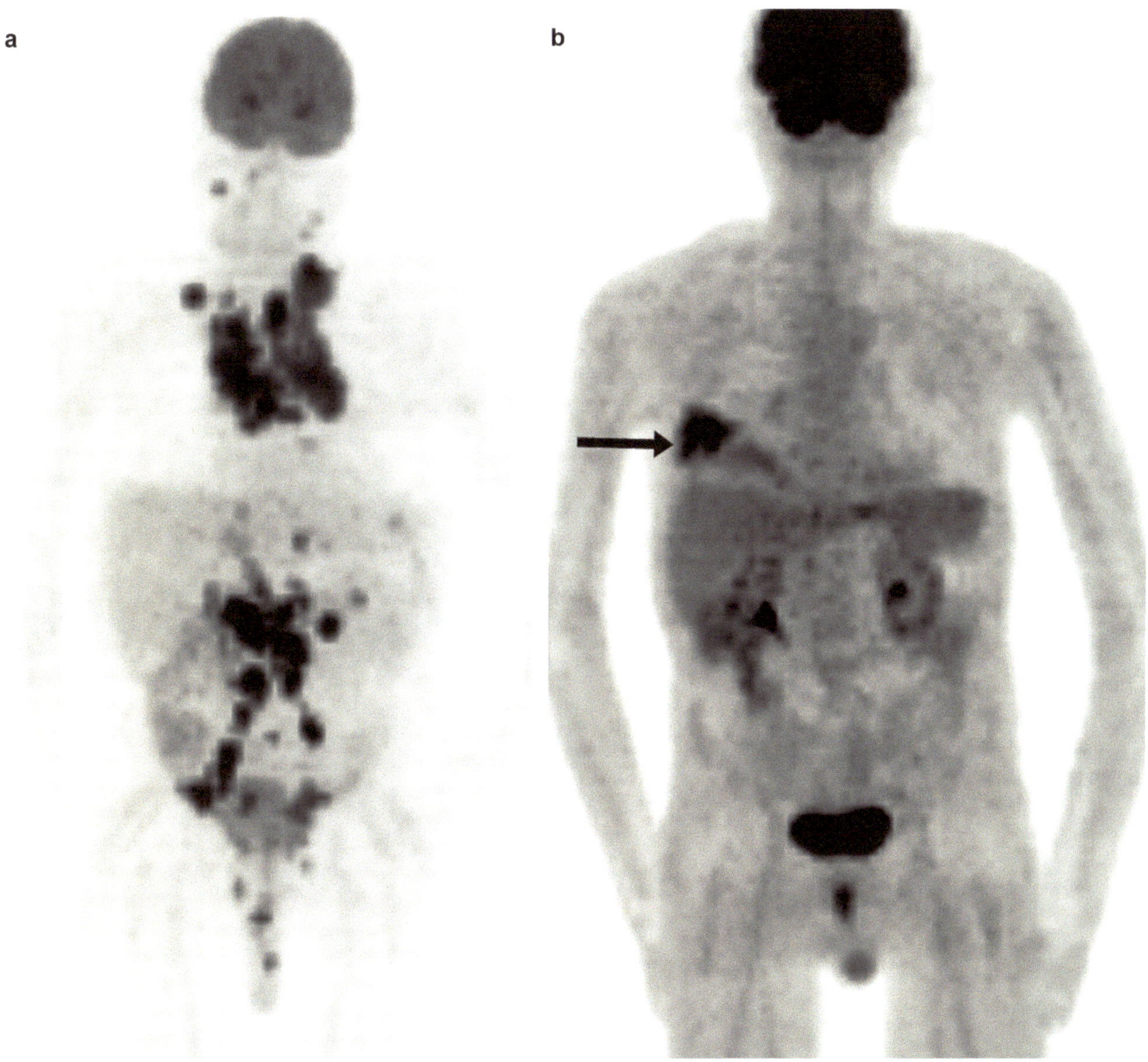

Fig. 7.30 MIP images before chemotherapy showed mediastinal and intraabdominal hypermetabolic lymph nodes (**a**), after the chemotherapy all of the hypermetabolic lymph nodes disappeared but focal increased FDG uptake at right lung was noticed (*arrow*) (**b**)

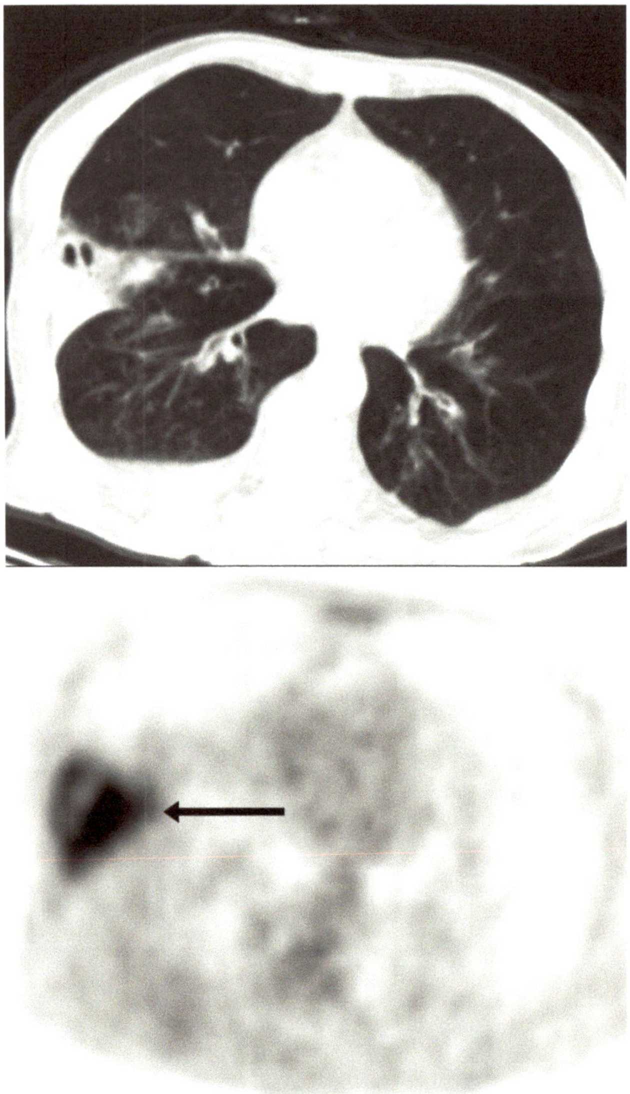

Fig. 7.31 Axial CT and PET images show moderately increased FDG uptake corresponding to infiltration area at lower lobe of right lung (*arrow*)

7.16 Case 16: Pulmonary Infection After Treatment of non-Hodgkin Lymphoma

History A 65-year-old female who was diagnosed to have NHL underwent ^{18}F-FDG PET/CT for pretreatment staging. Patient received chemotherapy and PET/CT scan was repeated 5 months after the first study. Second PET/CT scan showed complete resolution of hypermetabolic lymph nodes but hypermetabolism corresponding to an infiltration area at right lung was detected. The patient was treated with antibiotics and PET/CT scan was performed 2 months after the second study.

Findings

Interpretation Hypermetabolic lesion at lung appearing after complete remission of NHL is compatible with infection and resolution of the lesion after appropriate therapy confirms the inflammatory nature of the lesion.

Teaching Point Repeat ^{18}F-FDG PET/CT scan 2 months after antibiotherapy will be helpful in confirming the infectious process at lungs.

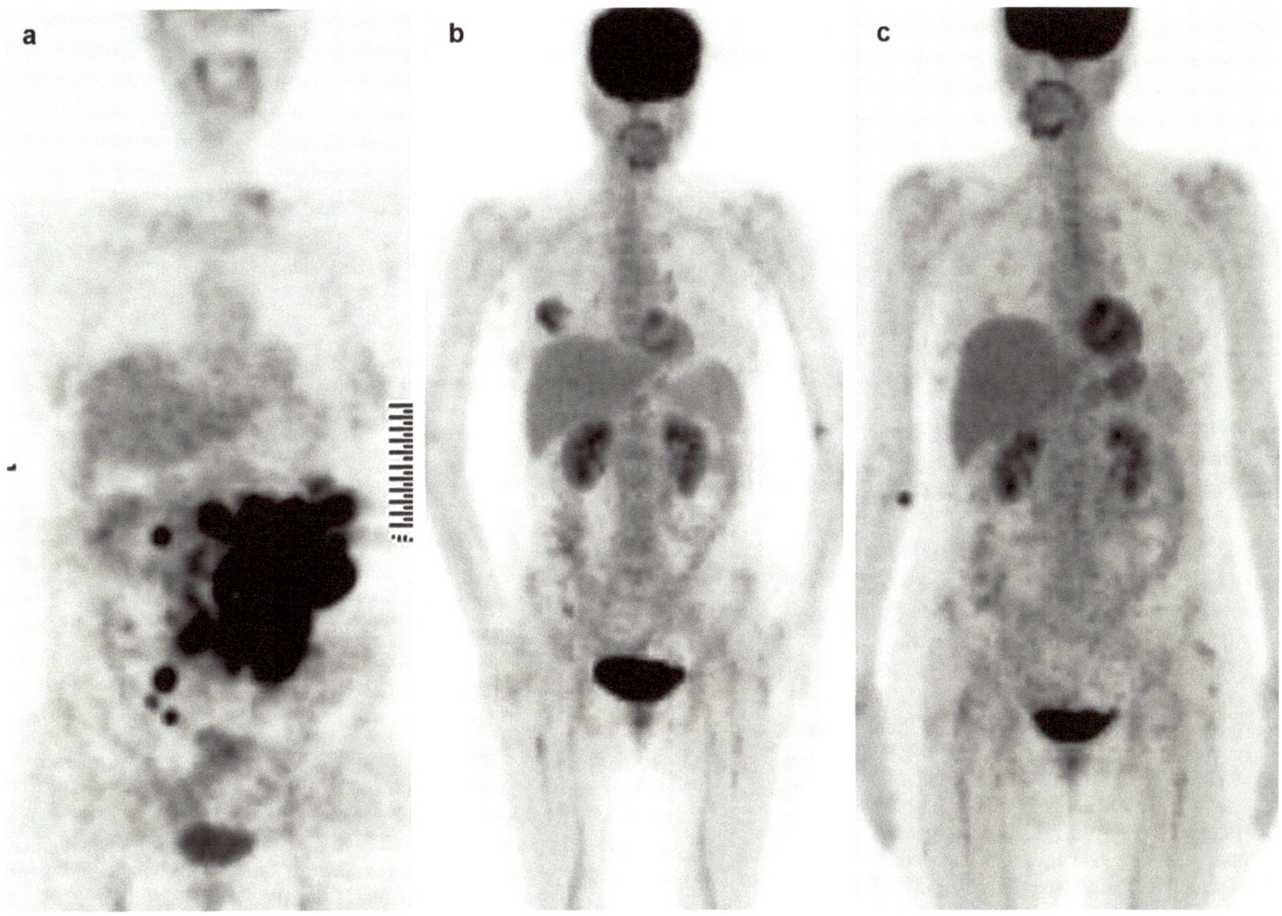

Fig. 7.32 MIP images before chemotherapy showed bulky intraabdominal hypermetabolic lymph nodes (**a**), after the chemotherapy all of the hypermetabolic lymph nodes disappeared but focal increased FDG uptake at right lung was noticed (**b**), following antibiotic therapy the lesion at right lung disappeared (**c**)

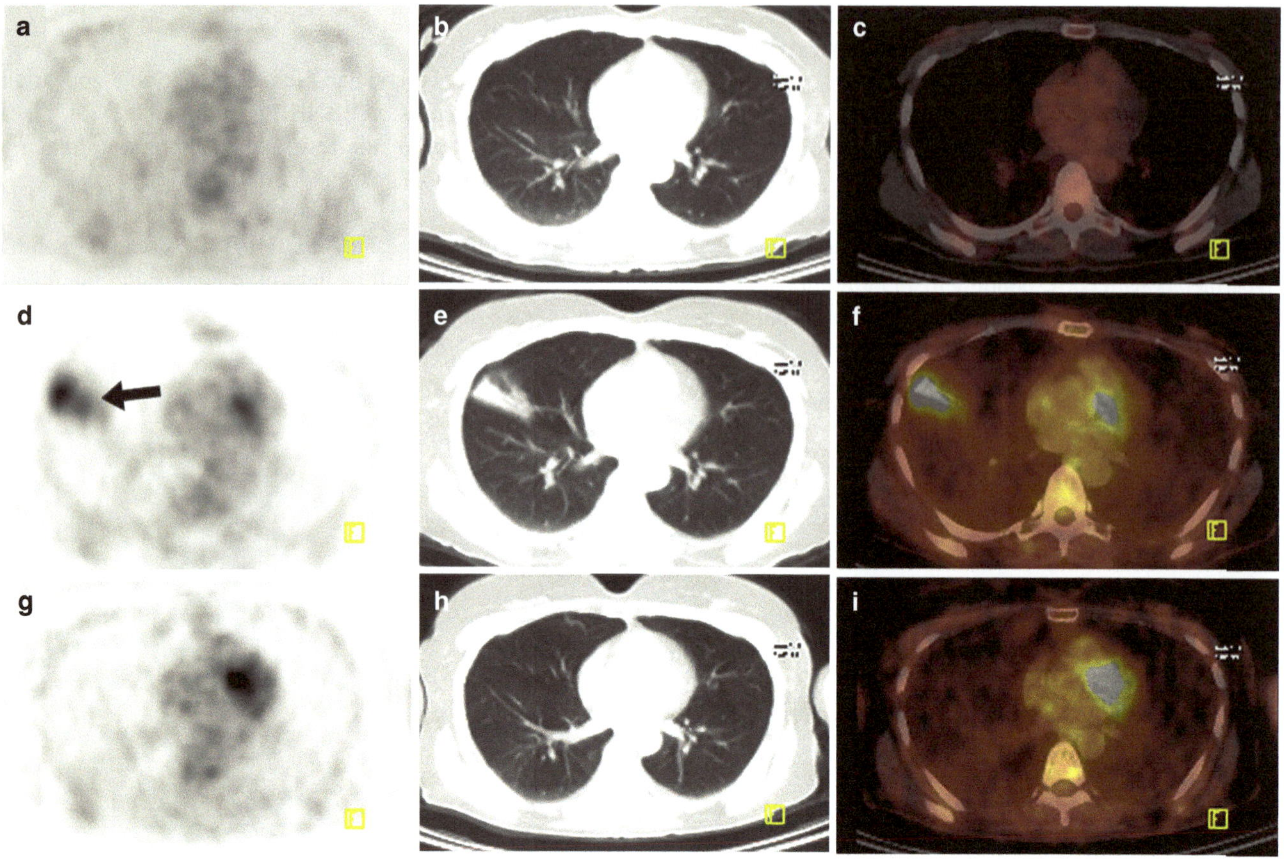

Fig. 7.33 Axial PET, CT and fusion images before (**a, b, c**), after (**d, e, f**) chemotherapy, and after antibiotic therapy (**g, h, i**) show moderately increased FDG uptake corresponding to infiltration area (*arrow*) at middle lobe of right lung and resolution of the lesion after antibiotherapy

Bibliography

1. Ahmad SS, Idris SF, Follows GA, Williams MV. Primary testicular lymphoma. Clin Oncol (R Coll Radiol). 2012;24:358–65. doi:10.1016/j.clon.2012.02.005.
2. Najem AZ, Porcaro JL, Rush Jr BF. Primary non-Hodgkin's lymphoma of the duodenum. Cancer. 1984;54:895–8.
3. Smith C, Kubicka RA, Thomas Jr CR. Non-Hodgkin lymphoma of the gastrointestinal tract. Radiographics. 1992;12:887–99.
4. Balikian JP, Nassar NT, Shammaya MH. Primary lymphomas of the small intestine including the duodenum. Am J Roentgenol Radium Ther Nucl Med. 1969;107:131–41.
5. Lee DY, Lee JJ, Kim JY, Park SH, Chae SY, Kim S, et al. (18) F-FDG PET in patients with primary systemic anaplastic large cell lymphoma: differential features according to expression of anaplastic lymphoma kinase. Nucl Med Mol Imaging. 2013;47:249–56. doi:10.1007/s13139-013-0224-6.
6. Ömür Ö, Baran Y, Oral A, Ceylan Y. Fluorine-18 fluorodeoxyglucose PET-CT for extranodal staging of non-Hodgkin and Hodgkin lymphoma. Diagn Interv Radiol. 2014;20:185–92. doi:10.5152/dir.2013.13174.
7. Özülker T, Özülker F, Eker Ö, Özpaçacı T, Karyağar S. A case of extranodal non-Hodgkin lymphoma with multiple organ involvement detected with 18F-FDG PET CT. Turk J Nucl Med. 2009;18:111–5.
8. Pakos EE, Fotopoulos AD, Ioannidis JP. 18F -FDG PET for evaluation of bone marrow infiltration in staging of lymphoma: a meta-analysis. J Nucl Med. 2005;46:958–63.
9. Radan L, Fischer D, Bar-Shalom R, Dann EJ, Epelbaum R, Haim N, et al. FDG avidity and PET/CT patterns in primary gastric lymphoma. Eur J Nucl Med Mol Imaging. 2008;35:1424–30. doi:10.1007/s00259-008-0771-8.
10. Rutherford C, Andemariam B, Philips SM, Elstrom RL, Chadburn A, Furman RR, et al. FDG-PET in prediction of splenectomy findings in patients with known or suspected lymphoma. Leuk Lymphoma. 2008;49:719–26. doi:10.1080/10428190801927387.
11. Schaefer NG, Hany TF, Taverna C, Seifert B, Stumpe KD, von Schulthess GK, et al. Non-Hodgkin lymphoma and Hodgkin disease: coregistered FDG PET and CT at staging and restaging—do we need contrast-enhanced CT? Radiology. 2004;232:823–9.
12. Spaepen K, Stroobants S, Verhoef G, Mortelmans L. Positron emission tomography with [(18)F]FDG for therapy response monitoring in lymphoma patients. Eur J Nucl Med Mol Imaging. 2003;30 Suppl 1:97–105.

8 Colorectal Cancer

8.1 Case 1: Incidentally Detected Villous Adenoma

History A 55-year-old female patient who is being followed up with the diagnosis of lung carcinoma underwent ^{18}F-FDG PET/CT scan for restaging.

Findings

Interpretation Increased FDG uptake at proximal rectal lesion in soft tissue density is suspicious for villous adenoma.

Result The lesion at rectum is resected and the histopathology revealed villous adenoma.

Teaching Point Colonic adenomas constitute 70–80 % of all colorectal polyps, and they are considered a precursor of colorectal cancer. In a study ^{18}F-FDG PET was found to have a true-positive rate of 83.3 % in detecting precancerous colonic adenomas.

T. Özülker, F. Özülker, *Atlas of PET-CT Imaging in Oncology: A Case-Based Guide to Image Interpretation*,
DOI 10.1007/978-3-319-18994-9_8

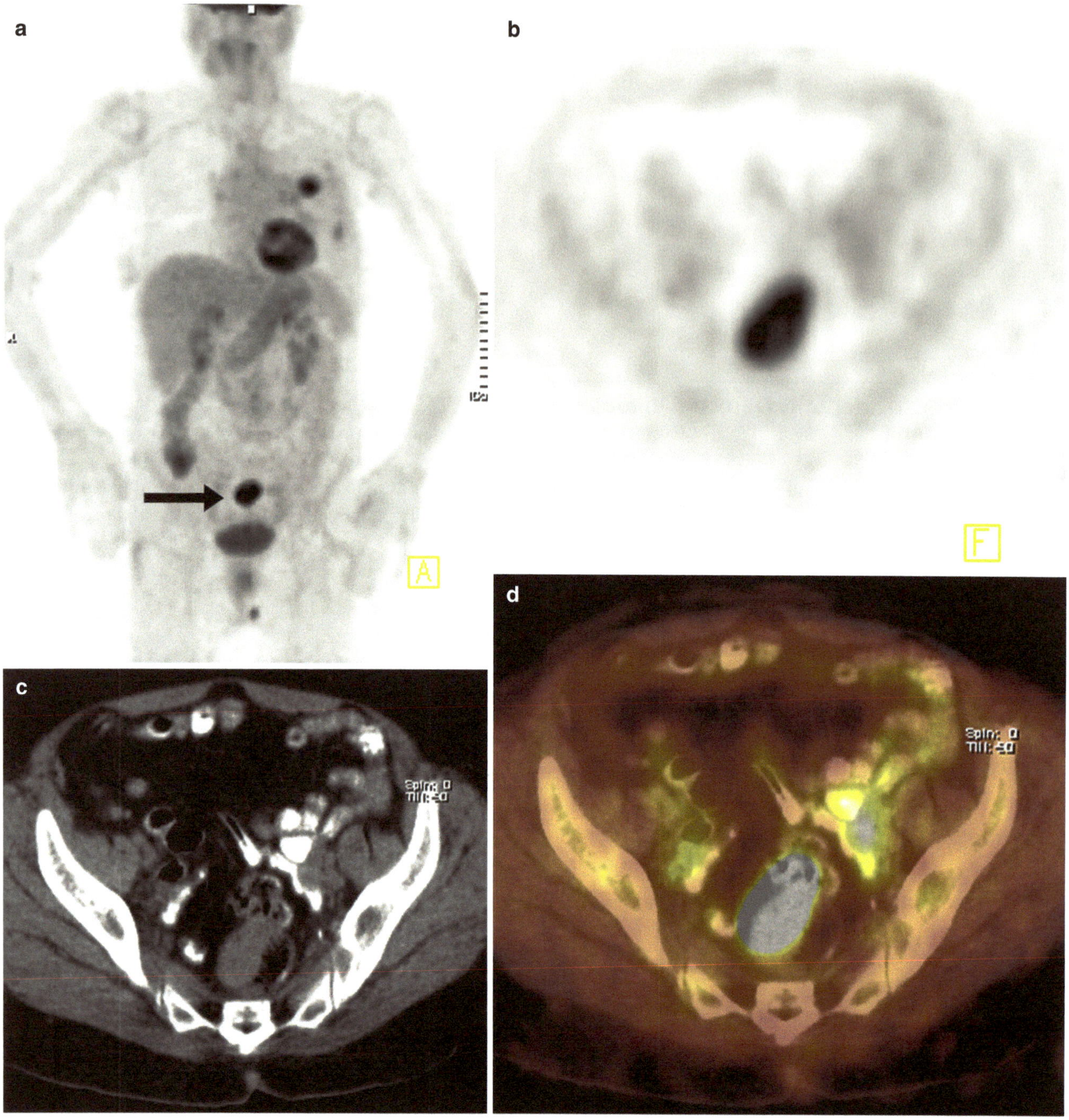

Fig. 8.1 MIP image (**a**) shows increased FDG uptake at left lung consistent with primary lung cancer. Axial slices of PET, CT, and fusion images (**b–d**) show hypermetabolic (SUVmax 7.4) soft tissue lesion at proximal rectum

8.2 Case 2: Metastatic Pulmonary Nodule and Villous Adenoma at Rectum in a Patient with Previous History of Lung Carcinoma

History A 54-year-old female patient who had been treated for NSCLC underwent ^{18}F-FDG PET/CT scan for restaging. Since a suspicious lung nodule was detected in the first procedure, ^{18}F-FDG PET/CT scan is repeated 6 months later.

Findings

Interpretation Hypermetabolic mass lesion in soft tissue density at rectum suspicious for villous adenoma. Pulmonary lung nodule is considered as a metastatic lesion.

Result The lesion at rectum is resected and the histopathology revealed tubulovillous adenoma.

Teaching Point Oral contrast agents provides better delineation of intestinal structures and mass lesions like villous adenomas. There is no significant difference between benign hyperplastic or precancerous lesions regarding SUVmax values, so when a hypermetabolic lesion causing filling defect is detected, colonoscopy should be performed.

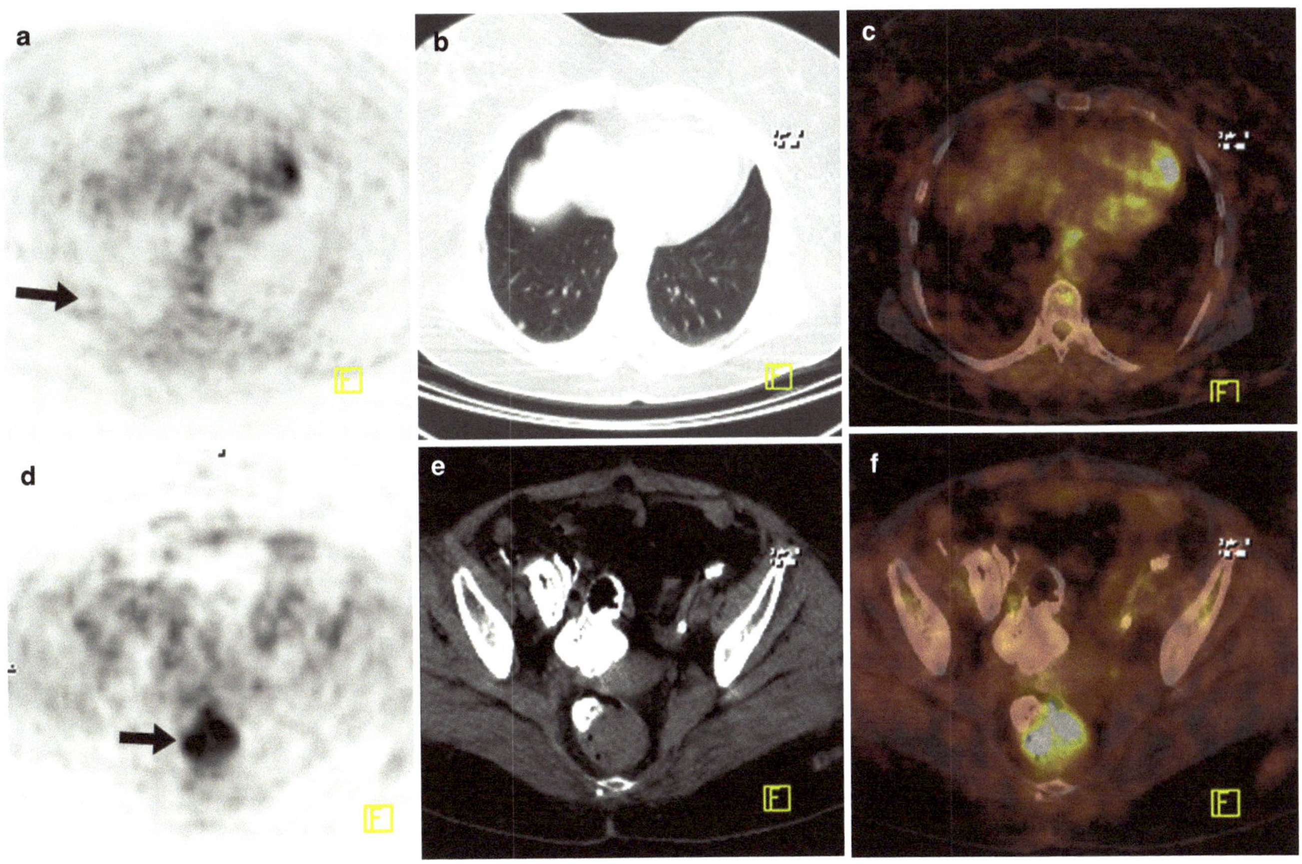

Fig. 8.2 Axial PET, CT, and fusion images (*upper row*) show a tiny pulmonary nodule at right lung located peripherally and showing subtle FDG uptake (*arrow*). There is a mass lesion at rectum (*arrow*) which creates a filling defect and exhibits significant FDG uptake (SUVmax 6.2) (*second row*)

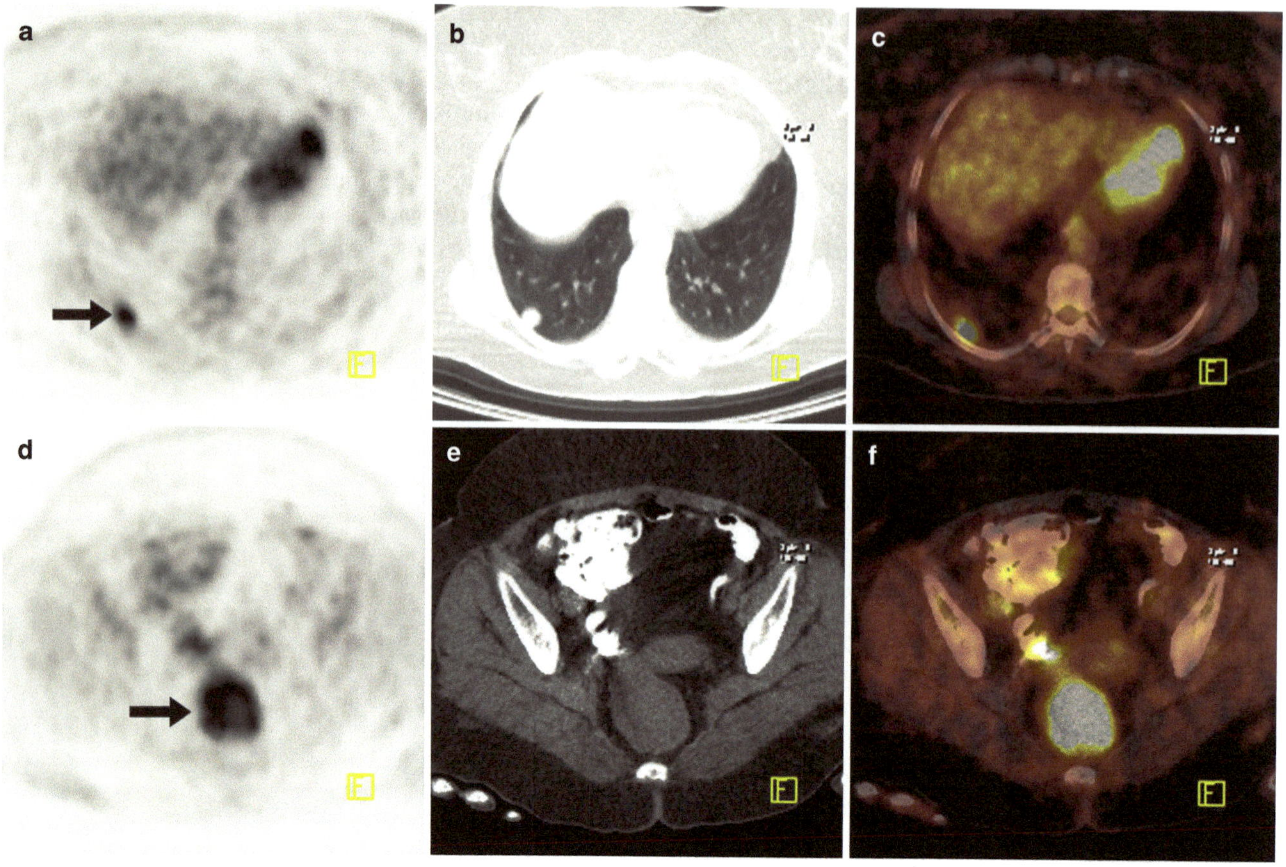

Fig. 8.3 (**a–c**)[18]F-FDG PET/CT scan repeated 6 months after the first one (**d–f**) shows progression at pulmonary nodule in terms of both size and metabolic activity. Mass lesion at rectum also shows progression (*arrows*)

8.3 Case 3: Initial Staging of Colorectal Carcinoma

History A 72-year-old male patient with adenocarcinoma at sigmoid colon was referred to ^{18}F-FDG PET/CT scanning for pretreatment staging.

Findings

Interpretation Hypermetabolic lesion at sigmoid colon consistent with primary malignancy and metastatic focus at right lobe of liver.

Teaching Point ^{18}F-FDG PET/CT is effective in the detection of liver metastases of colorectal carcinoma. On a per-patient basis the sensitivities of CT, MRI, and ^{18}F-FDG PET/CT are found as 83.6 %, 88.2 %, and 94.1 % respectively.

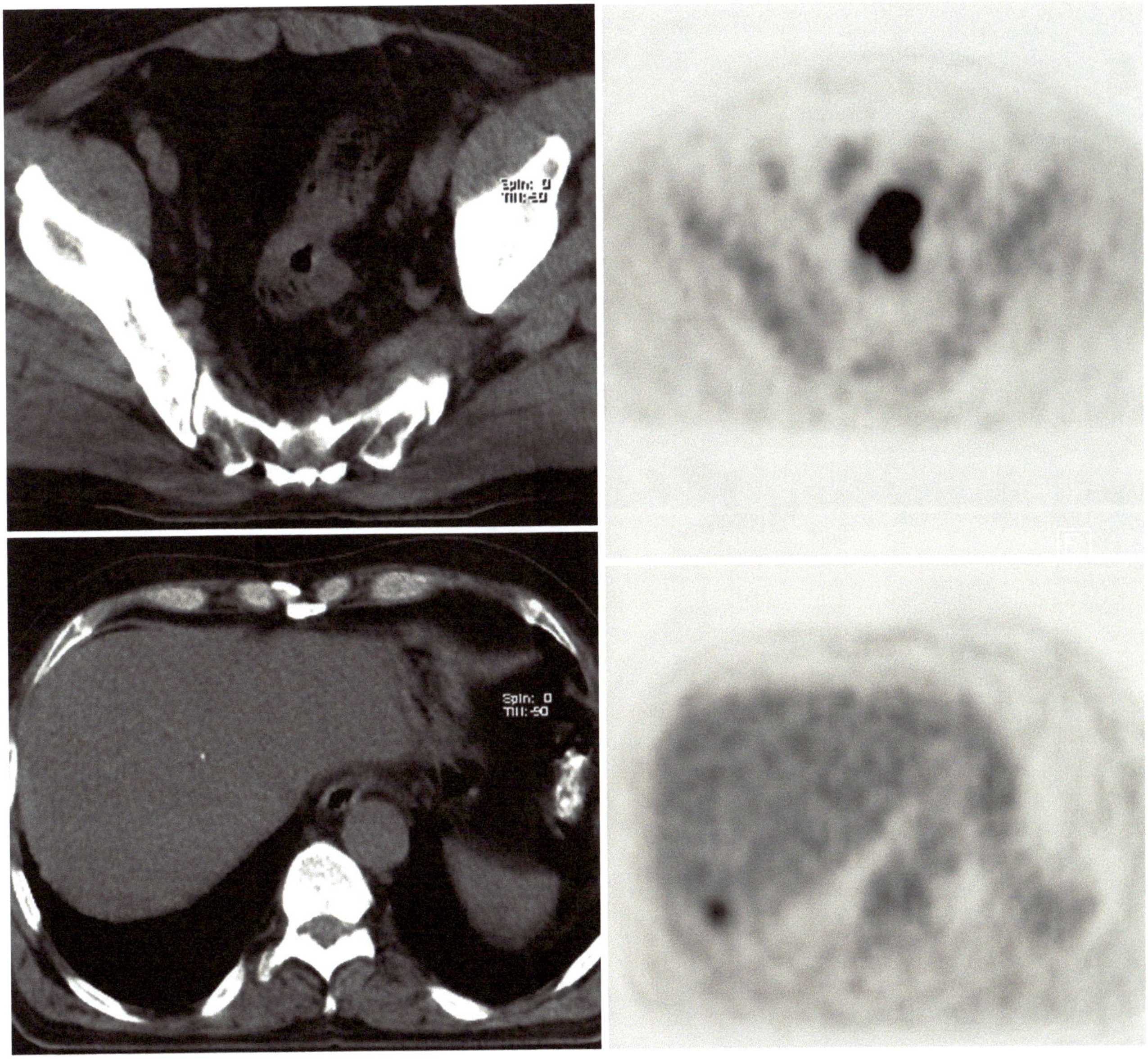

Fig. 8.4 Axial CT and PET images display intensely increased FDG uptake at sigmoid colon (*upper row*) and focal hypermetabolic lesion at right lobe of liver (*lower row*)

8.4 Case 4: Initial Staging of Colorectal Carcinoma

History A 74-year-old female patient who was diagnosed to have colorectal adenocarcinoma was referred to ^{18}F-FDG PET/CT scanning for initial staging.

Findings

Interpretation Primary malignant lesion at proximal ascending colon and multiple metastatic lung nodules.

Result The patient underwent operation for malignant lesion at colon.

Teaching Point ^{18}F-FDG PET/CT has limited role in diagnosis and initial staging of colorectal cancer. FDG PET is not effective in local and regional staging because of its limited spatial resolution. Current staging algorithms are mainly include surgical and pathologic data. Intense FDG uptake by the primary tumor, masks the pathological uptake at structures in vicinity resulting in a low sensitivity for detection of regional metastatic lymph nodes. ^{18}F-FDG PET/CT may only be effective in pretreatment staging of patients who bear high risk for surgery.

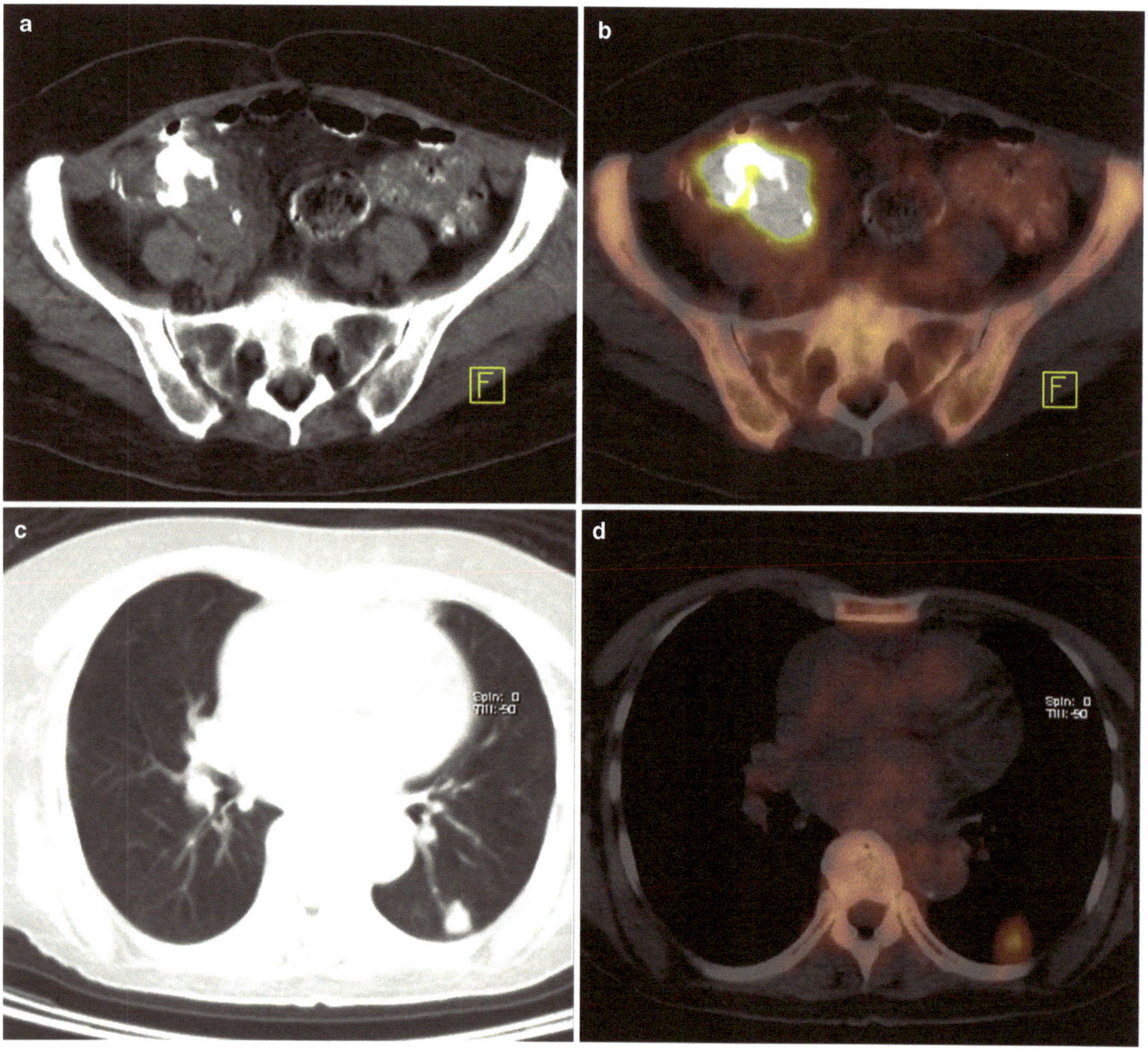

Fig. 8.5 Axial CT and fusion images show significantly hypermetabolic (SUVmax 14.3) mass lesion located at proximal ascending colon (*upper row*) and hypermetabolic lung nodule at lower zone of left lung (*lower row*)

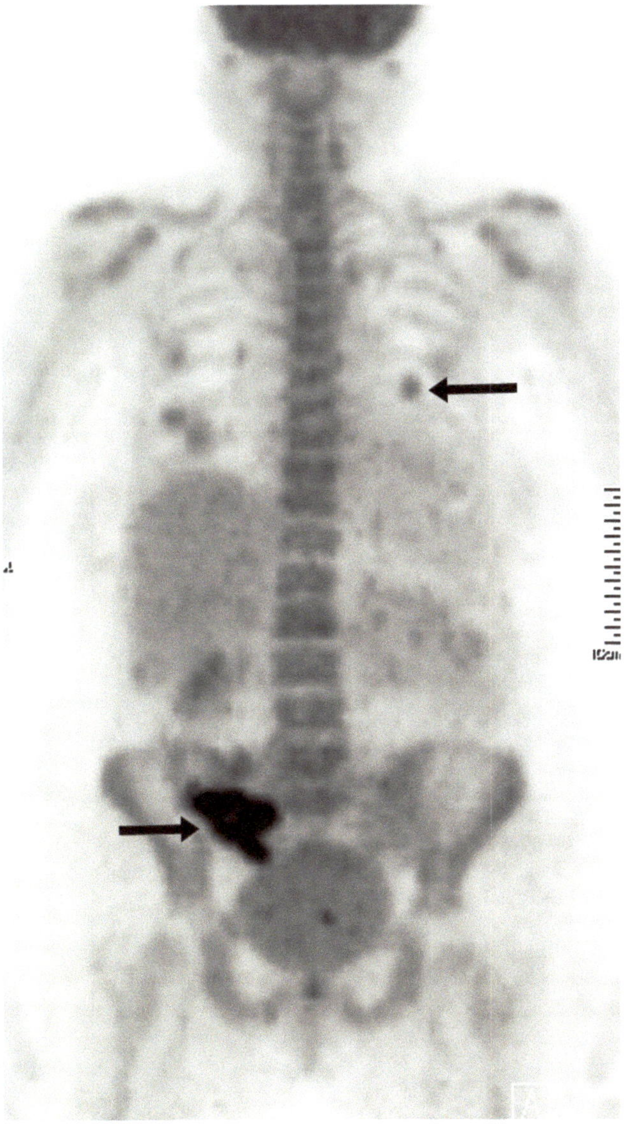

Fig. 8.6 MIP image shows intensely hypermetabolic mass lesion at right lower quadrant of abdomen and multiple hypermetabolic foci representing lung nodules (*arrows*)

8.5 Case 5: Initial Staging of Colorectal Carcinoma

History A 28-year-old female patient with colorectal adenocarcinoma was referred to ^{18}F-FDG PET/CT scanning for pretreatment staging.

Findings

Interpretation Primary malignant lesion at rectum. Pararectal lymph nodes are metastatically involved but they are not clearly identified on PET images.

Result The patient underwent operation for colorectal adenocarcinoma and lymph nodes turned out to be metastatically involved.

Teaching Point Pararectal lymph nodes are not very well documented on PET images due to low FDG uptake because of micrometastatic invasion and obscuring effect of primary tumor which is in close proximity.

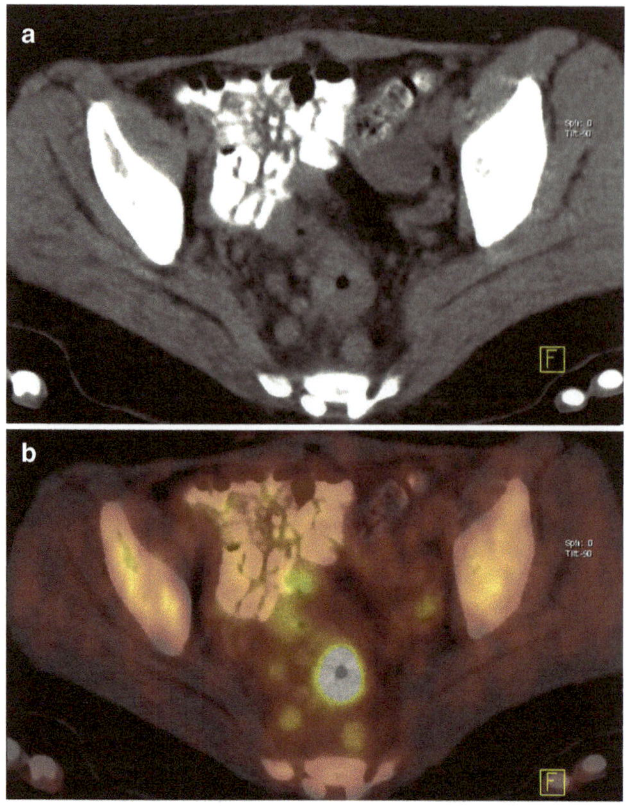

Fig. 8.7 Axial CT and fusion images (**a**, **b**) display intensely increased FDG uptake (SUVmax 16) at rectum and pararectal lymph nodes with mild FDG uptake (SUVmax 4)

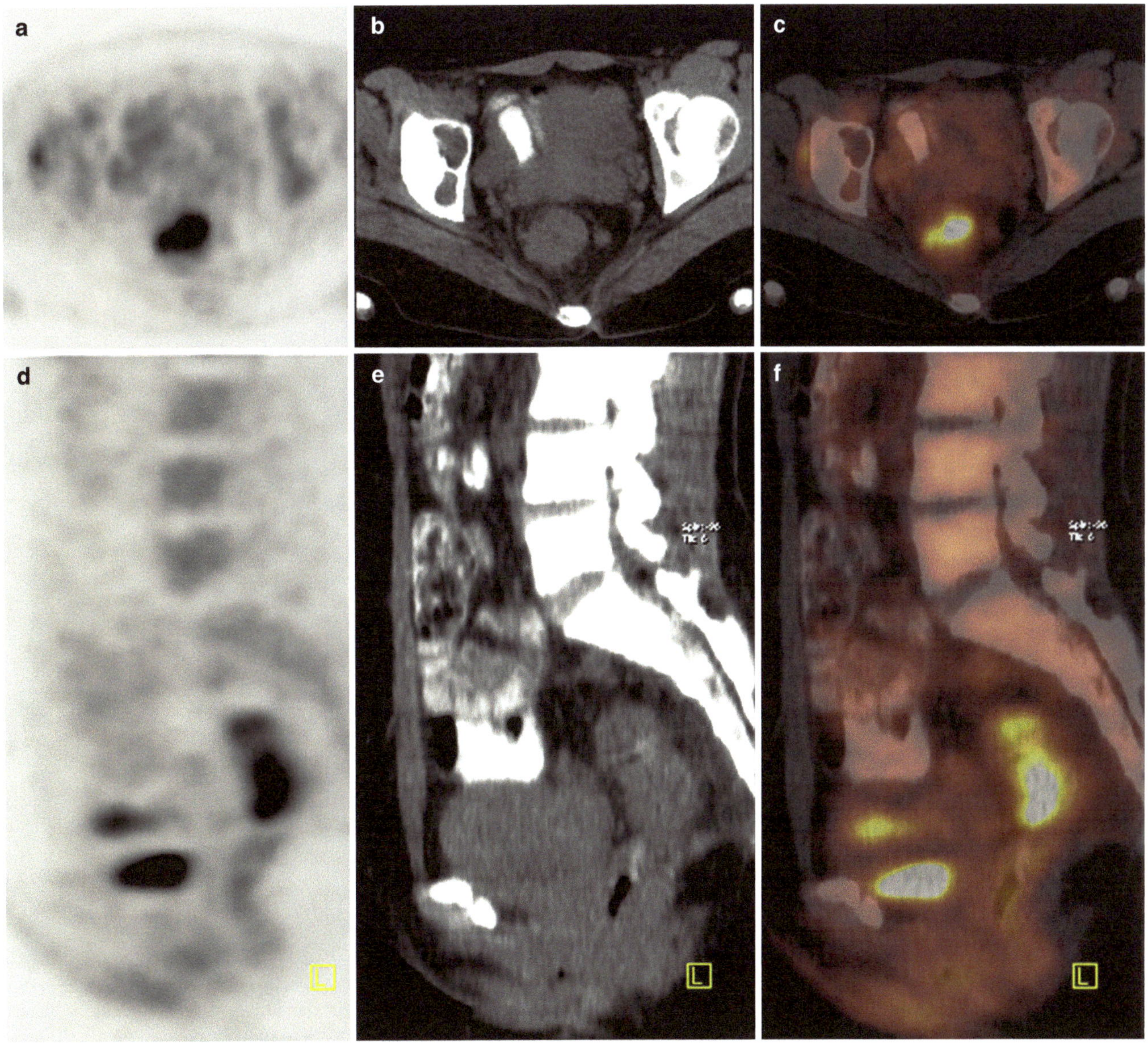

Fig. 8.8 Axial (**a–c**) and sagittal (**d–f**) PET, CT, and fusion images show intensely increased FDG uptake at rectum and pararectal lymph nodes showing mild FDG uptake and barely seen on PET images

8.6 Case 6: Anal Cancer with Inguinal Lymph Node Metastasis

History A 56-year-old male patient was diagnosed to have anal cancer and referred to ^{18}F-FDG PET/CT scanning for pretreatment staging.

Findings

Interpretation Primary malignancy at anal canal which show metastasis to left inguinal lymph node.

Teaching Point ^{18}F-FDG PET/CT is a useful imaging tool in the pretreatment staging of anal cancer. Size of the primary tumor, lymph node involvement, and distant metastases are three main determinants that TNM staging depends on and they can be evaluated effectively with ^{18}F-FDG PET/CT in a single whole-body imaging procedure.

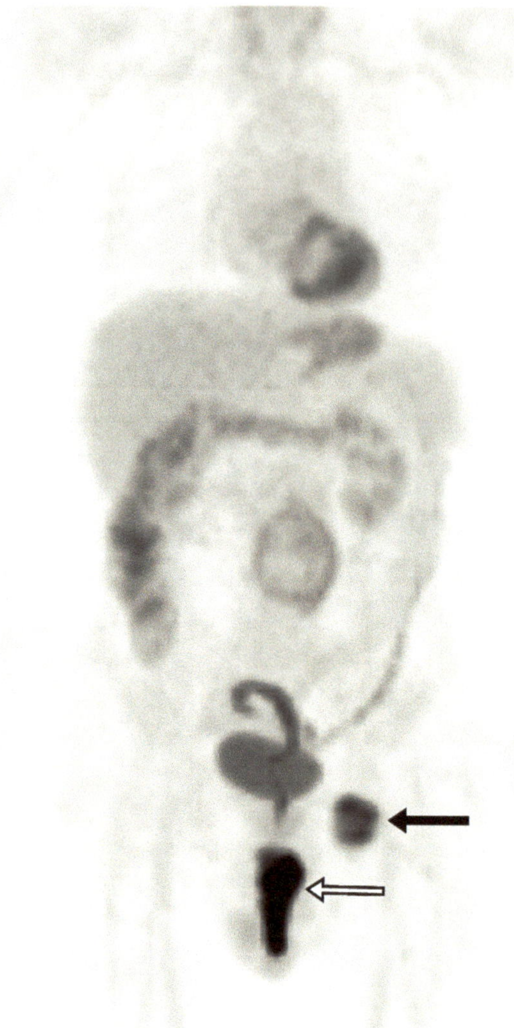

Fig. 8.9 MIP image shows hypermetabolism at anal canal (*empty arrow*), hypermetabolic focus at left inguinal area (*arrow*). There is also increased FDG uptake in circular fashion at upper middle abdomen reflecting an aortic aneurysm

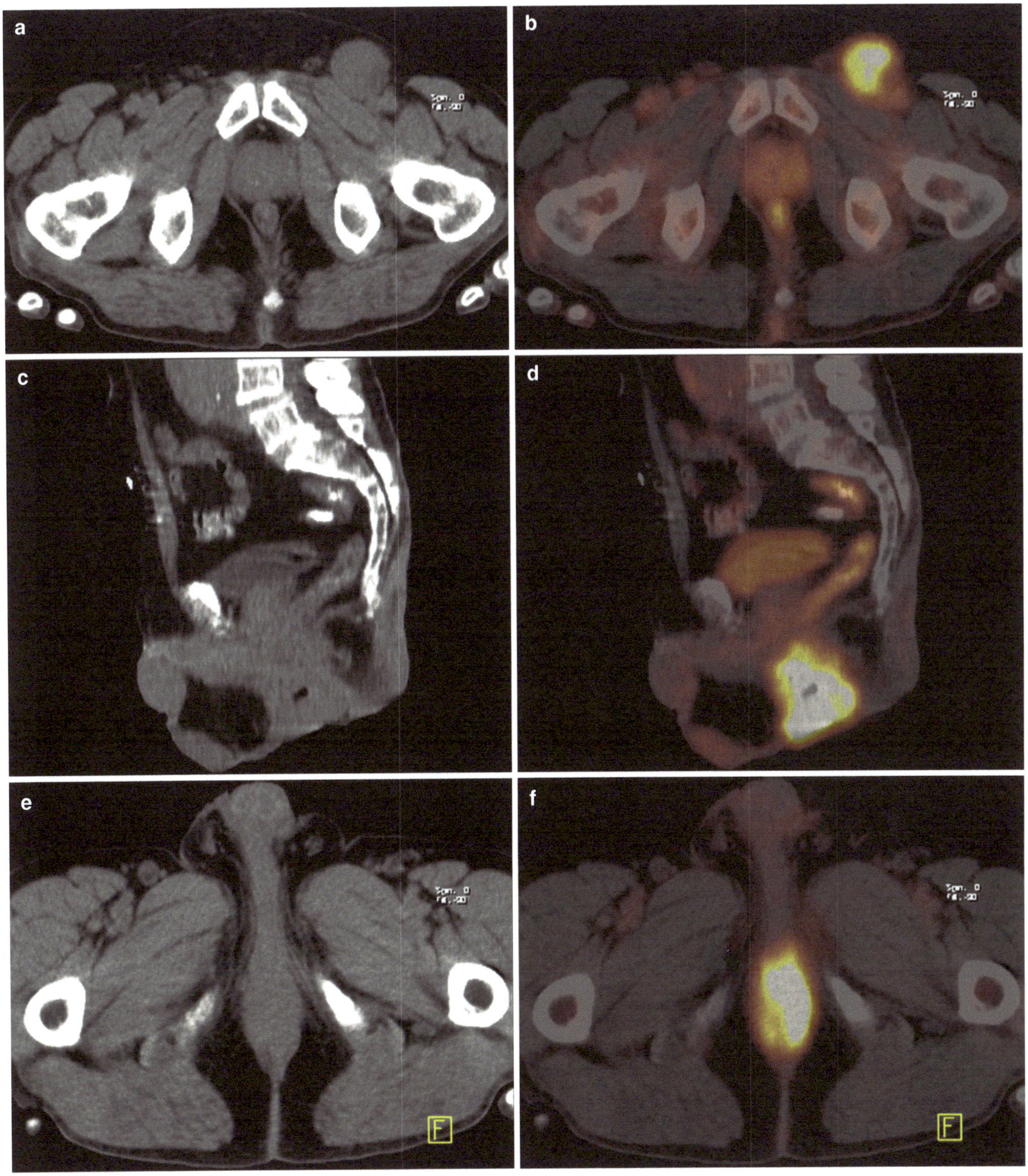

Fig. 8.10 Axial (**a**, **b**, **e**, **f**) and sagittal (**c**, **d**) CT and fusion images show a intensely hypermetabolic (SUVmax 26) mass lesion at anal canal. There is also a hypermetabolic lymph node at left inguinal area, with dimensions of 3.6×3.4 cm. There is not any other pathological FDG uptake that can be considered in favor of distant metastasis

8.7 Case 7: Rectum Cancer with Distant Metastasis

History A 62-year-old male patient who had been operated 4 years ago and diagnosed to have rectal adenocarcinoma underwent ^{18}F-FDG PET/CT scanning for restaging.

Findings

Interpretation Metastatic lesion at right lung. Metachronous cancer of lung should also be taken into account in differential diagnosis.

Teaching Point ^{18}F-FDG PET CT scan has an important role in restaging of colorectal carcinoma, as it excludes metastasis at other regions of body and enables treatment of solitary metastatic lesion at lung either by surgery and/or radiotherapy.

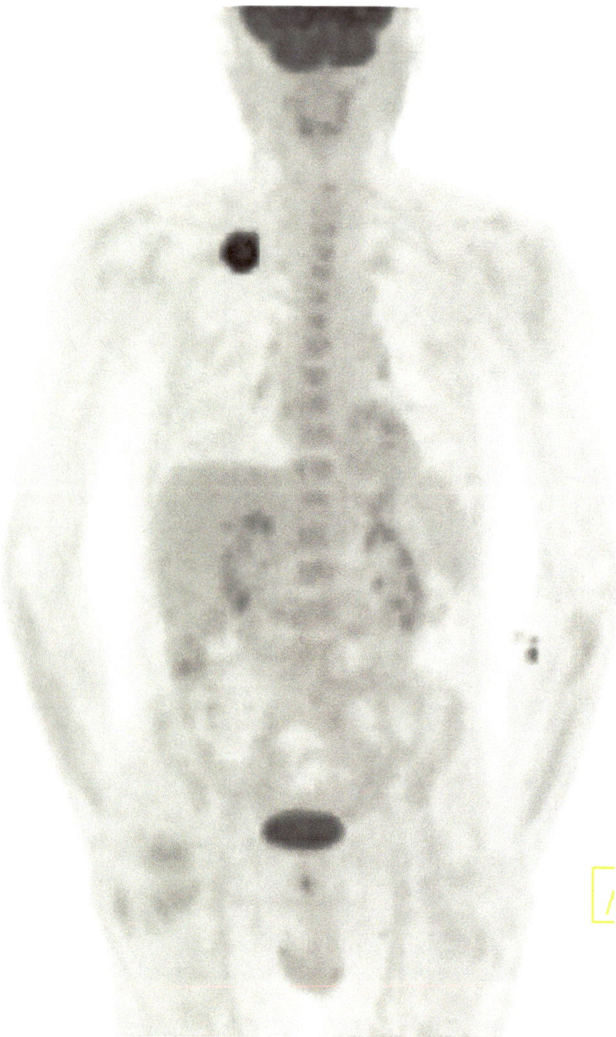

Fig. 8.11 MIP image

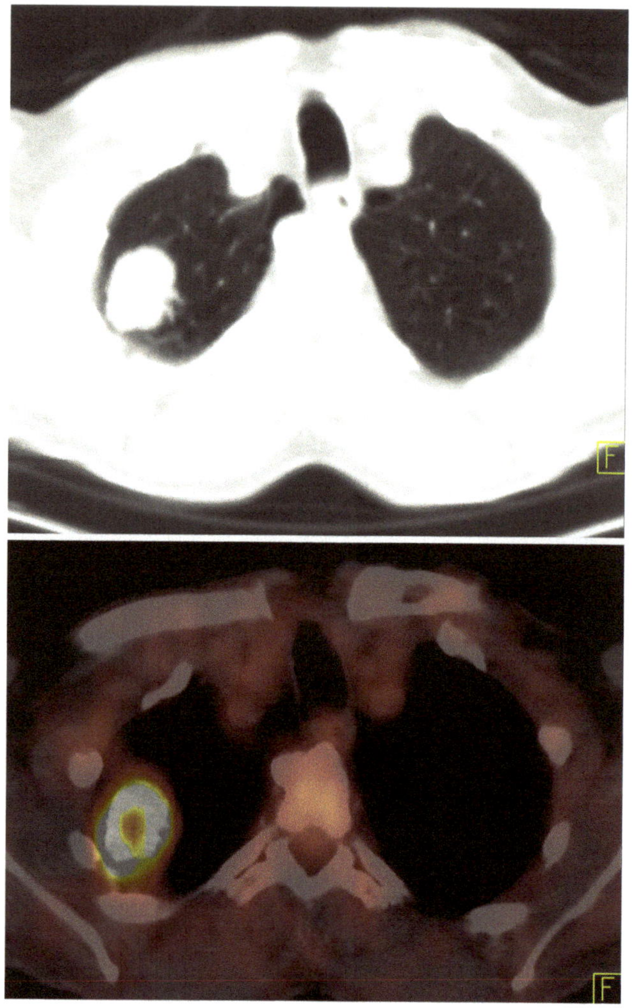

Fig. 8.12 Axial CT and fusion images show a intensely hypermetabolic (SUVmax 19.7), mass lesion at apical segment of right lung, which has a central hypometabolic necrotic area

8.8 Case 8: Discrimination of Local Recurrence from Postoperative Scar

History A 31-year-old female patient who had undergone operation for rectal carcinoma before was referred to ^{18}F-FDG PET/CT scanning for discrimination of local recurrence from fibrotic scar tissue.

Findings

Interpretation Absence of FDG uptake at the soft tissue lesion leads to diagnosis of benign fibrotic scar tissue.

Teaching Point Pelvic recurrence can be encountered in up to 30 % of the cases following primary curative surgery of colorectal carcinoma. Development of fibrotic presacral mass following operation is detected in as many as 39 % of the patients following anterior resection and in 19 % of the patients after abdominoperineal resection. In a metaanalysis, ^{18}F-FDG PET/CT showed a sensitivity of 94.5 % and specificity of 97.7 % in detecting local pelvic recurrence.

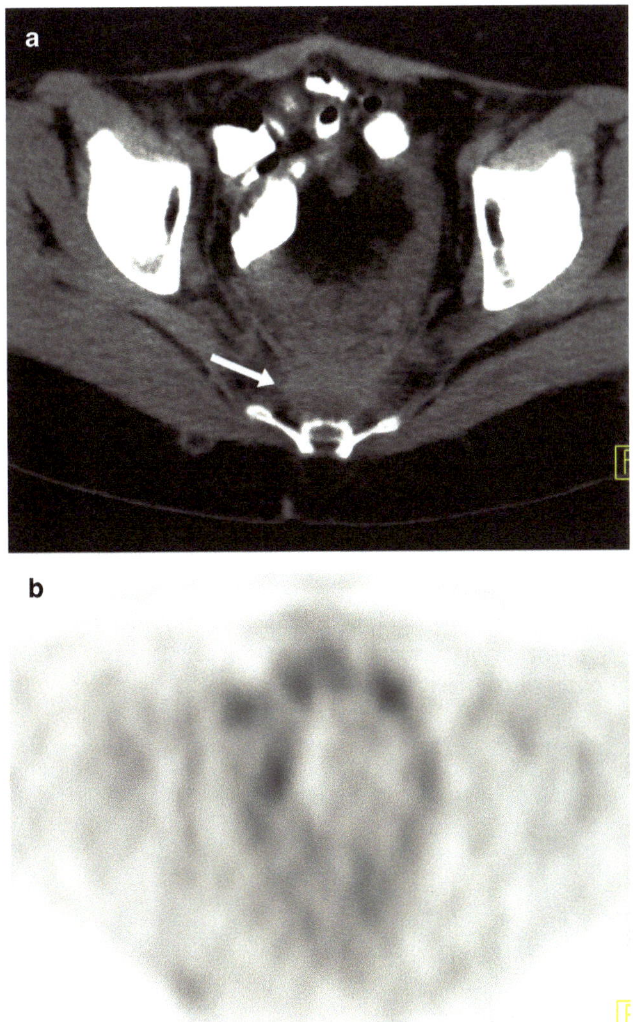

Fig. 8.13 Axial CT and PET images (**a**, **b**) show presacral lesion in soft tissue density (*arrow*) without any corresponding significant metabolic activity

8.9 Case 9: Recurrence at Colostomy Site in Colorectal Cancer

History A 32-year-old female patient who had undergone an abdominoperineal resection for rectal adenocarcinoma was referred to ^{18}F-FDG PET/CT scanning for restaging.

Findings

Interpretation The pattern and intensity of increased FDG uptake at colostomy site is consistent with recurrence. There is also metastatic involvement in lymph nodes at mediastinal, bilateral common iliac, and left inguinal lymph node stations.

Result The lesion at colostomy site is resected and histopathology revealed adenocarcinoma.

Teaching Point

- The synchronous and metachronous development of two or more primary adenocarcinomas accounts for 3–5 % of cases of colorectal cancer.
- There are several mechanisms responsible for occurrence of recurrences preferentially at colostomy site. Compression caused by clothing at the stoma site, presence of enterobacteria and bile acids in the stools can be accused. The mechanisms may be similar to that of recurrence of cancer in an old surgery scar. ^{18}F-FDG PET/CT scan has higher accuracy in detecting recurrence at colostomy site than conventional imaging, the CT performed simultaneously missed the recurrent lesion at colostomy site in our case.

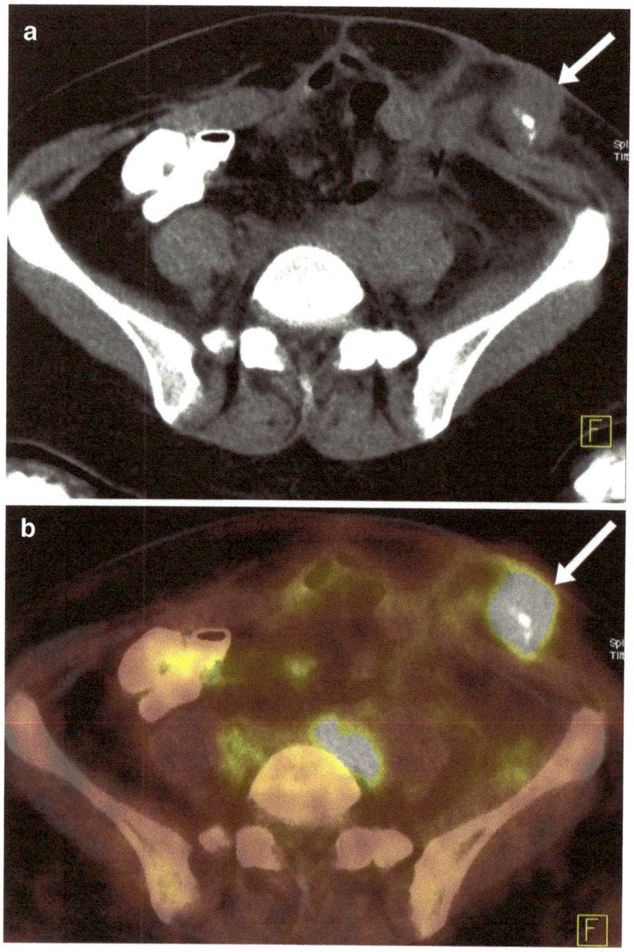

Fig. 8.14 Axial CT and fusion images (**a**, **b**) show significantly hypermetabolic (SUVmax 7.5) lesion in soft tissue density at colostomy site at the left lower quadrant of abdomen (*arrow*) and hypermetabolic lymph nodes at left common iliac area

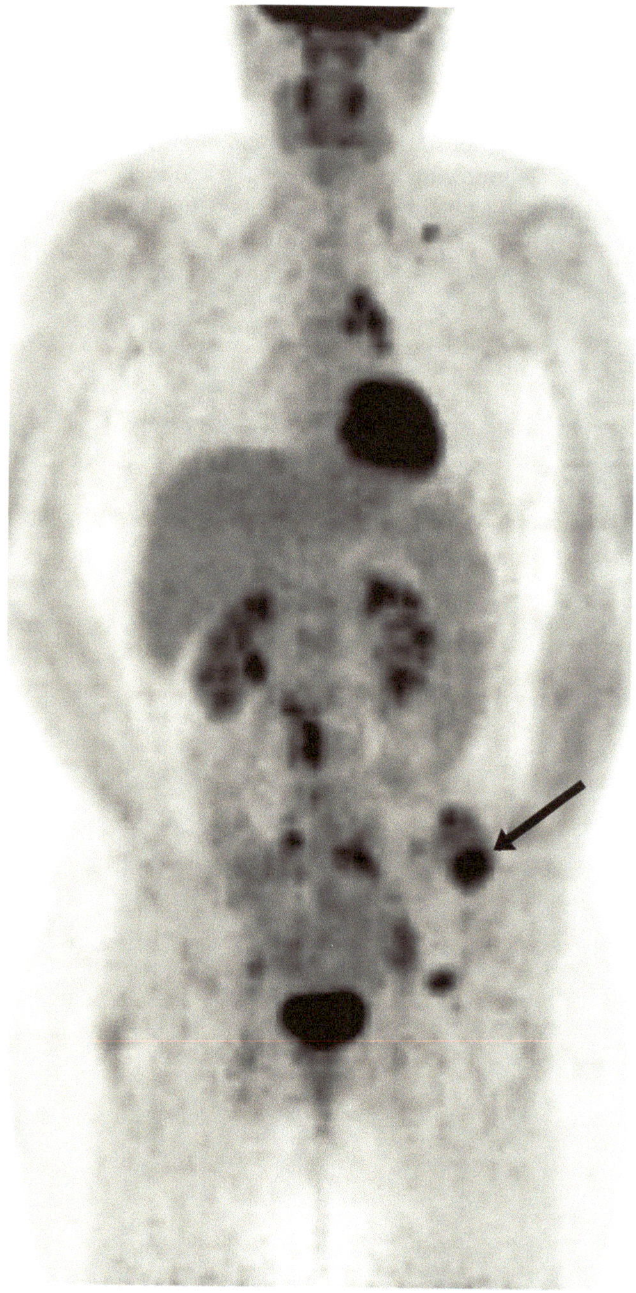

Fig. 8.15 MIP image shows intense hypermetabolism at colostomy site (*arrow*), and apart from this pathological uptake at mediastinal, bilateral common iliac, and left inguinal lymph nodes is detected

8.10 Case 10: Restaging of Colorectal Carcinoma

History A 73-year-old male patient who has been treated with chemotherapy for rectum carcinoma is referred to ^{18}F-FDG PET/CT scanning for detection of recurrence.

Findings

Interpretation Local recurrence at sigmoid colon and rectum together with a metastatic lymph node at left internal iliac region. Focal lung lesions can be either metastatic or inflammatory.

Teaching Point CT cannot always differentiate between fibrotic masses and soft tissue recurrences since it relies on size and morphology. ^{18}F-FDG PET/CT scan is an efficient tool in making the discrimination between benign fibrotic tissue and recurrence.

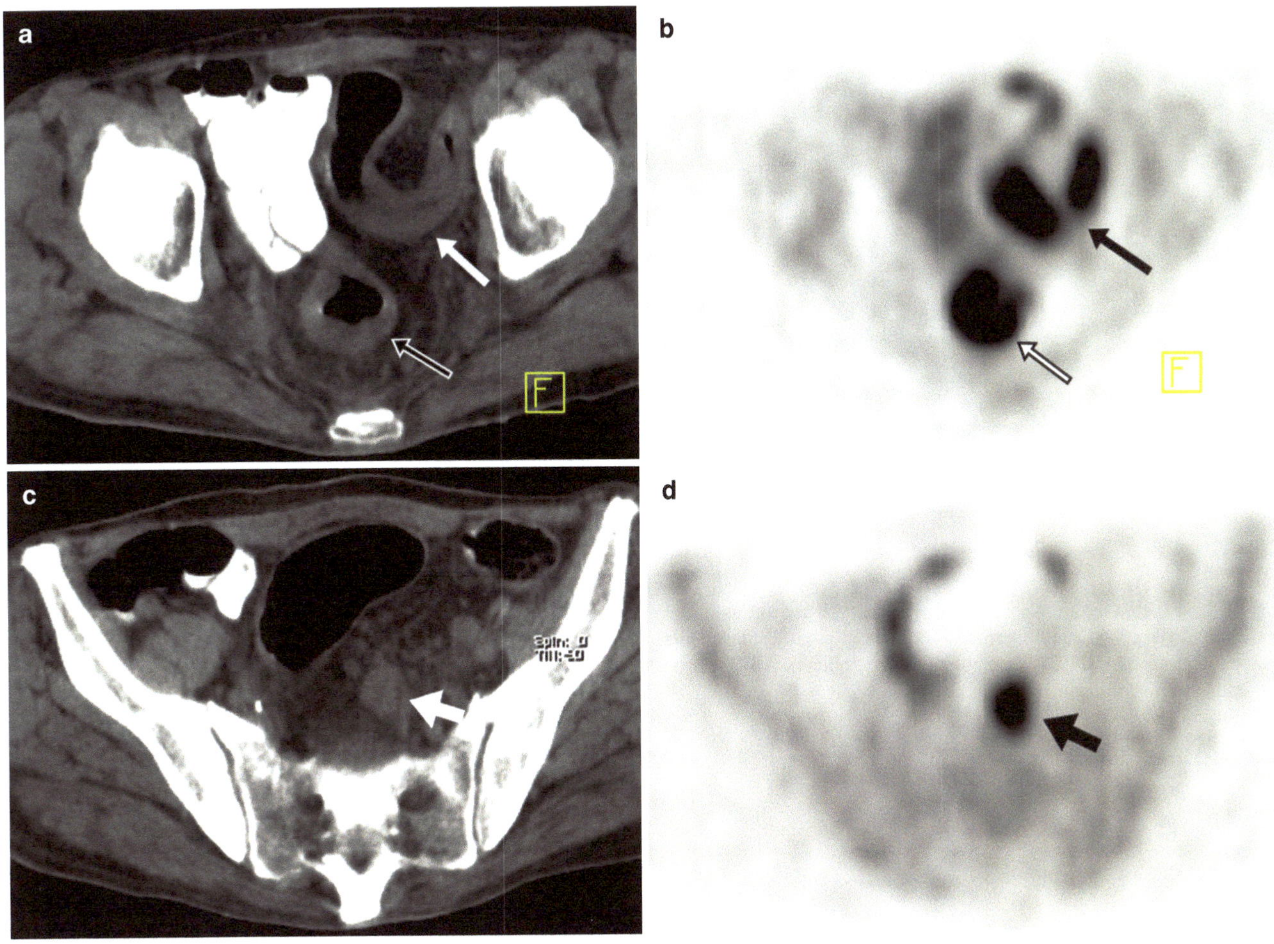

Fig. 8.16 Axial, CT, and PET (**a–d**) images show pathologically increased FDG uptake at sigmoid colon (*arrow*) and rectum (*empty arrow*). Apart from these, a hypermetabolic lymph node at left internal iliac area is detected (*short arrow*)

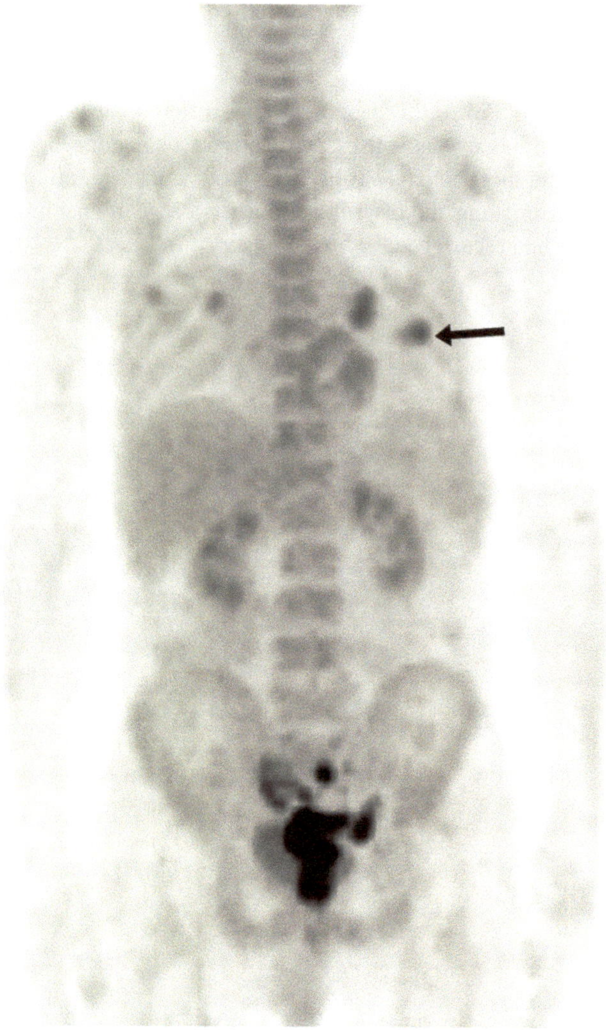

Fig. 8.17 MIP image shows increased FDG uptake corresponding to lesions at distal colon and hypermetabolic foci adjacent to these mass lesions. There are focal FDG accumulations at both lungs, which can be either due to metastatic or inflammatory lesions (*arrow*)

8.11 Case 11: Carcinoma of Unknown Primary

History A 68-year-old male patient with hypodense lesions at liver detected on CT which are suspicious for metastatic disease is referred to ^{18}F-FDG PET/CT scanning for identification of primary malignancy and evaluation of the extent of the disease.

Findings

Interpretation Primary malignant lesion at sigmoid colon. Multiple hypermetabolic lesions at liver compatible with metastases.

Teaching Point Empiric treatment regimens might be effective for some of the occult primary sites, but they are not successful for patients with advanced colorectal carcinoma. So accurate identification of carcinoma of unknown primary site (CUP) in patients with colorectal sites of origin may give better results by directing colorectal chemotherapy instead of empiric chemotherapy.

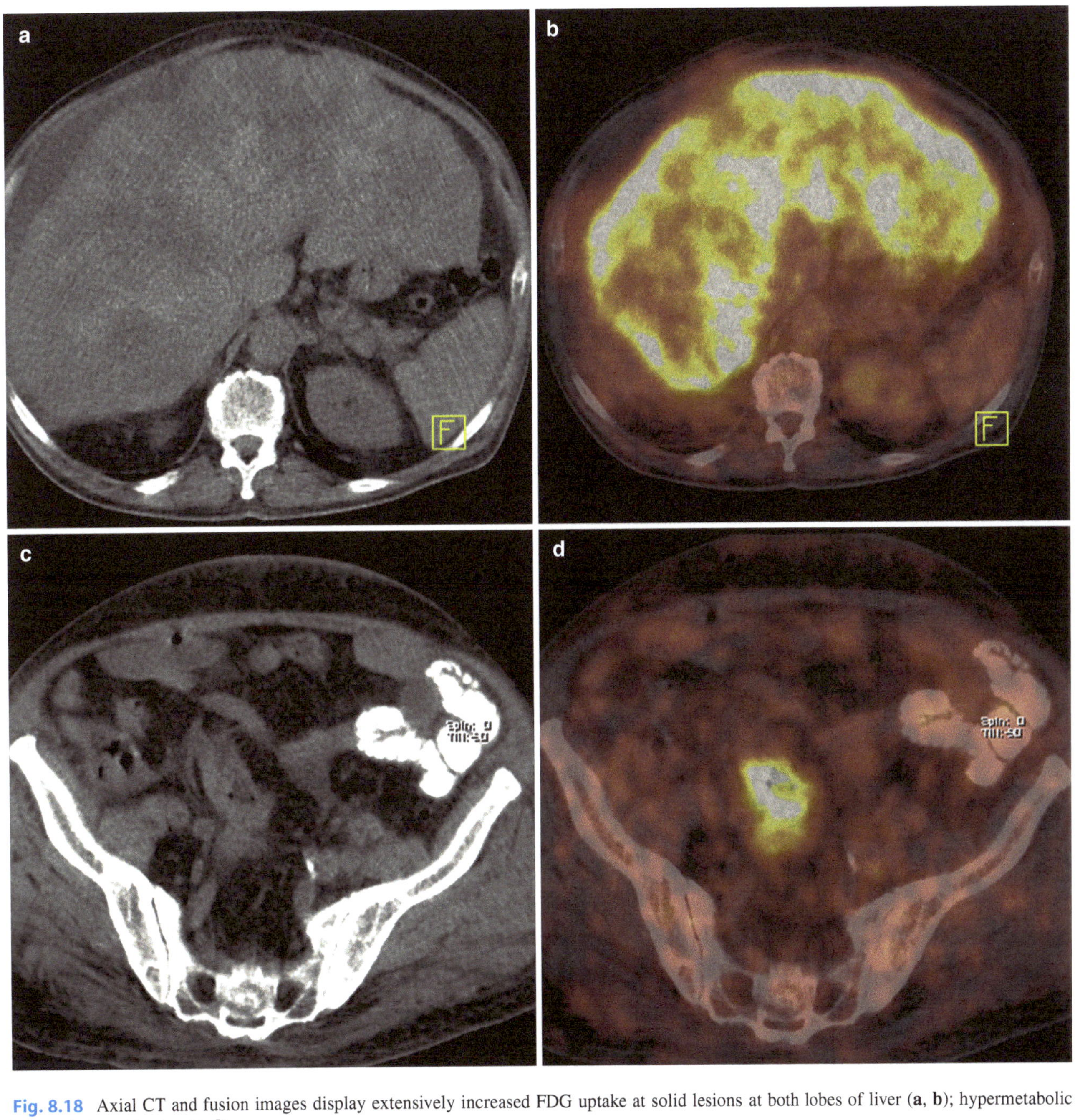

Fig. 8.18 Axial CT and fusion images display extensively increased FDG uptake at solid lesions at both lobes of liver (**a**, **b**); hypermetabolic lesion at sigmoid colon (**c**, **d**)

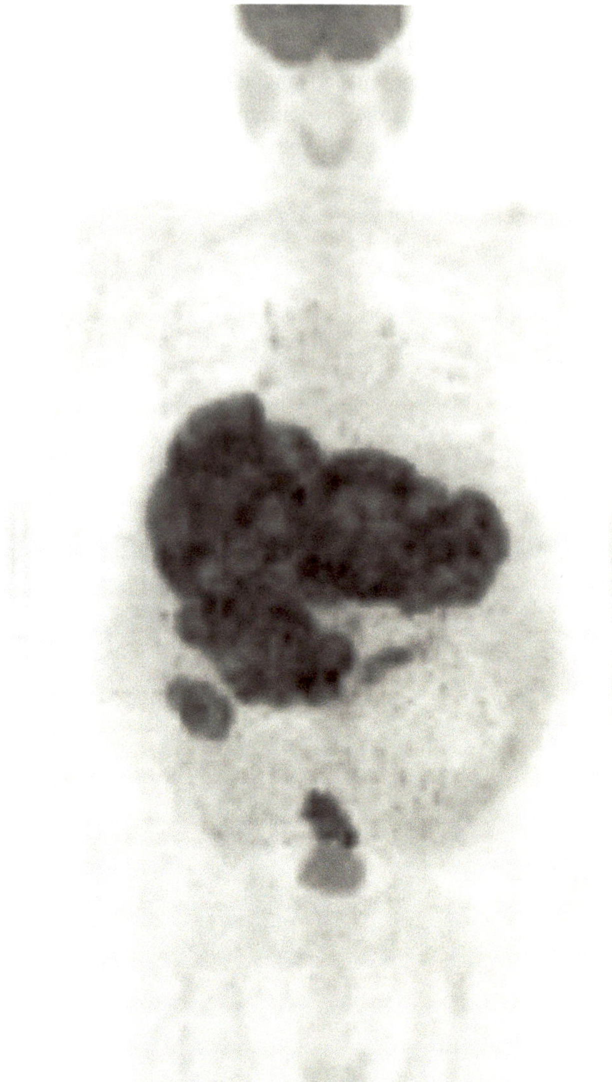

Fig. 8.19 MIP image

Bibliography

1. Abdel-Nabi H, Doerr RJ, Lamonica DM, Cronin VR, Galantowicz PJ, Carbone GM, et al. Staging of primary colorectal carcinomas with fluorine-18 fluorodeoxyglucose whole-body PET: correlation with histopathologic and CT findings. Radiology. 1998;206:755–60.
2. Arslan N, Dehdashti F, Siegel BA. FDG uptake in colonic villous adenomas. Ann Nucl Med. 2005;19:331–4.
3. Bond JH. Polyp guideline: diagnosis, treatment, and surveillance for patients with colorectal polyps. Practice Parameters Committee of the American College of Gastroenterology. Am J Gastroenterol. 2000;95:3053–63.
4. Chintamani, Singhal V, Bansal A, Bhatnagar D, Saxena S. Isolated colostomy site recurrence in rectal cancer-two cases with review of literature. World J Surg Oncol. 2007;5:52.
5. Greco F, Lennington W, Spigel D, Varadhachary G, Hainsworth J. Carcinoma of unknown primary site: outcomes in patients with a colorectal molecular profile treated with site specific chemotherapy. J Cancer Ther. 2012;3:37–43. doi:10.4236/jct.2012.31005.
6. Grigsby PW. FDG-PET/CT: new horizons in anal cancer. Gastroenterol Clin Biol. 2009;33:456–8.
7. Gutman F, Alberini JL, Wartski M, Vilain D, Le Stanc E, Sarandi F, et al. Incidental colonic focal lesions detected by FDG PET/CT. AJR Am J Roentgenol. 2005;185(2):495–500.
8. Huebner RH, Park KC, Shepherd JE, Schwimmer J, Czernin J, Phelps ME, et al. A meta-analysis of the literature for whole-body FDG PET detection of recurrent colorectal cancer. J Nucl Med. 2000;41:1177–89.
9. Huguier M, Houry S, Barrier A. Local recurrence of cancer of the rectum. Am J Surg. 2001;182:437–9.
10. Mukai M, Sadahiro S, Yasuda S, Ishida H, Tokunaga N, Tajima T, et al. Preoperative evaluation by whole-body 18F-fluorodeoxyglucose positron emission tomography in patients with primary colorectal cancer. Oncol Rep. 2000;7:85–7.
11. Nguyen BD, Ram PC, Roarke MC. F-18 FDG PET/CT imaging of anal canal squamous cell carcinoma. Clin Nucl Med. 2007;32:234–6.
12. Niekel MC, Bipat S, Stoker J. Diagnostic imaging of colorectal liver metastases with CT, MR imaging, FDG PET, and/or FDG PET/CT: a meta-analysis of prospective studies including patients who have not previously undergone treatment. Radiology. 2010;257:674–84. doi:10.1148/radiol.10100729.
13. O'Connor OJ, McDermott S, Slattery J, Sahani D, Blake MA. The use of PET-CT in the assessment of patients with colorectal carcinoma. Int J Surg Oncol. 2011. doi:10.1155/2011/846512.
14. Ohta J, Araki Y, Morodomi T, Shirouzu K, Isomoto H, Kakegawa T. A case of metachronous multiple carcinomas arising at the colostomy site after Miles operation. J Jpn Soc Coloproctol. 1991;44:481–4.
15. Purandare NC, Dua SG, Arora A, Shah S, Rangarajan V. Colorectal cancer – patterns of locoregional recurrence and distant metastases as demonstrated by FDG PET/CT. Indian J Radiol Imaging. 2010;20:284–8. doi:10.4103/0971-3026.73545.
16. Trautmann TG, Zuger JH. Positron emission tomography for pre-treatment staging and posttreatment evaluation in cancer of the anal canal. Mol Imaging Biol. 2005;7:309–13.
17. Tziris N, Dokmetzioglou J, Giannoulis K, Kesisoglou I, Sapalidis K, Kotidis E, et al. Synchronous and metachronous adenocarcinomas of the large intestine. Hippokratia. 2008;12:150–2.

9 Gastric and Esophageal Tumors

9.1 Case 1: Gastric Poorly Differentiated Adenocarcinoma

History A 40-year-old male who was diagnosed to have gastric poorly differentiated adenocarcinoma after endoscopic biopsy underwent ^{18}F-FDG PET/CT for staging.

Findings

Interpretation Primary gastric malignancy with multiple metastatic lesions at skeletal system.

Teaching Point The role of ^{18}F-FDG PET/CT in pretreatment staging of gastric cancer is limited due to its low sensitivity for primary tumor and lymph node metastasis but it has the advantage of detecting distant solid organ and skeletal metastases by evaluating whole-body at one time.

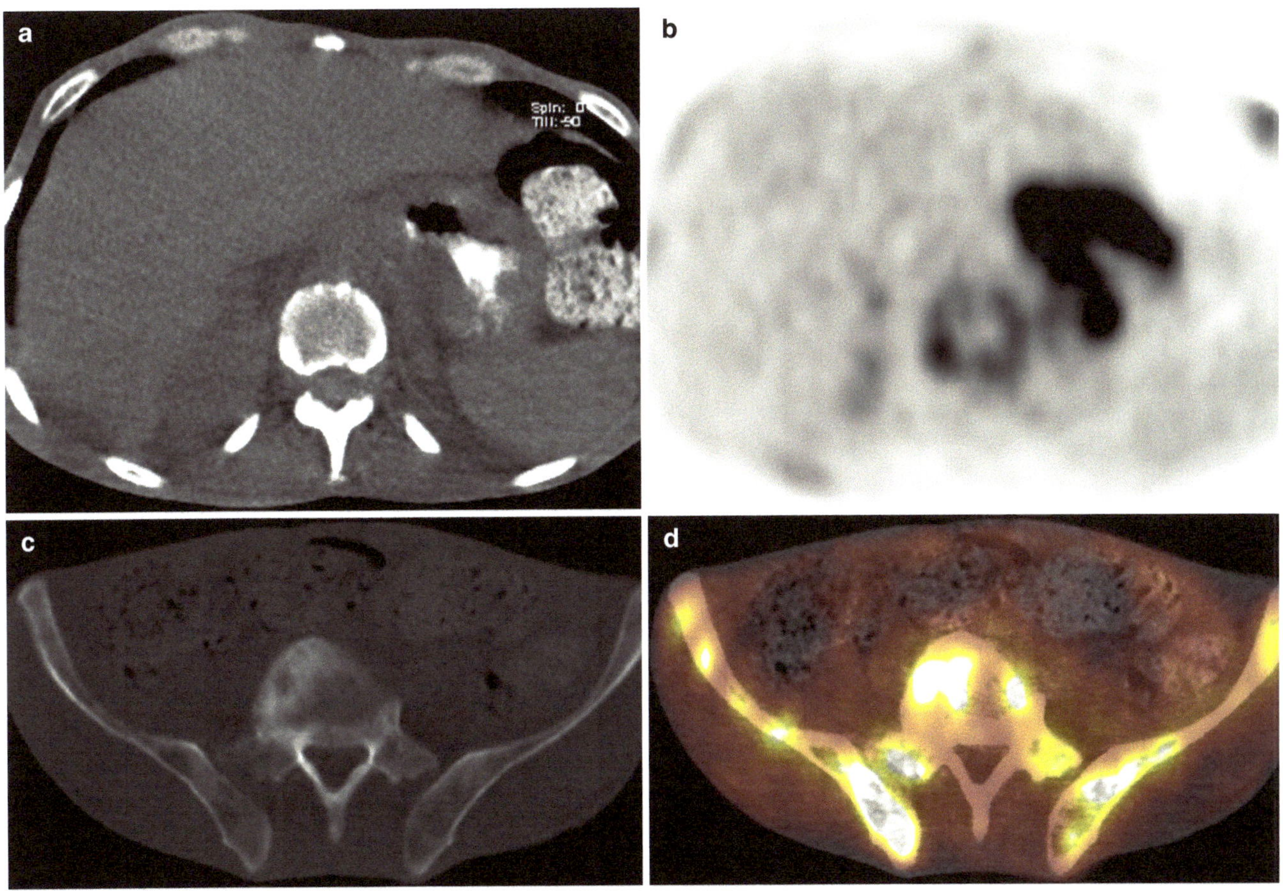

Fig. 9.1 Axial CT and PET images show intensely increased FDG uptake at gastric wall thickening (SUVmax 17.7) (**a**, **b**), hypermetabolic sclerotic lesions at pelvic bones are seen on CT and fusion images (SUVmax 5.9) (**c**, **d**)

T. Özülker, F. Özülker, *Atlas of PET-CT Imaging in Oncology: A Case-Based Guide to Image Interpretation*,
DOI 10.1007/978-3-319-18994-9_9

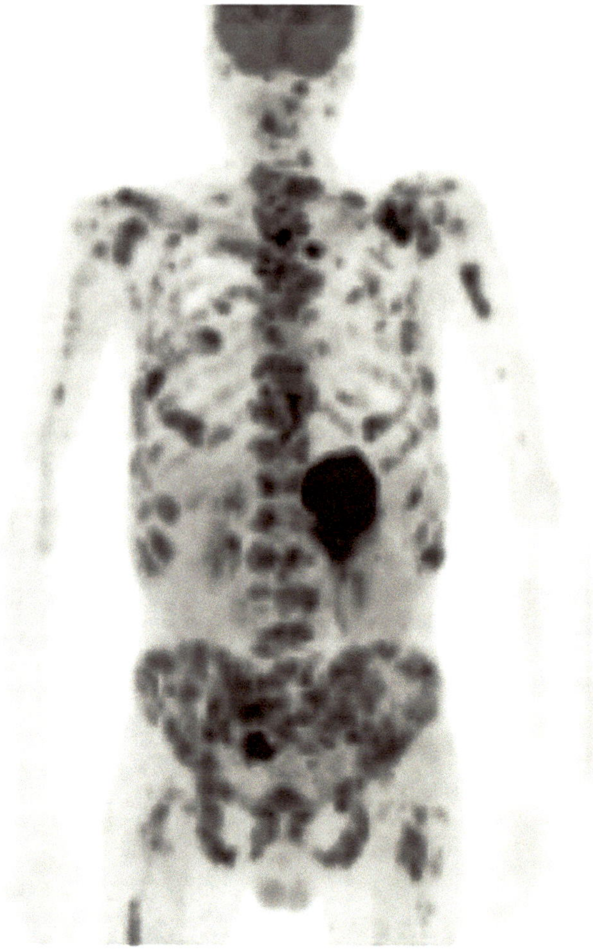

Fig. 9.2 MIP image show widespread hypermetabolic lesions at skeletal system as well as increased FDG uptake at gastric wall

9.2 Case 2: Gastric Adenocarcinoma and Virchow's Node

History A 60-year-old male who was diagnosed to have gastric adenocarcinoma after endoscopic biopsy underwent ^{18}F-FDG PET/CT for staging.

Findings

Interpretation Primary gastric malignancy with metastatic involvement of multiple lymph nodes. There is Virchow's node at left supraclavicular area which is characteristically involved in gastric malignancies.

Teaching point Although ^{18}F-FDG PET/CT is not effective in the detection of lymph node involvement in gastric adenocarcinoma with a sensitivity of 60 %, its specificity is higher (85 %). Demonstration of involvement of Virchow's node might be pathognomonic.

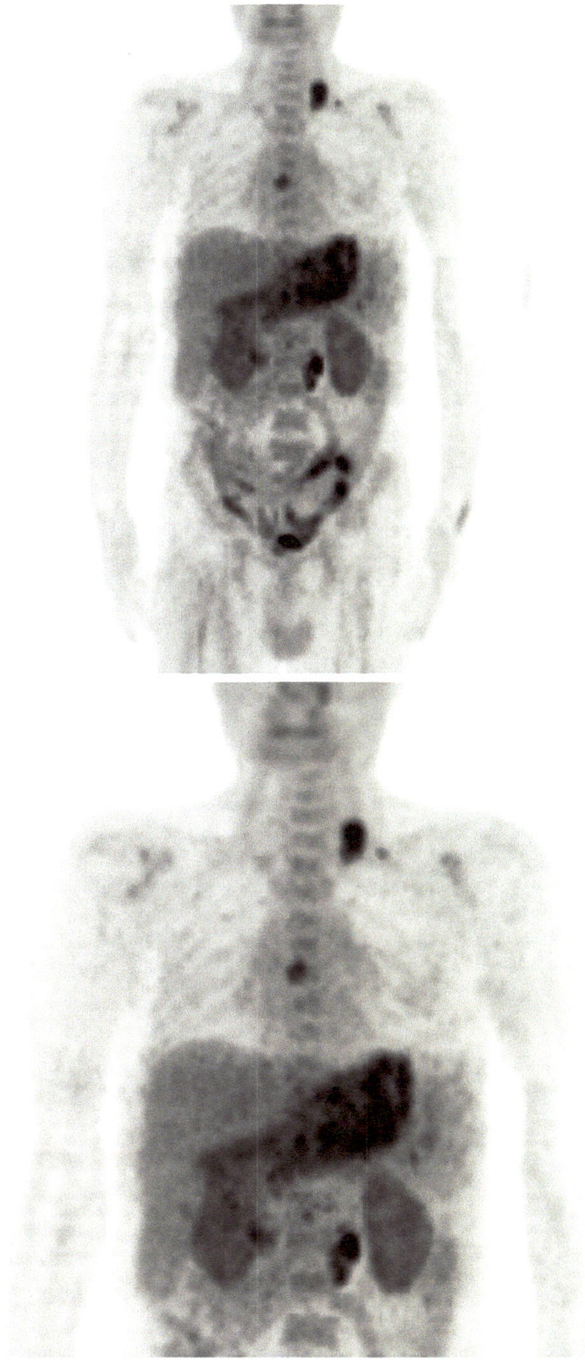

Fig. 9.3 MIP image shows moderately increased FDG uptake at stomach. There are hypermetabolic lymph nodes at subcarinal (SUVmax 6.4), left supraclavicular (SUVmax 8.8), paragastric, hepatogastric, and paraaortic (SUVmax 7.4) lymph node stations

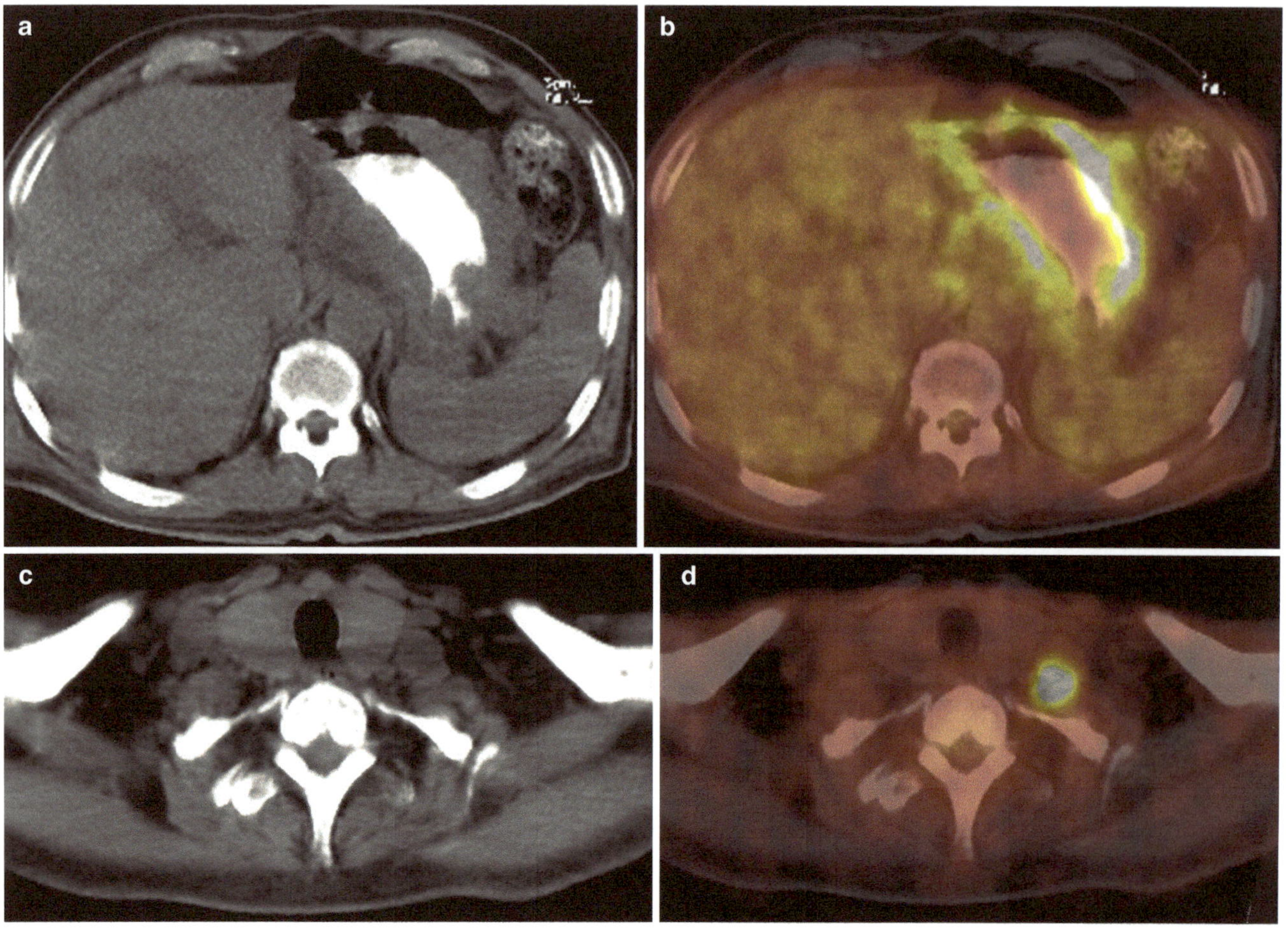

Fig. 9.4 Axial CT and fusion images show moderately increased FDG uptake at gastric walls (**a**, **b**), hypermetabolic lymph node at left supraclavicular area (**c**, **d**)

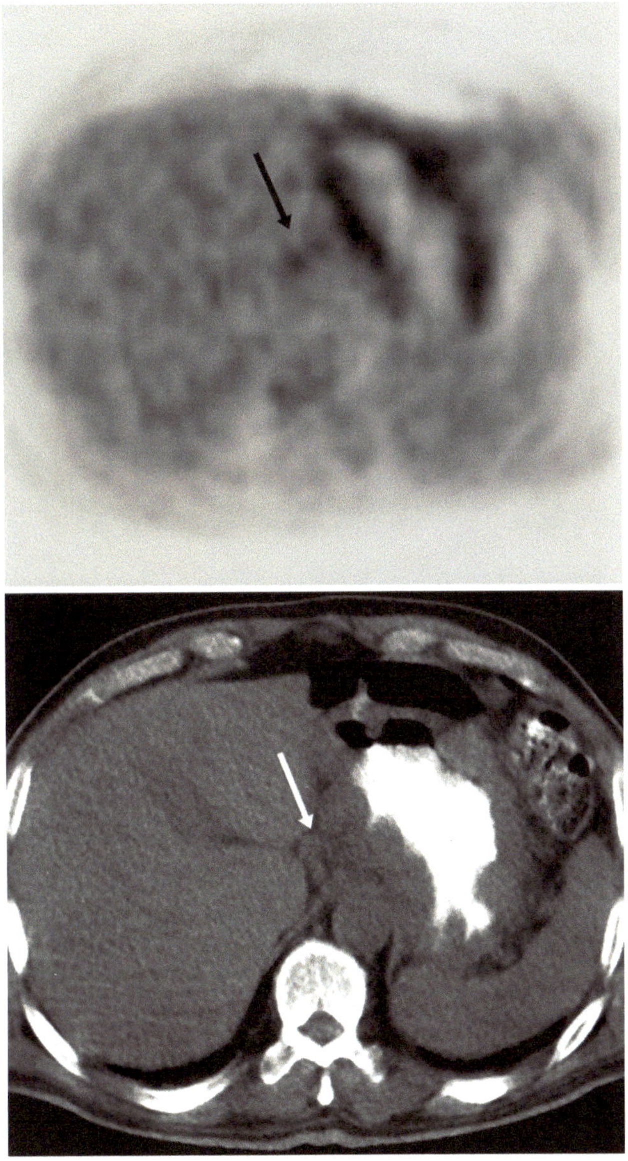

Fig. 9.5 Axial PET and CT images show mildly increased FDG uptake at hepatogastric lymph nodes (*arrow*)

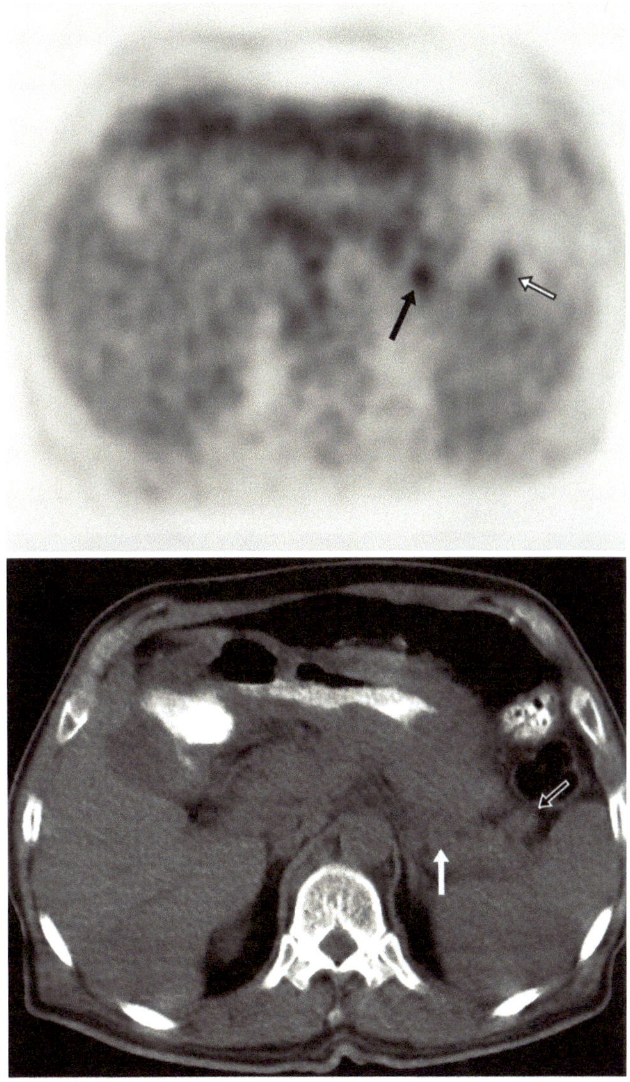

Fig. 9.6 Axial PET and CT images show mildly increased FDG uptake at paragastric lymph nodes (*arrows*)

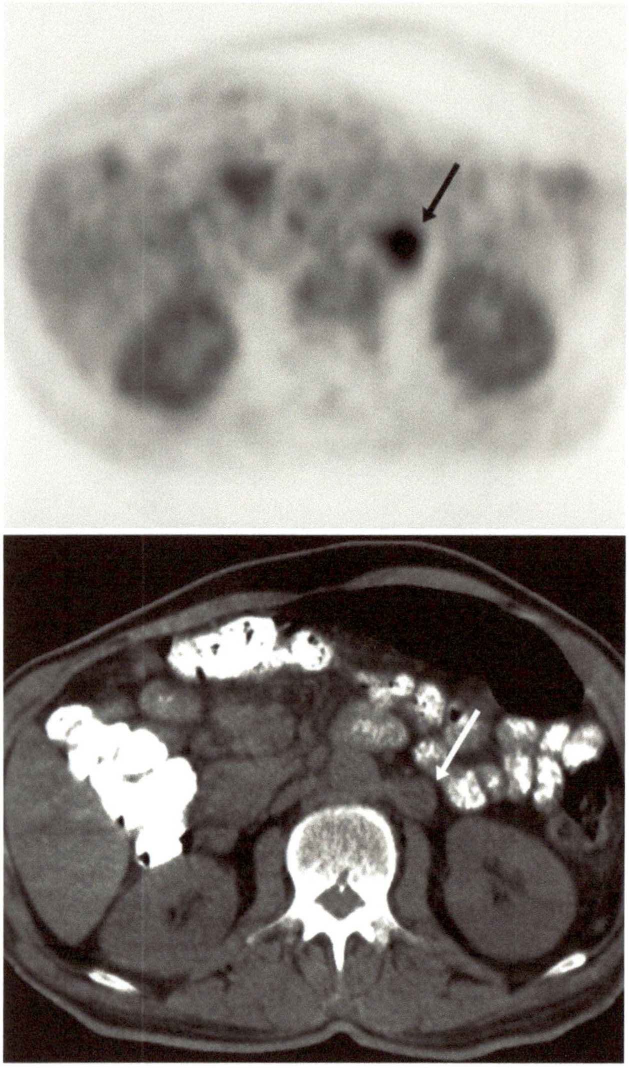

Fig. 9.7 Axial PET and CT images show significantly increased FDG uptake at left paraaortic lymph node (*arrow*)

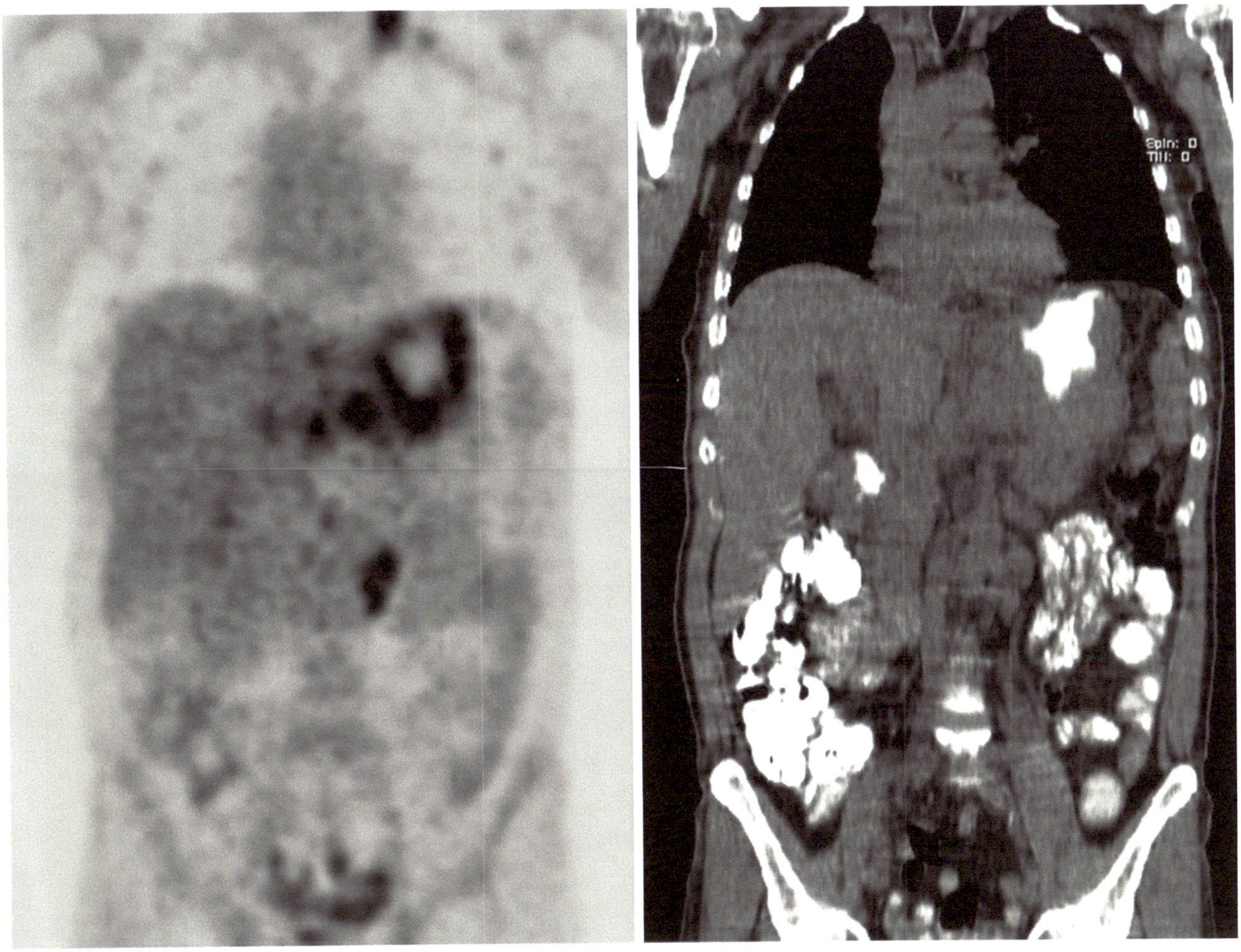

Fig. 9.8 Coronal PET and CT images show increased FDG uptake at stomach and intraabdominal lymph nodes

9.3 Case 3: Gastric Adenocarcinoma Found Incidentally

History A 65-year-old female who has been followed up with the diagnosis of colorectal carcinoma for 3 years, underwent ^{18}F-FDG PET/CT for staging.

Findings

Interpretation Second primary gastric malignancy and lung metastasis either due to colorectal cancer or gastric malignancy.

Result Biopsy from the lesion at stomach revealed adenocarcinoma involving 50 % mucinous component and no signet cell ring component.

Teaching Point The sensitivity of ^{18}F-FDG PET/CT is low in detecting lesions with high mucinous component but in this case although there is 50 % mucinous component, significant FDG uptake is noted.

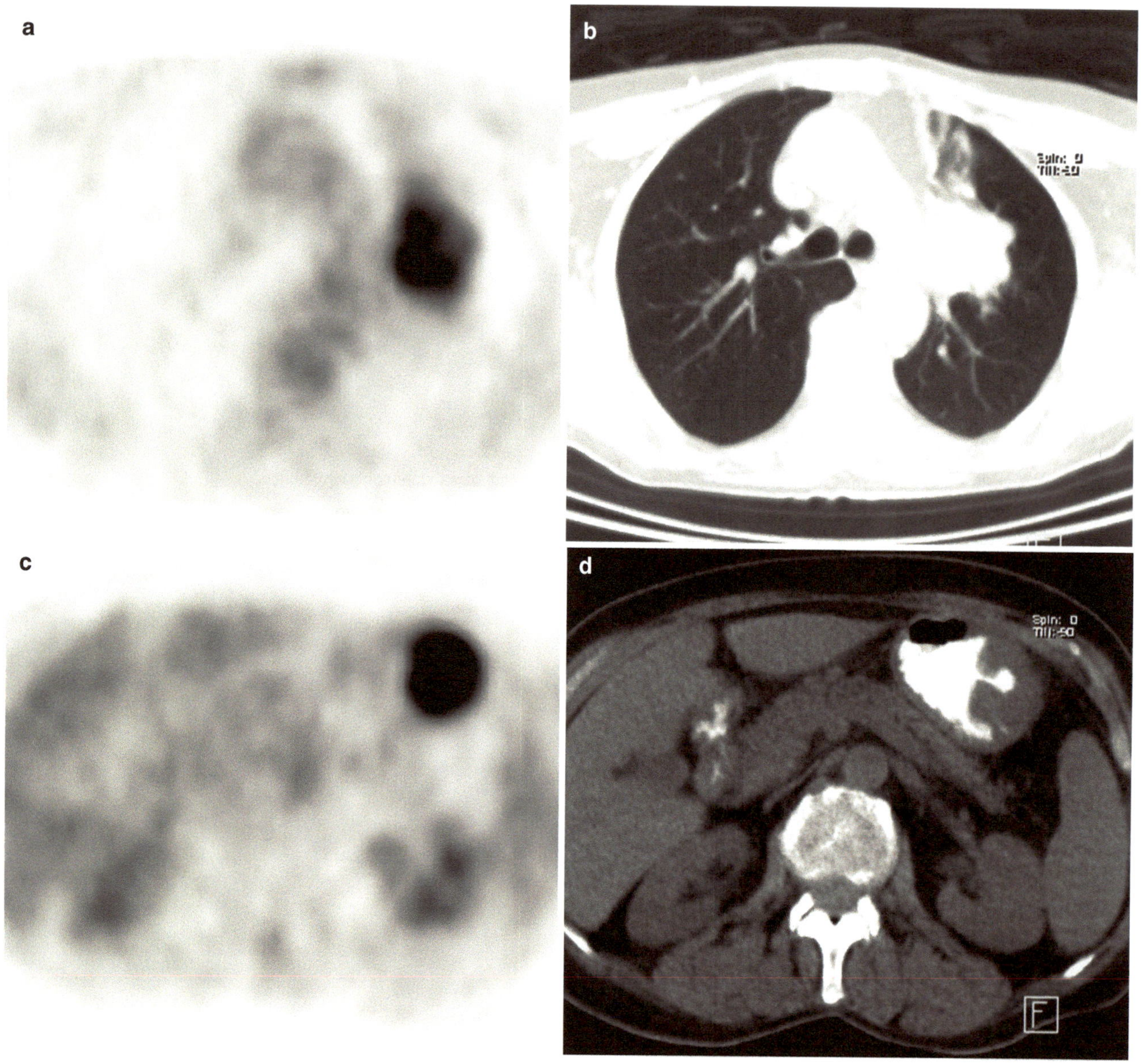

Fig. 9.9 Axial PET and CT images show mass lesion at anterior segment of upper lobe of left lung showing significantly increased FDG uptake (SUVmax 11.9) (**a**, **b**), intensely increased FDG uptake at greater curvature of corpus of stomach corresponding to the thickening at gastric wall (SUVmax 22.7) (**c**, **d**)

9.4 Case 4: Gastric Adenocarcinoma with Signet Ring Cell Component

History A 69-year-old female who had the diagnosis of Gastric Adenocarcinoma with Signet Ring Cell Component underwent ^{18}F-FDG PET/CT for staging.

Findings

Interpretation Although there is not any pathologically increased FDG uptake at stomach, when the histologic subtype of the malignancy concerned, primary evaluation with ^{18}F-FDG PET/CT is not satisfactory.

Teaching Point The FDG affinity is extremely low in signet ring cell type gastric malignancies and ^{18}F-FDG PET/CT is not effective in the management of the disease in this histologic subtype.

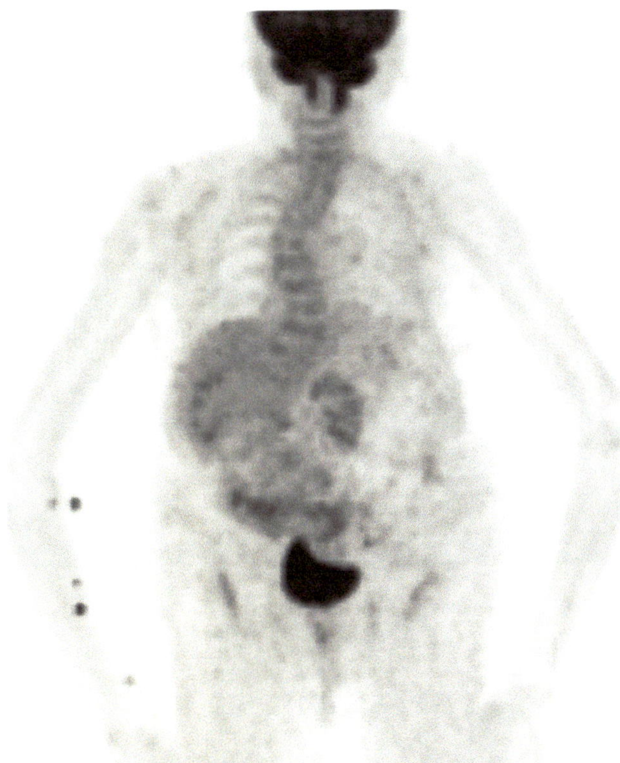

Fig. 9.10 MIP image does not display any significant pathologically increased FDG uptake

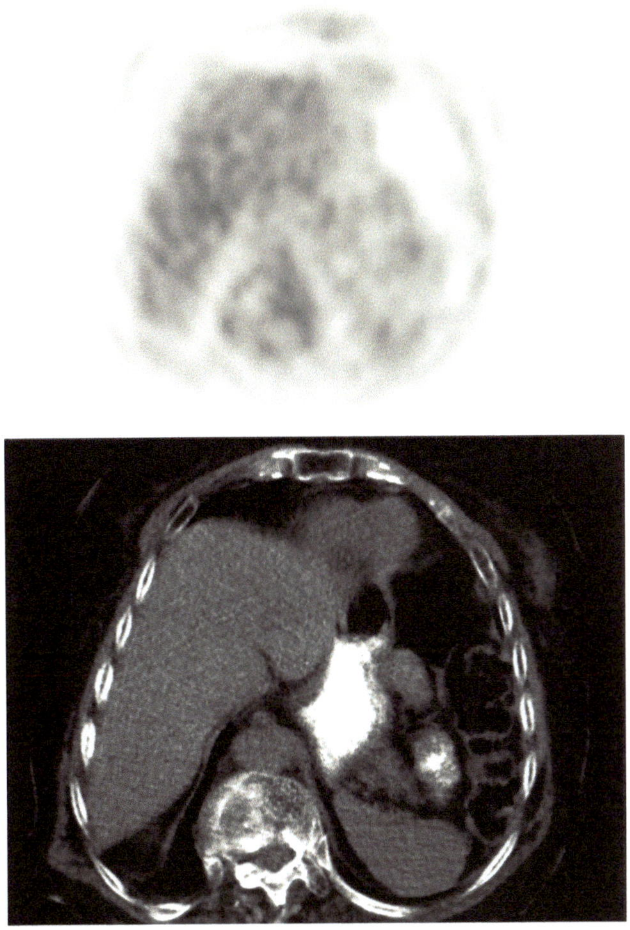

Fig. 9.11 Axial slices PET and CT images does not show any pathological activity other than subtle FDG uptake at gastric walls

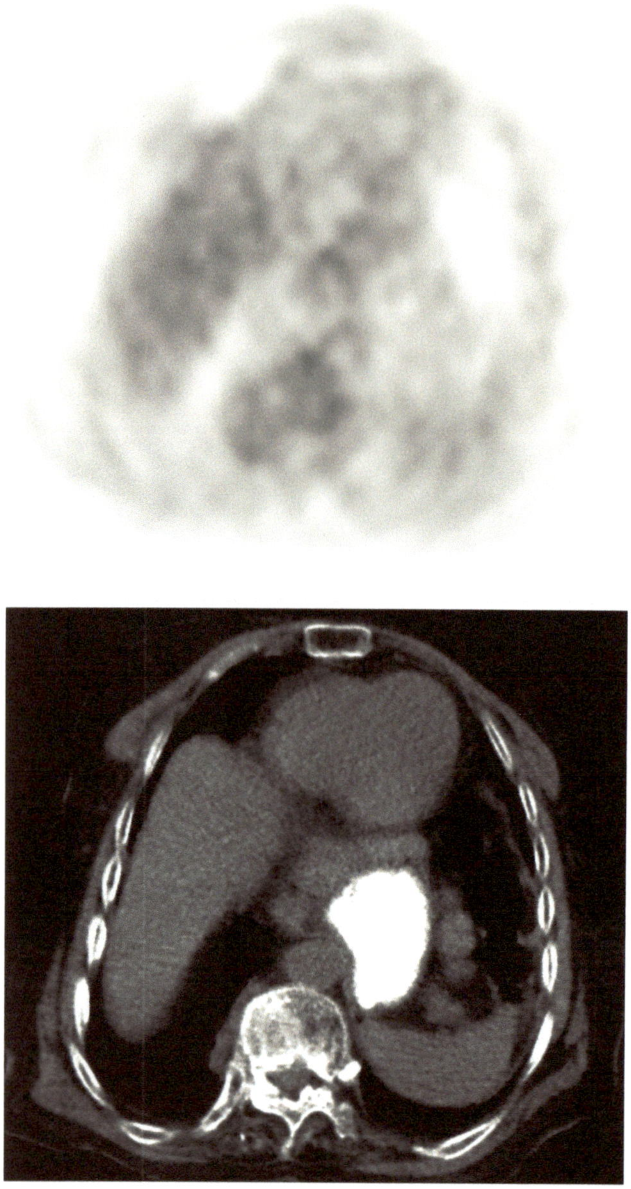

Fig. 9.12 Axial slices PET and CT images

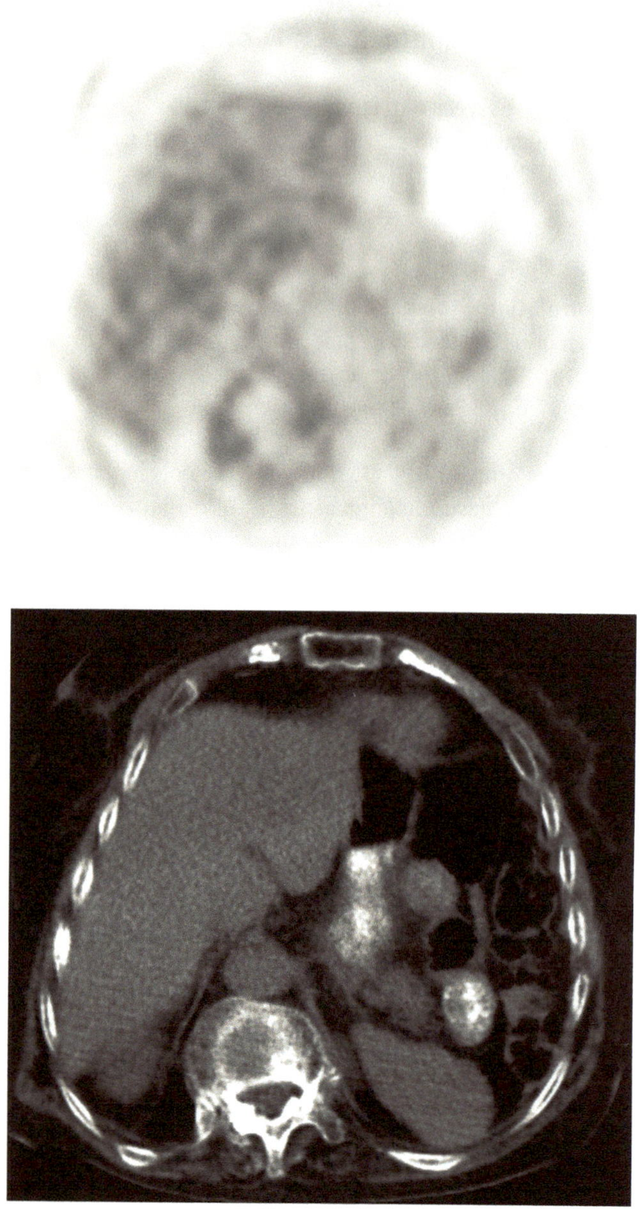

Fig. 9.13 Axial slices PET and CT images

9.5 Case 5: Restaging of Esophagus Squamous Cell Carcinoma

History A 65-year-old female who had undergone total esophagectomy 3 years ago and diagnosed to have esophagus squamous cell carcinoma underwent ^{18}F-FDG PET/CT for restaging.

Findings

Interpretation Local recurrence at pharyngogastrostomy anastamosis, metastatic deposits at mesentery, and metastatic nodule at parenchyma of right lung.

Teaching Point In one study, the sensitivity and specificity of PET were found as 94 % and 82 % for the diagnosis of regional and distant recurrences of esophageal cancer; 100 % and 57 % for the diagnosis of a perianastomotic recurrence. The specificity of FDG PET for local recurrences is not high as its sensitivity but in this case there is little doubt about the malignant nature of the local hypermetabolic lesion.

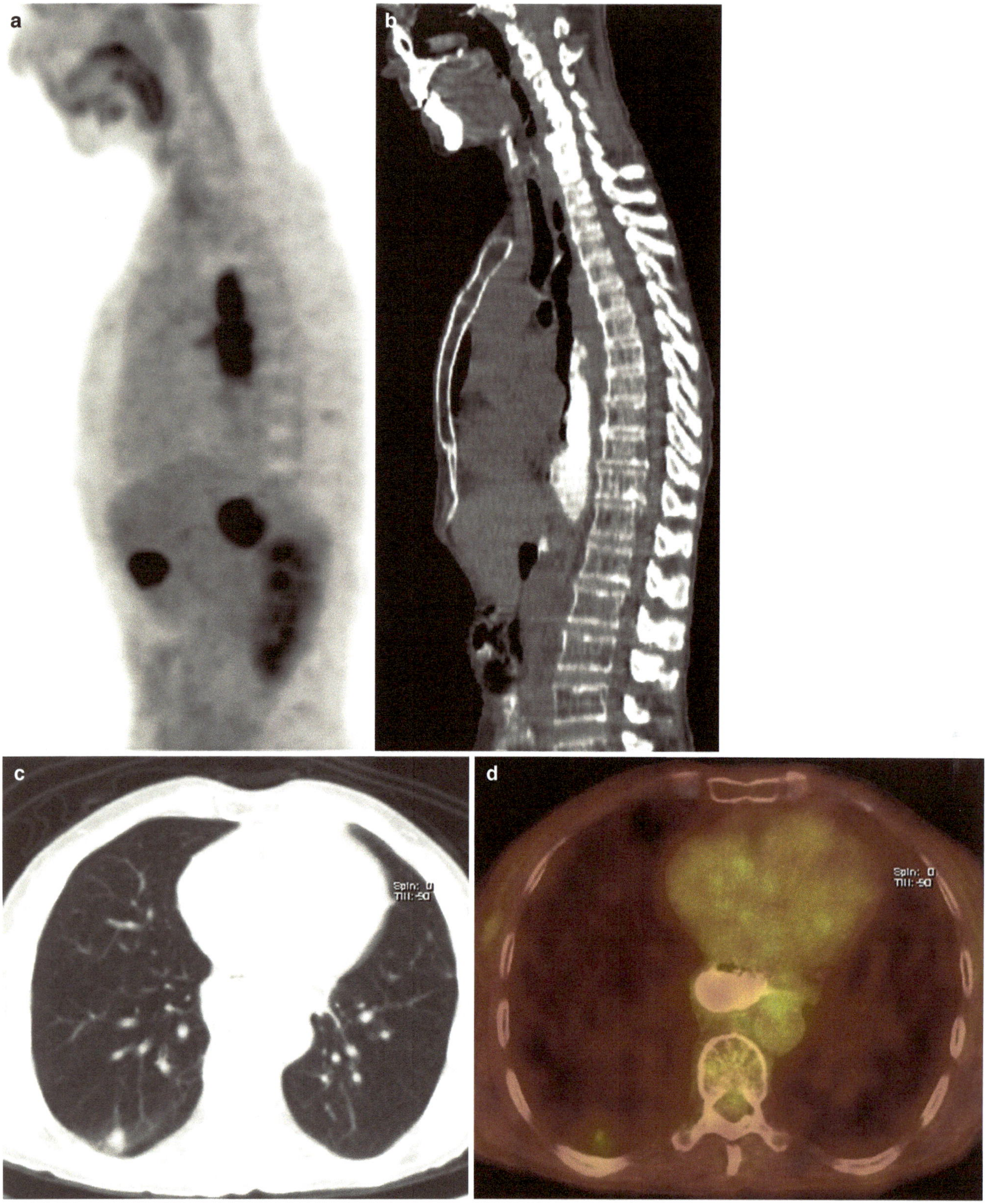

Fig. 9.14 Sagittal PET and CT images (**a**, **b**) and axial CT and fusion images (**c**, **d**) show intensely hypermetabolic lesion posterior to pharyngogastrostomy anastamosis (SUVmax 8.3) and two additional foci showing increased FDG uptake in upper abdomen. There is also a tiny nodule showing subtle FDG uptake at posterobasal segment of lower lobe of right lung (SUVmax 1.5)

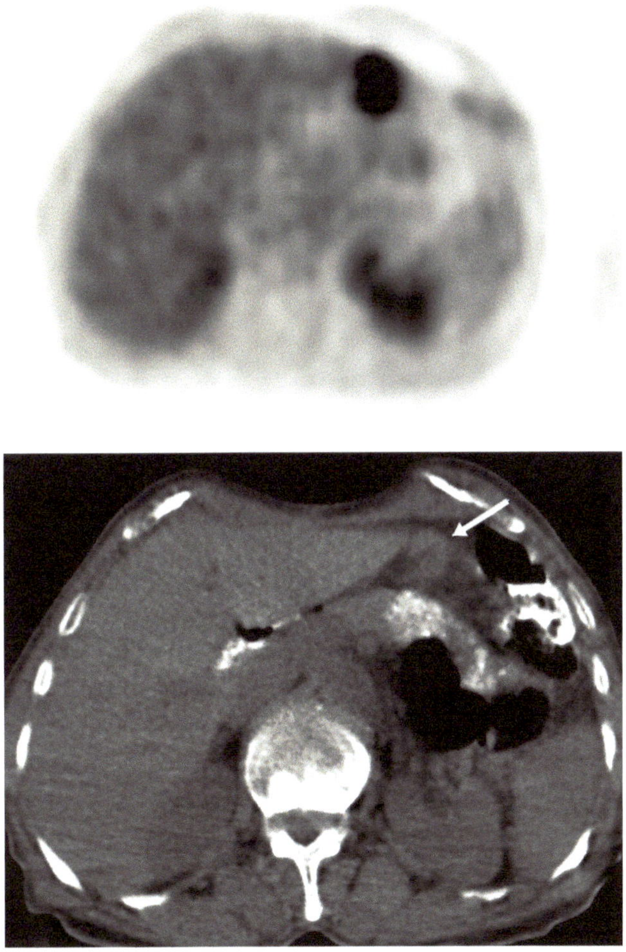

Fig. 9.15 Axial slices of PET and CT images show hypermetabolism at soft tissue lesion located adjacent to the left lobe of liver (*arrow*)

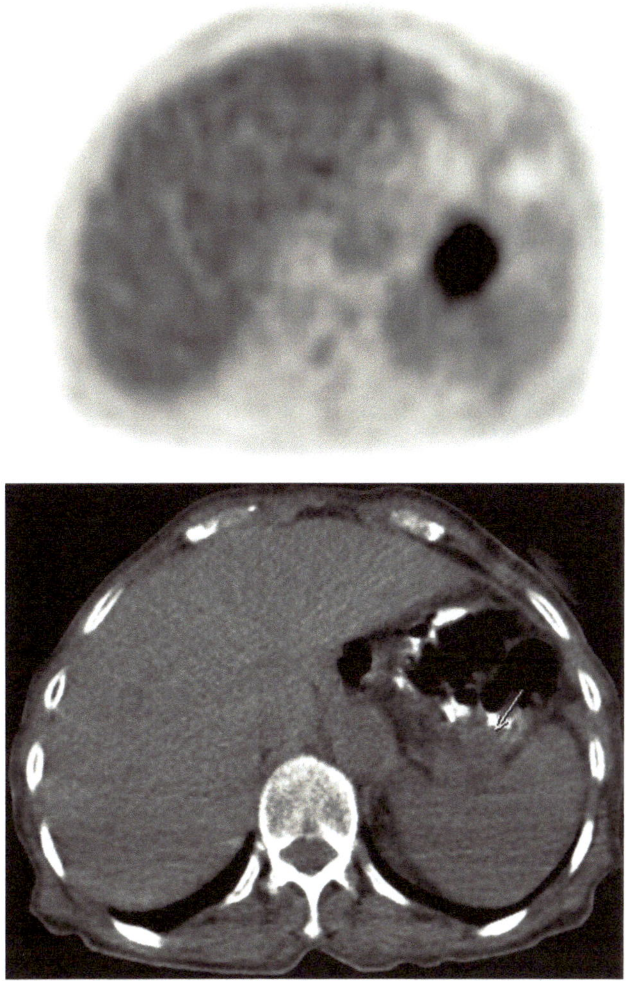

Fig. 9.16 Axial slices of PET and CT images show hypermetabolism at soft tissue lesion located adjacent to spleen (*arrow*)

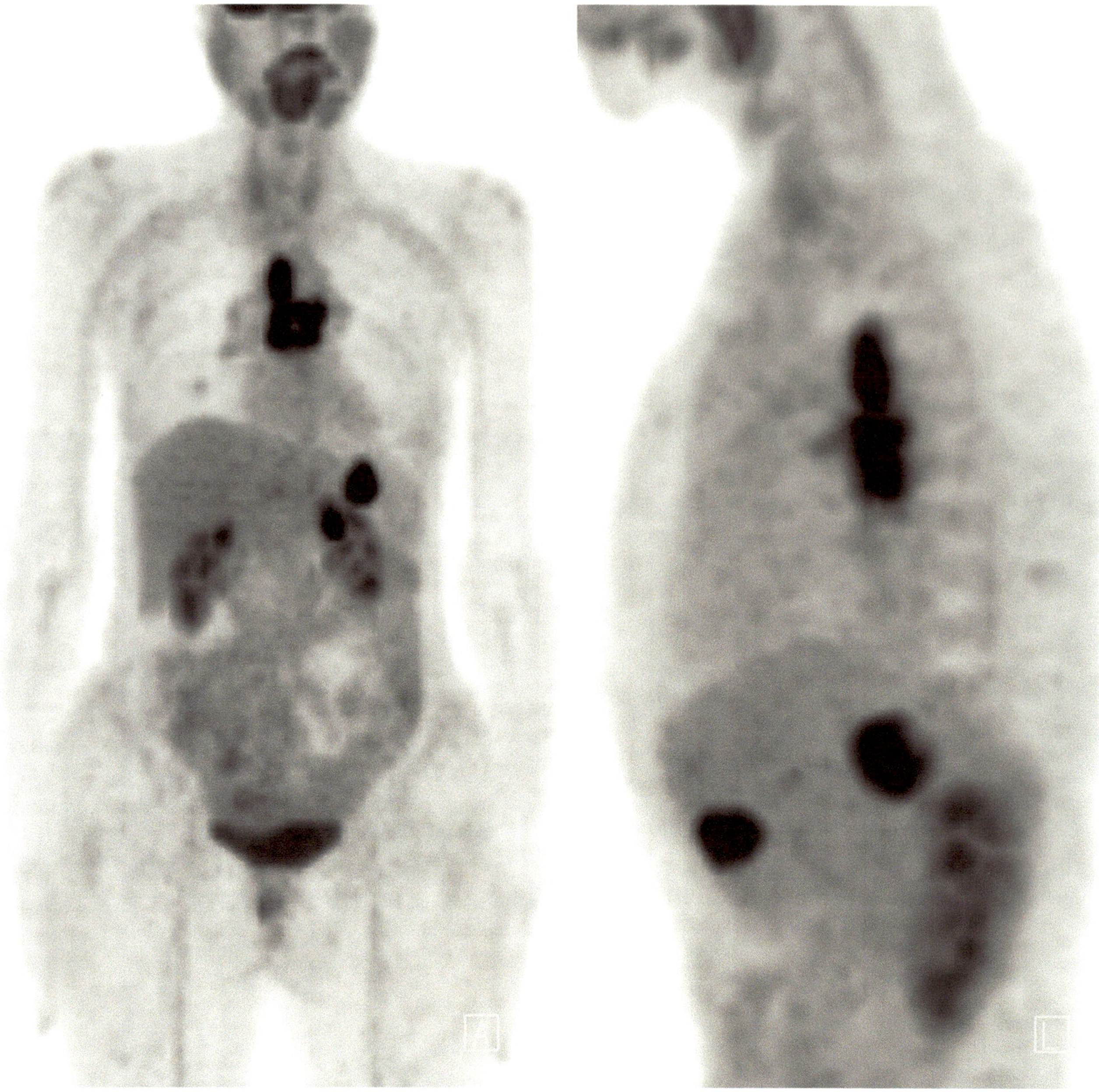

Fig. 9.17 Anterior and lateral MIP images

Bibliography

1. Flamen P, Lerut A, Van Cutsem E, Cambier JP, Maes A, De Wever W, et al. The utility of positron emission tomography for the diagnosis and staging of recurrent esophageal cancer. Thorac Cardiovasc Surg. 2000;120:1085–92.
2. McAteer D, Wallis F, Couper G, Norton M, Welch A, Bruce D, et al. Evaluation of ^{18}F-FDG positron emission tomography in gastric and oesophageal carcinoma. Br J Radiol. 1999;72:525–9.

Liver Tumors

10

10.1 Case 1: Staging of Hepatocellular Carcinoma

History A 66-year-old male underwent ^{18}F-FDG PET/CT after having diagnosed as hepatocellular carcinoma (HCC).

Findings

Interpretation Hypermetabolism at liver is compatible with primary hepatic malignancy.

Teaching Point HCC exhibit variations in FDG accumulation for unknown reasons. Low or absent FDG uptake can be seen in low-grade hepatocarcinoma, and this fact is attributed to the presence of a higher glucose-6-phosphatase activity resulting in a low FDG uptake.^{18}F-FDG PET CT may give additional information in the routine staging as a complementary imaging tool to dynamic CT of liver and chest x-ray.

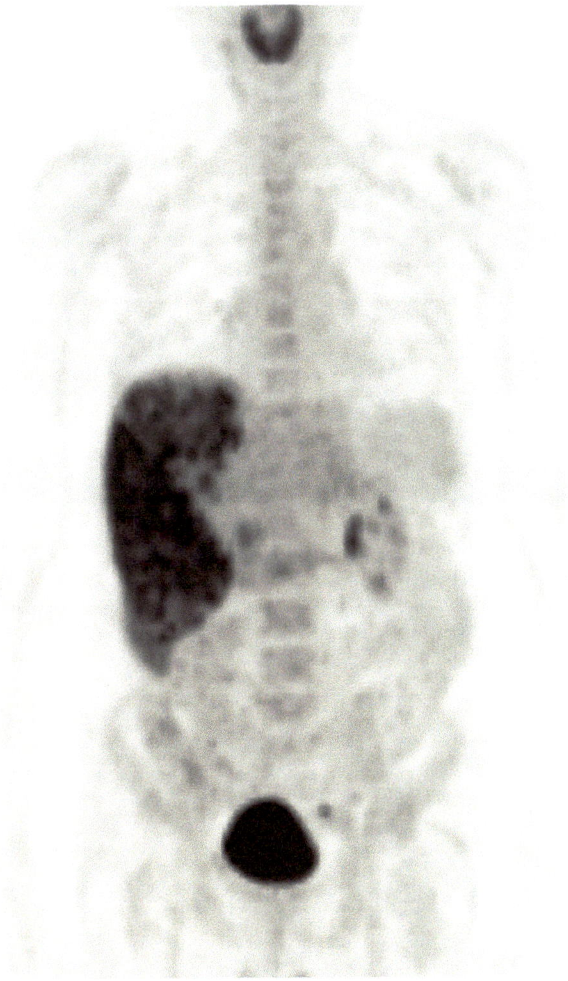

Fig. 10.1 MIP image shows heterogenously increased FDG uptake at liver. There is not any other pathological FDG uptake detected at rest of the body

T. Özülker, F. Özülker, *Atlas of PET-CT Imaging in Oncology: A Case-Based Guide to Image Interpretation*,
DOI 10.1007/978-3-319-18994-9_10

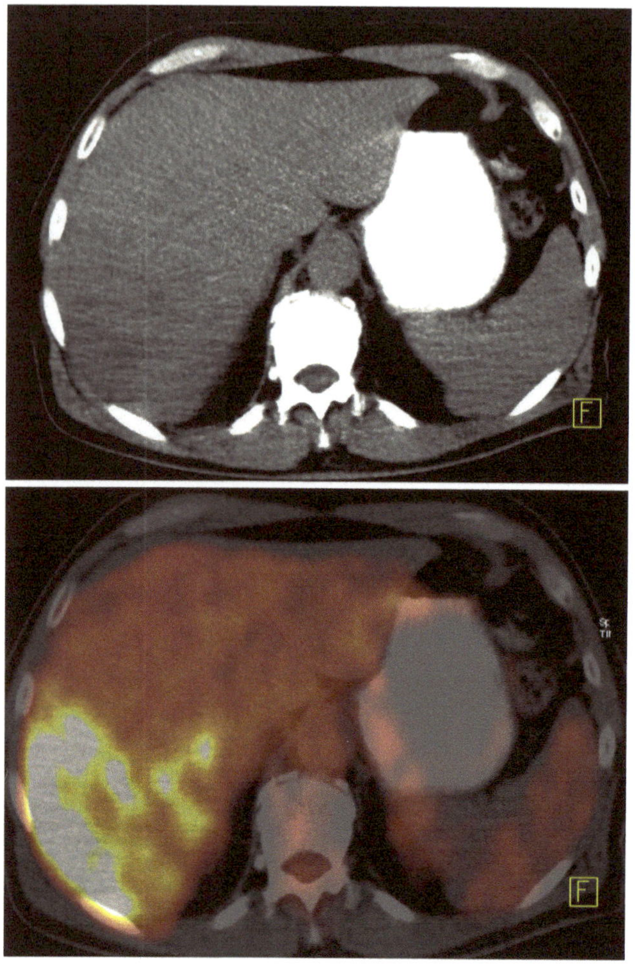

Fig. 10.2 Axial CT and fusion images show heterogenous hypermetabolism at right lobe of liver

10.2 Case 2: Restaging of Hepatocelular Carcinoma

History A 63-year-old male who had undergone hepatic resection for HCC 1 year ago underwent ^{18}F-FDG PET/CT for restaging.

Findings

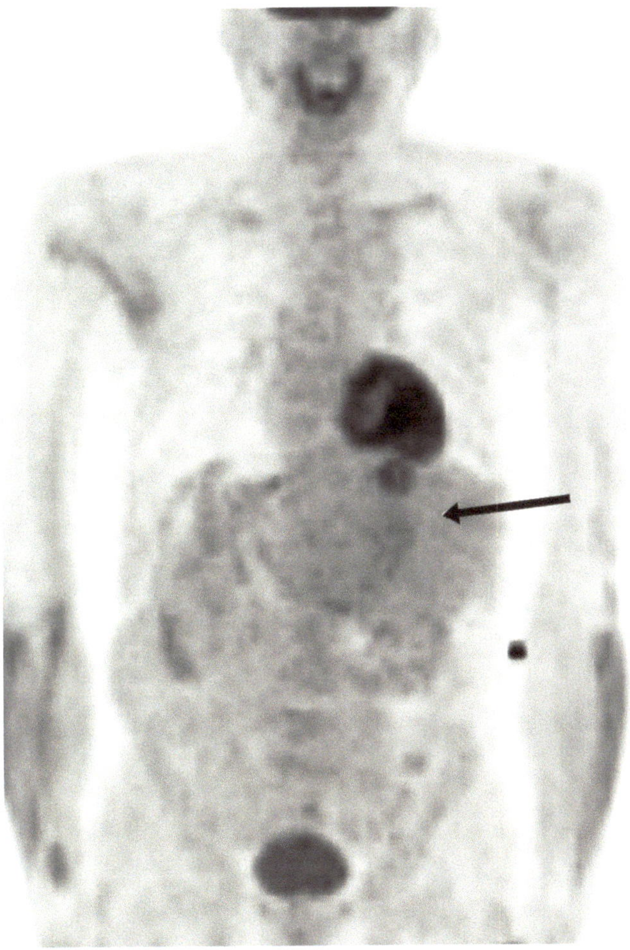

Fig. 10.3 MIP image shows focal FDG uptake at liver. Displacement of liver to left side of abdomen is also noted (*arrow*)

Interpretation Focus of increased FDG uptake at hepatic remnant represents recurrent disease.

Teaching Point ^{18}F-FDG PET CT may be useful in the early evaluation of residual, intrahepatic recurrent, or extra-hepatic metastatic lesions and able to provide valuable information for the management of HCC recurrence.

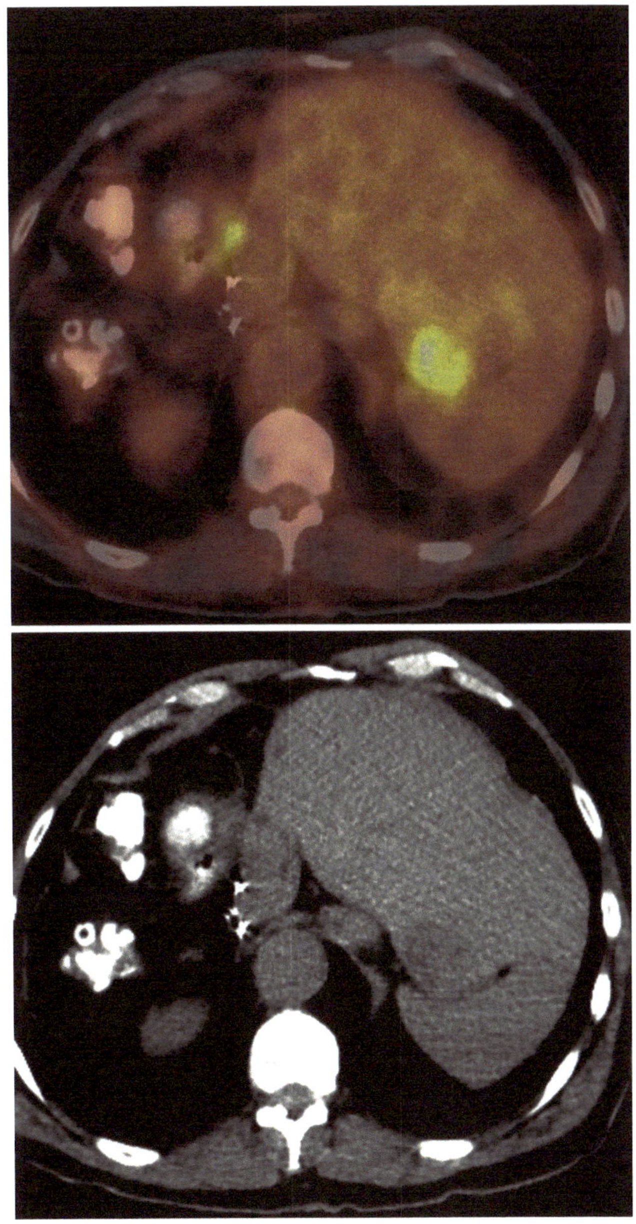

Fig. 10.4 Axial CT and fusion images show focal hypermetabolic lesion at left lobe of liver (SUVmax 5). The liver is displaced to left after resection

10.3 Case 3: Radiofrequency Ablation in Hepatocelular Carcinoma

History A 60-year-old male who has been followed up with the diagnosis colorectal carcinoma had metastasis at liver detected on ^{18}F-FDG PET/CT study. The patient underwent radiofrequency ablation (RFA) and then ^{18}F-FDG PET/CT scan was repeated 7 and 16 months after the therapy.

Findings

Interpretation Metastatic lesion at segment 6 of the liver responded well to RFA but recurrence is detected at the FDG PET/CT study performed 17 months after the end of therapy.

Teaching Point Evaluation of treatment response after RFA used in the treatment of primary and secondary hepatic malignancies can be done with conventional imaging modalities but they have limitations of differentiation between viable tumor from post-RFA changes. ^{18}F-FDG PET/CT can be used for response evaluation and restaging after RFA in liver tumors.

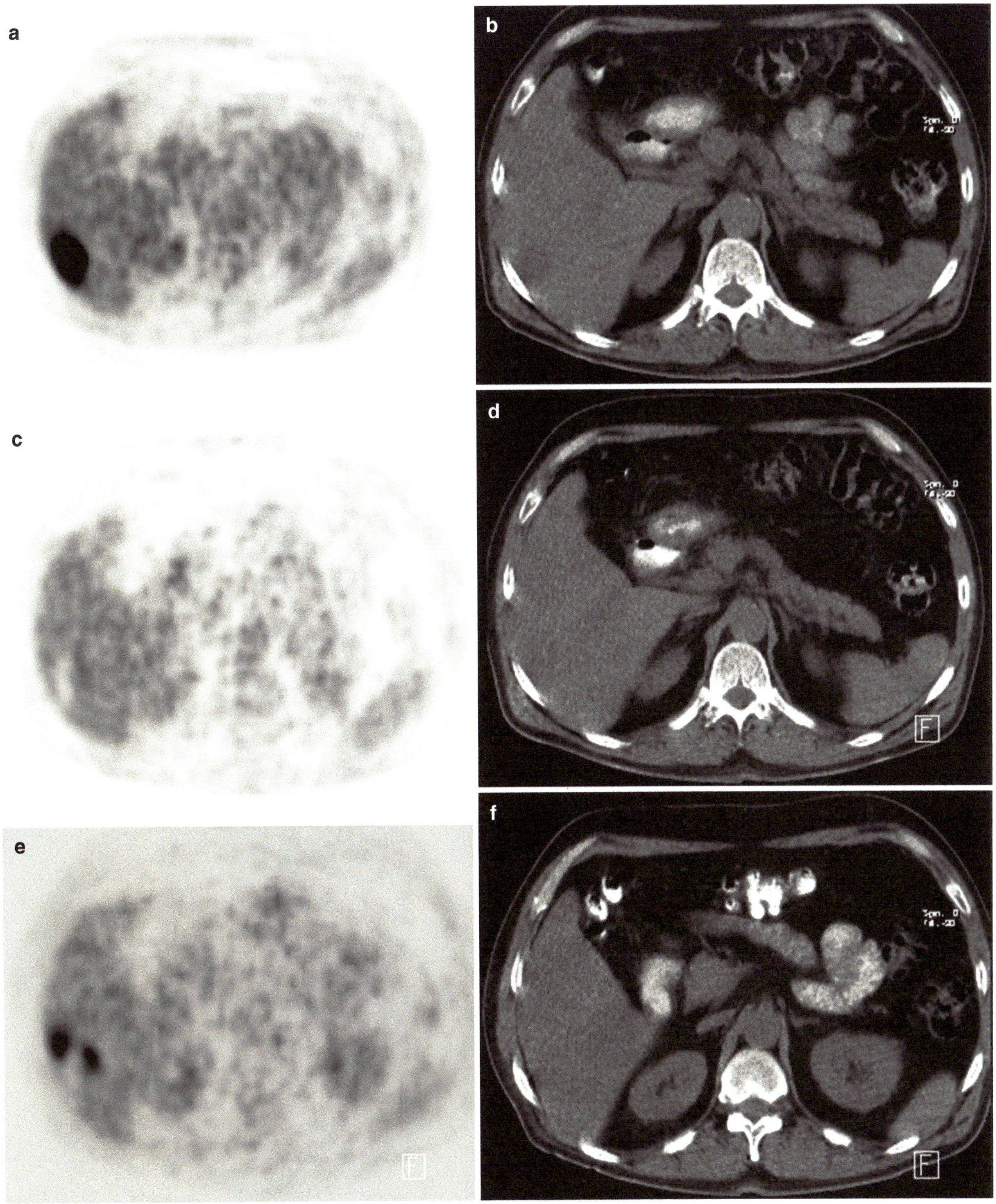

Fig. 10.5 Axial PET and CT images show focal hypermetabolic lesion at segment 6 of liver (**a**, **b**), disappearance of the lesion at the image obtained 6 months after the therapy (**c**, **d**), and focal hypermetabolic lesion at segment 6 of the liver at the image obtained 17 months after the therapy (**e**, **f**)

Bibliography

1. Cho Y, Lee DH, Lee YB, Lee M, Yoo JJ, Choi WM, et al. Does ^{18}F-FDG positron emission tomography-computed tomography have a role in initial staging of hepatocellular carcinoma? PLoS One. 2014. doi:10.1371/journal.pone.0105679.
2. Lee Z, Luo G. Issues pertaining to PET imaging of liver cancer. J Fasting Health. 2014;2:62–4.
3. Sun L, Guan YS, Pan WM, Luo ZM, Wei JH, Zhao L, et al. Metabolic restaging of hepatocellular carcinoma using whole-body F-FDG PET/CT. World J Hepatol. 2009;1:90–7. doi:10.4254/wjh.v1.i1.90.
4. Thulkar S, Chawla M, Sharma P, Malhotra A, Kumar R. ^{18}F-FDG PET/CT in evaluation of radiofrequency ablation of liver metastasis. Clin Nucl Med. 2012;37:498–501. doi:10.1097/RLU.0b013e31824d24e2.

11 Pancreas Tumors

11.1 Case 1: Pancreas Adenocarcinoma

History A 73.-year-old female underwent tru-cut biopsy from mass lesion at liver and histopathology revealed metastasis of adenocarcinoma. A ^{18}F-FDG PET/CT scan was performed in order to determine the primary malignancy.

Findings

Interpretation Hypermetabolic lesions at liver representing metastases from primary malignant lesion at head of pancreas.

Teaching Point In a metaanalysis, primary tumor detection rate of ^{18}F-FDG PET/CT was reported as 37 %. The most frequently reported unknown primary tumor locations include the lung, pancreas, and oropharynx. ^{18}F-FDG PET/CT has high rates of sensitivity (85–100 %) and specificity (67–99 %) for distinguishing benign from malignant pancreatic masses.

T. Özülker, F. Özülker, *Atlas of PET-CT Imaging in Oncology: A Case-Based Guide to Image Interpretation*,
DOI 10.1007/978-3-319-18994-9_11

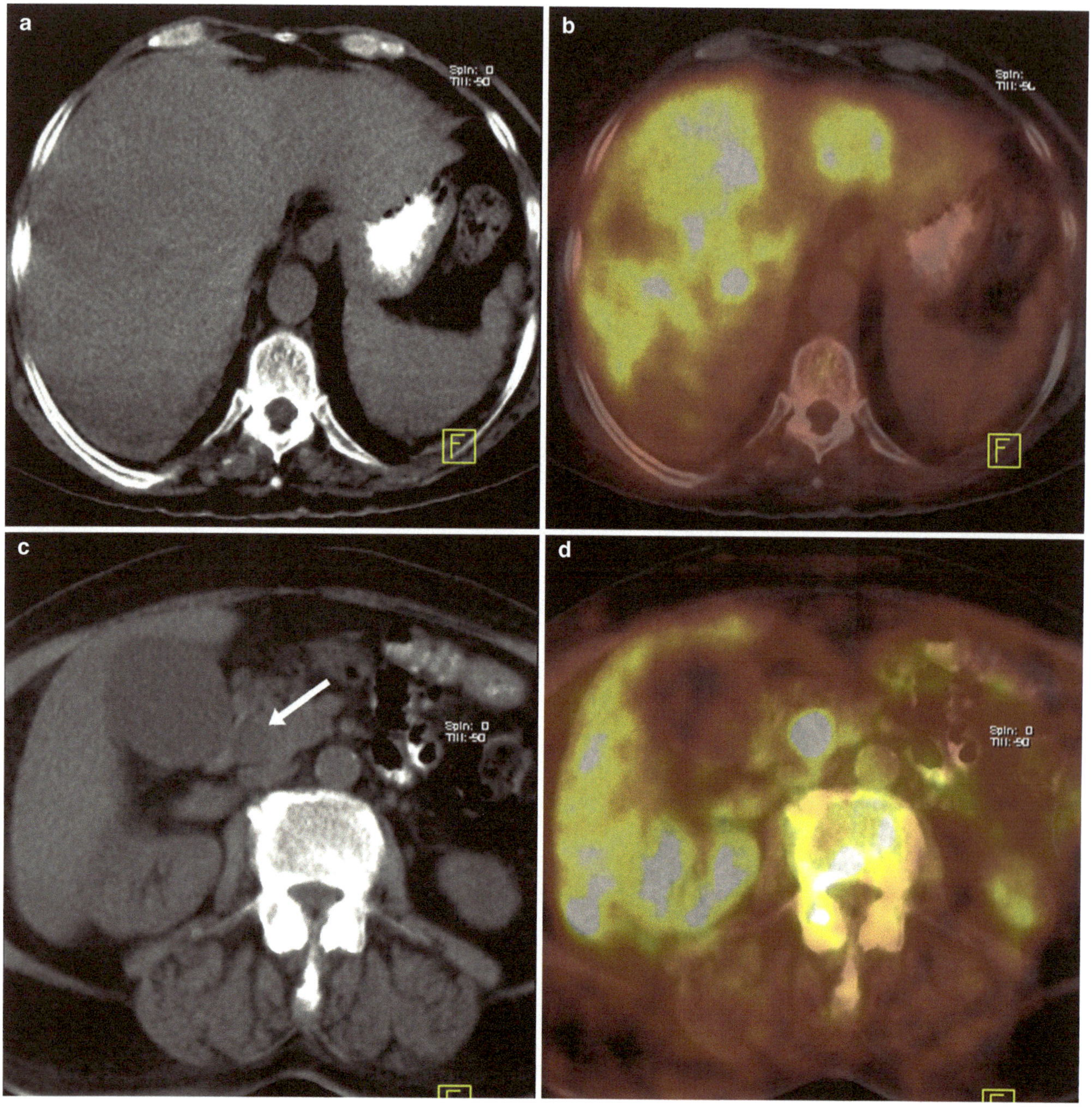

Fig. 11.1 Axial CT and fusion images show multiple hypermetabolic mass lesions at both lobes of liver (SUVmax 10) (**a**, **b**) and a focal hypermetabolic lesion at the head of the pancreas (*arrow*) (SUVmax 8.7) (**c**, **d**)

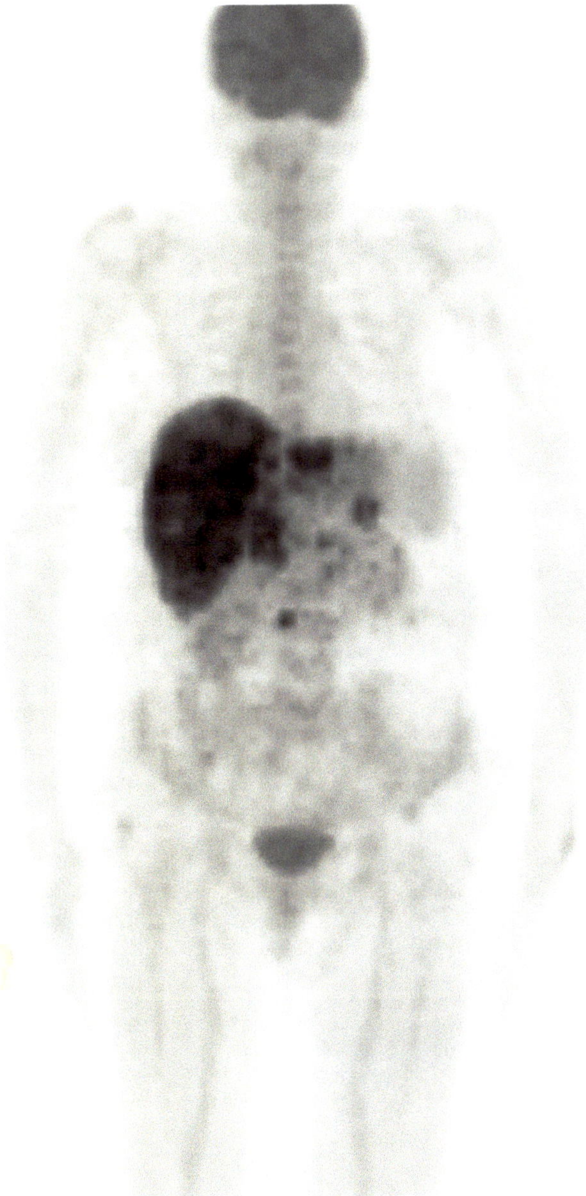

Fig. 11.2 MIP image

11.2 Case 2: Pancreas Neuroendocrine Tumor

History A 47-year-old female was referred to ^{18}F-FDG PET/CT study after an increase in tumor markers was detected incidentally on laboratory tests.

Findings

Interpretation Although FDG uptake at mass lesion is not at malignancy level, the lesion is suspicious for malignancy.

Result Biopsy from lesion revealed neuroendocrine tumor of pancreas.

Teaching Point Although ^{18}F-FDG PET/CT is not effective in imaging of gastropancreatic neuroendocrine tumors, tumors with high proliferative activity and low differentiation shows an increased FDG uptake.

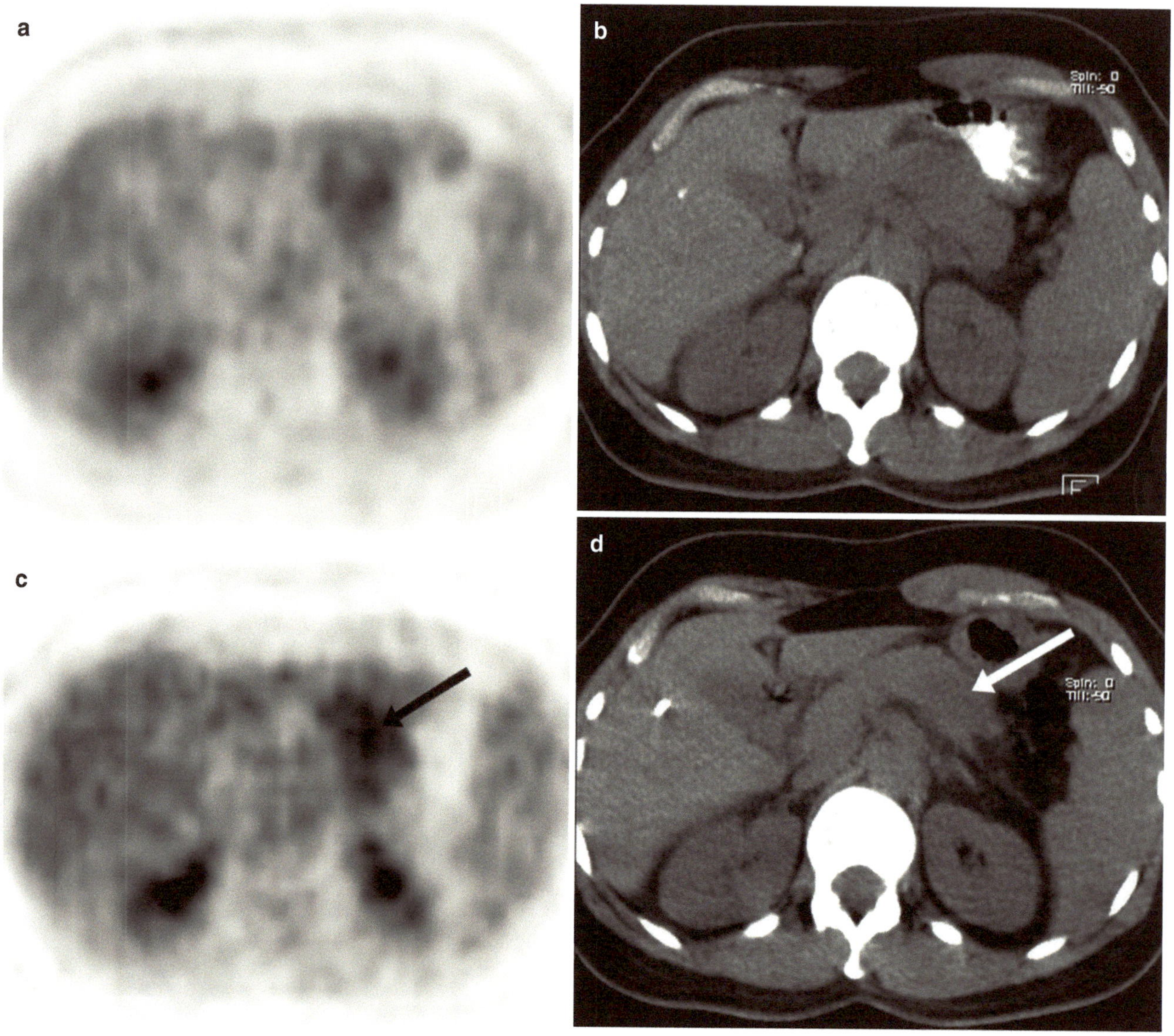

Fig. 11.3 Axial PET and CT images show hypodense lesion occupying tail and body of pancreas showing mildly increased FDG uptake (*arrow*) (SUVmax 3.2) (**a**–**d**)

Bibliography

1. Delbeke D, Martin WH. PET and PET/CT for pancreatic malignancies. Surg Oncol Clin N Am. 2010;19:235–54.
2. Kwee TC, Basu S, Alavi A. PET and PET/CT for unknown primary tumors. Methods Mol Biol. 2011;727:317–33. doi:10.1007/978-1-61779-062-1_17.

12 Gastrointestinal Stromal Tumors

12.1 Case 1: Gastrointestinal Stromal Tumor Progression

History A 33-year-old male status post biopsy from a mass lesion in abdomen was diagnosed to have gastrointestinal stromal tumor (GIST) 5 months ago. The patient has been treated with imatinib mesylate (Gleevec) and referred to ^{18}F-FDG PET/CT scan for evaluation of therapy response.

Findings

Interpretation The increase in size and metabolic activity of lesion is consistent with progression.

Teaching Point ^{18}F-FDG PET/CT scan is effective in assessment of response to Gleevec therapy in GIST. Although regression is detected on PET, these tumors might become larger within the few months following the therapy, because of hemorrhage, edema, or myxoid degeneration. In this case the lesion became larger but since there is also increase in metabolic activity, the case is accepted as progression.

T. Özülker, F. Özülker, *Atlas of PET-CT Imaging in Oncology: A Case-Based Guide to Image Interpretation*,
DOI 10.1007/978-3-319-18994-9_12

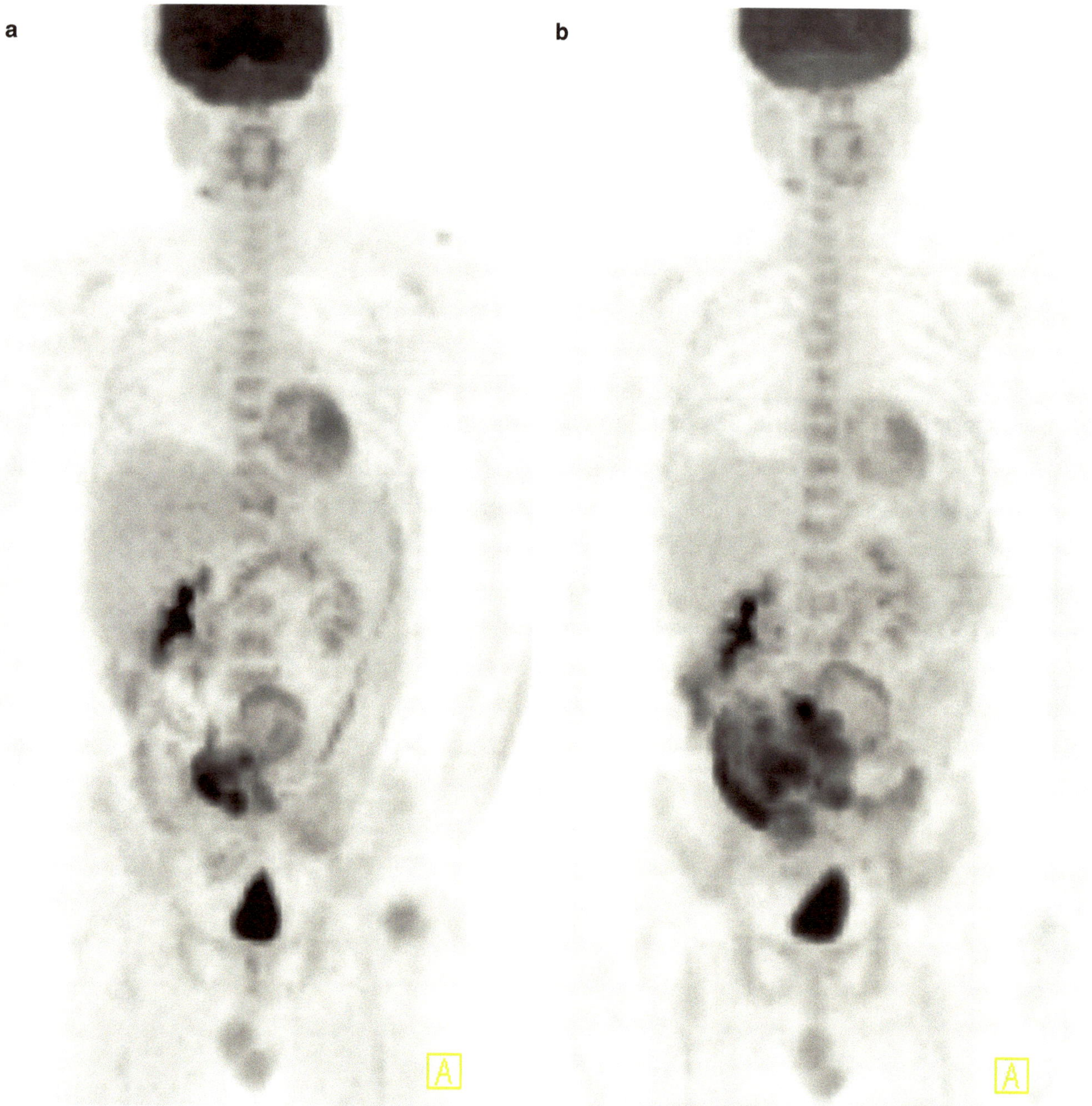

Fig. 12.1 MIP images show heterogenously hypermetabolic mass lesion located at lower abdomen (**a**), increase in size and metabolic activity of lesion 5 months after treatment (**b**)

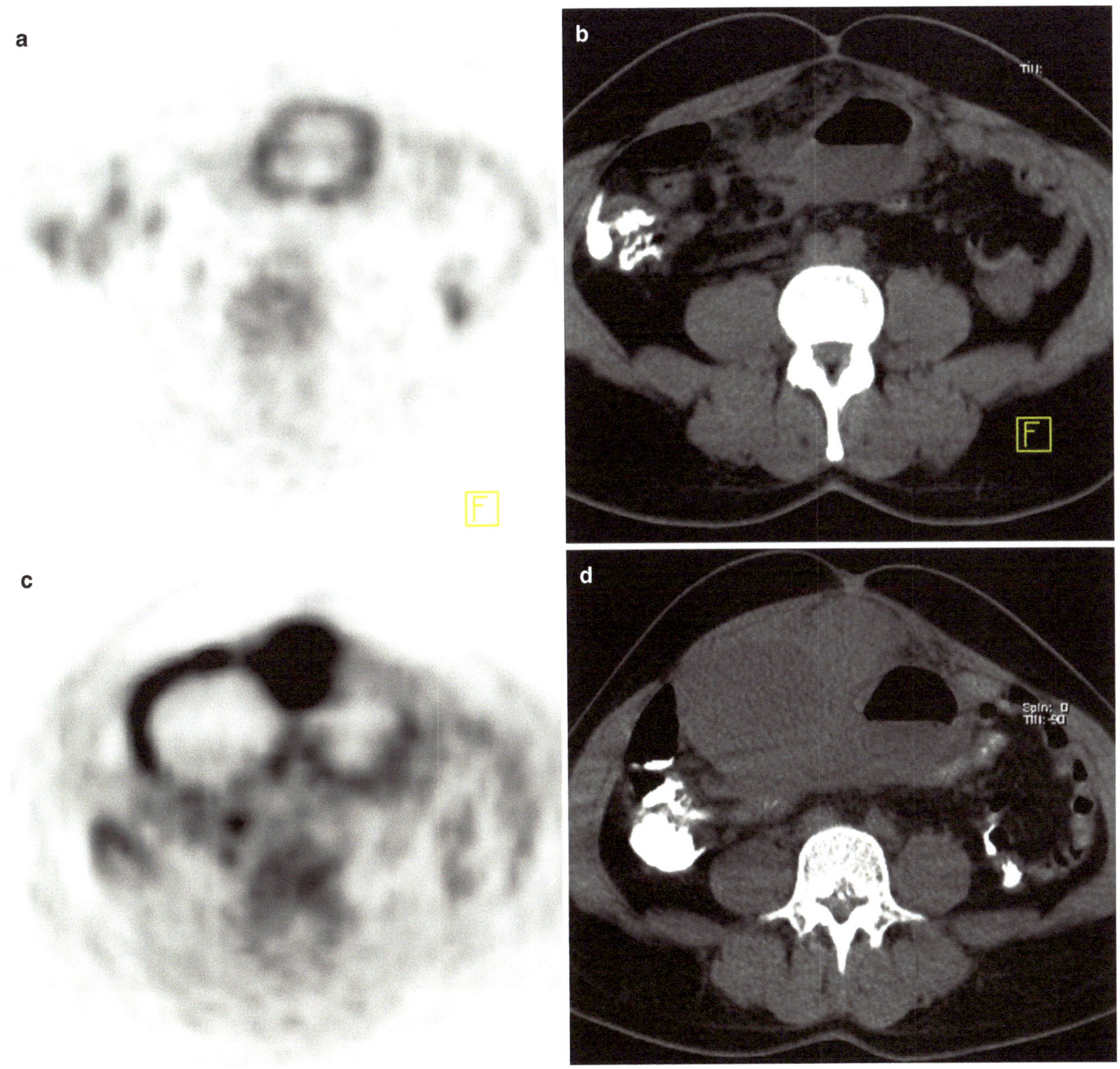

Fig. 12.2 Axial PET and CT images show mass lesion with intensely increased FDG uptake in circular fashion, located adjacent to anterior wall of abdomen (SUVmax 13.5) (**a**, **b**). After Gleevec therapy the lesion increased in size with the inner side being more hypodense and intensity of FDG uptake increased at periphery of mass with a newly appearing solid component (SUVmax 14.7) (**c**, **d**)

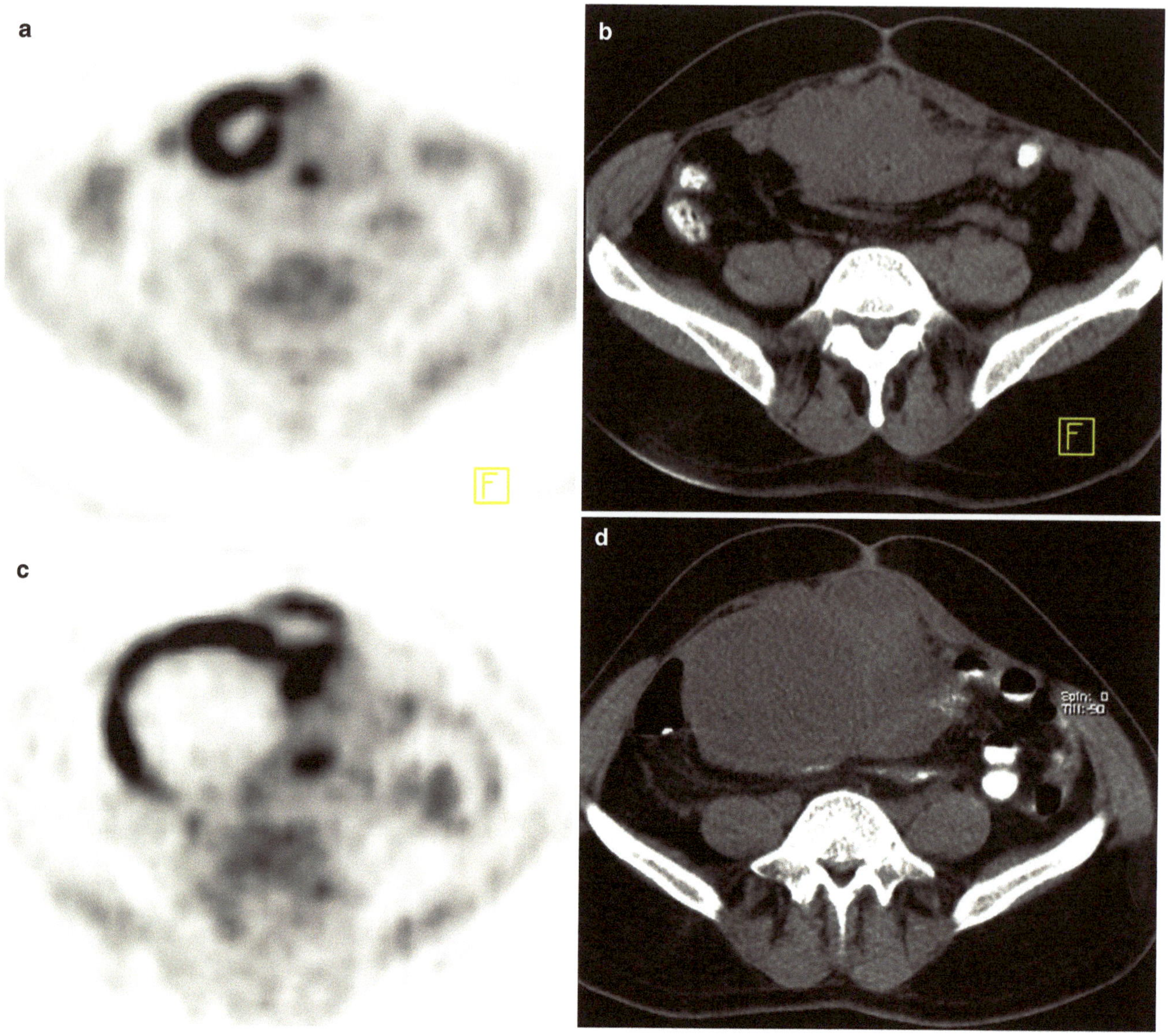

Fig. 12.3 Axial PET and CT images showing hypermetabolic mass lesion at the entrance of pelvis before (**a**) and after (**b**) Gleevec therapy (**c, d**)

12.2 Case 2: Gastrointestinal Stromal Tumor Progression

History A 57-year-old male who had the diagnosis of GIST after excision of a tumoral lesion from small intestine, underwent chemotherapy with Gleevec, and the efficacy of the therapy is being assessed with ^{18}F-FDG PET/CT at regular intervals.

Findings

Interpretation The second study shows mild regression but the disease showed significant progression at third study.

Teaching Point The liver and peritoneum are common sites of distant GIST lesions, whereas lung metastases are infrequent, accounting for 7 % of all lesions.

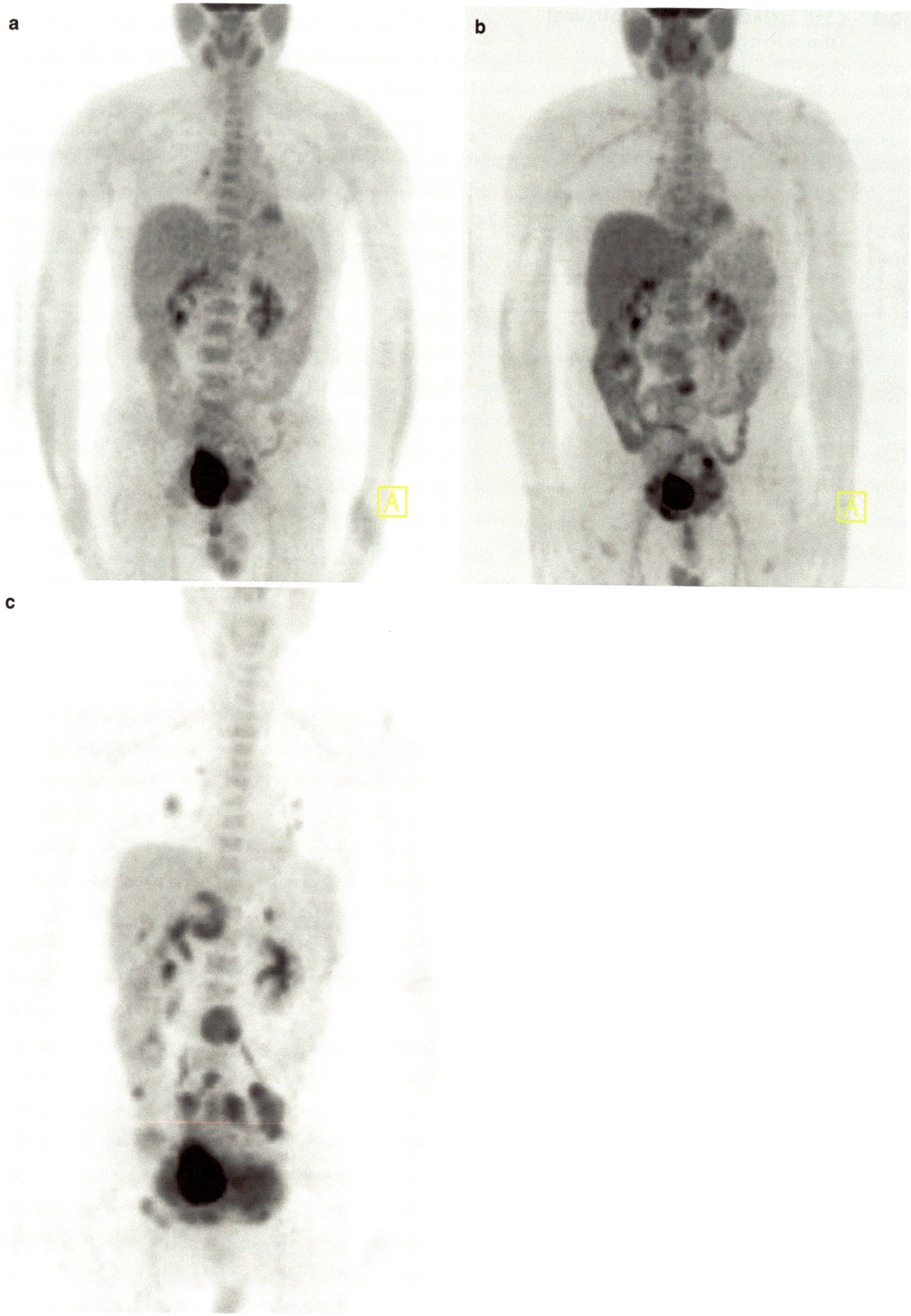
a
A
b
A
c

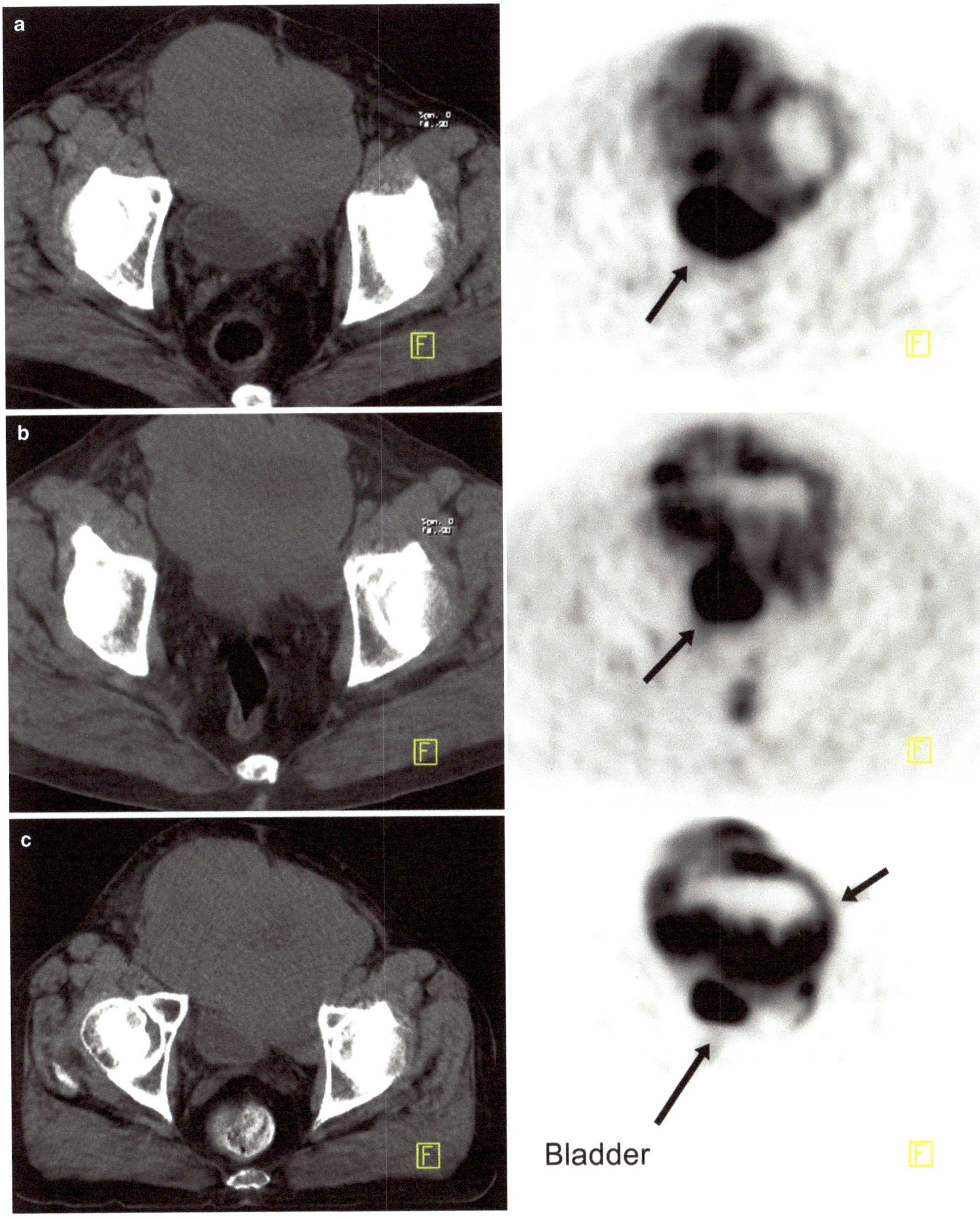

Fig. 12.5 Axial slices of CT and PET images show heterogenously increased FDG uptake at mass lesion in front of the bladder (**a**), 10 months after the first study (**b**), 7 months after the second study (**c**) (*arrows*)

Fig. 12.4 MIP images show intensely increased FDG uptake at mass lesion in front of the bladder (SUVmax 7.2) (**a**), 10 months later slight regression at the lesion is seen (SUVmax 6.6) but there is a mildly hypermetabolic newly developed lesion at level of L3 (**b**), 7 months after the second study there is progression at the lesion (SUVmax 9.5) and newly developed numerous hypermetabolic lesions in abdomen and both lungs are noted (**c**)

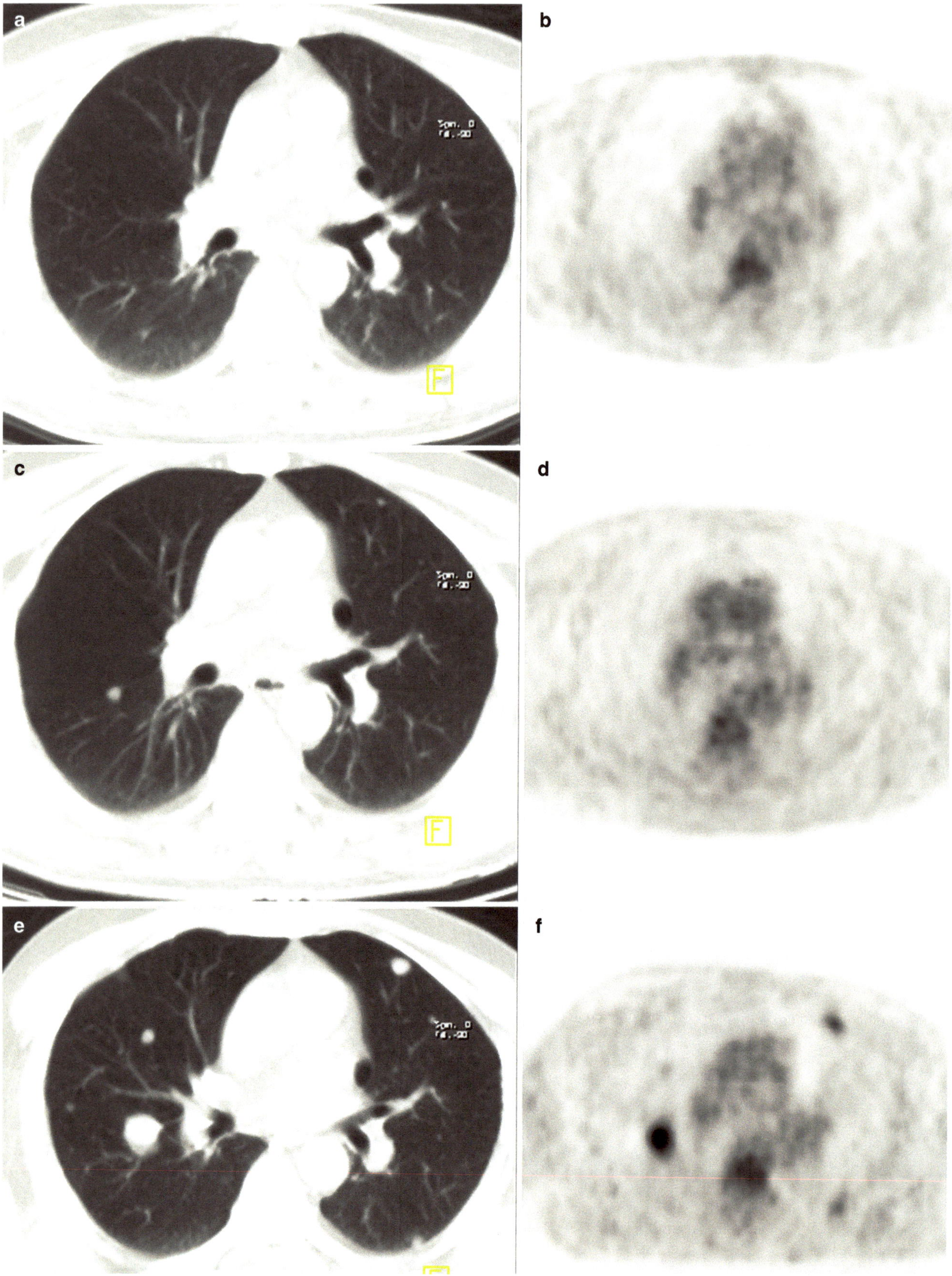

Fig. 12.6 Axial slices of CT and PET images from thorax show no pathological FDG uptake site at first study (**a**, **b**), 10 months after the first study focal hyperdense nodule at right lung without corresponding FDG uptake (**c**, **d**), 7 months after the second study moderately hypermetabolic nodules at both lung parenchyma (SUVmax 6.2) (**e**, **f**)

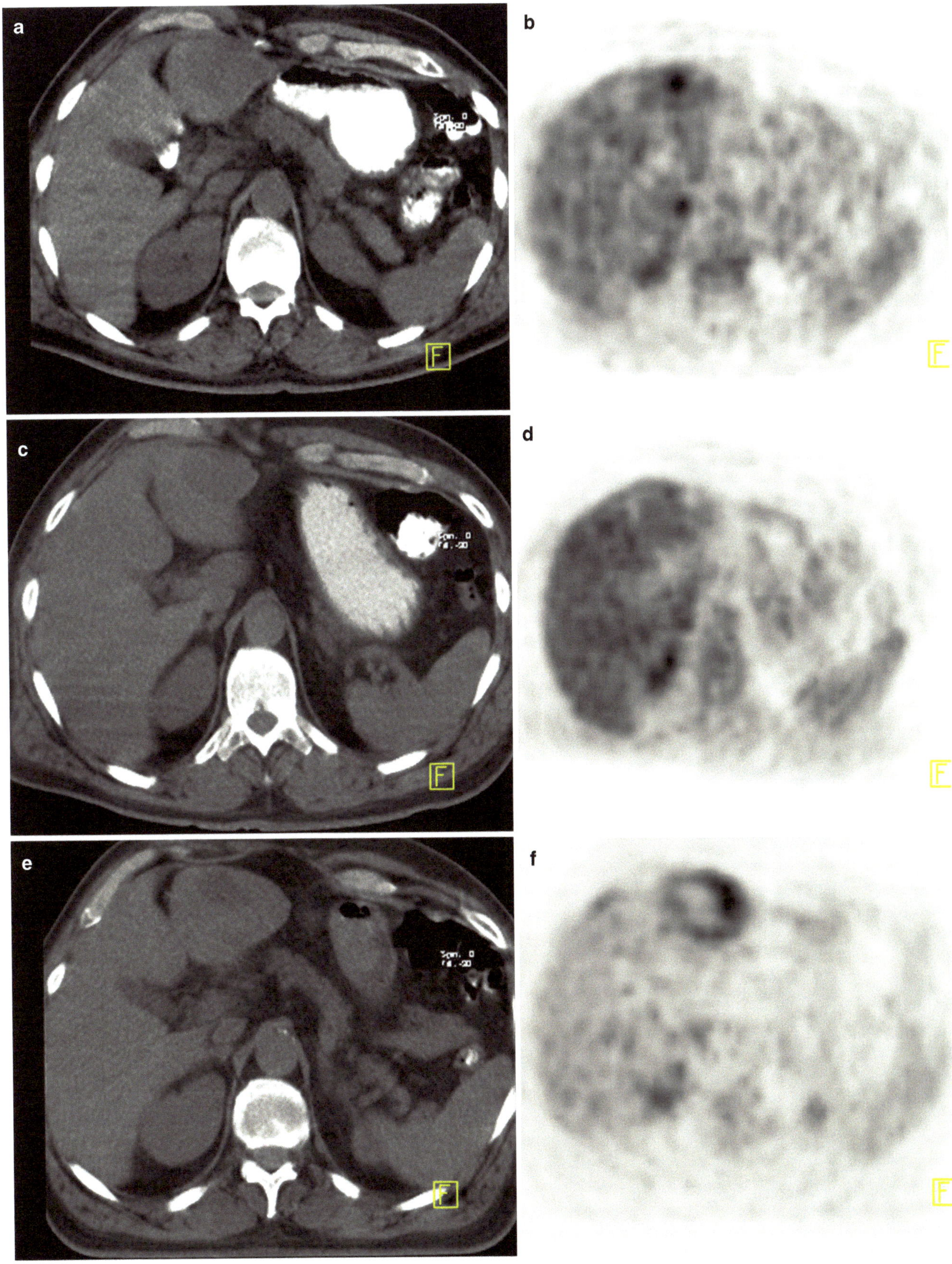

Fig. 12.7 Axial slices of CT and PET images from liver show hypermetabolic focus at a hypodense lesion at segment 3 of liver (**a**, **b**), 10 months after the first study hypodense lesion at CT still exists but hypermetabolic focus is not seen (**c**, **d**), 7 months after the second study hypermetabolism at segment 3 is detected again despite the decrease in size of hypodense lesion at CT (**e**, **f**)

12.3 Case 3: Gastrointestinal Stromal Tumor Progression

History A 44-year-old female who is being followed-up with the diagnosis of GIST underwent ^{18}F-FDG PET/CT scan before and 6 months after Gleevec therapy.

Findings

Interpretation The increase in size and metabolic activity represents progressive disease.

Teaching Point Enlargement of the lesion together with an increase in metabolic activity reflects progression. The HU of the lesions remained same before and after the therapy. Approximately 20 % of the lesions detected on CT do not have any FDG uptake, and in these cases a decrease in HU may be evaluated in favor of regression.

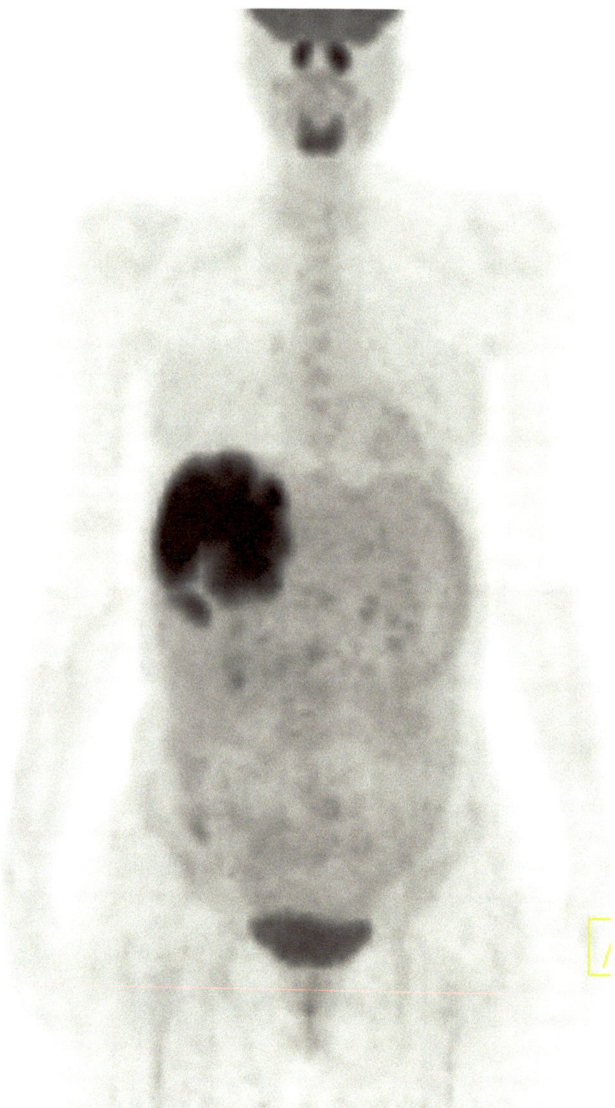

Fig. 12.8 MIP image shows intensely increased FDG uptake at mass lesion at liver (SUVmax 7.7)

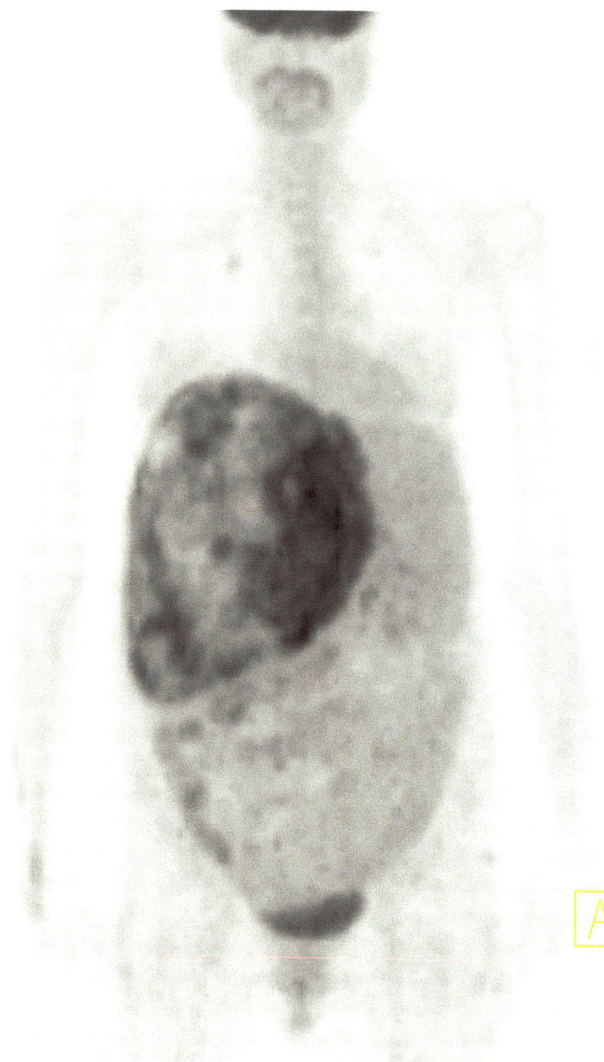

Fig. 12.9 Six months after the beginning of treatment with Gleevec the lesion at liver increased in size and metabolic activity (SUVmax 11.4)

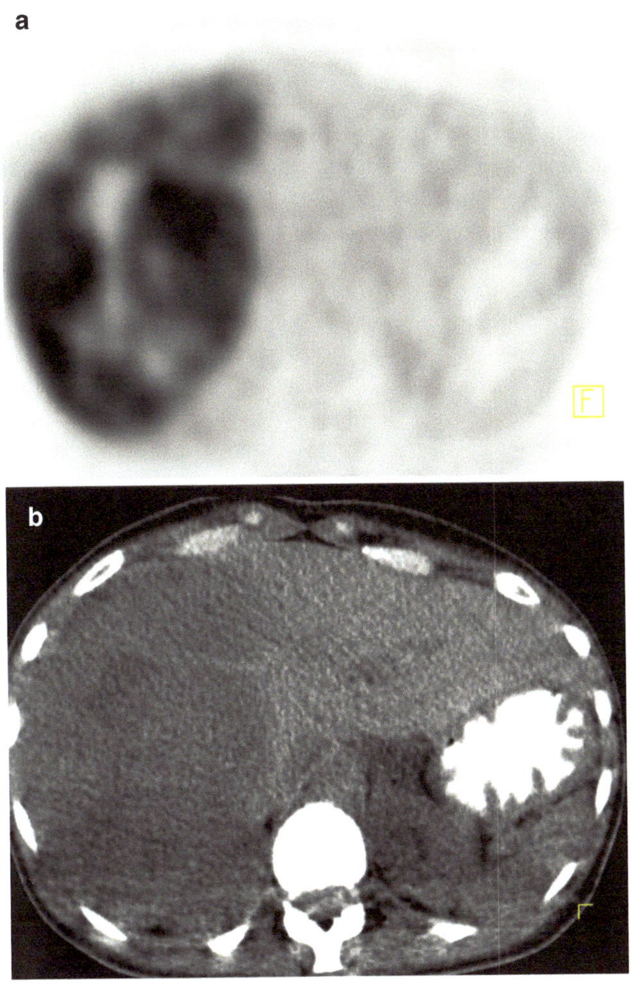

Fig. 12.10 Axial slices of PET and CT images show intensely and heterogenously increased FDG uptake at mass lesion occupying right lobe and segment 4 of liver (HU 17.2) (**a**, **b**)

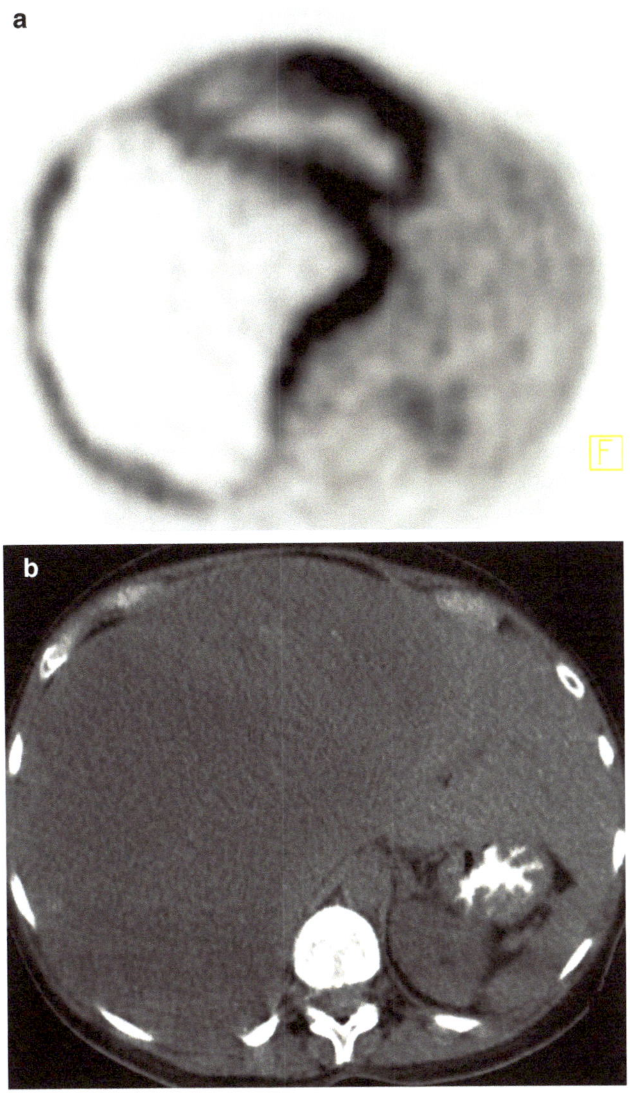

Fig. 12.11 6 months after therapy the lesion increases in size with hypodense center and increased metabolic activity in comparison with the previous study (HU 18) (**a**, **b**)

12.4 Case 4: Gastrointestinal Stromal Tumor with Complete Response to Therapy

History A 23-year-old male underwent operation for a mass lesion at omentum which was thought to be originated from gastric wall. The lesion turned out to be GIST and the patient was referred to ^{18}F-FDG PET/CT for staging. After completion of chemotherapy the ^{18}F-FDG PET/CT scan was repeated for evaluation of response.

Findings

Interpretation There is complete response to therapy.

Teaching Point Primary GIST can be originated from anywhere along GI tract but most commonly seen at stomach (60–70 %), small intestine (20–25 %), and rarely rectum, esophagus, colon, and appendix.

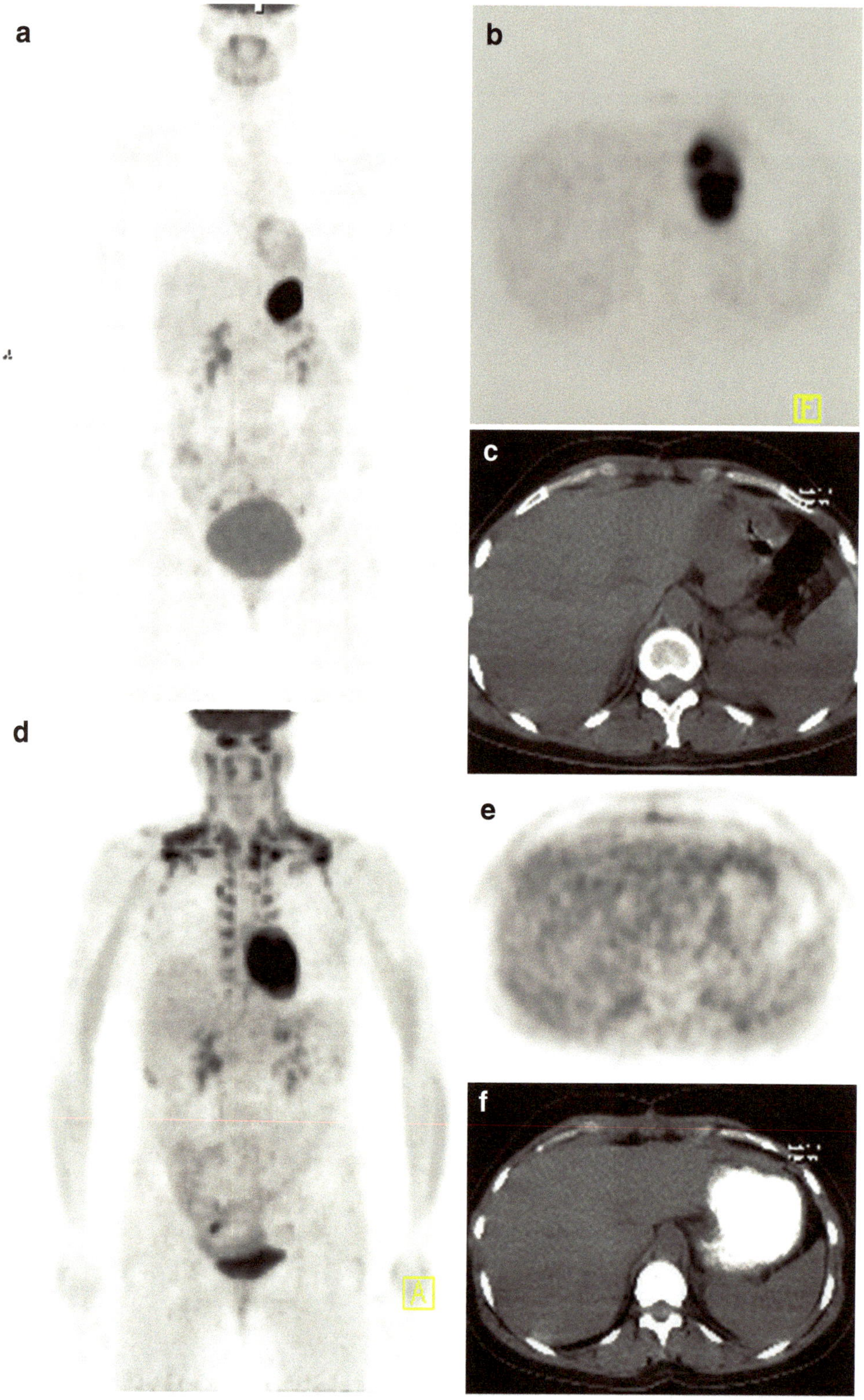

Fig. 12.12 MIP (**a**), axial PET, and CT images (**b**, **c**) show intensely increased FDG uptake at mass lesion at stomach (SUVmax 44.3), disappearance of the lesion after completion of chemotherapy (**d**–**f**). The FDG uptake at cervical, supraclavicular, and mediastinal area reflects physiological accumulation of FDG due to sympathetic activation at BAT

Bibliography

1. Eugene CL, Alavi A. Gastric, esophageal, and gastrointestinal tumors. In: Eugene CL, Alavi A, editors. PET and PET/CT: a clinical guide. 2nd ed. New York: Thieme; 2009. p. 170.
2. Nannini M, Biasco G, Di Scioscio V, Di Battista M, Zompatori M, Catena F, et al. Clinical, radiological and biological features of lung metastases in gastrointestinal stromal tumors (case reports). Oncol Rep. 2011;25:113–20.

Surrenal Tumors

13

13.1 Case 1: Surrenal Adenoma

History A 52-year-old male without any known primary malignancy underwent ^{18}F-FDG PET/CT after a left adrenal incidentaloma was detected by abdominal MRI.

Findings

Interpretation This finding is diagnostic of a benign adrenal incidentaloma.

Teaching Point Adrenal adenomas are neoplasms which are either functional or not and incidentally detected on conventional anatomic imaging. They are typically less than 3 cm in diameter, well marginated, and of uniform and less than 10 HU attenuation at unenhanced CT. Approximately 30 % of adenomas are lipid poor with an attenuation greater than 10 HU. They show marked contrast material washout at delayed imaging at contrast enhanced CT and drop in signal intensity on out of phase chemical shift MR imaging.

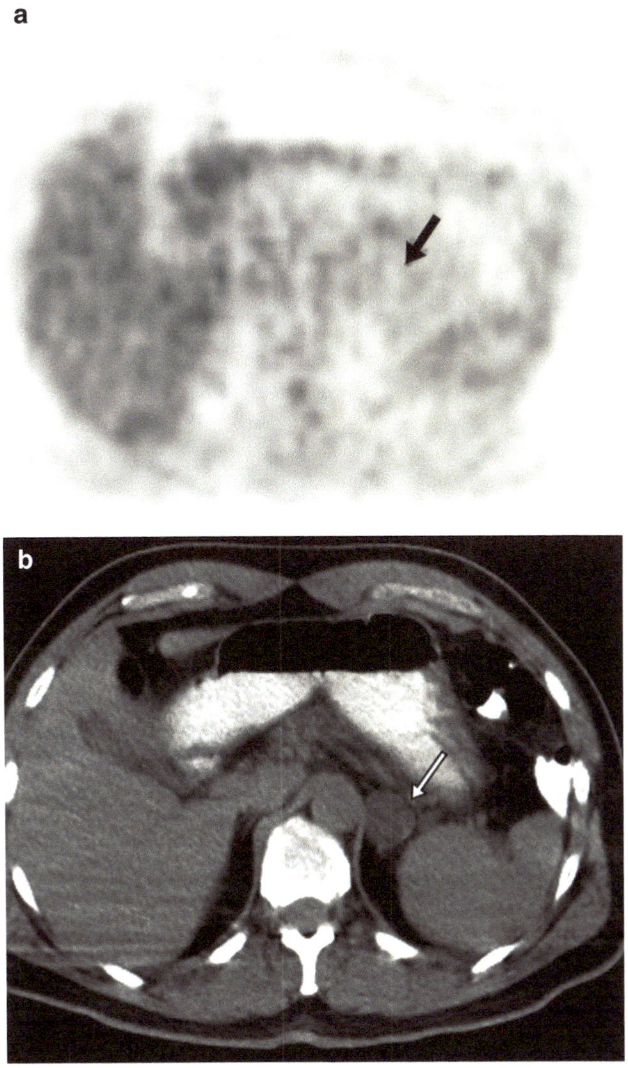

Fig. 13.1 Axial slices of CT and PET (**a**, **b**) show homogeneous, well-defined, 5.4-HU round mass with dimensions of 4.5 × 4 × 3.5 cm in the left adrenal gland without any significant FDG uptake (*arrow*). MRI (not shown here) displayed a drop in signal intensity on out of phase imaging

T. Özülker, F. Özülker, *Atlas of PET-CT Imaging in Oncology: A Case-Based Guide to Image Interpretation*,
DOI 10.1007/978-3-319-18994-9_13

13.2 Case 2: Surrenal Adenoma

History A 55-year-old male without any known primary malignancy underwent ^{18}F-FDG PET/CT for evaluation of a left adrenal incidentaloma.

Findings

Interpretation This finding is indicative of likelihood for a benign adrenal incidentaloma.

Teaching Point It has been proposed that identification of malignancy at surrenal gland can be accomplished by applying an SUVmax cutoff of greater than 3.1 and SUV ratio of greater than 1.0. Combined PET/CT with mean attenuation >10 HU and SUV(max) >3.1 had 97.3 % sensitivity and 86.2 % specificity in identification of malignancy, and combined PET/CT with mean attenuation >10 HU and SUV ratio >1.0 had 97.3 % sensitivity and 74.1 % specificity.

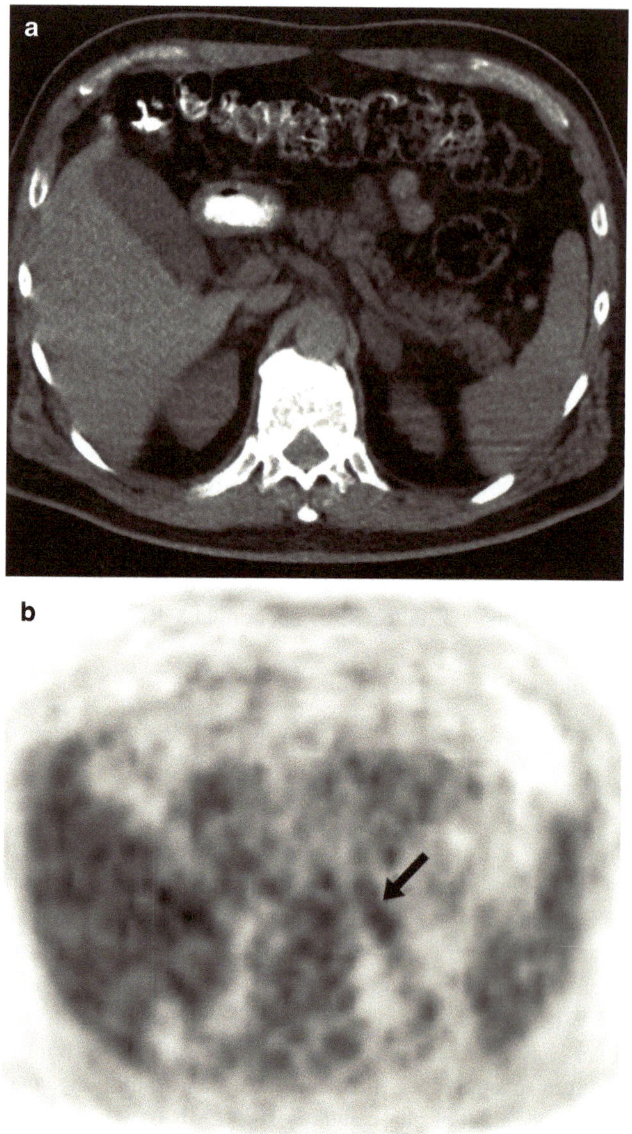

Fig. 13.2 Axial slices of CT and PET (**a**, **b**) show mildly increased FDG uptake at left oval surrenal mass measuring 2×2 cm (SUVmax 3) (*arrow*). SUV ratio (nodule SUV(max)/liver SUV(avg)) is 3/2.7=1.1. MRI (not shown here) displayed a drop in signal intensity on out of phase imaging. The lesion had a mean HU of −13 on CT images

13.3 Case 3: Adrenal Schwannoma

History A 32-year-old woman was incidentally found to have a left adrenal mass of 4×8×10 cm on abdominal ultrasonography. The patient underwent ^{18}F-FDG PET/CT and then left adrenalectomy was performed.

Findings

Interpretation Metabolic activity of the lesion is at the level of malignancy, and when the size and the imaging characteristics of the lesion is taken into account, the lesion is strongly suspicious of a malignant adrenal neoplasm.

Result Histological examination revealed the diagnosis of schwannoma. This diagnosis was supported by immunohistochemistry of S-100 and vimentin positivity.

Teaching Point Although adrenal lesions with a SUVmax >3 are thought to be malignant, benign lesions like schwannoma can cause false positive results.

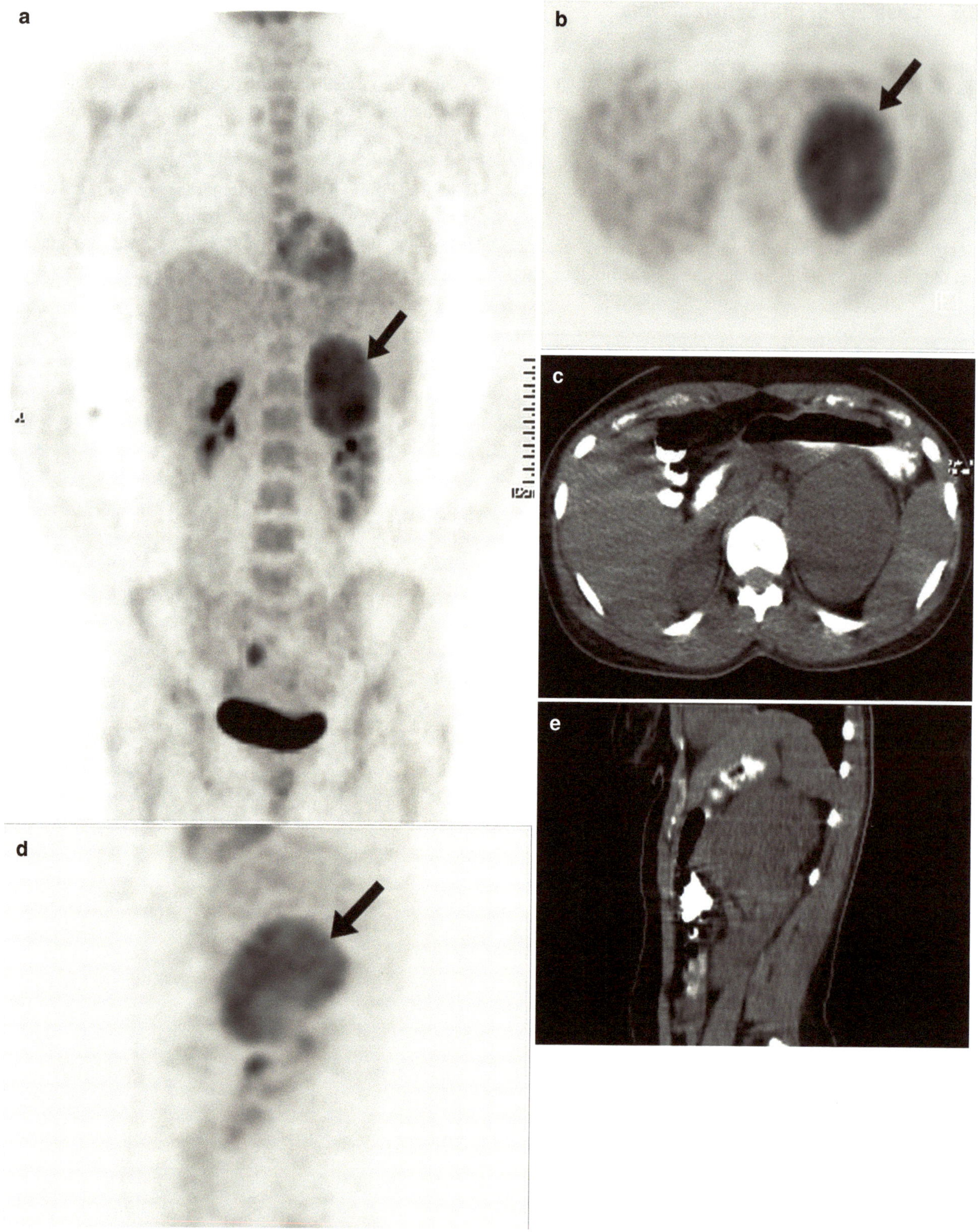

Fig. 13.3 MIP (**a**), axial (**b**, **c**), and sagittal (**d**, **e**) PET and CT images show intense uptake within the left adrenal mass (*arrows*)

13.4 Case 4: Adrenal Ganglioneuroma

History A 18-year-old male patient underwent CT, which showed a relatively homogenous left adrenal tumor measuring 5.2×4.3×7.1 cm. ^{18}F-FDG PET/CT scan was performed to rule out malignancy at primary lesion and detect any possible metastases.

Findings

Interpretation Metabolic activity of the lesion is at the level of malignancy, when the SUVmax threshold for malignancy is accepted as 3.

Result The patient underwent left adrenalectomy and histological examination revealed the diagnosis of ganglioneuroma (GN).

Teaching Point GN is a benign neoplasm that originates from neural crest cells of sympathetic ganglia or adrenal medulla. Although FDG PET has high accuracy in distinguishing benign surrenal lesions from malignant ones, it may give misleading results.

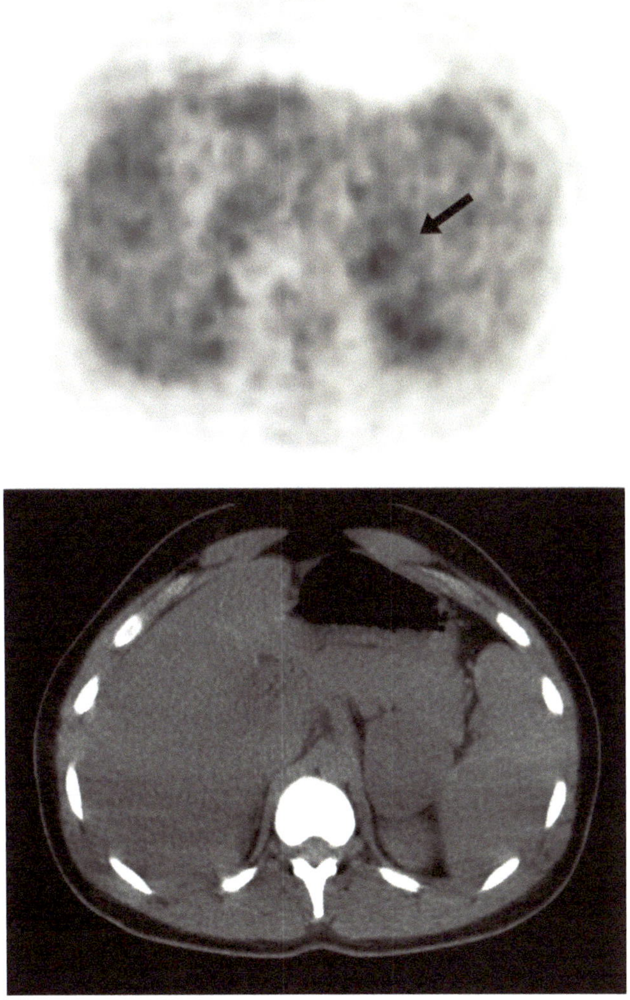

Fig. 13.4 Axial slices of PET and CT images show mild uptake at left adrenal mass (*arrow*) (SUVmax 4.1)

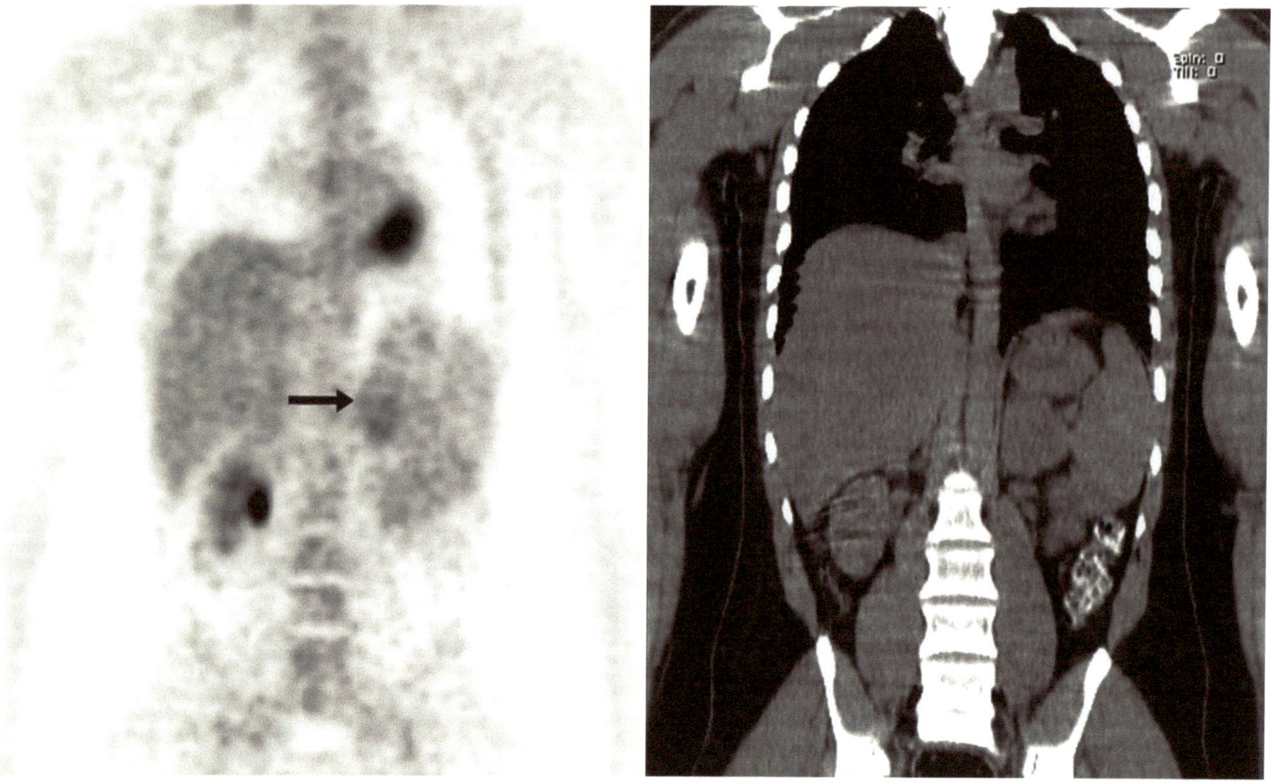

Fig. 13.5 Coronal PET and CT images show mass lesion at left adrenal gland with subtle FDG uptake (*arrow*)

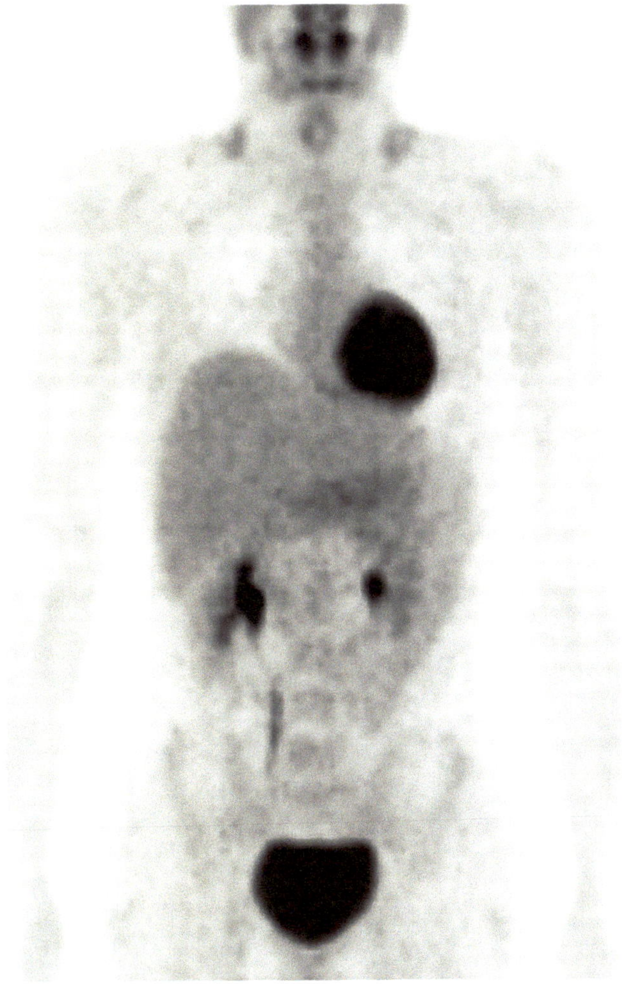

Fig. 13.6 MIP image

13.5 Case 5: Surrenal Cyst

History A 45-year-old female underwent ^{18}F-FDG PET/CT for evaluation of a right adrenal incidentaloma which was detected on USG.

Findings

Interpretation This finding is compatible with primary cystic lesion of adrenal gland.

Teaching Point Cystic lesions of the adrenal gland are rare findings, and although they are mostly benign entities, they may be associated with neoplasms. There are several distinct histopathological entities like endothelial cysts, epithelial cysts, and pseudocysts. Pseudocysts might be associated with adrenal neoplasms like adrenal cortical carcinomas, adrenal cortical adenomas, and pheochromocytomas.

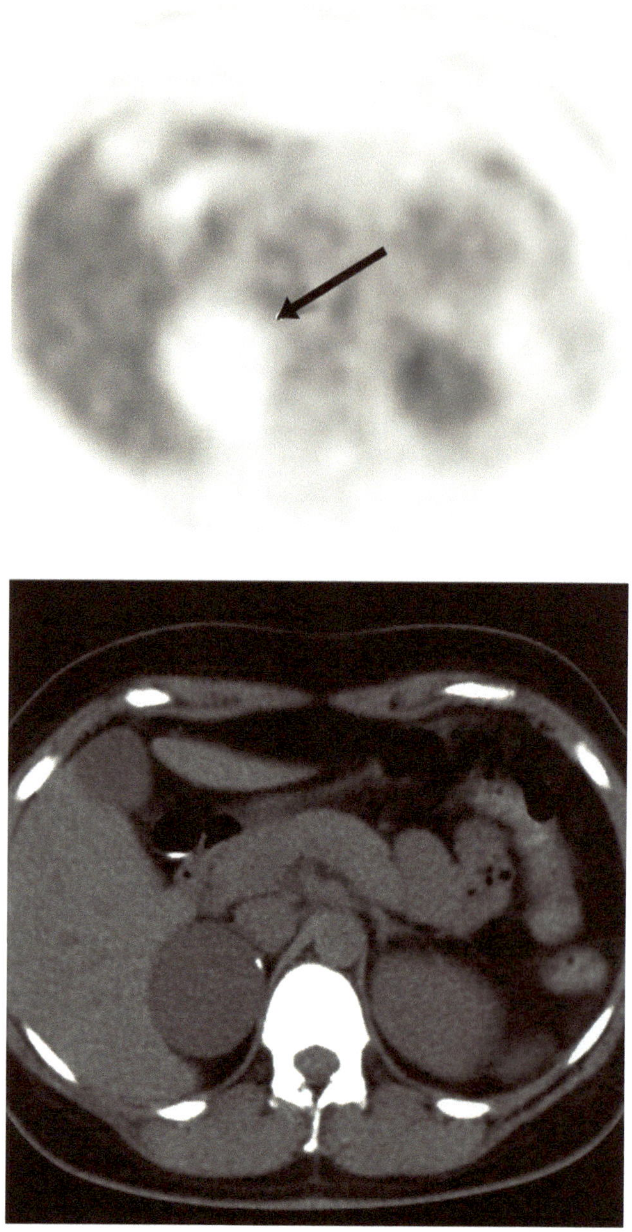

Fig. 13.7 Axial slices of PET and CT images show hypodense mass lesion at right adrenal gland which is ametabolic (*arrow*) on PET images

13.6 Case 6: Imaging of Brown Fat due to Bilateral Pheochromocytoma

History A 52-year-old male with a history of poorly controlled hypertension presented with a hypertensive crisis. Abdominal imaging revealed bilateral adrenal mass lesions with dimensions of 3.6×4×7 cm at left and 1.2×1.2 cm at right. The patient underwent ^{18}F-FDG PET/CT scan for evaluation of adrenal masses and laboratory investigations. A 24-h urinary collection revealed markedly elevated catecholamines (particularly norepinephrine), confirming the diagnosis of pheochromocytoma.

Findings

Interpretation Hypermetabolism detected at deep cervical, supraclavicular, interscapular, and paravertebral regions represent uptake at BAT and hypermetabolic lesions at both surrenal glands are compatible with pheochromocytoma.

Teaching Point Increased FDG uptake at BAT can be seen as a result of activation of sympathetic nervous system by cold stimulation. In this case, catecholamine-secreting pheochromocytoma is the cause of BAT activation. Pheochromocytomas show high FDG avidity but the imaging characteristics of malignant adrenal masses and pheochromocytomas are similar.

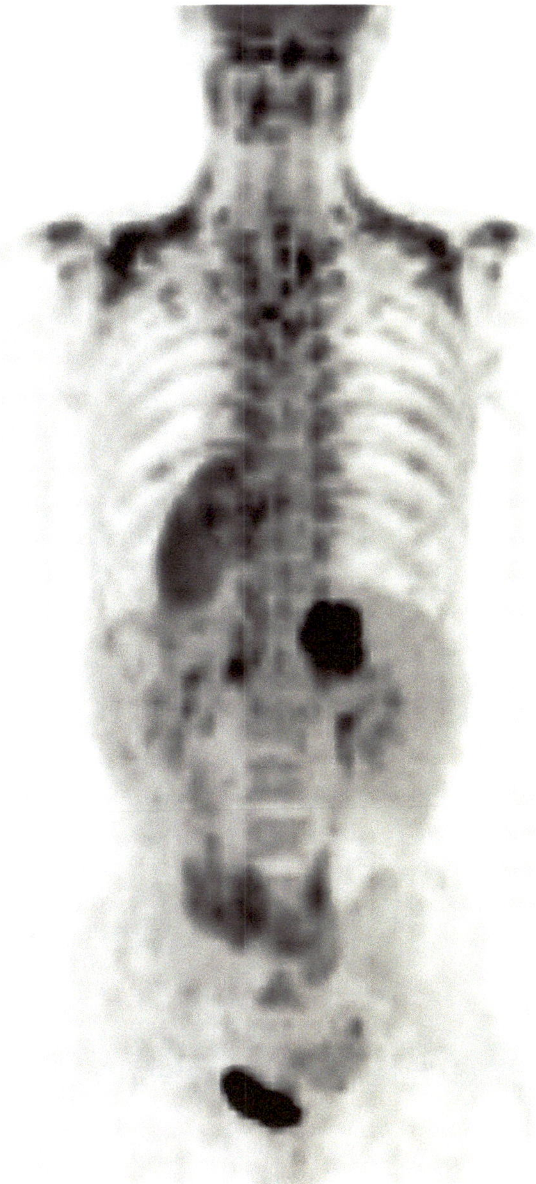

Fig. 13.8 MIP image shows intensely increased FDG uptake at left (SUVmax 15) and right adrenal glands (SUVmax 10). There is remarkably increased FDG uptake at deep cervical, supraclavicular, interscapular, and paravertebral regions without any corresponding lesion at CT component, representing uptake at BAT. The patient also has Kartagener syndrome, characterized by situs inversus totalis with myocardium at right hemithorax and liver at left side of abdomen

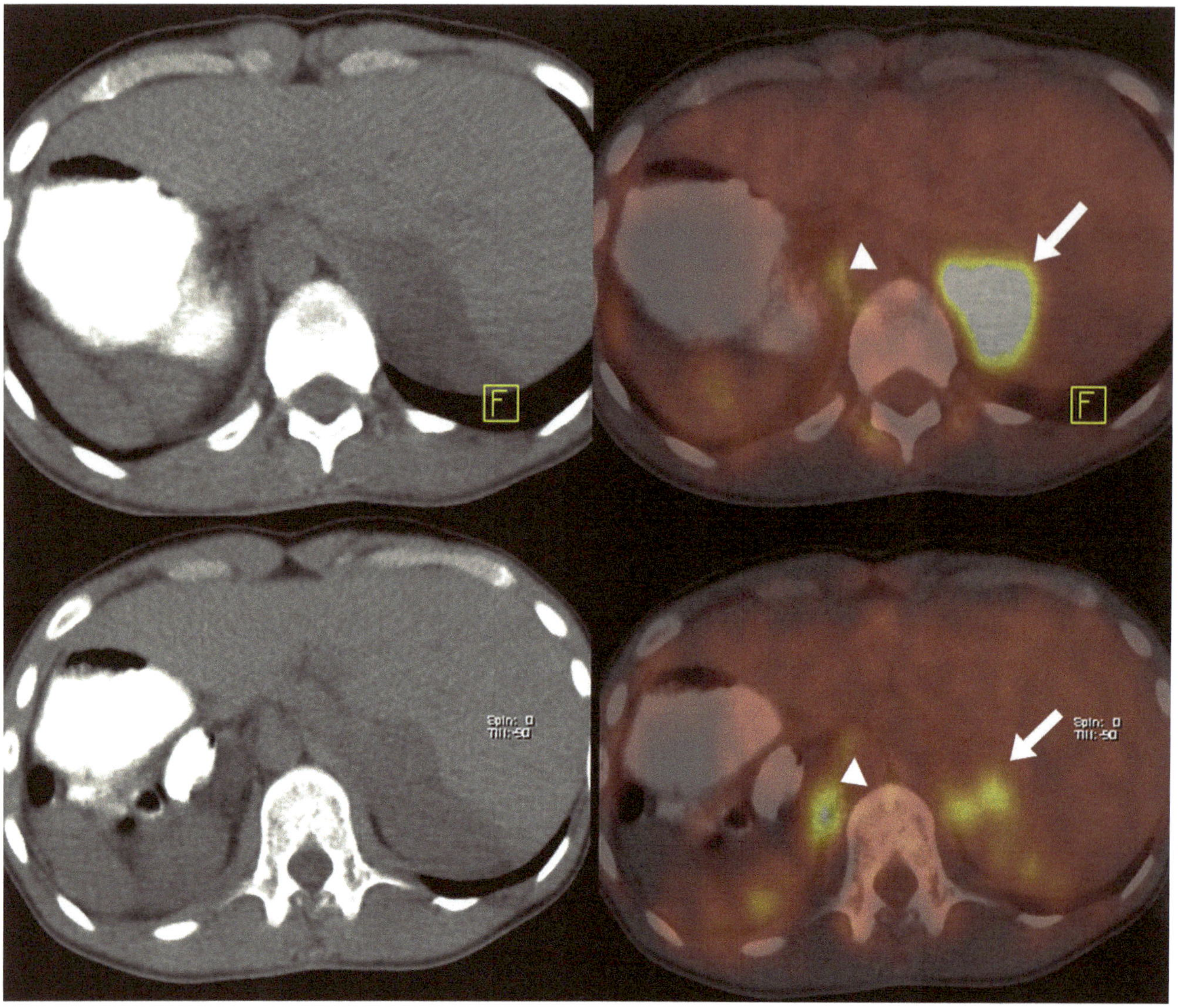

Fig. 13.9 Axial CT and fusion images show intensely increased FDG uptake at left (*arrow*) and right (*arrow head*) adrenal masses. Localization of FDG at retroperitoneal area due to BAT activation is also noted

13.7 Case 7: Adrenocortical Carcinoma

History A 56-year-old male, who had the diagnosis of lung cancer underwent ^{18}F-FDG PET/CT for restaging.

Findings

Interpretation This finding is suggestive for a malignant surrenal lesion.

Result The patient underwent right adrenalectomy and histopathology revealed adrenocortical carcinoma.

Teaching Point Adrenocortical carcinoma (ACC) is an aggressive cancer originating in the cortex (steroid hormone-producing tissue) of the adrenal gland. PET is useful for the identification of primary adrenal carcinomas in patients with equivocal tumors on computed tomography (CT) scan. It can also provide prognostic information and the intensity of FDG uptake has been shown to correlate with survival in ACC. Its use for restaging purposes is recommended in patients with high clinical suspicion for recurrence or metastases.

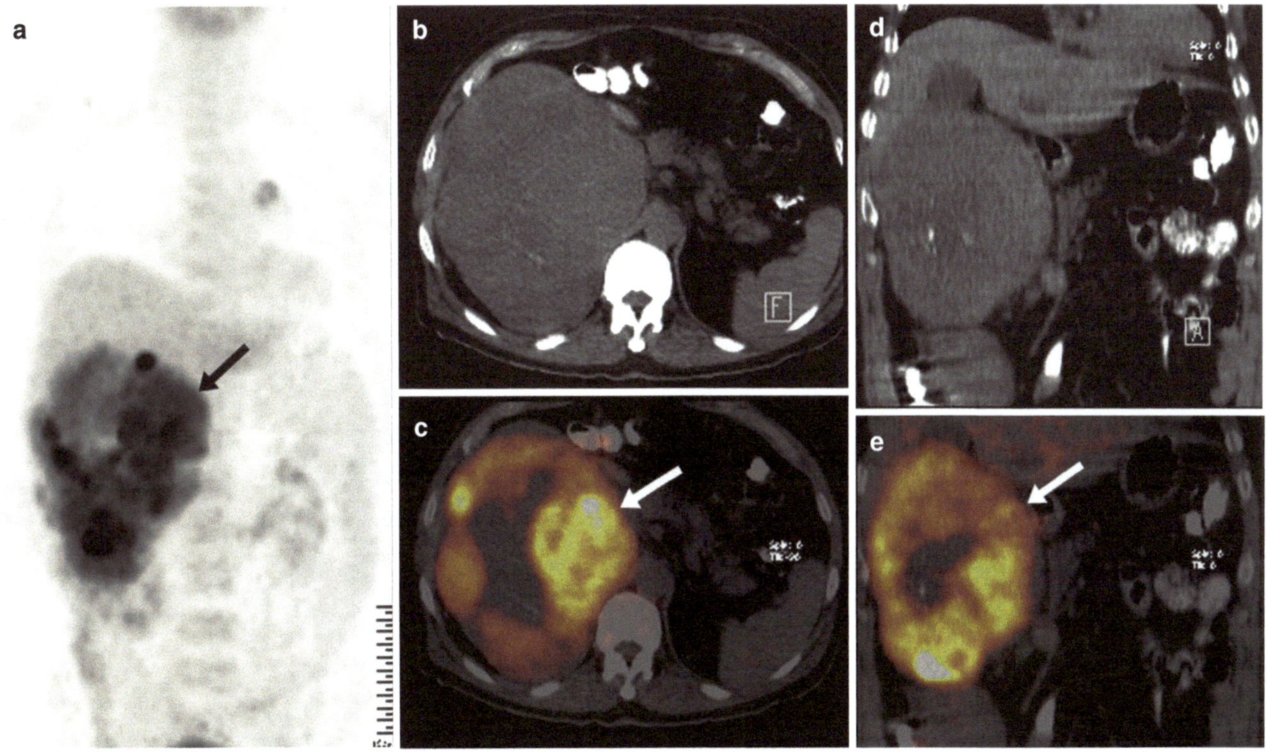

Fig. 13.10 MIP image (**a**), axial (**b**, **c**), and coronal (**d**, **e**) slices of CT and fusion images show intensely hypermetabolic mass lesion originating from right adrenal gland (*arrow*). There are hypometabolic necrotic areas in the lesion

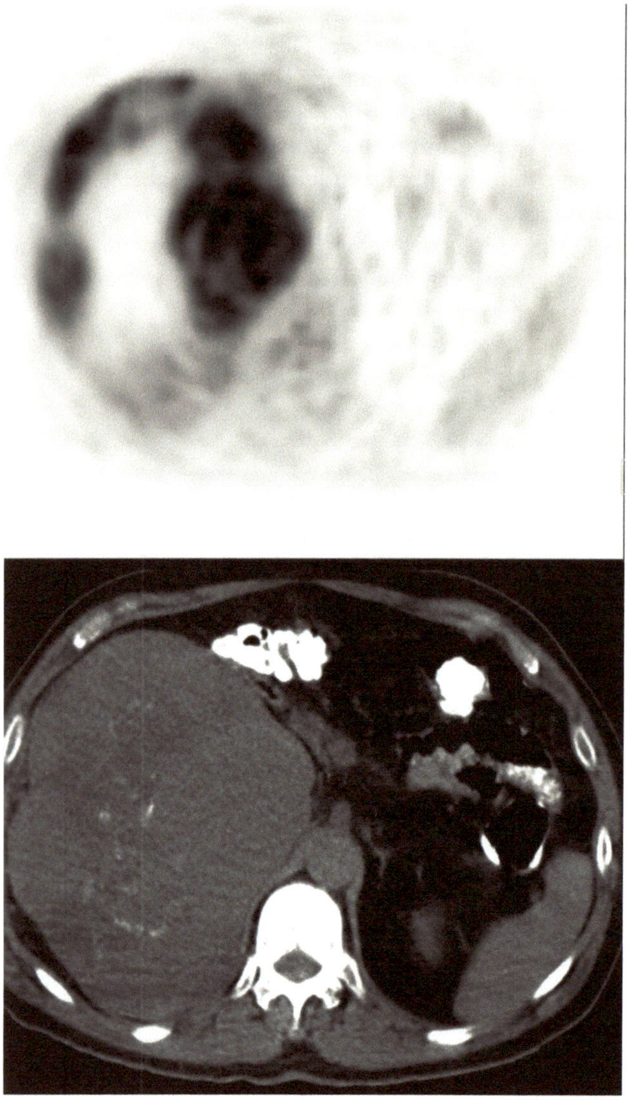

Fig. 13.11 Axial PET and CT images

Bibliography

1. Adas M, Koc B, Adas G, Ozulker F, Aydin T. Ganglioneuroma presenting as an adrenal incidentaloma: a case report. J Med Case Rep. 2014;8:131. doi:10.1186/1752-1947-8-131.
2. Adas M, Ozulker F, Adas G, Koc B, Ozulker T, Sahin IM. A rare adrenal incidentaloma: adrenal schwannoma. Case Rep Gastroenterol. 2013;7:420–7. doi:10.1159/000355871.
3. Boland GW, Lee MJ, Gazelle GS, Halpern EF, McNicholas MM, Mueller PR. Characterization of adrenal masses using unenhanced CT: an analysis of the CT literature. AJR Am J Roentgenol. 1998;171:201–4.
4. Brady MJ, Thomas J, Wong TZ, Franklin KM, Ho LM, Paulson EK. Adrenal nodules at FDG PET/CT in patients known to have or suspected of having lung cancer: a proposal for an efficient diagnostic algorithm. Radiology. 2009;250:523–30. doi:10.1148/radiol.2502080219.
5. Caoili EM, Korobkin M, Francis IR, Cohan RH, Platt JF, Dunnick NRA, et al. Adrenal masses: characterization with combined unenhanced and delayed enhanced CT. Radiology. 2002;222:629–33.
6. Elaini AB, Shetty SK, Chapman VM, Sahani DV, Boland GW, Sweeney AT, et al. Improved detection and characterization of adrenal disease with PET-CT. Radiographics. 2007;27:755–67.
7. Erickson LA, Lloyd RV, Hartman R, Thompson G. Cystic adrenal neoplasms. Cancer. 2004;101:1537–44.
8. Leboulleux S, Dromain C, Bonniaud G, Aupérin A, Caillou B, Lumbroso J, et al. Diagnostic and prognostic value of fluorodeoxyglucose positron emission tomography in adrenocortical carcinoma: A prospective comparison with computed tomography. J Clin Endocrinol Metab. 2006;91:920–5.
9. Nunes ML, Rault A, Teynie J, Valli N, Guyot M, Gaye D, et al. 18F-FDG PET for the identification of adrenocortical carcinomas among indeterminate adrenal tumors at computed tomography scanning. World J Surg. 2010;34:1506–10. doi:10.1007/s00268-010-0576-3.
10. Taïeb D, Sebag F, Barlier A, Tessonnier L, Palazzo FF, Morange I, et al. 18F-FDG avidity of pheochromocytomas and paragangliomas: a new molecular imaging signature? J Nucl Med. 2009;50:711–7. doi:10.2967/jnumed.108.060731.
11. Yun M, Kim W, Alnafisi N, Lacorte L, Jang S, Alavi A. 18F-FDG PET in characterizing adrenal lesions detected on CT or MRI. J Nucl Med. 2001;42:1795–9.

14 Gynecologic Tumors

14.1 Case 1: Restaging of Uterine Carcinosarcoma

History A 62-year-old female who is status post total hysterectomy and bilateral salphyngoopherectomy had the diagnosis of malignant mixed Müllerian tumor and is now being evaluated for restaging with ^{18}F-FDG PET/CT.

Findings

Interpretation Local residual malignant tissue at pelvis and lymph nodes at among both iliac lymphatic chain showing metastatic involvement.

Teaching Point Carcinosarcomas (malignant mixed Müllerian tumors) are rarely encountered malignancies, representing less than 5 % of all uterine tumors. ^{18}F-FDG PET/CT has shown 87.5 % sensitivity of and 97.5 % specificity for detecting disease in asymptomatic patients, and 92.9 % and 100 %, respectively, for patients suspected of recurrence on CT.

T. Özülker, F. Özülker, *Atlas of PET-CT Imaging in Oncology: A Case-Based Guide to Image Interpretation*,
DOI 10.1007/978-3-319-18994-9_14

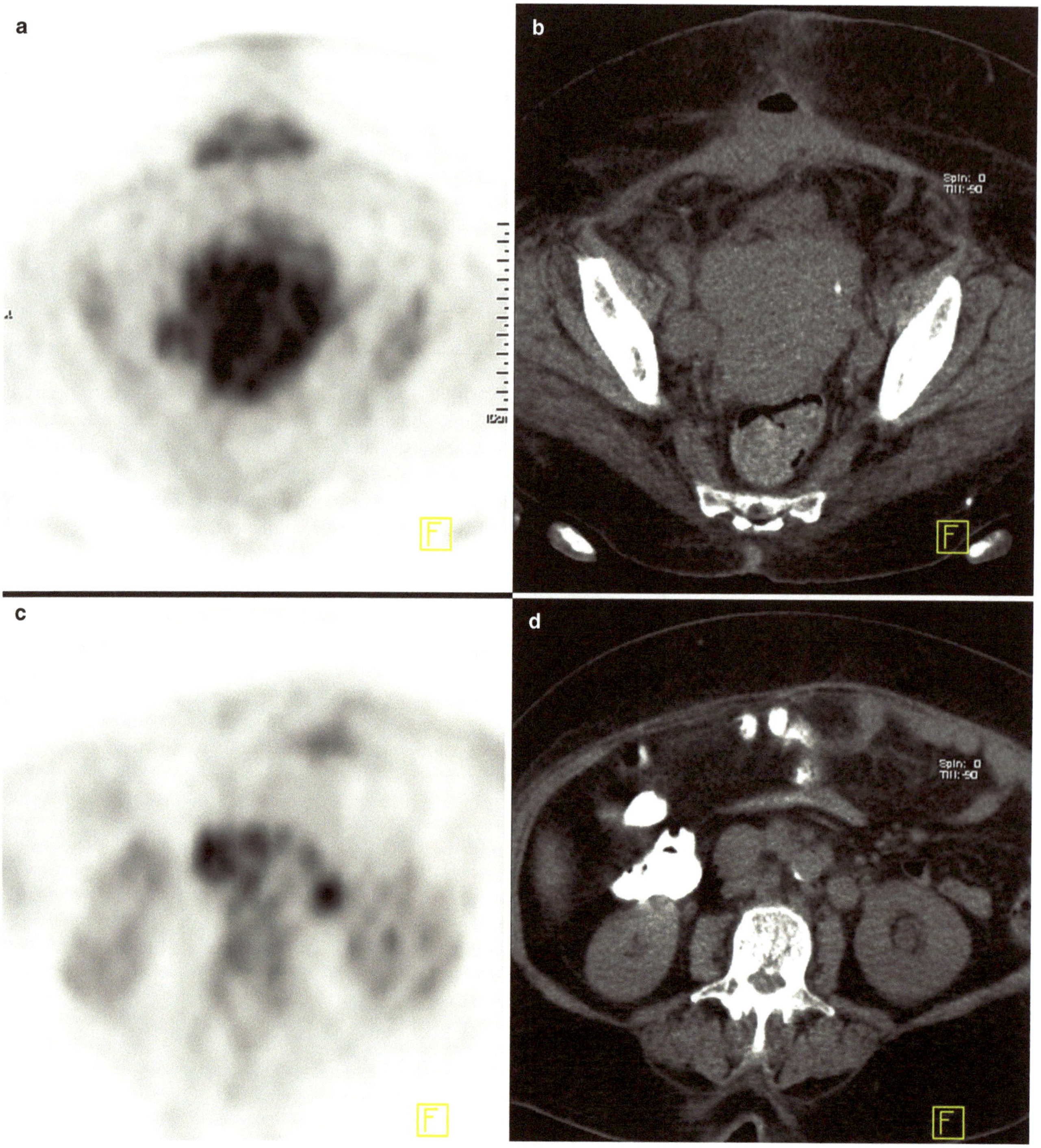

Fig. 14.1 Axial PET and CT images (**a**, **b**) show pelvic mass lesion with intense FDG uptake (SUVmax 16.6) and hypermetabolic lymph nodes at bilateral internal iliac region. There are lymph nodes at paraaortic, paracaval, and interaortocaval areas showing increased FDG uptake (SUVmax 6.6) (**c**, **d**). FDG accumulation at anterior wall of pelvis consistent with postoperative inflammation is also noticed

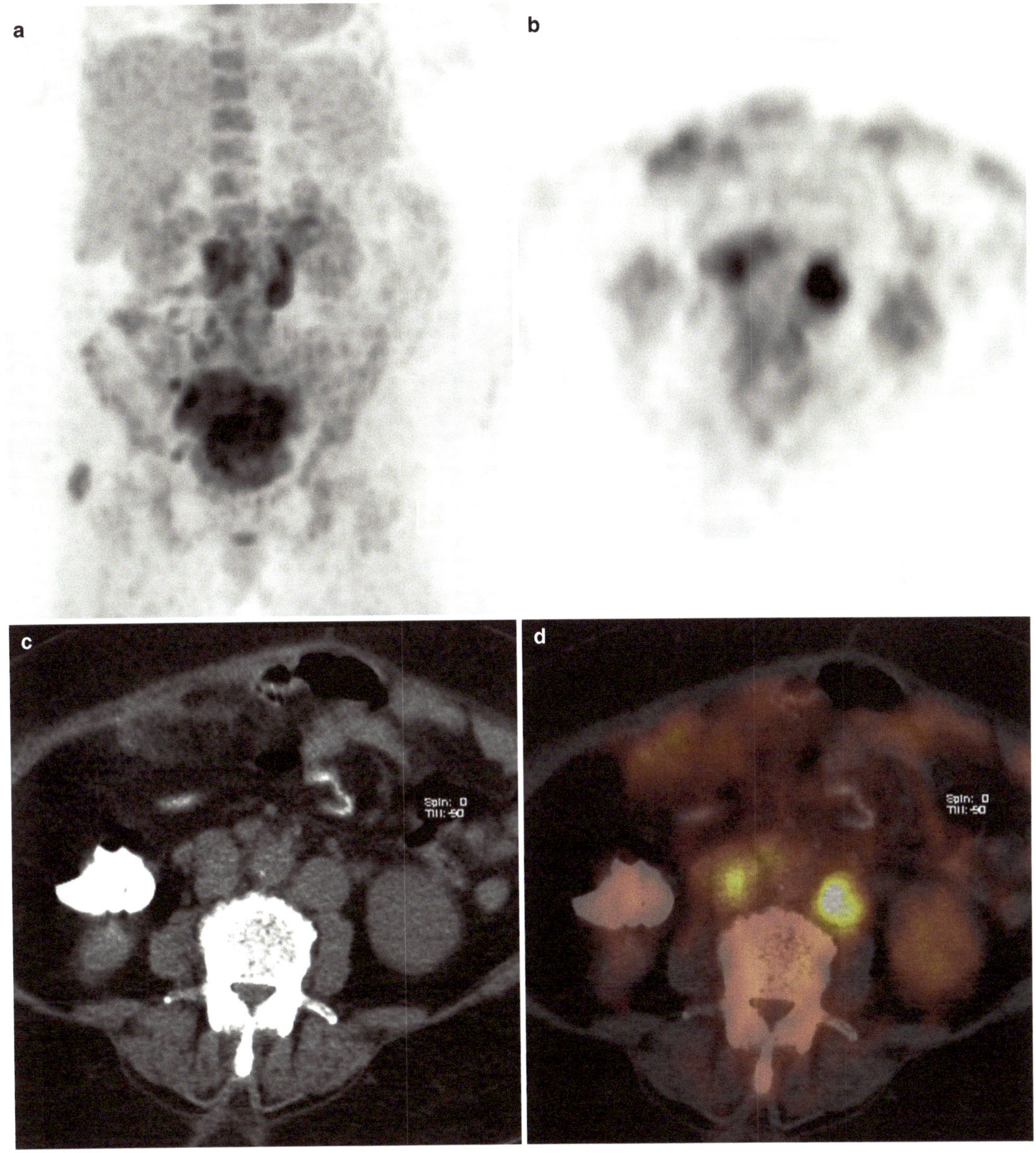

Fig. 14.2 MIP image (**a**), axial PET, CT, and fusion images (**b–d**) show hypermetabolic lymph nodes at paraaortic and paracaval areas

14.2 Case 2: Restaging of Uterine Carcinosarcoma

History A 51-year-old female who had undergone total hysterectomy and bilateral salphyngooopherectomy was being followed up with the diagnosis of malignant mixed Müllerian tumor. Patient received chemotherapy following the operation. Seven months after the operation ^{18}F-FDG PET/CT scan is performed for restaging.

Findings

Interpretation There is local recurrence and rapid progression of malignancy despite therapy which indicates bad prognosis.

Teaching Point FDG PET/CT scan is effective in evaluating therapy response and predicting the prognosis in uterine sarcomas.

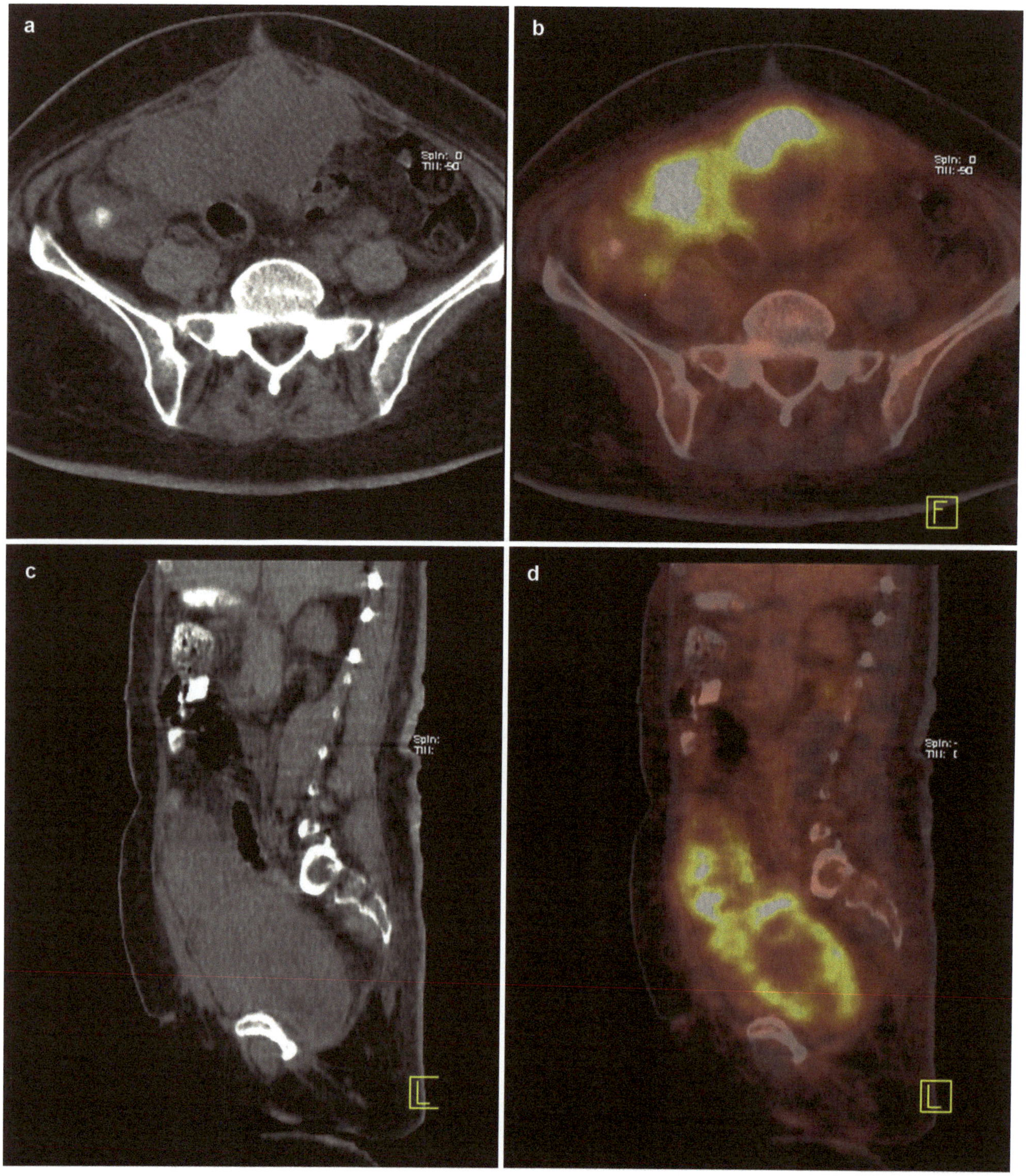

Fig. 14.3 Axial (**a**, **b**) and sagittal (**c**, **d**) CT and fusion images show intensely hypermetabolic (SUVmax 15.3) mass lesion with centrally necrotic hypometabolic areas. The lesion invades peritoneal surfaces and omental fat tissue

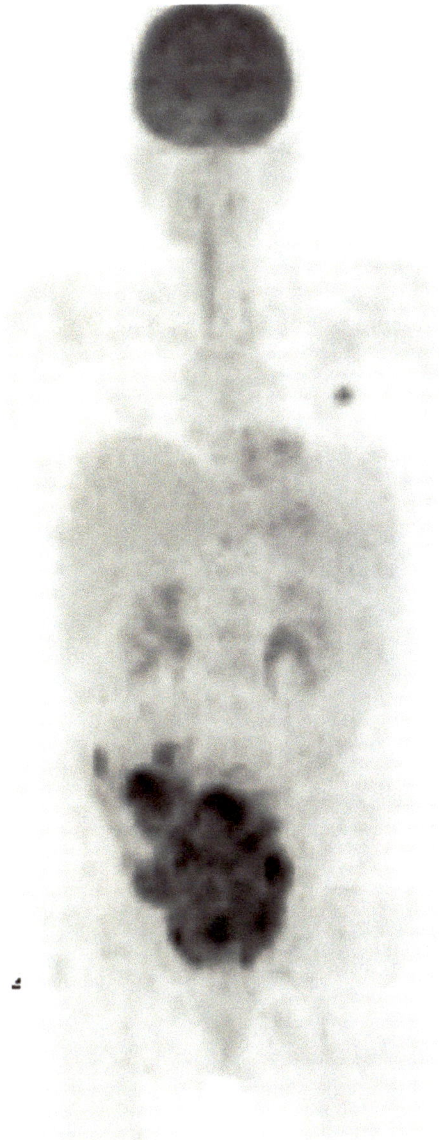

Fig. 14.4 MIP image

14.3 Case 3: Restaging of Uterine Endometrioid Adenocarcinoma

History A 68-year-old female who is status post total hysterectomy, bilateral salphyngoopherectomy, and pelvic lymphadenectomy had the diagnosis of endometrioid adenocarcinoma and underwent ^{18}F-FDG PET/CT scan for restaging.

Findings

Interpretation Lower limb lymphedema is caused by pelvic lymph node dissection. There is still left pelvic lymph node with metastatic involvement.

Teaching Point Lymphedema occurs as a result of an obstruction or interruption of the lymphatic system, generally in proximal limb segments at lymph nodes, due to surgery, infection, malignancy, or scar tissue. Obstruction is frequently seen at pelvic and inguinal groups of nodes in the lower limbs.

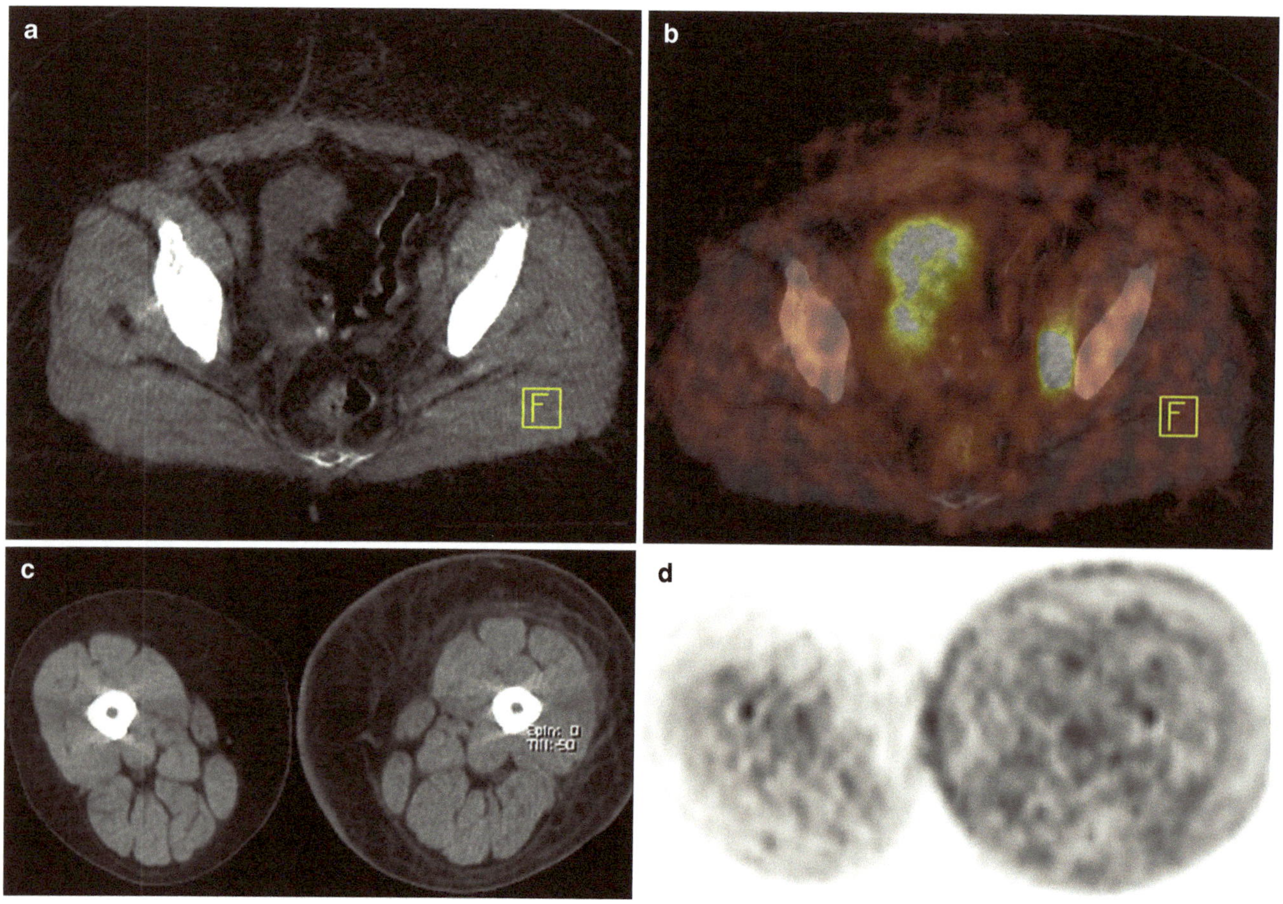

Fig. 14.5 Axial CT and fusion images (**a**, **b**) show lymph node at left internal iliac area with extensive FDG uptake (SUVmax 13). Swelling at left lower extremity with mild diffuse increased FDG uptake is compatible with lymphedema (**c**, **d**)

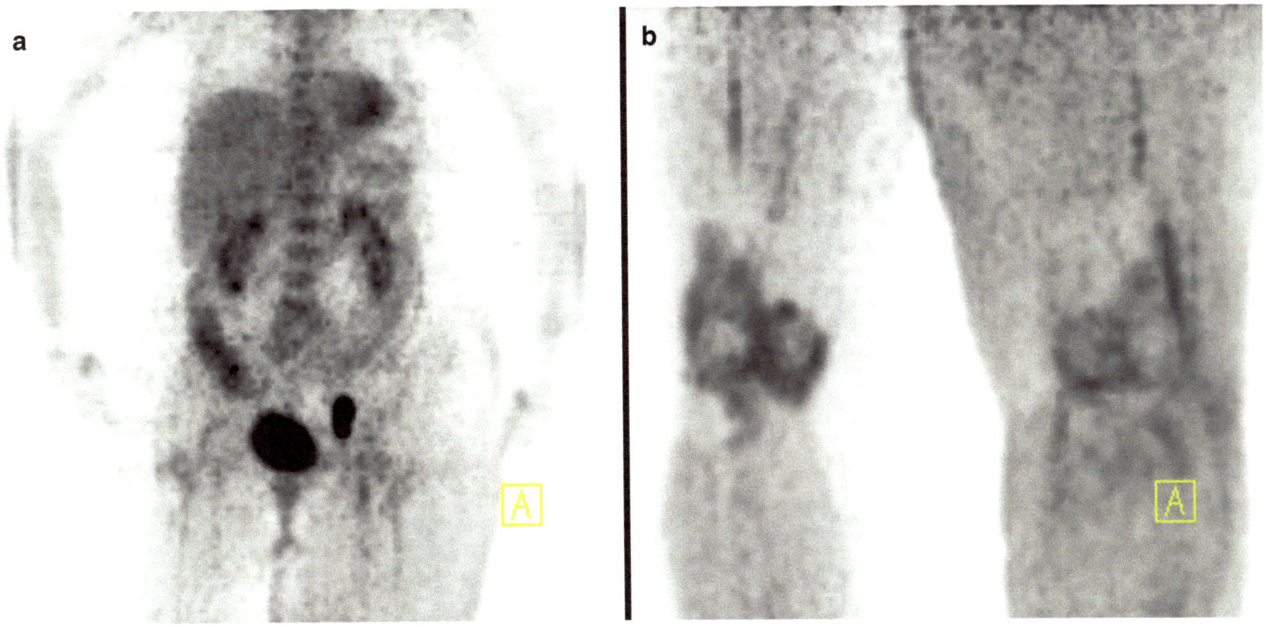

Fig. 14.6 MIP image (**a**) show hypermetabolic lymph node at left pelvic region, and swelling at left lower extremity (**b**)

14.4 Case 4: Ovarian Papillary Serous Adenocarcinoma

History A 78-year-old female patient had ovarian papillary serous adenocarcinoma (PSAC) and had undergone total abdominal hysterectomy and bilateral salpingoophorectomy 2 years ago. Histopathology revealed PSAC with psammoma bodies within papillary tumor cells. Her CA 125 cerum level was 110.9 units (normal 0–35 units) and a calcified lesion at 6th segment of liver suspicious for metastasis was detected on CT. The patient was referred to us for further evaluation with ^{18}F-FDG PET/CT.

Findings

Interpretation Hypermetabolic calcified lesions consistent with metastases of ovarian PSAC.

Teaching point PSAC accounts for approximately 40 % of all cancers of the ovary and are the most common malignant ovarian tumor. Extensive calcification of PSAC is due to high content of nearly spherical, concentrically laminated psammoma bodies.

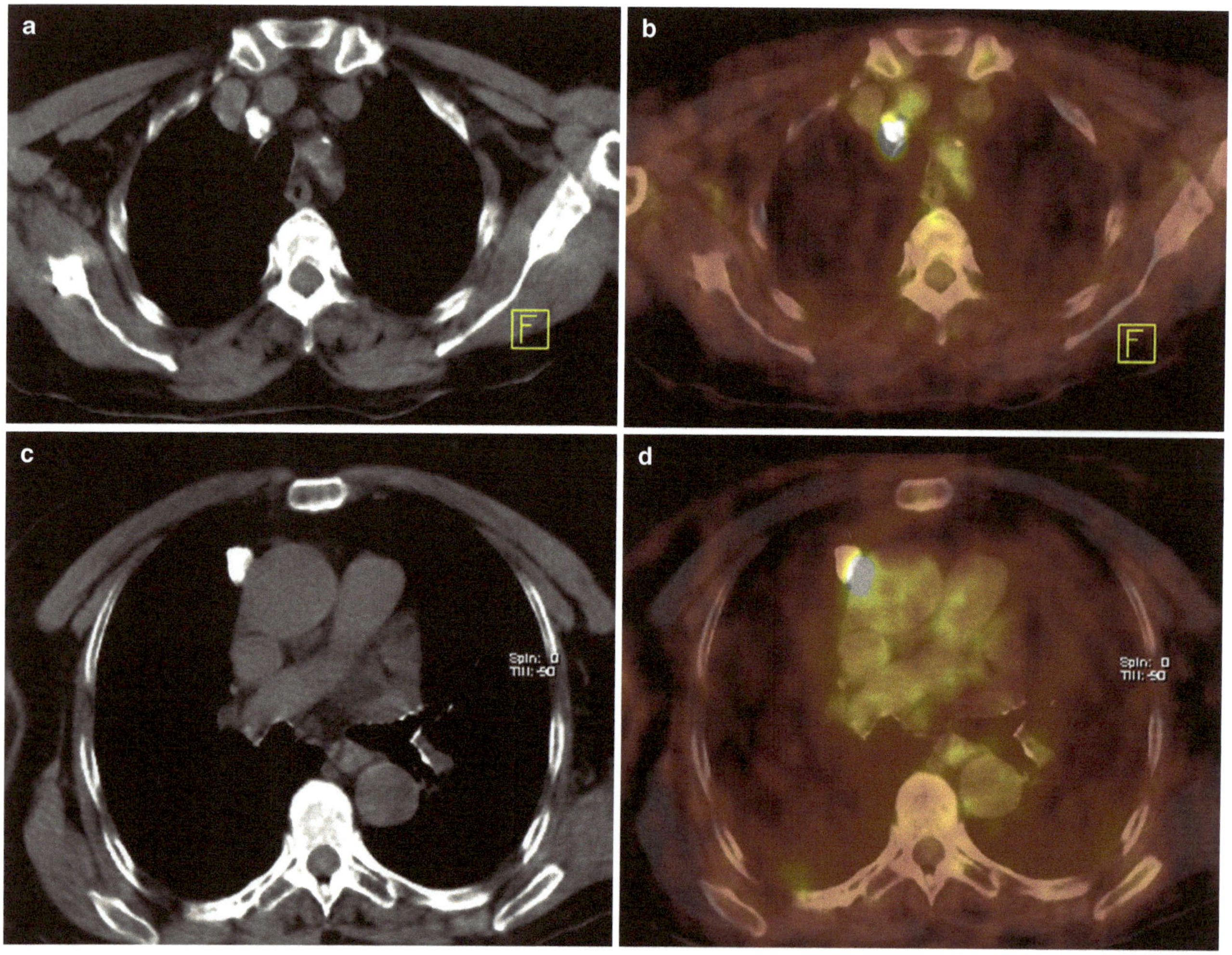

Fig. 14.7 Axial CT and fusion images show calcified lesion at right upper paratracheal and paracardiac regions that exhibit moderate FDG uptake

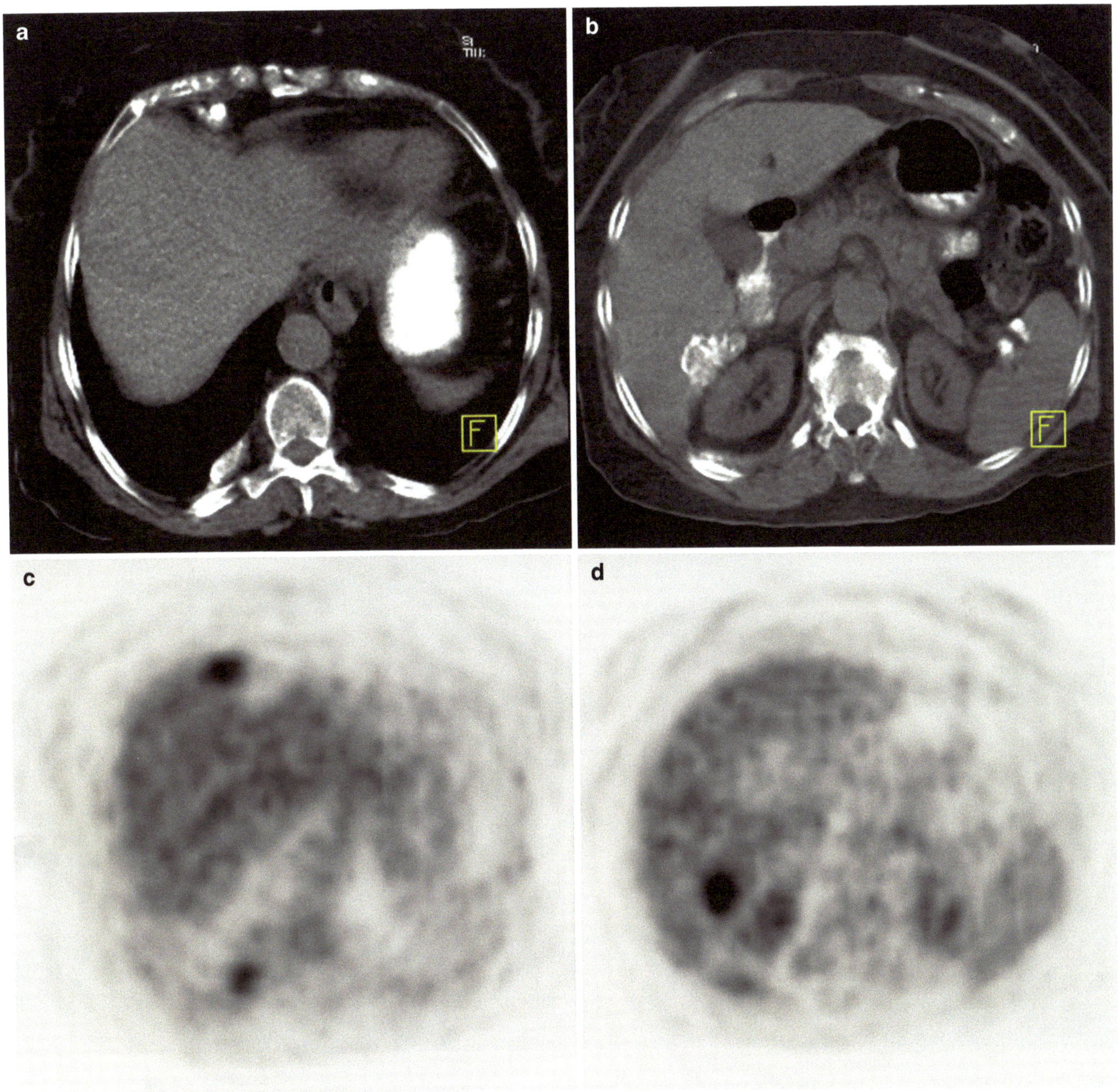

Fig. 14.8 Axial PET and CT images show hypermetabolic calcified lesions at right anterior diaphragmatic area and adjacent to right lobe of liver

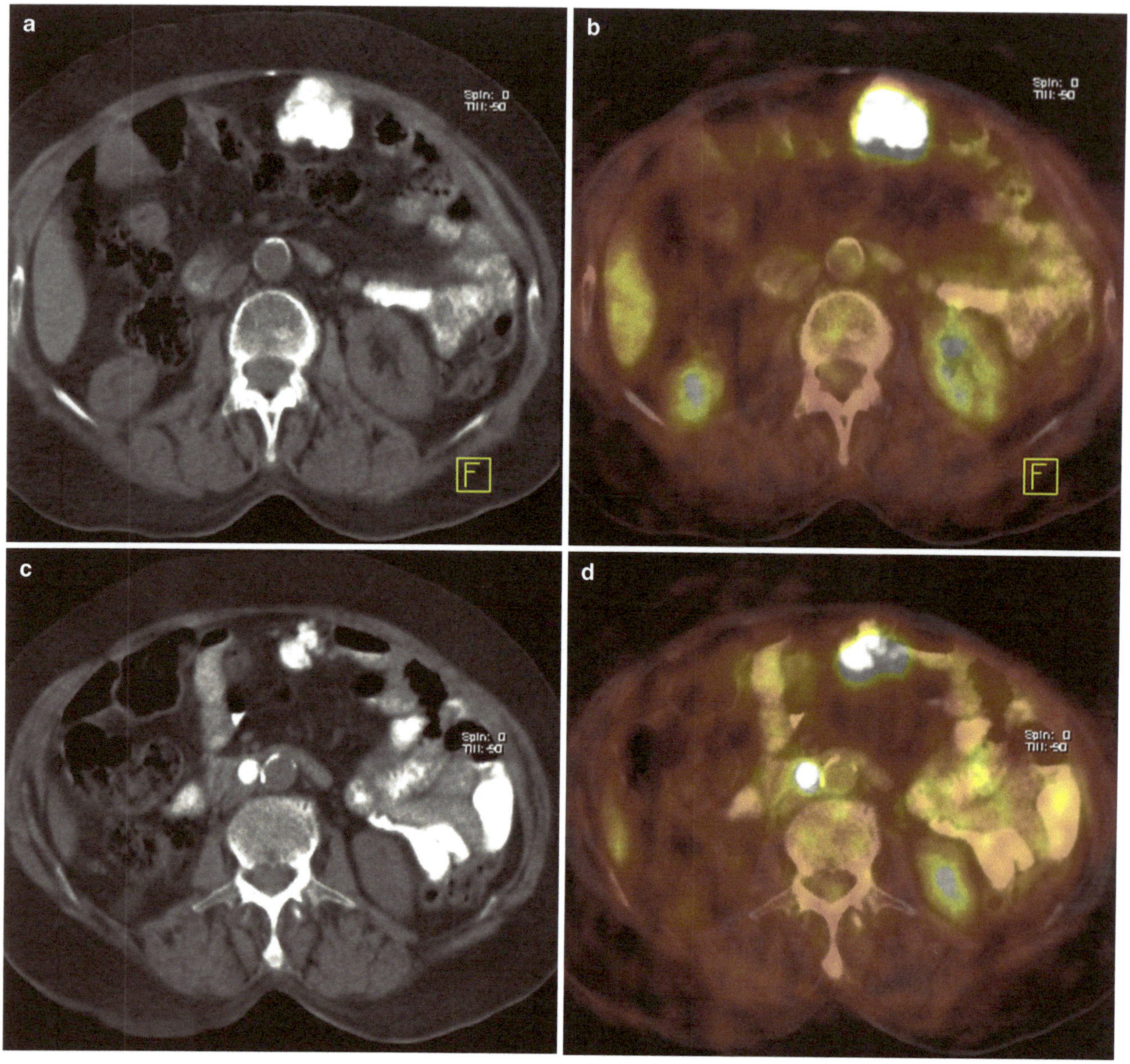

Fig. 14.9 Axial CT and fusion images show hypermetabolic calcified lesions at mesenteric fatty tissues

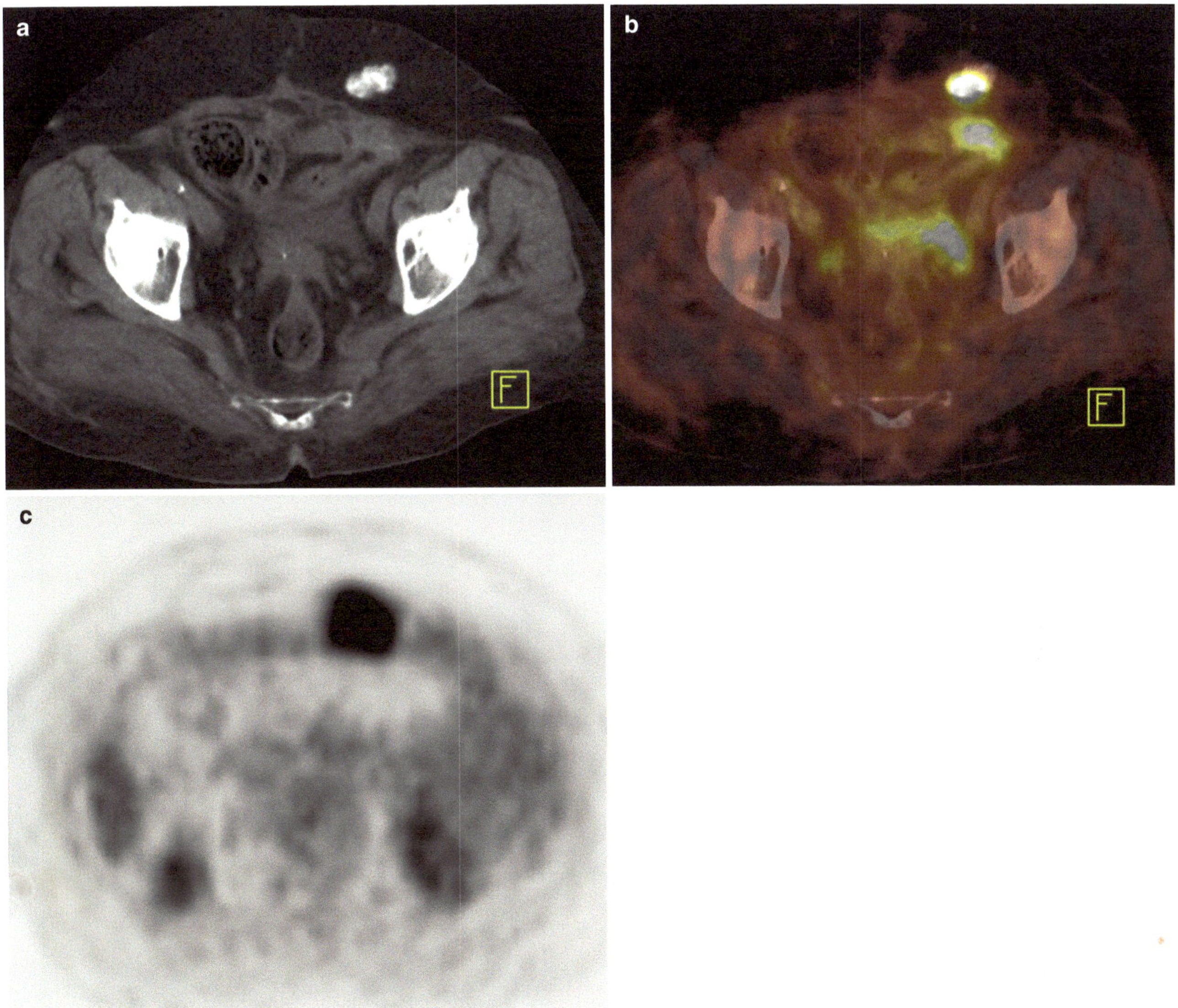

Fig. 14.10 Axial PET, CT, and fusion images show hypermetabolic calcified lesion at subcutaneous fatty tissues

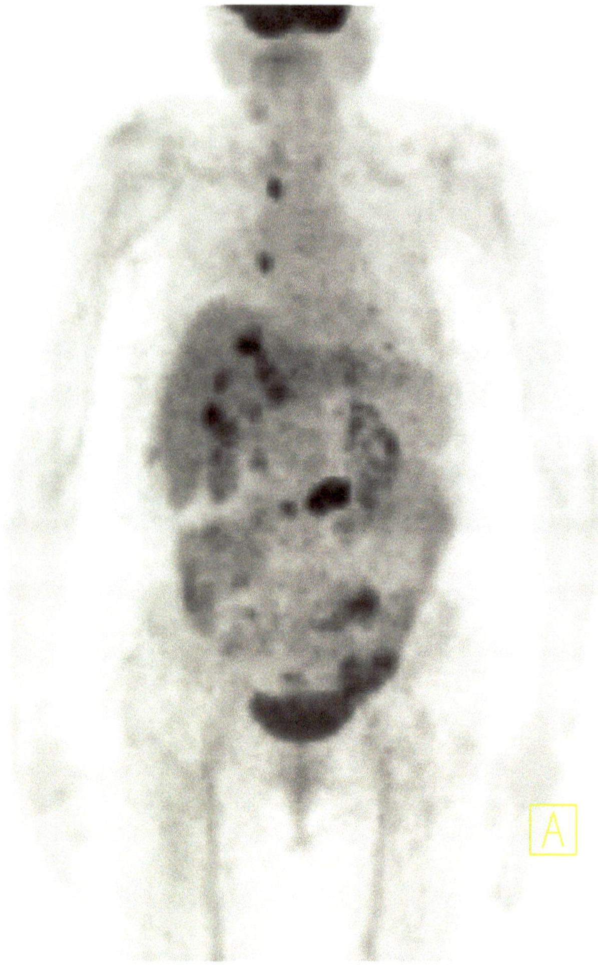

Fig. 14.11 MIP image

14.5 Case 5: Therapy Response Evaluation in Ovary Carcinoma

History A 68-year-old female status post hysterectomy and bilateral salpingoophorectomy for ovarian cancer underwent ^{18}F-FDG PET/CT and metastatic lesions were detected. Two months after chemotherapy a control PET/CT scan was performed.

Findings

Interpretation Local recurrence at left upper quadrant of abdomen and left obturator region gave complete response to chemotherapy. Decrease in the metabolic activity at hypermetabolic lymph node at right lower paratracheal region is suggestive of partial response to chemotherapy.

Teaching Point PET is advised for assessing suspected or diagnosed recurrence only when cytoreductive surgery is planned. Currently there are no strong evidence supporting the role of ^{18}F-FDG PET or PET/CT in therapy monitoring. Neoadjuvant chemotherapy followed by surgical debulking is effective in improving outcome. A higher rate of complete tumor resections was achieved in metabolic responders than in nonresponders. When a SUVmax cutoff of 3.8 is chosen for differentiating between responders and nonresponders after therapy, ^{18}F-FDG PET showed a sensitivity of 90 % and a specificity of 63.6 %.

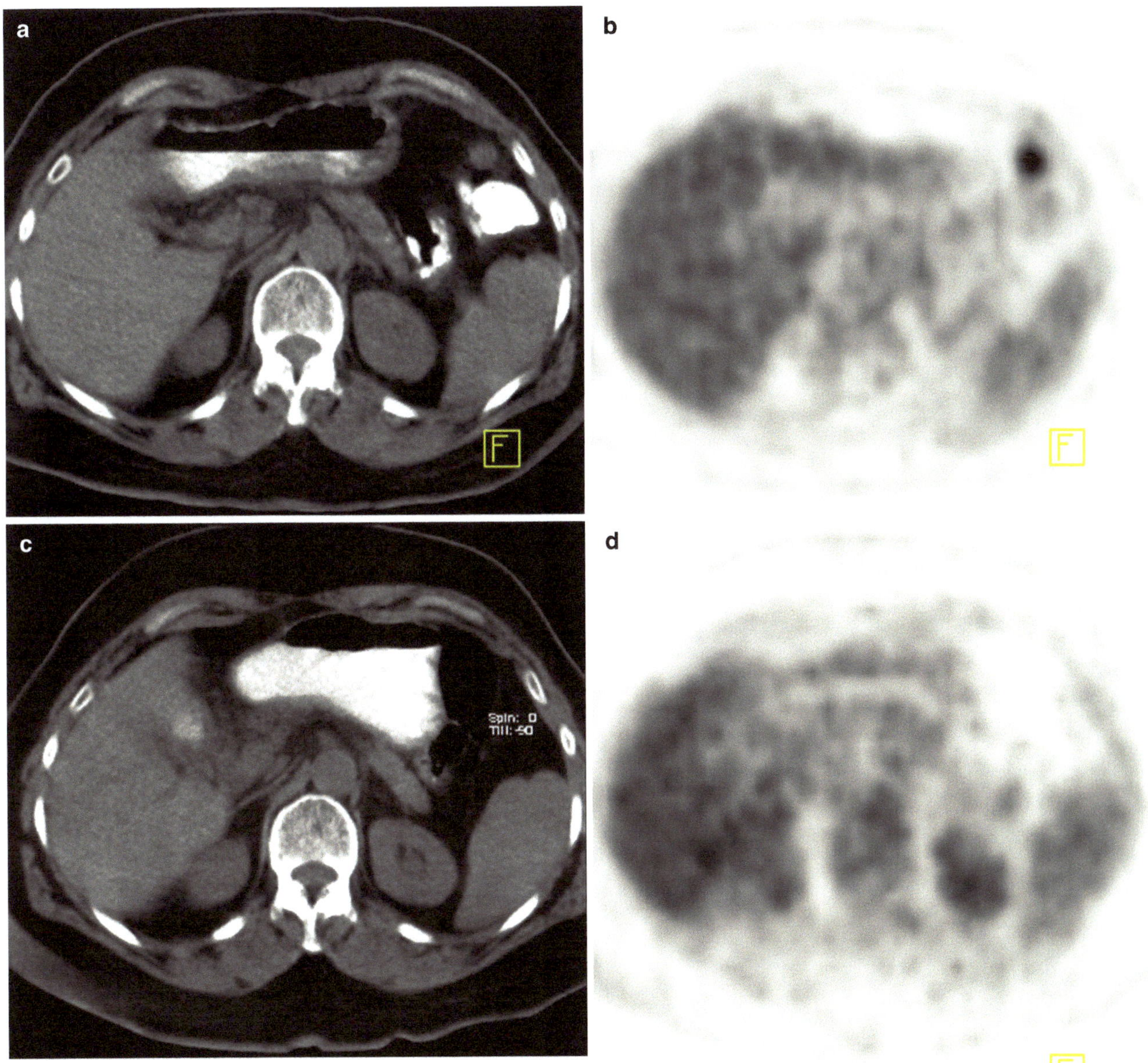

Fig. 14.12 Axial CT and PET images before (**a**, **b**) and after chemotherapy (**c**, **d**) showed focal intense FDG uptake at left upper quadrant of abdomen (SUVmax 8.6) and clearance of activity after chemotherapy

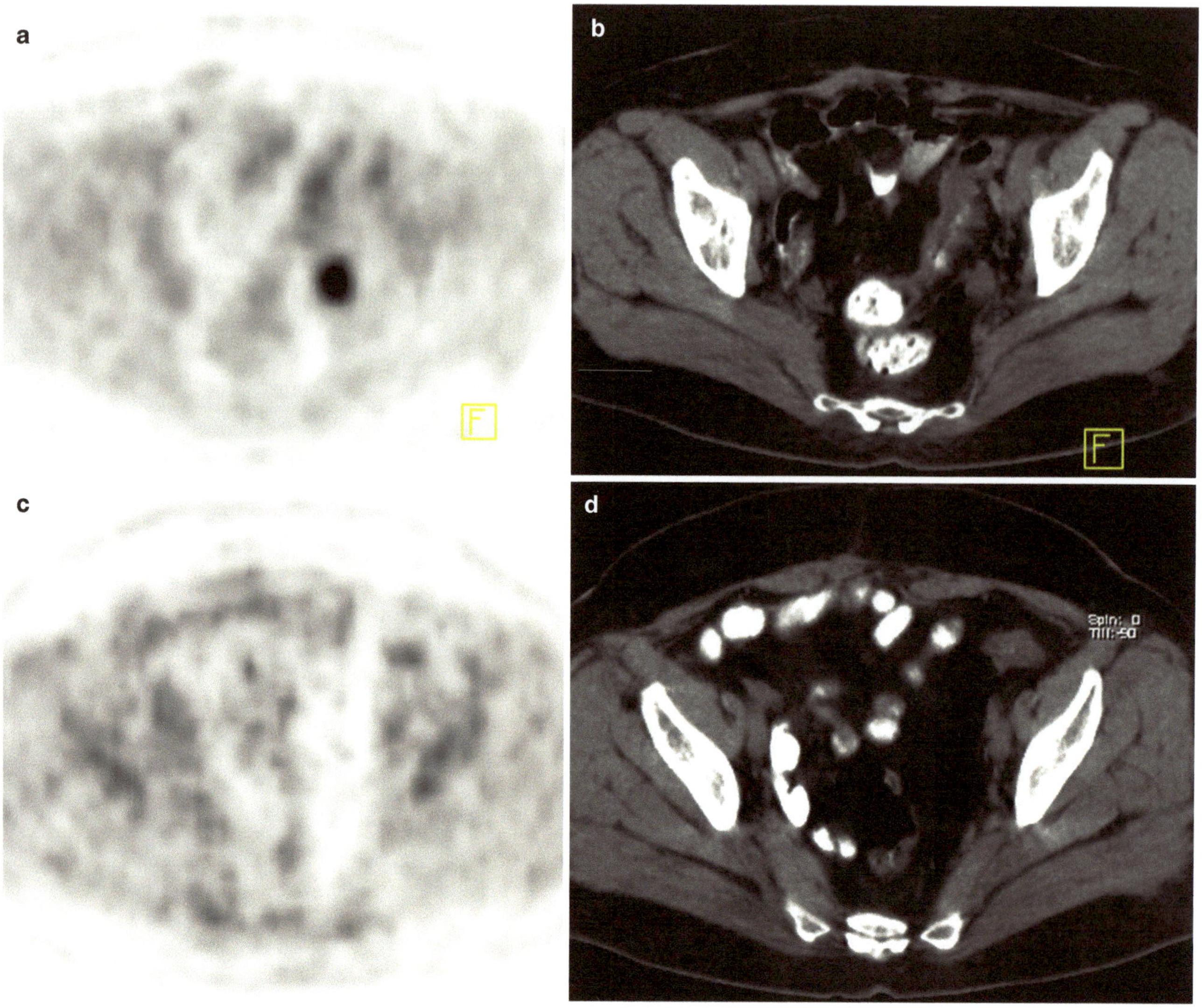

Fig. 14.13 Axial PET and CT images before (**a**, **b**) and after chemotherapy (**c**, **d**) show focal intense FDG uptake at left obturator region (SUVmax 7.5) and clearance of activity after chemotherapy

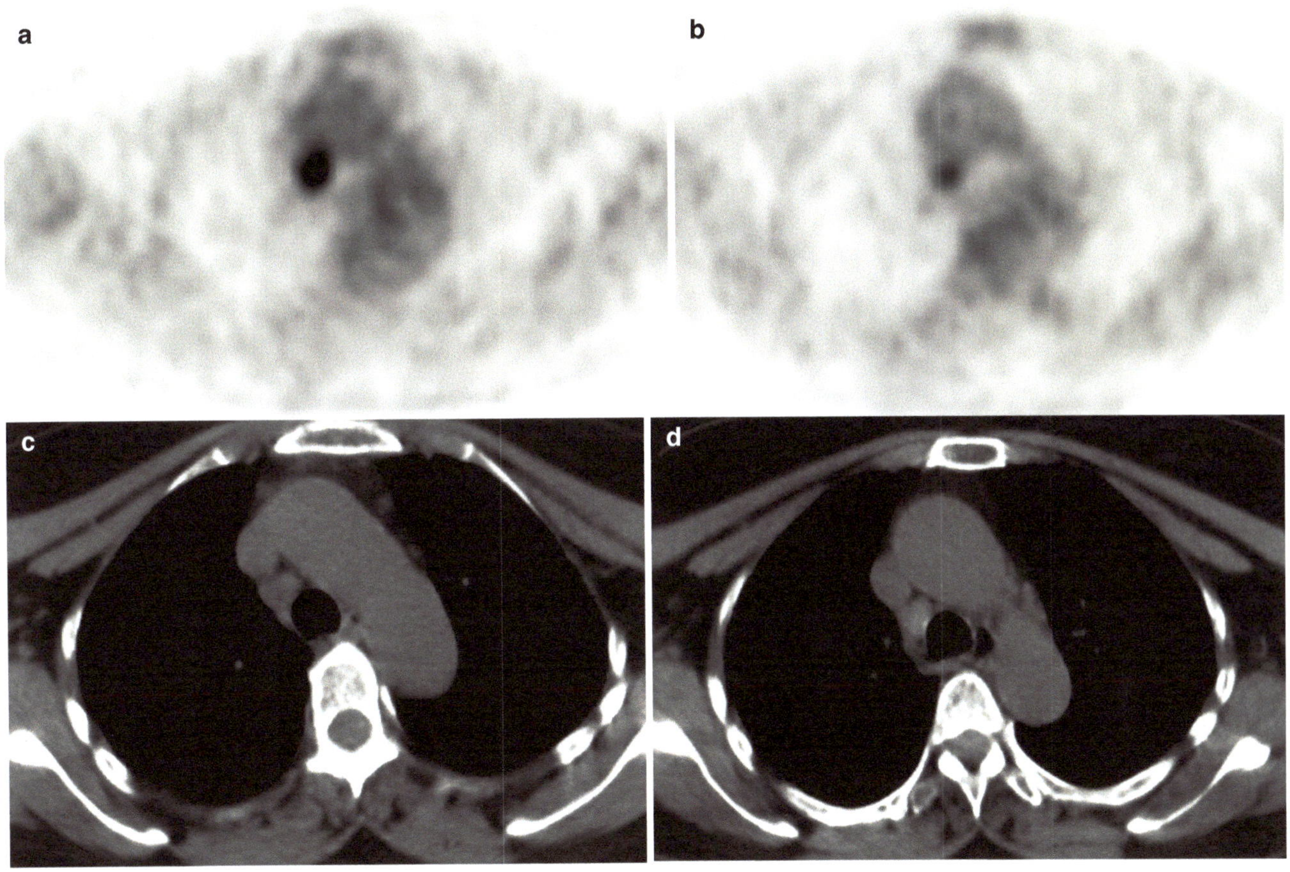

Fig. 14.14 Axial PET and CT images before (**a**, **b**) and after chemotherapy (**c**, **d**) show focal intense FDG uptake at right lower paratracheal region (SUVmax 7.8) and decrease in intensity of activity after chemotherapy (SUVmax 6)

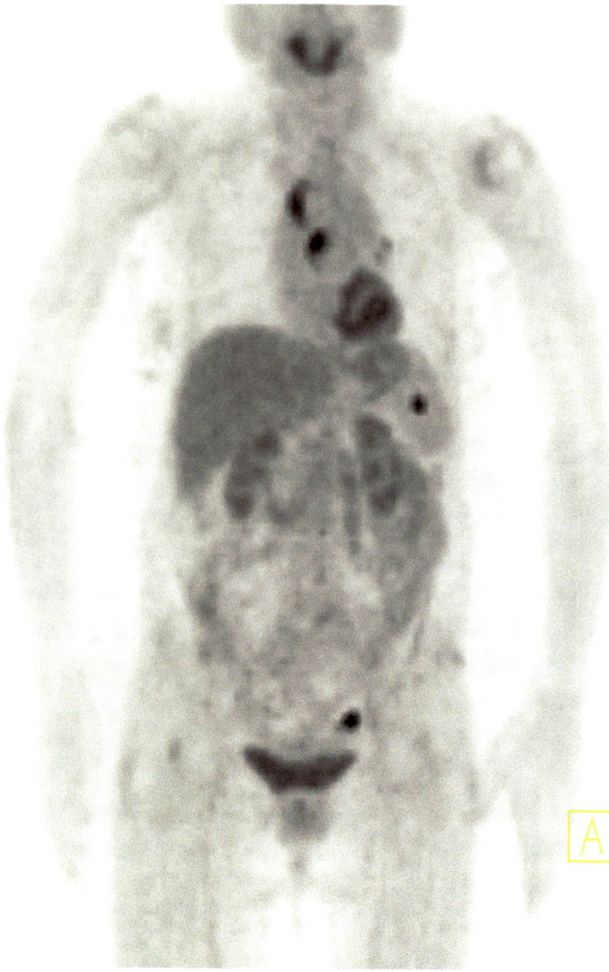

Fig. 14.15 MIP image before chemotherapy

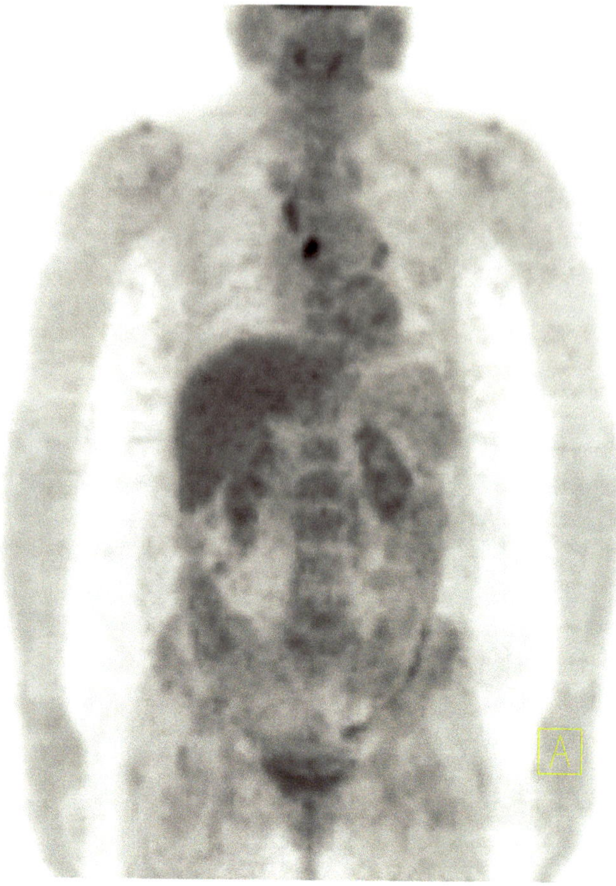

Fig. 14.16 MIP image after chemotherapy

14.6 Case 6: Peritonitis Carcinomatosa in Ovary Carcinoma

History A 68-year-old female was admitted to the hospital with the complaints of anorexia and progressive abdominal distension. The abdomen and pelvis CT revealed massive ascites and thickening of greater omentum and peritoneum. The findings were consistent with omental caking. Cytology of the fluid from paracentesis and biopsy from omentum showed metastatic ovarian carcinoma. Patient underwent ^{18}F-FDG PET/CT.

Findings

Interpretation Peritoneal carcinomatosis due to tumor infiltration of the omentum and metastatic invasion of the mediastinal lymph nodes.

Teaching Point The peritoneum is a preferred site of metastasis of several primary malignancies, principally carcinoma from colorectum in men and ovary in women, as well as stomach, pancreas, and adrenocortex. In one study sensitivity and specificity for the diagnosis of peritoneal carcinomatosis were 96.2 % and 90 %, respectively, for ^{18}F-FDG PET/CT and 88.5 % and 65 %, respectively, for enhanced abdominal CT. In another study multi detector computed tomography is reported as the technique of choice in the diagnosis of peritoneal seeding but ^{18}F-FDG PET/CT, also shows similar accuracy.

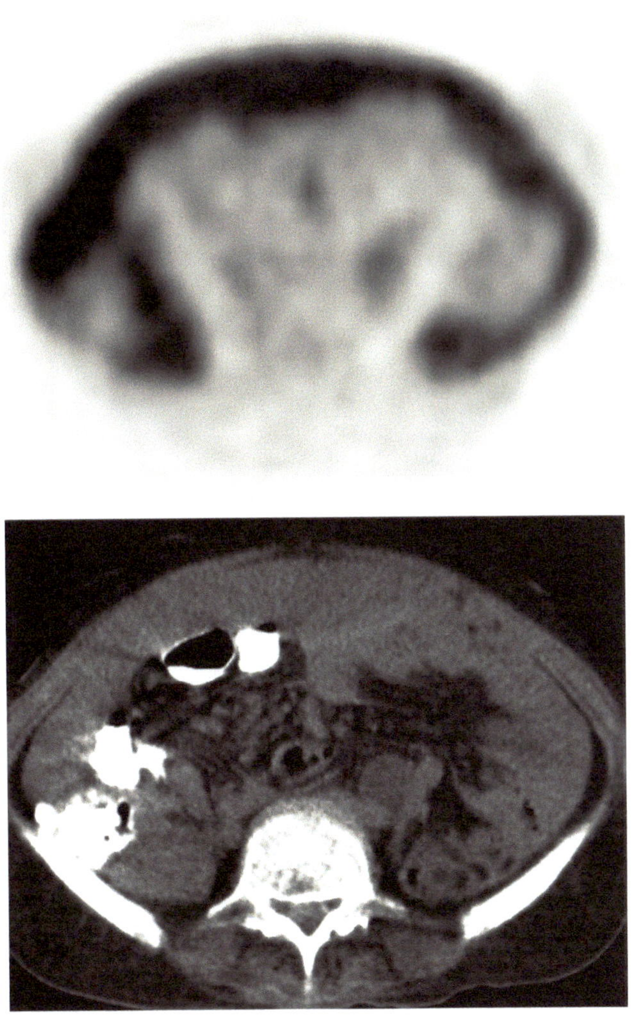

Fig. 14.17 Axial PET and CT images show intensely increased FDG uptake at peritoneum and gross thickening of the omentum (SUVmax 6.4)

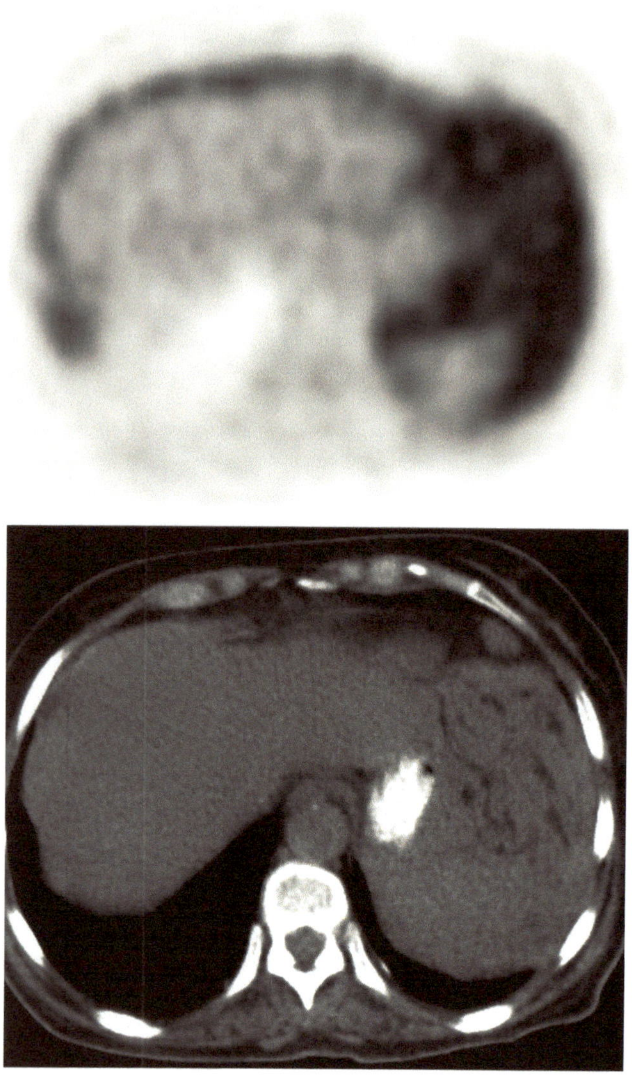

Fig. 14.18 Axial PET and CT images

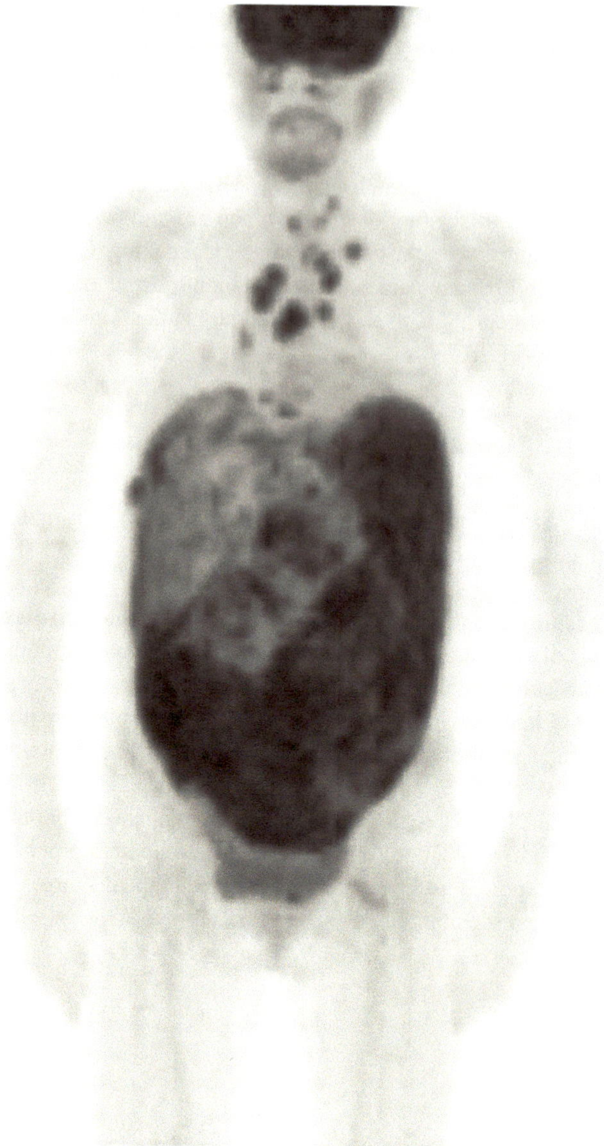

Fig. 14.19 MIP image demonstrates widespread accumulation of FDG in the peritoneum and omentum as well as mediastinal lymph nodes

14.7 Case 7: Peritonitis Carcinomatosa in Ovary Carcinoma

History A 64-year-old female who is being followed up with the diagnosis of ovarian carcinoma underwent ^{18}F-FDG PET/CT for the evaluation of her abdominal distension.

Findings

Interpretation Peritoneal carcinomatosis due to tumor infiltration of the omentum.

Teaching Point Although the metabolic activity at peritoneal surfaces and omentum is not as high as the patient in the previous case, when the metabolic activity at peritoneal and omental fat tissues is at the same level with liver FDG uptake, peritoneal carcinomatosis is the likely diagnosis.

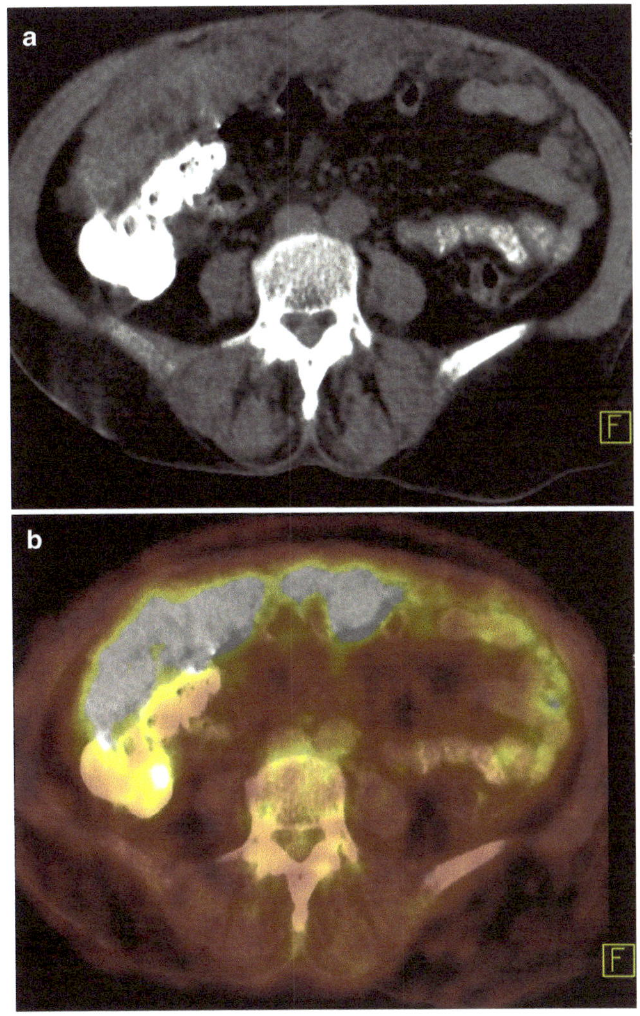

Fig. 14.20 Axial CT and fusion (**a**, **b**) images show increased FDG uptake at peritoneal surfaces and at nodular thickenings of the omentum

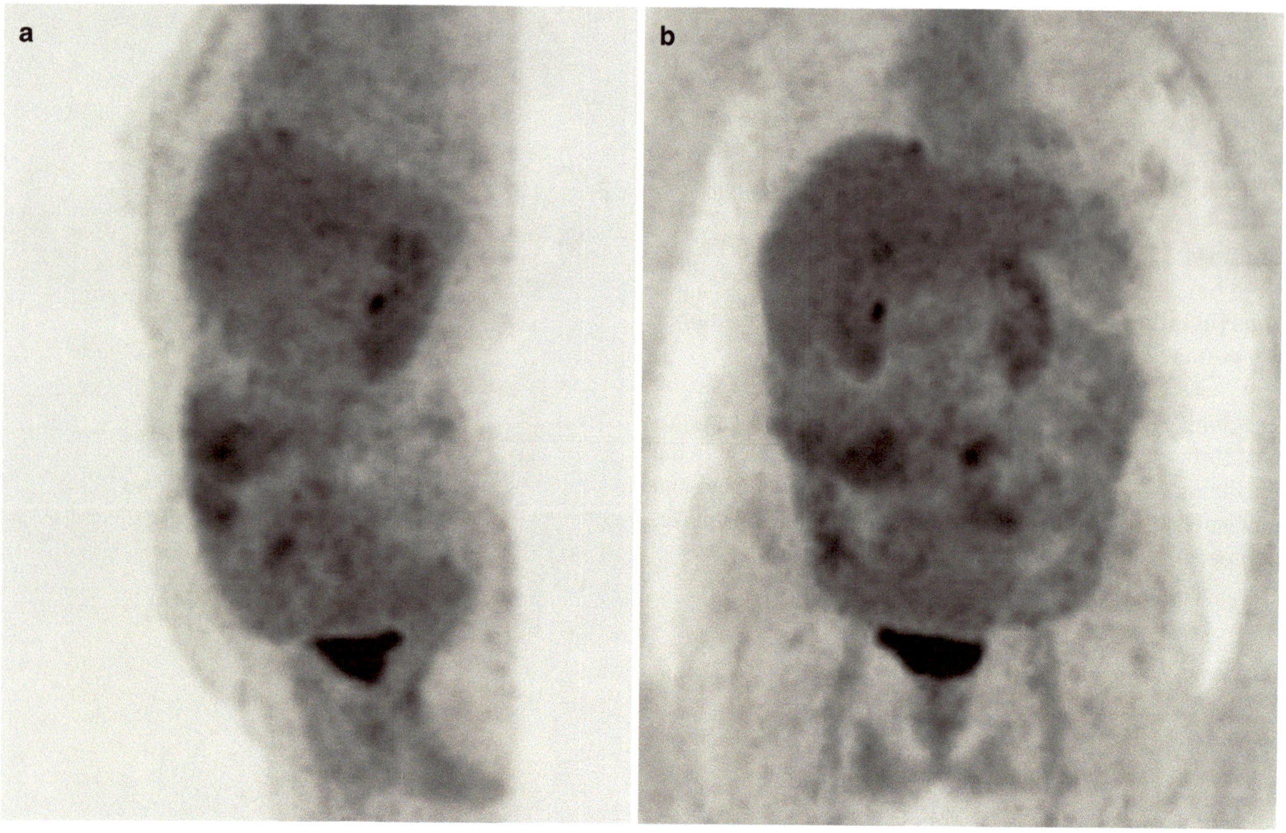

Fig. 14.21 Lateral (**a**) and anterior (**b**) MIP images demonstrate moderately increased diffuse FDG uptake at abdomen

14.8 Case 8: Restaging of Cervical Carcinoma

History A 65-year-old female who has a history of cervical cancer treated 25 years ago with radiotherapy is now being evaluated for recurrence with ^{18}F-FDG PET/CT

Findings

Interpretation Local recurrence at cervix and multiple metastatic hypermetabolic lesions

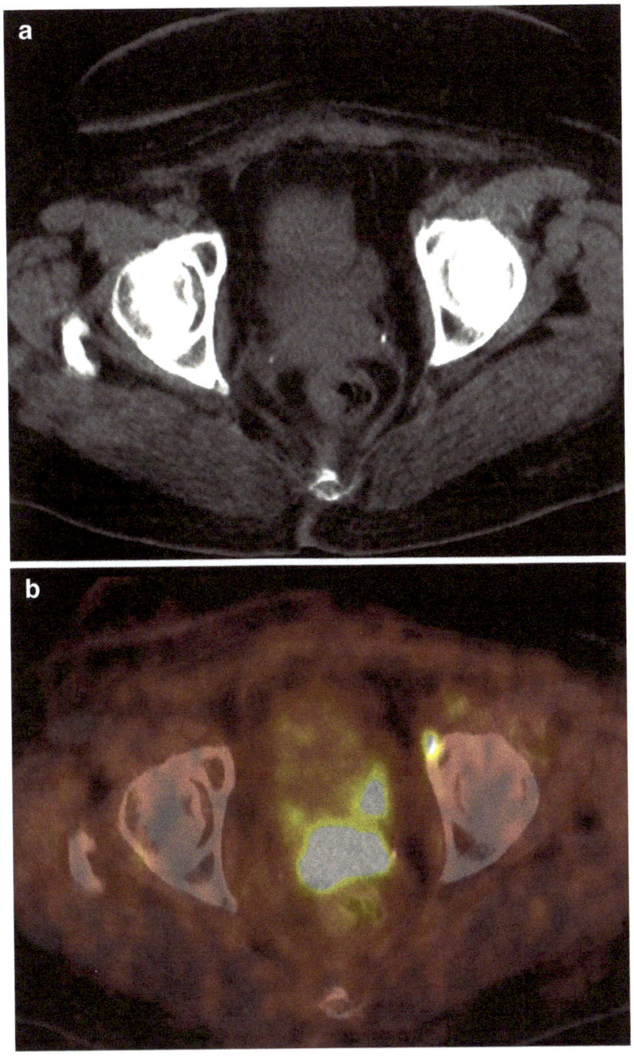

Fig. 14.22 Axial CT and fusion images (**a**, **b**) show intense FDG uptake at cervix (SUVmax 12) and a hypermetabolic lymph node at left external iliac region

Teaching Point One third of patients with locally advanced cervical cancer will have disease recurrence, usually within 2 years of completing treatment. The sensitivity and specificity of ^{18}F-FDG PET for detection of early recurrence were 90.3 % and 76.1 %, respectively.

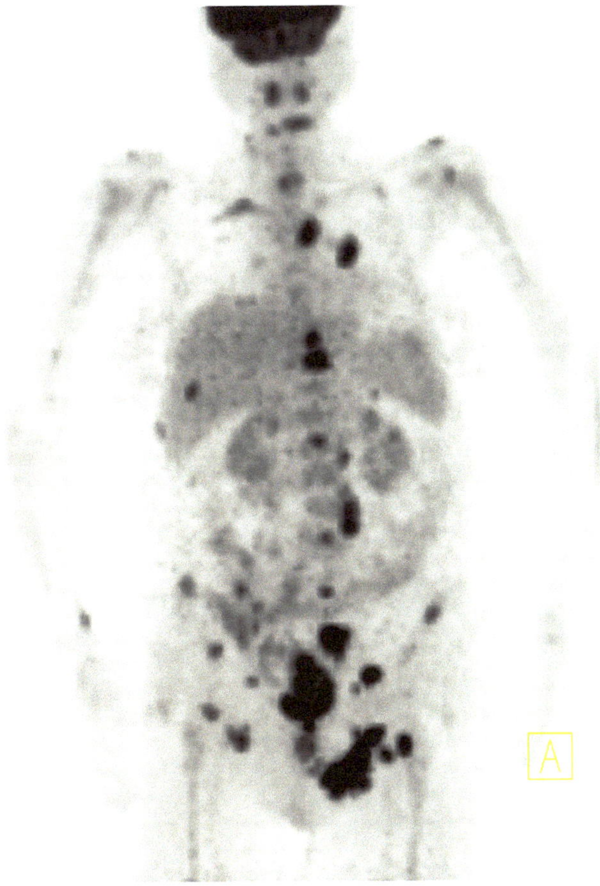

Fig. 14.23 MIP image shows multiple hypermetabolic foci involving vertebral colon, liver, pelvic, paraortic, and mediastinal lymph nodes

14.9 Case 9: Restaging of Cervical Carcinoma

History A 67-year-old female who has a history of cervical cancer treated 2 years ago with radiotherapy underwent ^{18}F-FDG PET/CT imaging with the purpose of restaging.

Findings

Interpretation Local recurrence at cervix with extension to uterus and metastatic hypermetabolic lesions at D8 vertebra and right femur head.

Teaching Point ^{18}F-FDG PET/CT is found to be more accurate than CT in lymph node staging. In early stage disease, ^{18}F-FDG PET/CT has a sensitivity of 53–73 %, and a specificity of 90–97 % for the detection of lymph node involvement. In advanced cervical cancer, the detection rate of ^{18}F-FDG PET/CT further increases. In one study, ^{18}F-FDG PET/CT reported to have a sensitivity of 75 % and a specificity of 92 % in locally advanced cervical cancer.

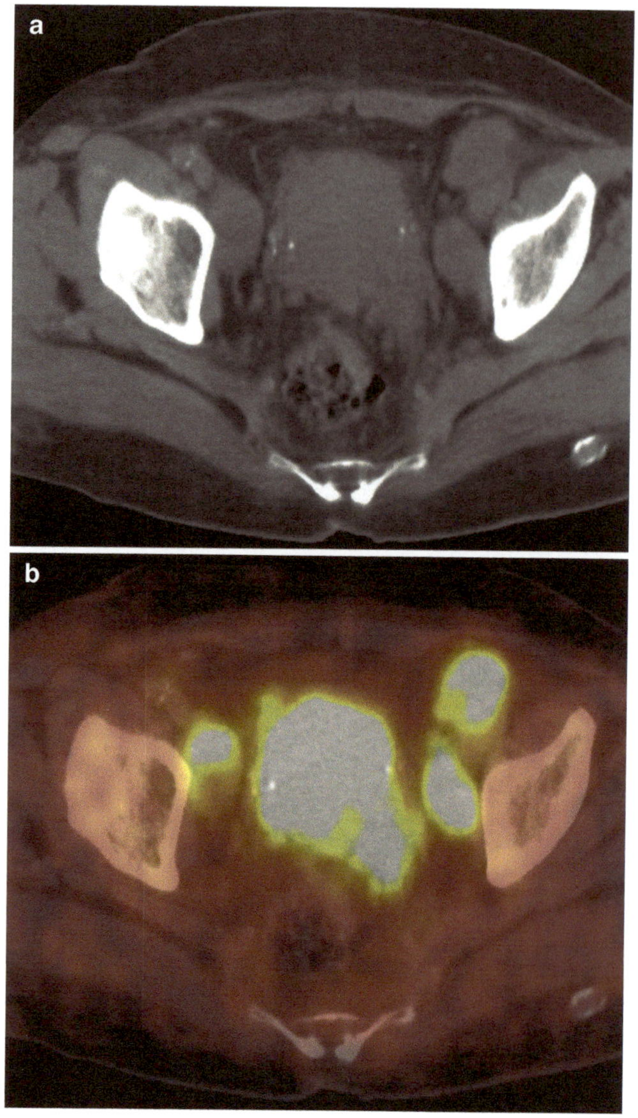

Fig. 14.24 Axial CT and fusion images showed intense FDG uptake at cervix (SUVmax 12) and there is extension of tumor into the endometrial cavity. Lymph nodes showing hypermetabolism are detected at bilateral external iliac lymph node stations (**a**, **b**)

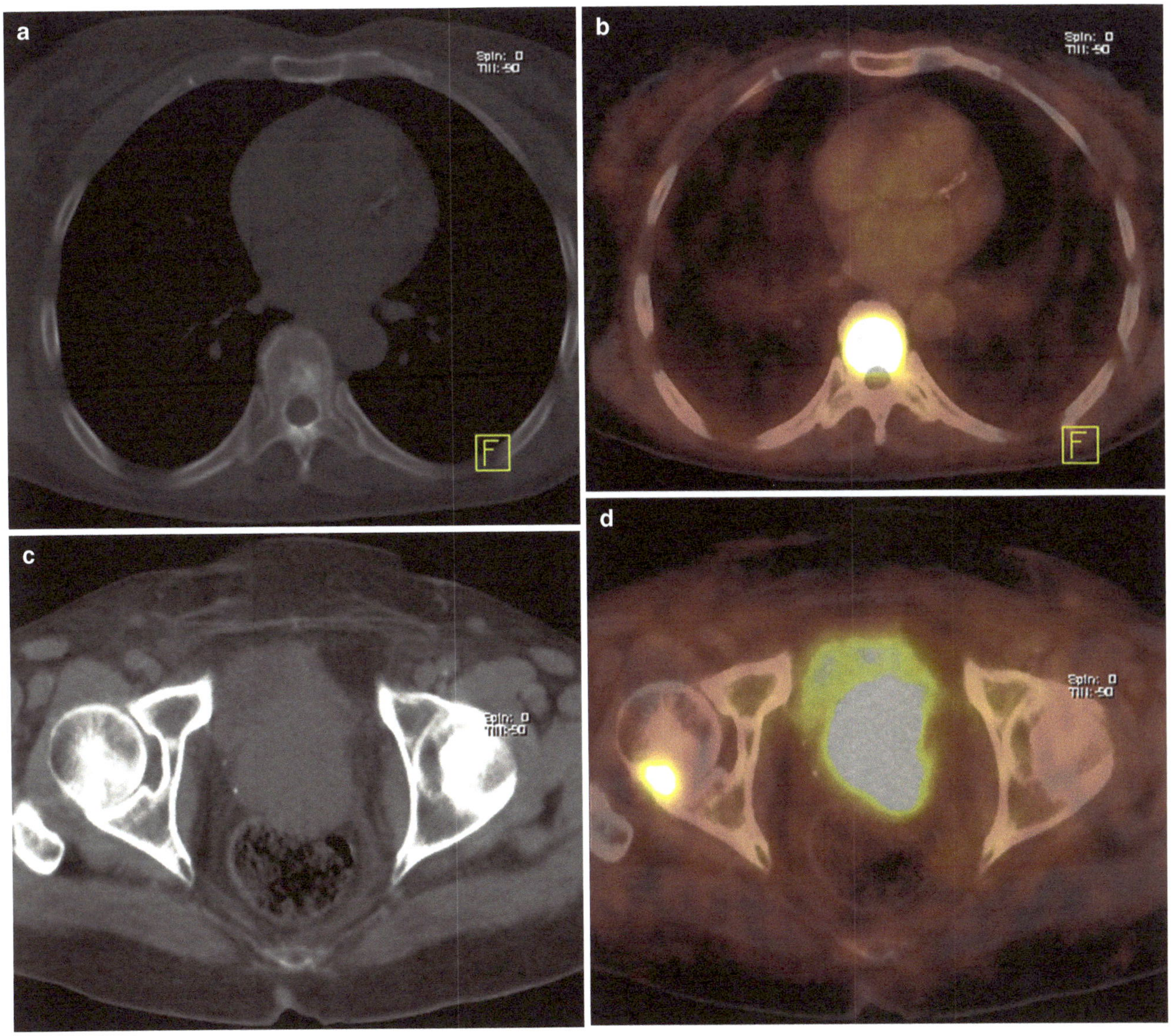

Fig. 14.25 Axial CT and fusion images showing increased FDG uptake at D8 vertebra (**a**, **b**), and right femur head and uterus (**c**, **d**)

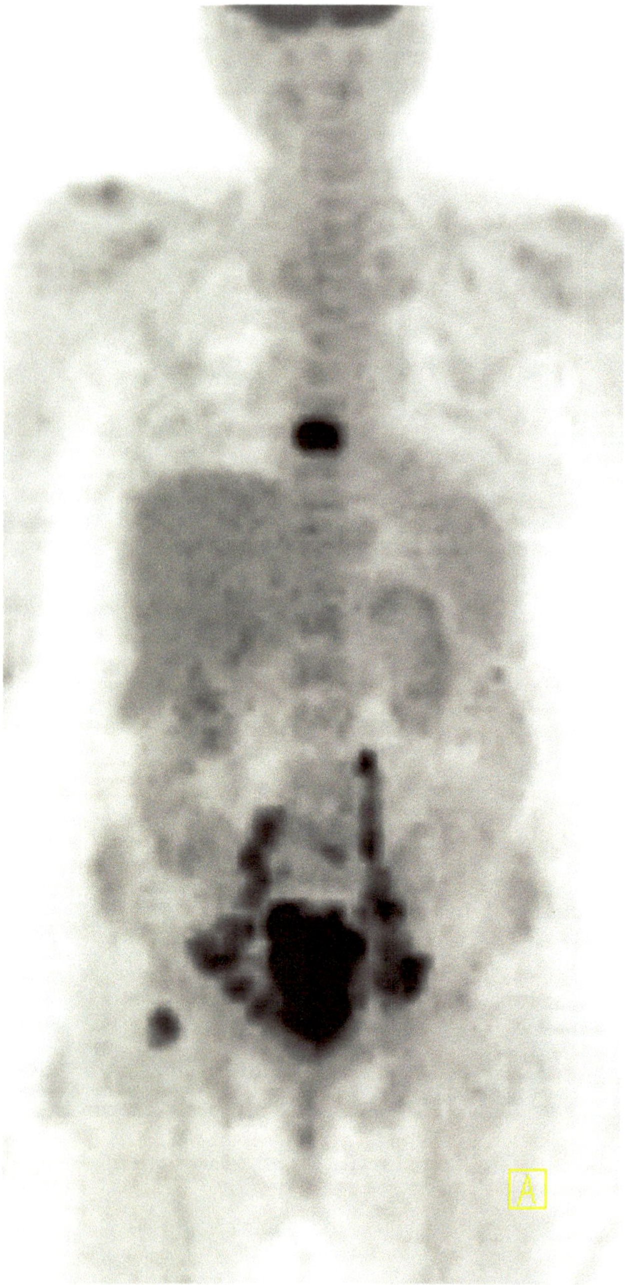

Fig. 14.26 MIP image

Bibliography

1. Avril N, Sassen S, Schmalfeldt B, Naehrig J, Rutke S, Weber WA, et al. Prediction of response to neoadjuvant chemotherapy by sequential F-18-fluorodeoxyglucose positron emission tomography in patients with advanced-stage ovarian cancer. J Clin Oncol. 2005;23:7445–53.
2. Bhoil A, Kashyap R, Bhattacharya A, Mittal BR. F-18 fluorodeoxyglucose positron emission tomography/computed tomography in a rare case of recurrent malignant mixed mullerian tumor. World J Nucl Med. 2014;13:64–6. doi:10.4103/1450-1147.138578.
3. Brennan MJ. Lymphedema following the surgical treatment of breast cancer: a review of pathophysiology and treatment. J Pain Symptom Manage. 1992;7:110–6.
4. Chou HH, Chang TC, Yen TC, Ng KK, Hsueh S, Ma SY, et al. Low value of [18F]-fluoro-2-deoxy-D-glucose positron emission tomography in primary staging of early-stage cervical cancer before radical hysterectomy. J Clin Oncol. 2006;24:123–8.
5. Funicelli L, Travaini LL, Landoni F, Trifirò G, Bonello L, Bellomi M. Peritoneal arcinomatosis from ovarian cancer: the role of CT and [^{18}F]FDG-PET/CT. Abdom Imaging. 2010;35:701–7. doi:10.1007/s00261-009-9578-8.
6. Herrera FG, Prior JO. The role of PET/CT in cervical cancer. Front Oncol. 2013;3:34. doi:10.3389/fonc.2013.00034.
7. Kanthan R, Senger JL. Uterine carcinosarcomas (malignant mixed müllerian tumours): a review with special emphasis on the controversies in management. Obstet Gynecol Int. 2011;2011:470795 doi:10.1155/2011/470795
8. Kidd EA, Siegel BA, Dehdashti F, Rader JS, Mutch DG, Powell MA, et al. Lymph node staging by positronemission tomography in cervical cancer: relationship to prognosis. J Clin Oncol. 2010;28:2108–13.
9. Kim HW, Won KS, Zeon SK, Ahn BC, Gayed IW. Peritoneal carcinomatosis in patients with ovarian cancer: enhanced CT versus 18F-FDG PET/CT. Clin Nucl Med. 2013;38:93–7. doi:10.1097/RLU.0b013e31826390ec.
10. Mortimer PS. The pathophysiology of lymphedema. Cancer. 1998;83:2798–802.
11. Nishiyama Y, Yamamoto Y, Kanenishi K, Ohno M, Hata T, Kushida Y, et al. Monitoring the neoadjuvant therapy response in gynecological cancer patients using FDG PET. Eur J Nucl Med Mol Imaging. 2008;35:287–95.
12. Ozulker T, Ozulker F, Ozpacaci T. 99mTc-MDP and 18F-FDG uptake in calcified metastatic lesions from ovarian papillary serous adenocarcinoma. Hell J Nucl Med. 2009;12:287–8.
13. Park JY, Kim EN, Kim DY, Suh DS, Kim JH, Kim YM, et al. Role of PET or PET/CT in the post-therapy surveillance of uterine sarcoma. Gynecol Oncol. 2008;109:255–62.
14. Reinhardt MJ, Ehritt-Braun C, Vogelgesang D, Ihling C, Högerle S, Mix M, et al. Metastatic lymph nodes in patients with cervical cancer:detection with MR imaging and FDG PET. Radiology. 2001;218:776–82.
15. Roh JW, Seo SS, Lee S, Kang KW, Kim SK, Sim JS, et al. Role of positron emission tomography in pretreatment lymph node staging of uterine cervical cancer: a prospective surgicopathologic correlation study. Eur J Cancer. 2005;41:2086–92.
16. Rong-Hsin Yang, Yum-Kung Chu. 18F-FDG PET/CT findings of omental cake: a case report. Ann Nucl Med Sci. 2010;23:93–7.
17. Rose PG, Adler LP, Rodriguez M, Faulhaber PF, Abdul-Karim FW, Miraldi F. Positron emission tomography for evaluating paraaortic nodal metastasis in locally advanced cervical cancer before surgical staging: a surgicopathologic study. J Clin Oncol. 1999;17:41–5.
18. Ryu SY, Kim MH, Choi SC, Choi CW, Lee KH. Detection of early recurrence with 18F-FDG PET in patients with cervical cancer. J Nucl Med. 2003;44:347–52.
19. Schwarz JK, Grigsby PW, Dehdashti F, Delbeke D. The role of 18F-FDG PET in assessing therapy response in cancer of the cervix and ovaries. J Nucl Med. 2009;50 Suppl 1:64–73. doi:10.2967/jnumed.108.057257.
20. Sironi S, Buda A, Picchio M, Perego P, Moreni R, Pellegrino A, et al. Lymph node metastasis in patients with clinical early-stage cervical cancer: detection with integrated FDG PET/CT. Radiology. 2006;238:272–9.
21. Tada H, Teramukai S, Fukushima M, Sasaki H. Risk factors for lower limb lymphedema after lymph node dissection in patients with ovarian and uterine carcinoma. BMC Cancer. 2009;9:47. doi:10.1186/1471-2407-9-47.
22. Wright JD, Dehdashti F, Herzog TJ, Mutch DG, Huettner PC, Rader JS, et al. Preoperative lymph node staging of early stage cervical carcinoma by [18F]-fluoro-2-deoxy-D-glucose-positron emission tomography. Cancer. 2005;104:2484–91.

Urologic Tumors

15

15.1 Case 1: Diagnosis of Renal Cell Carcinoma

History A 51-year-old female is currently being evaluated for an incidentally detected right kidney mass. Patient underwent ^{18}F-FDG PET/CT imaging before undergoing an operation.

Findings

Interpretation Low level of FDG uptake at the lesion was suggestive of a benign lesion.

Result Histopathological evaluation after operation revealed renal cell carcinoma (RCC).

Teaching Point PET should have limited role in the characterization of primary renal tumors with its low sensitivity found as 62 % in a metaanalysis.

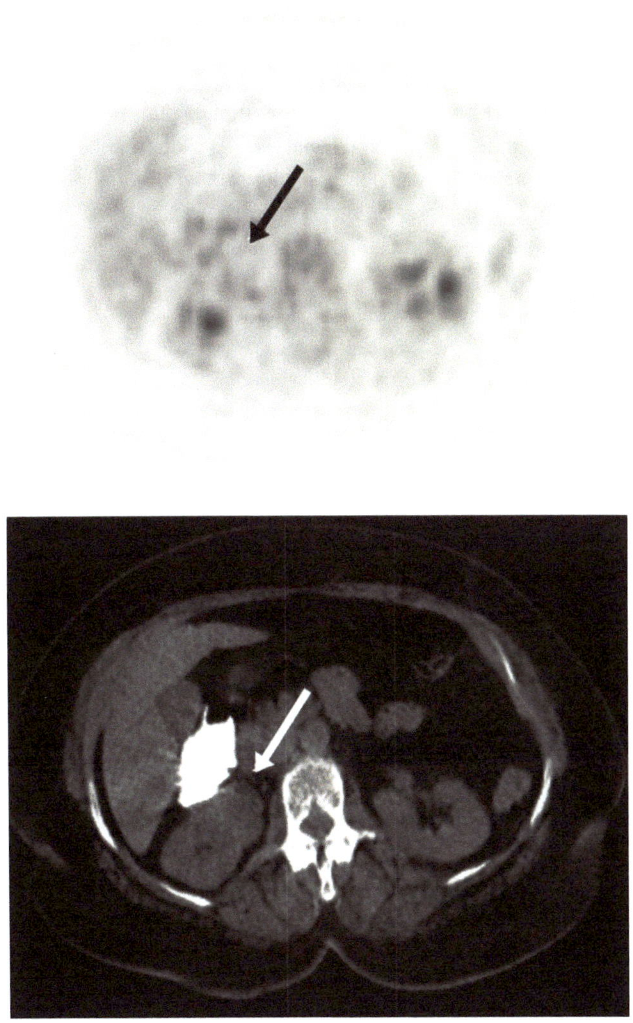

Fig. 15.1 Axial PET and CT images showed an anteromedially located cortical mass lesion with 2 cm diameter at right kidney (*arrow*). The lesion showed mild FDG uptake with a SUVmax of 2, which is not higher than renal parenchyma

T. Özülker, F. Özülker, *Atlas of PET-CT Imaging in Oncology: A Case-Based Guide to Image Interpretation*,
DOI 10.1007/978-3-319-18994-9_15

15.2 Case 2: False Positive Finding: Oncocytoma

History A 59-year-old female is currently being evaluated for a mass lesion at left kidney detected on USG. The patient was scheduled for operation and meanwhile she underwent ^{18}F-FDG PET/CT imaging.

Findings

Interpretation The lesion was suspicious for malignancy with its moderate FDG uptake.

Result After operation the lesion turned out to be an oncocytoma.

Teaching Point The pooled specificity of ^{18}F-FDG PET/CT is found to be 88 % in the determination of malignant nature of kidney masses in a metaanalysis. Besides oncocytoma, there are several other benign lesions causing false positive FDG uptake like renal angiomyolipoma, renal pericytoma, nephroblastoma, renal tuberculosis, and xanthogranulomatous nephritis.

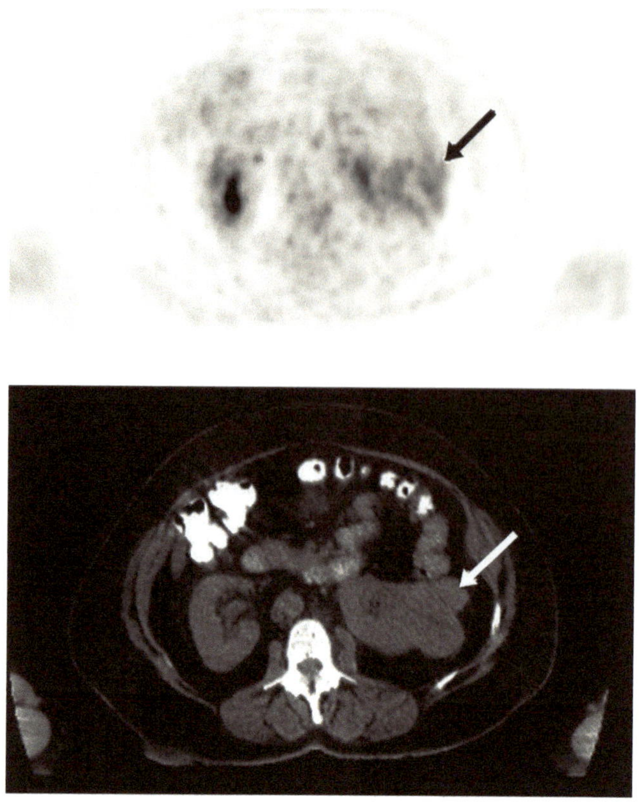

Fig. 15.2 Axial PET and CT images showed a lobulated mass lesion with 6.5 cm diameter, located at lateral cortex of left kidney (*arrow*). The lesion showed moderate FDG uptake with a SUVmax of 6.5

15.3 Case 3: Renal Cell Carcinoma Invading the Renal Vein

History A 52-year-old female with a mass lesion originating from left kidney underwent ^{18}F-FDG PET/CT imaging.

Findings

Interpretation Malignant lesion originating from left kidney and showing invasion to left renal vein.

Result The patient underwent operation and histopathology revealed RCC invading left renal vein.

Teaching Point ^{18}F-FDG PET/CT localizes RCC more efficiently in larger masses. One study showed an increase in sensitivity of FDG PET/CT from 76 to 92.9 % when the lesion size increased from more than 1–2 cm. RCC has a propensity to invade the venous system, with extension into the renal vein.

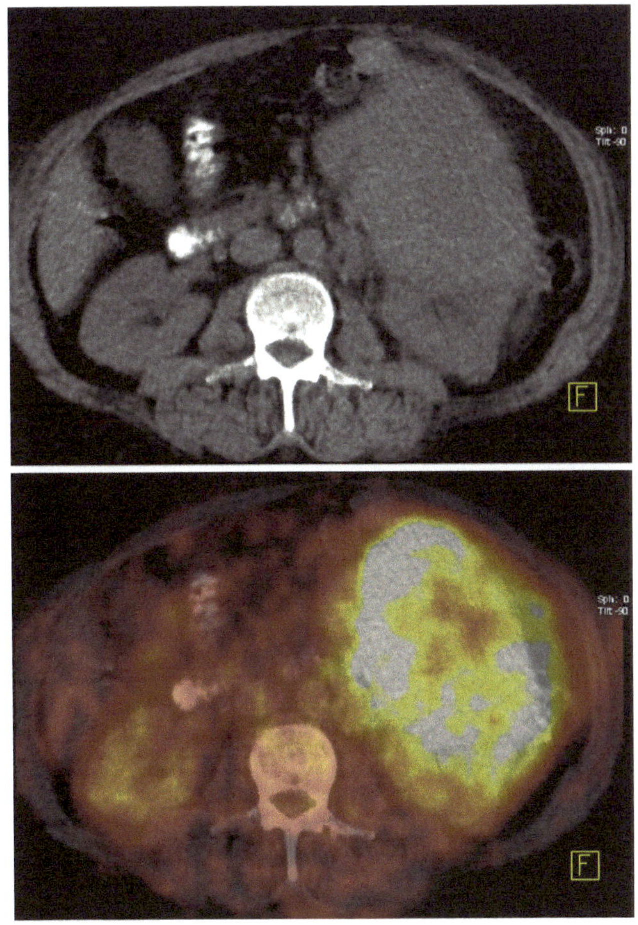

Fig. 15.3 Axial CT and fusion images showed a mass lesion with the dimensions of 11 × 12 × 14 cm originating from anterior cortex of left kidney (SUVmax 13.7)

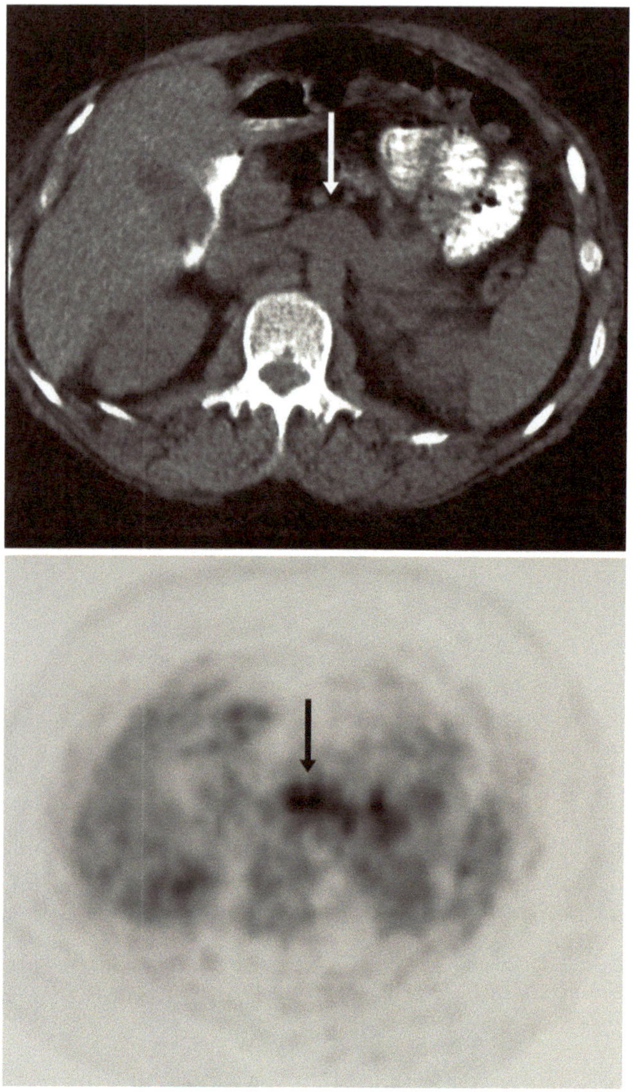

Fig. 15.4 Axial CT and PET images showing pathologically increased FDG uptake at left renal vein (*arrow*)

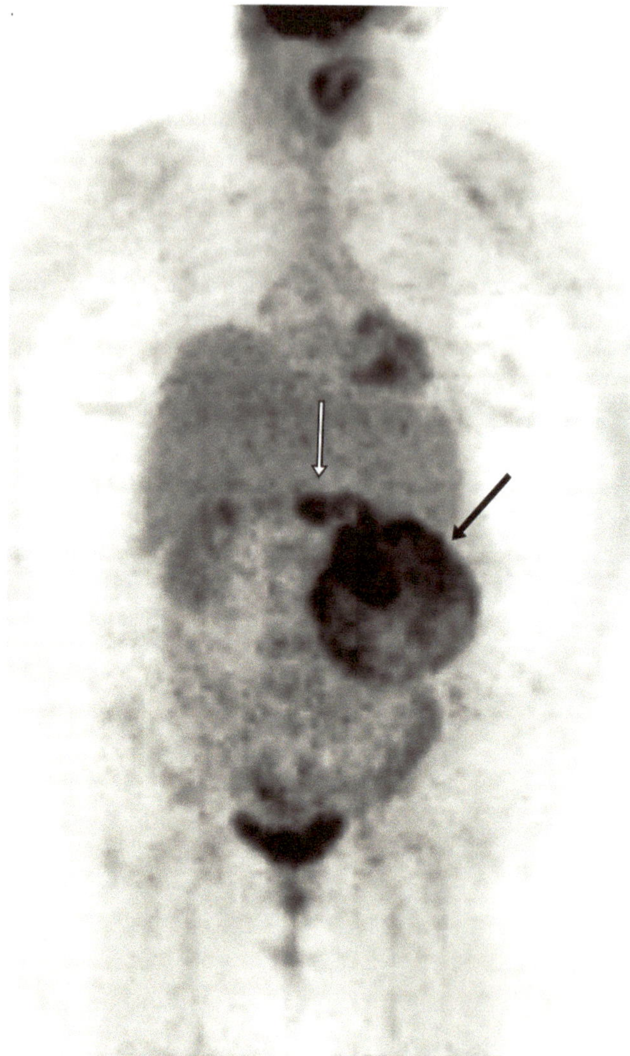

Fig. 15.5 MIP image showing intensely hypermetabolic left renal mass (*black arrow*), pathologically increased FDG uptake at left renal vein (*white arrow*)

15.4 Case 4: Renal Cell Carcinoma Invading the Inferior Vena Cava and Right Atrium

History A 52-year-old female suffering from weakness, weight loss, right-sided flank pain, and hematuria for 2 months. When she consulted with these symptoms, tenderness in the right flank region and hepatomegaly was detected on physical examination. The patient underwent CT scan with iv contrast, and besides the mass lesion at right kidney, a filling defect in IVC extending to the right atrium, which was strongly suggestive of tumor thrombus was detected. ^{18}F-FDG-PET/CT scan was performed in order to make metabolic characterization of the right renal mass together with the thrombus in IVC.

Findings

Interpretation FDG avid malignant lesion originating from right kidney and intensely hypermetabolic tumor thrombus in IVC extending into right atrium.

Result The patient underwent right nephrectomy and biopsy was obtained from tumor thrombus in the IVC. The histopathology of the mass from the right kidney and thrombus in the IVC revealed RCC.

Teaching Point RCC has a propensity to invade IVC occurring in 4–10 % of all patients with RCC. Among these patients, 2–16 % have tumors extending into the right atrium.

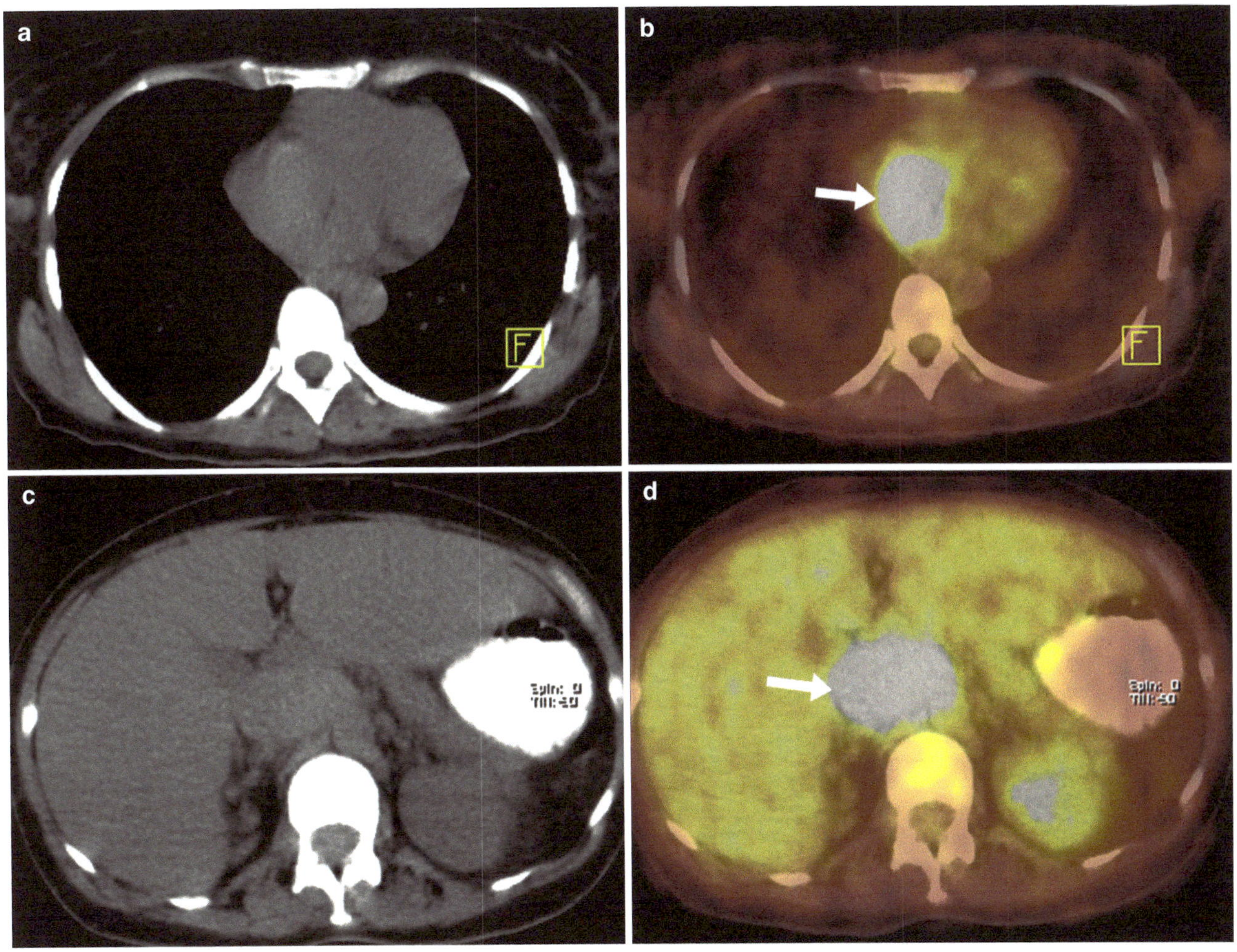

Fig. 15.6 Axial CT and fusion images show pathologically increased FDG uptake at right atrium (*arrow*) (**a**, **b**) and the thrombus at IVC (*arrow*) (**c**, **d**)

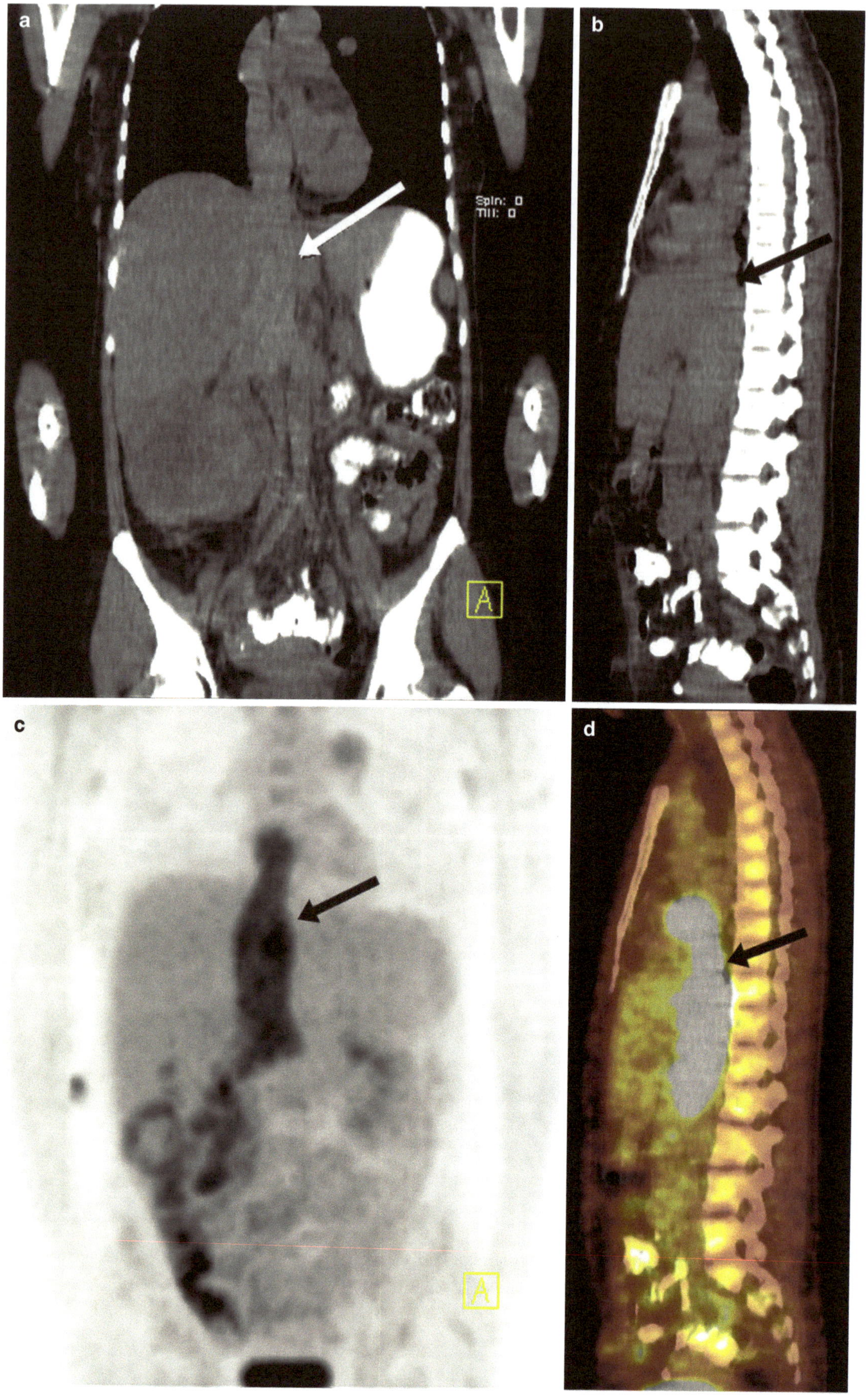

Fig. 15.7 Coronal CT and PET images of ^{18}F-FDG-PET/CT study showed intense FDG uptake in tumor thrombus in IVC (*arrows*) extending into right atrium and moderate FDG uptake in circular fashion in the right renal mass (**a**, **b**); sagittal CT and PET images show intense FDG uptake at thrombus in IVC (*arrows*) (**c**, **d**)

15.5 Case 5: Renal Cell Carcinoma Metastasis to Maxillary Sinus

History A 52-year-old male who has a history of renal cell carcinoma status post left nephrectomy and chemotherapy suffered from intermittent episodes of epistaxis and sinusitis. The patient underwent nasal endoscopy that diagnosed a tumor in the left maxillary sinus and biopsy was performed. Further evaluation with ^{18}F-FDG PET/CT imaging was done to determine the extent of metastatic disease.

Findings

Interpretation Metastatic lesion at left maxillary sinus and left nasal cavity.

Result The biopsy from left maxillary sinus showed clear cell carcinoma

Teaching Point Paranasal sinuses are rare metastatic sites for RCC, but the most frequent primary tumor that metastasizes to paranasal sinuses is the RCC. Approximately 50 cases of nasal recurrences of RCC have been reported in the literature. Tumor involvement of the paranasal sinuses and nasal cavity seems to occur via the hematogenous route through the Batson's paravertebral venous plexus.

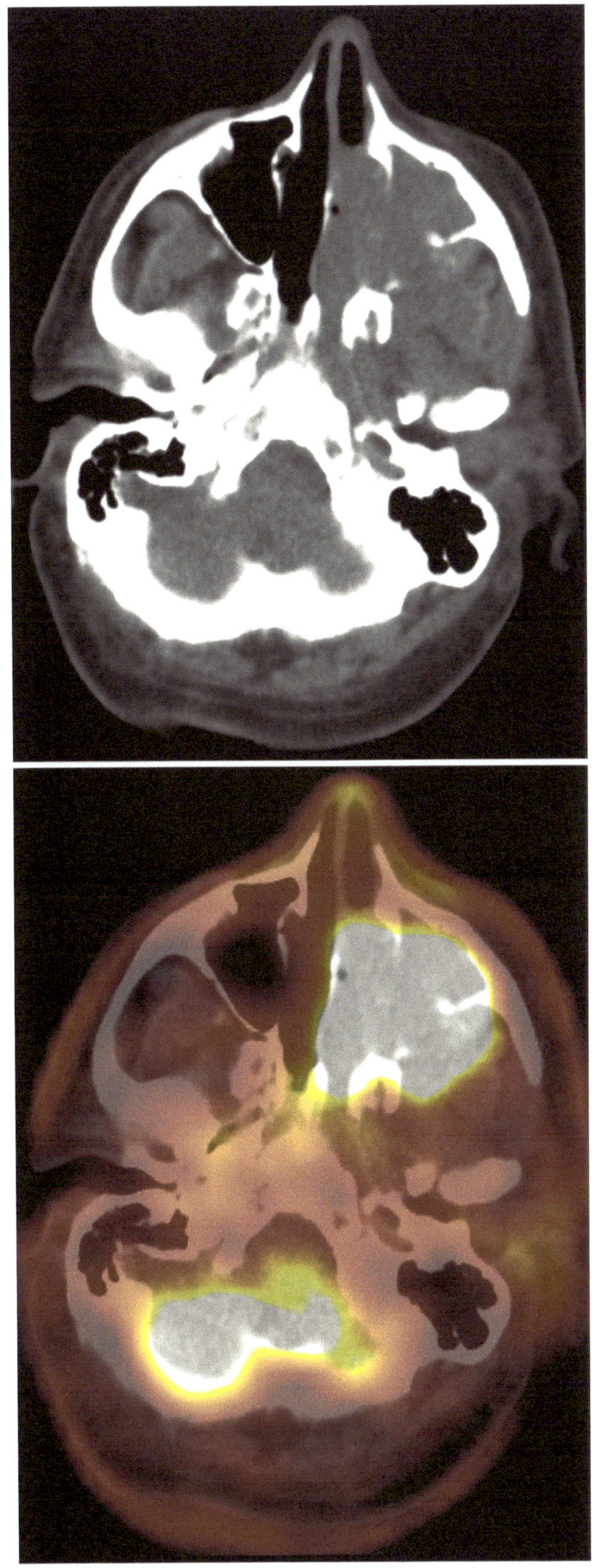

Fig. 15.8 Axial CT and fusion images showed an intensely hypermetabolic mass lesion filling left maxillary sinus and left nasal cavity (SUVmax 23)

15.6 Case 6: Renal Cell Carcinoma Bone Metastases

History A 60-year-old male underwent ^{18}F-FDG PET/CT imaging while he was being evaluated for the mass lesion at proximal diaphysis of left humerus.

Findings

Interpretation Mass lesion at left kidney was suspicious for malignancy. The hypermetabolism at left proximal humerus, right femur, and right iliac bone was indicating likelihood for metastases.

Result Biopsy of left humerus lesion revealed giant cell tumor of bone. Patient underwent left nephrectomy and histopathology was RCC.

Teaching Point One study reported that among all metastatic sites, ^{18}F-FDG PET/CT is most sensitive for bone metastases of RCC. PET is superior to bone scan in detecting active osseous metastasis of RCC. Sensitivity and specificity ^{18}F-18 FDG PET/CT reaches up to 100 % for the detection of bone metastases of RCC but there may be false positive findings like benign tumors of bone as in this case.

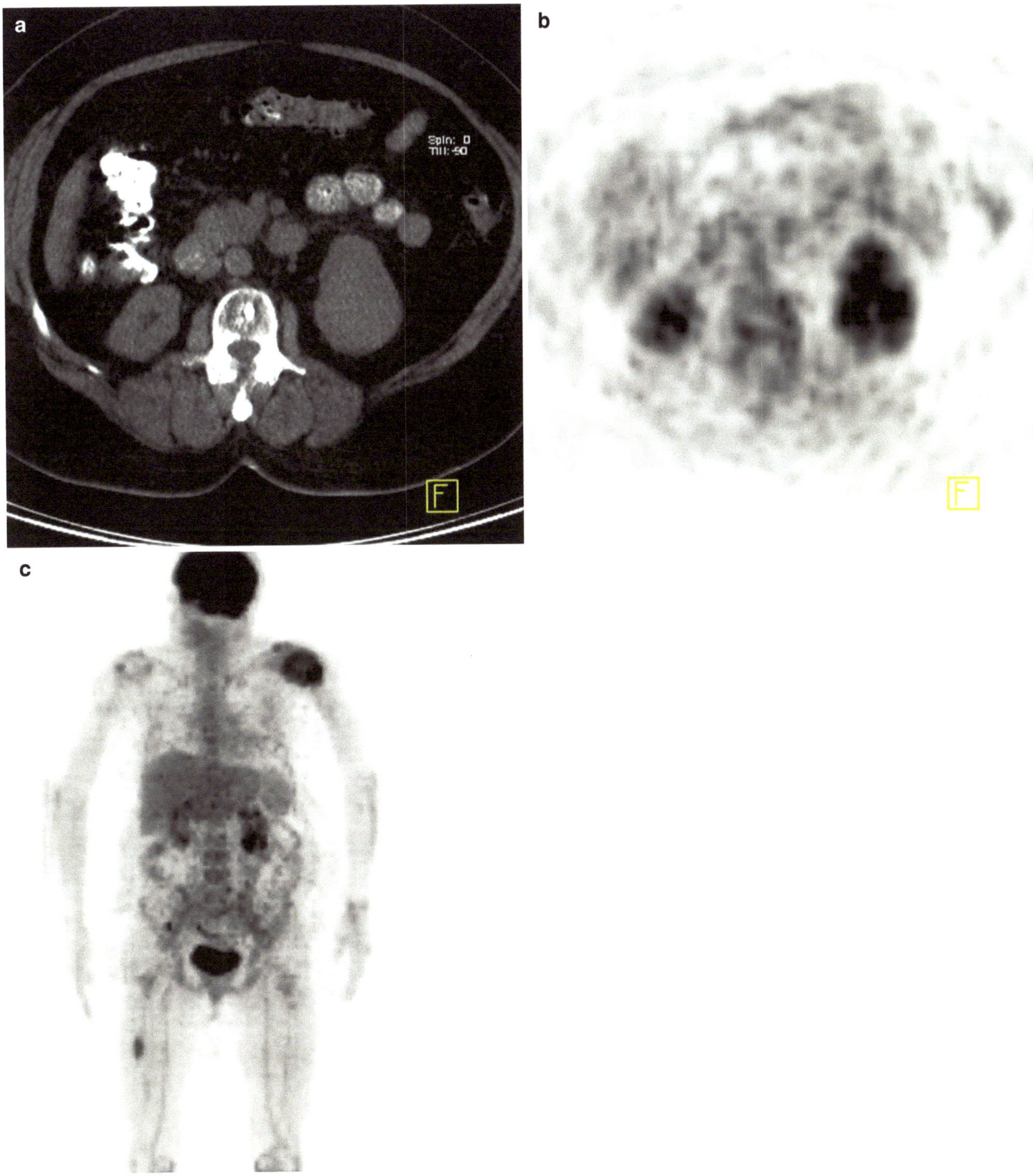

Fig. 15.9 Axial CT and PET images showed mass lesion at lower pole of left kidney exhibiting moderately increased FDG uptake (SUVmax 6.8) (**a**, **b**), MIP image showed intensely increased FDG uptake at proximal left humerus and focal uptake at proximal diaphysis of right femur (**c**)

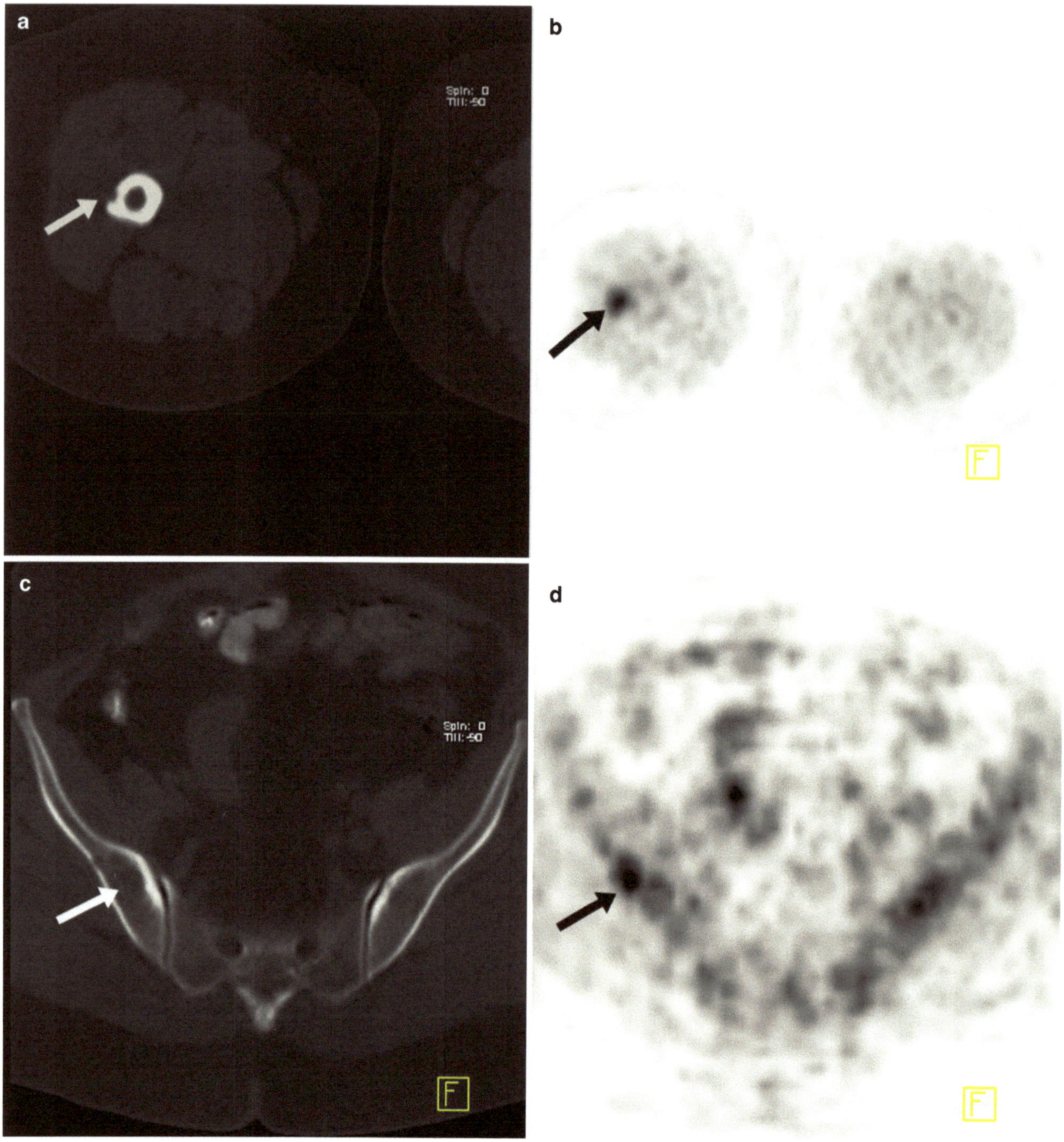

Fig. 15.10 Axial CT and PET images show lytic lesions at cortex of proximal diaphysis of right femur (**a**, **b**) and right iliac bone (**c**, **d**) both of which showed increased FDG uptake (SUVmax 4.4) (*arrows*)

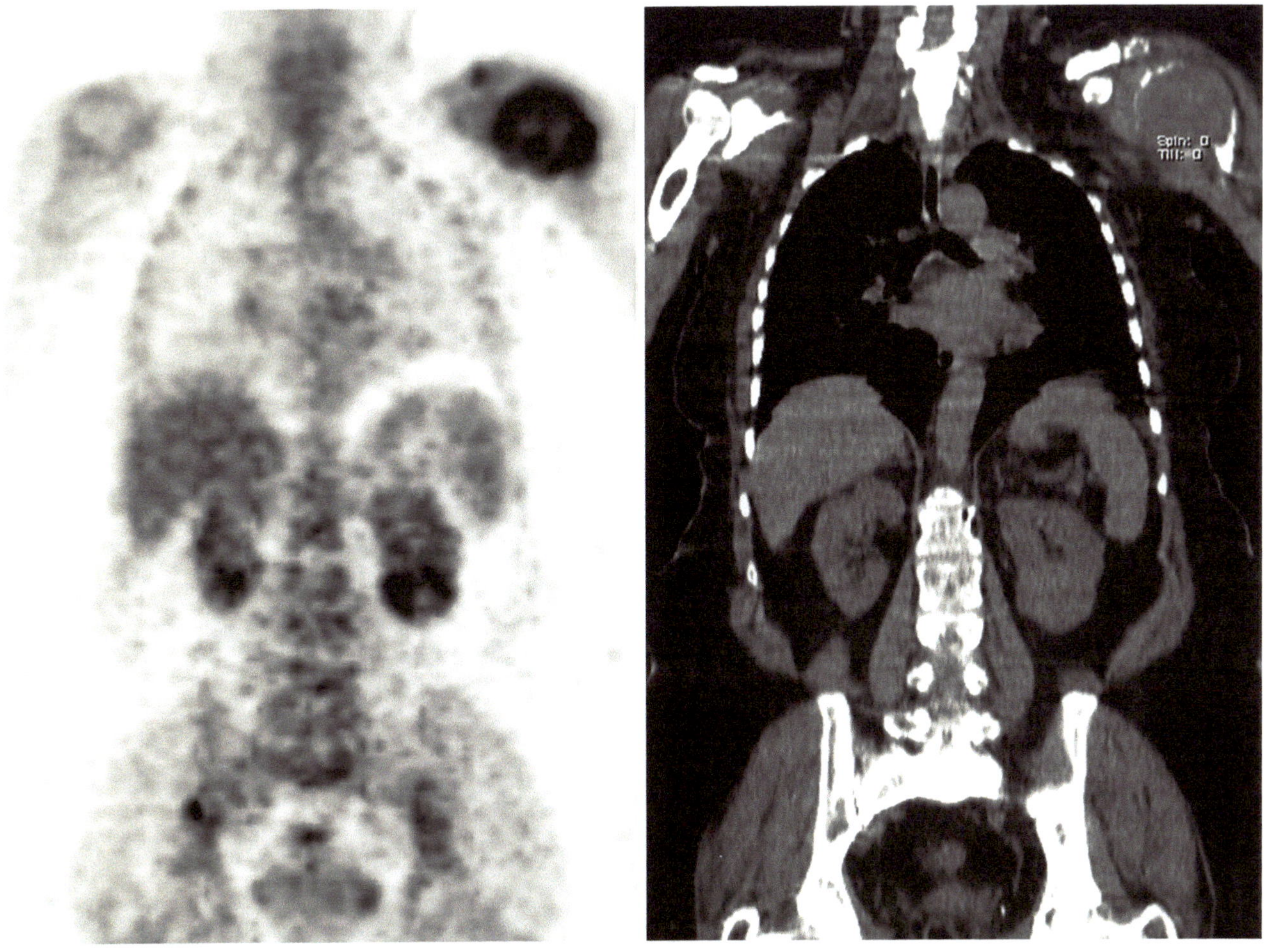

Fig. 15.11 Coronal PET and CT images show mass lesion at lower pole of left kidney with increased FDG uptake

15.7 Case 7: Renal Cell Carcinoma with Widespread Metastases

History A 62-year-old male underwent ^{18}F-FDG PET/CT imaging upon detection of a mass lesion at left kidney with anatomical imaging methods.

Findings

Interpretation Mass lesion at left kidney was strongly suspicious for malignancy. Highly FDG avid lesions at liver, bony structures, and lymph node stations were compatible with metastases.

Result Resection of the lesion in left kidney revealed RCC.

Teaching Point ^{18}F-FDG PET/CT can be helpful in ruling out metastasis in cystic lesions of kidney.

- ^{18}F-FDG PET/CT is better able to detect extrarenal rather than renal RCCs.

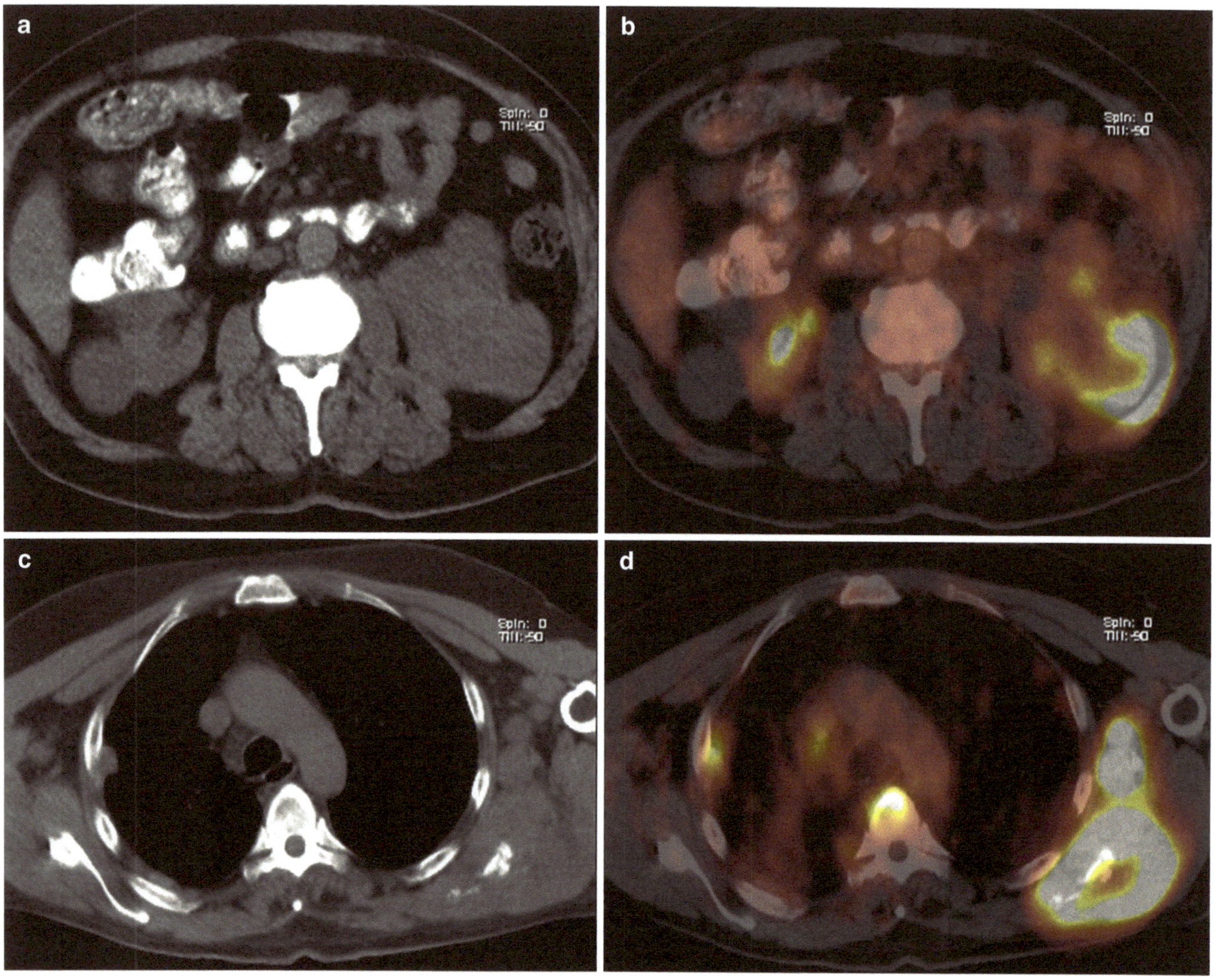

Fig. 15.12 Axial CT and fusion images showed mass lesion exhibiting intense FDG uptake, located posterolaterally at left kidney exhibiting moderately increased FDG uptake (SUVmax 19.3); hypodense cystic lesion at right kidney showing no FDG uptake (**a**, **b**), hypermetabolic lesion at left scapula extending into muscular structures and left axillary fossa (**c**, **d**)

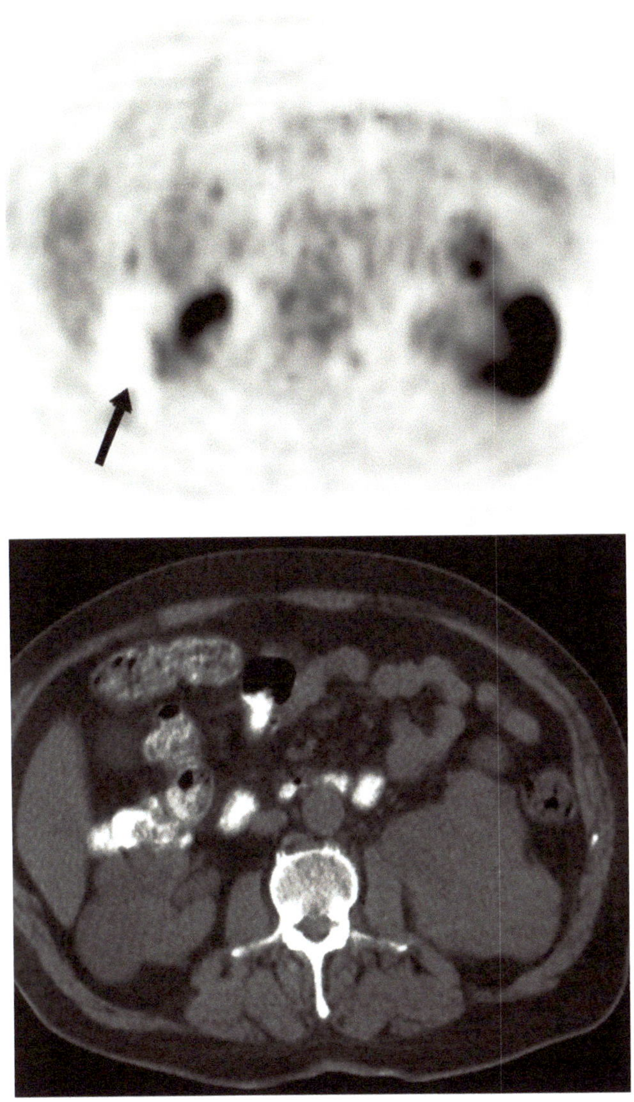

Fig. 15.13 Axial PET and CT images showed hypermetabolic lesion at left kidney and hypodense cystic lesion located at right kidney which shows no FDG uptake (*arrow*)

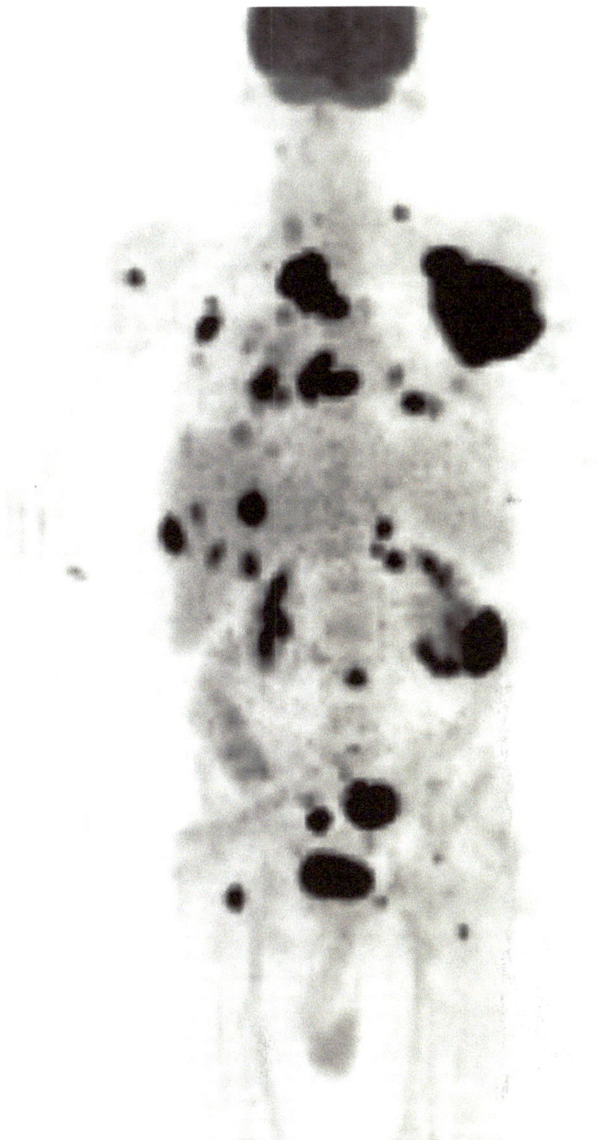

Fig. 15.14 MIP image showed widespread hypermetabolic lesions involving visceral organs and lymphatic and skeletal system

15.8 Case 8: Therapy Response Evaluation in Seminoma

History A 30-year-old male status post left orchiectomy and diagnosed with seminoma is currently being evaluated with ^{18}F-FDG PET/CT for therapy response after radiotherapy.

Findings

Interpretation ^{18}F-FDG PET/CT demonstrated that radiotherapy provided complete cure.

Teaching Point ^{18}F-FDG PET/CT is good predictor of viable residual tumor in postchemotherapy seminoma residuals with a sensitivity of 80 % and specificity of 100 %.

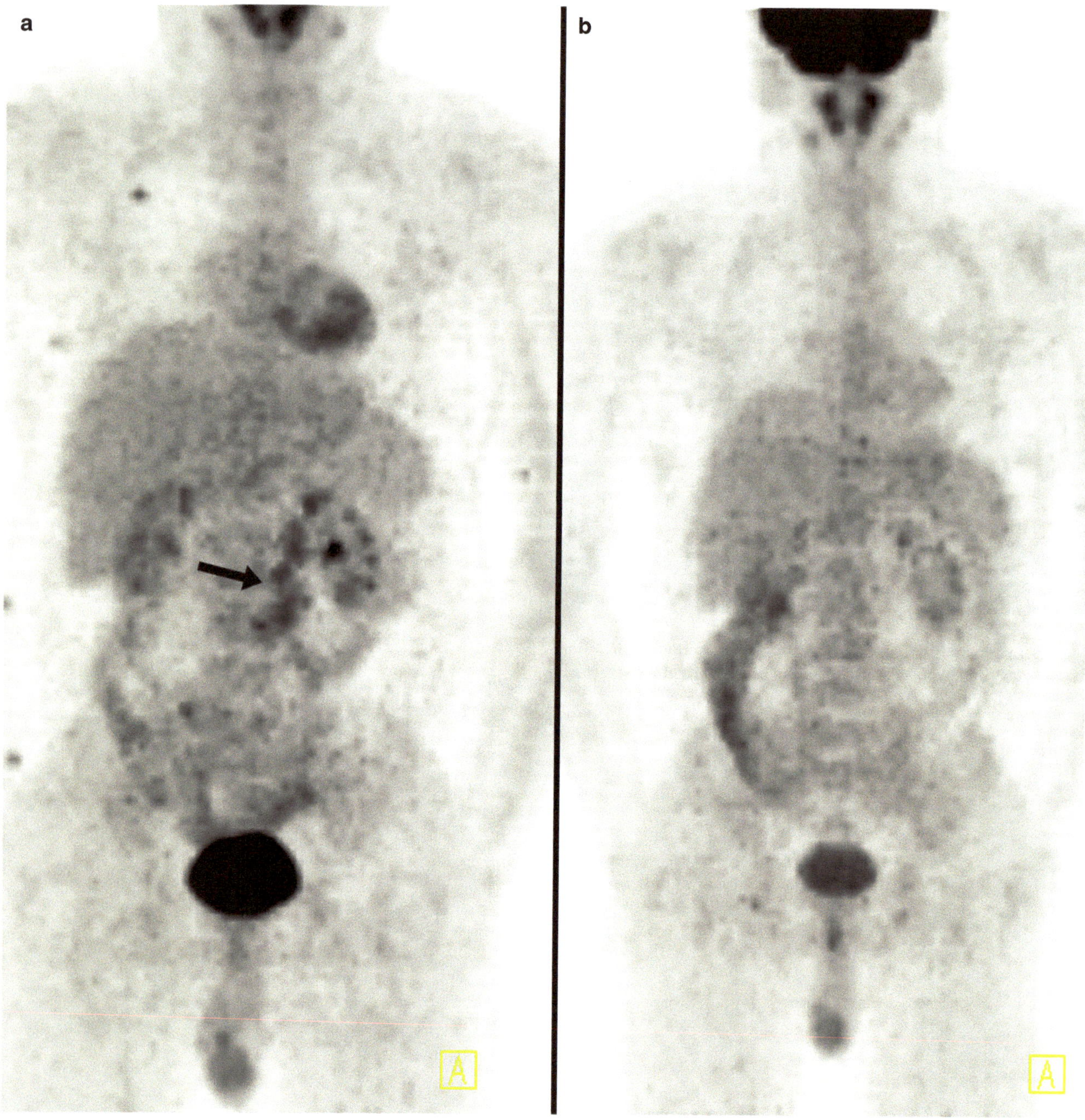

Fig. 15.15 MIP images show increased FDG uptake at abdominal paraaortic lymph nodes before therapy (**a**) (*arrow*), clearance of lymph nodes with pathological FDG uptake 4 months after chemotherapy (**b**)

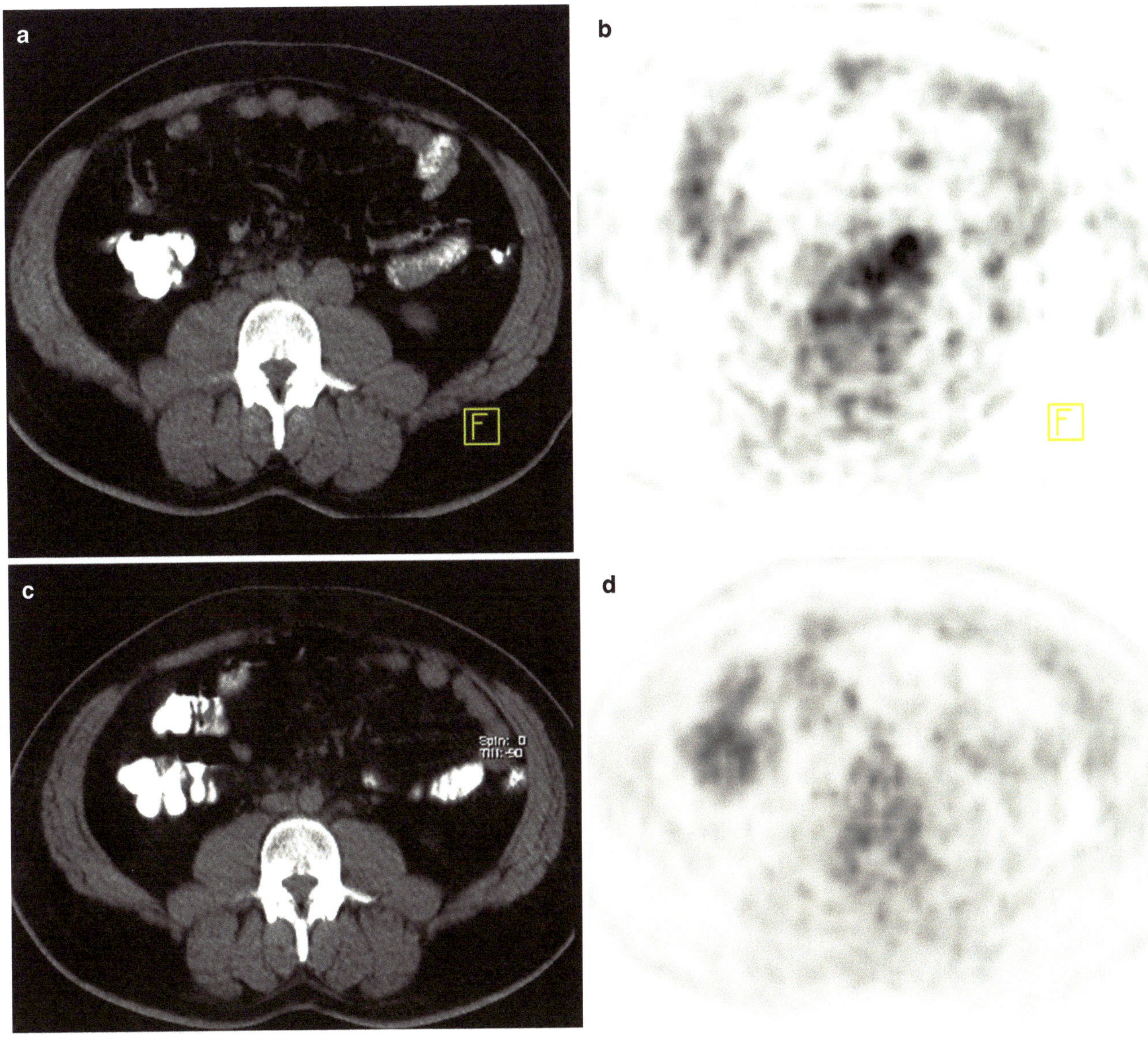

Fig. 15.16 Axial CT and PET images showing increased FDG uptake at left abdominal paraaortic lymph nodes before therapy (**a**, **b**), clearance of lymph nodes with pathological FDG uptake 4 months after chemotherapy (**c**, **d**)

15.9 Case 9: Preperative Evaluation in Mature Teratoma

History A 21-year-old male underwent ^{18}F-FDG PET/CT for treatment planning, after detection of multiple abdominal lymphadenopathies on CT.

Findings

Interpretation Enlarged abdominal lymph nodes without FDG uptake in a young male is suspicious for metastases of mature teratoma.

Teaching Point ^{18}F-FDG PET/CT has no role in management of mature teratoma which has a low glucose metabolic rate. Mature teratoma is a benign tumor that does not show any hypermetabolism on ^{18}F-FDG PET/CT, but it can undergo malignant transformation which causes FDG uptake.

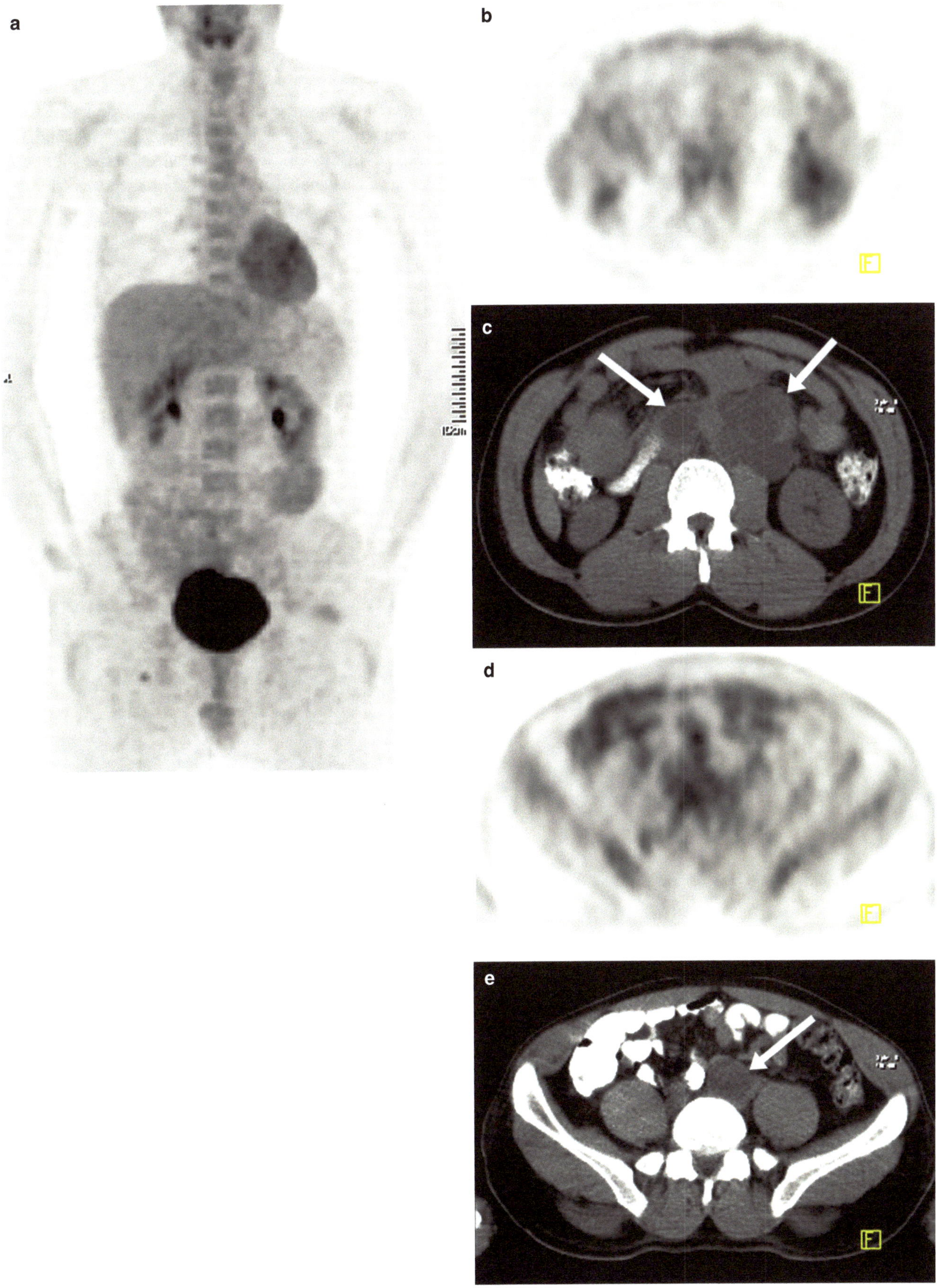

Fig. 15.17 MIP image (**a**) and axial PET and CT images show multiple enlarged hypodense lymph nodes without any FDG uptake at paraaortic, interaortocaval (**b**, **c**), and common iliac (**d**, **e**) lymph node stations (*arrows*)

15.10 Case 10: Yolk Sac Tumor in Mediastinum

History An 18-year-old male was diagnosed to have yolk sac tumor when a biopsy was made from a 10×9×5 cm mass lesion in mediastinum 4 months ago. The patient received chemotherapy and 3 week later underwent ^{18}F-FDG PET/CT for therapy response evaluation.

Findings

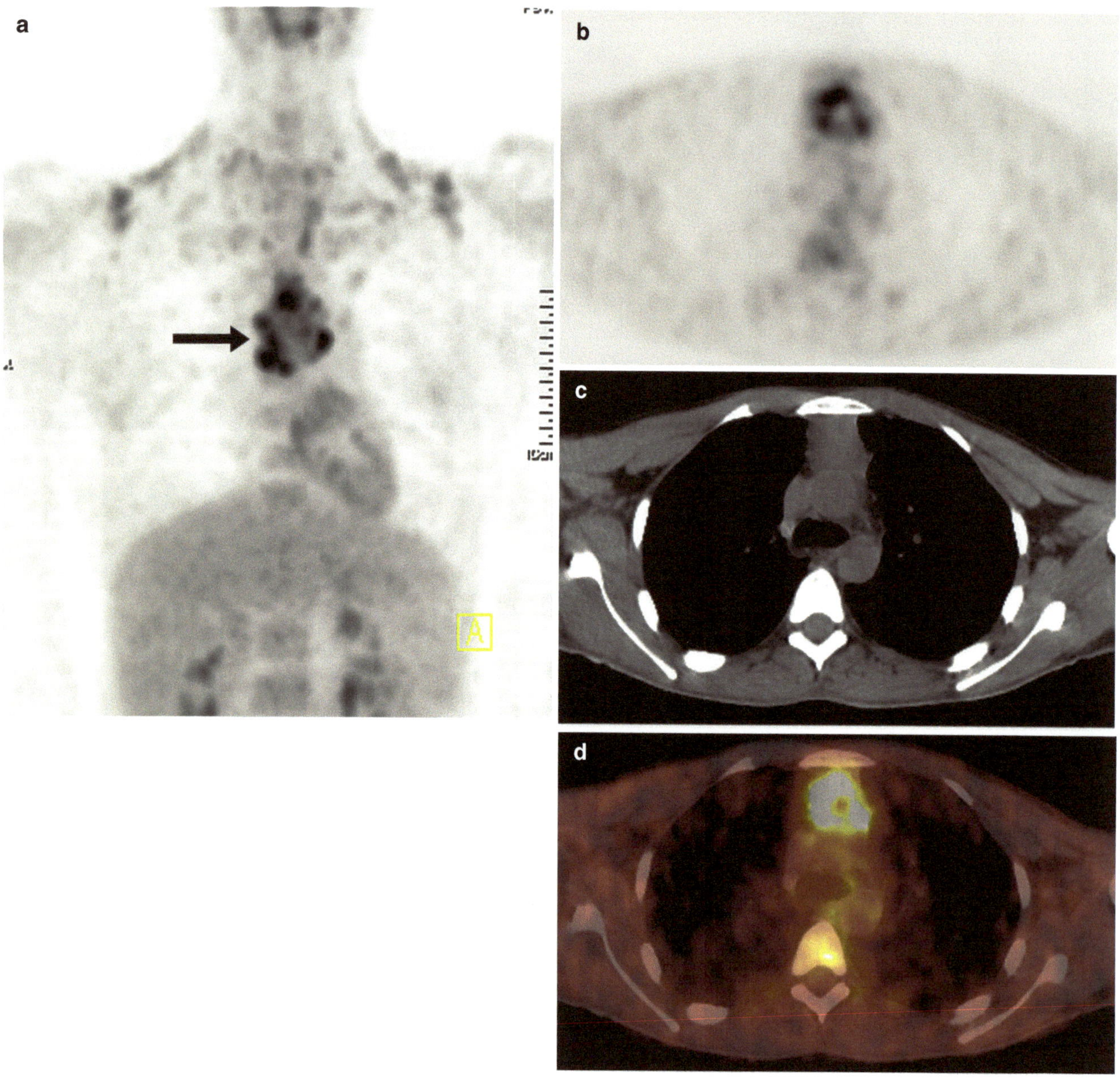

Fig. 15.18 MIP image (**a**), axial PET, CT, and fusion images (**b–d**) show moderately hypermetabolic (SUVmax 6) mass lesion at anterior mediastinum with a central necrotic area in it (*arrow*). There is physiologic FDG uptake at both testis (not shown here) and no any other pathological uptake elsewhere. Symmetrical FDG uptake at both cervical and supraclavicular area is consistent with physiological brown fat uptake

Interpretation Residual malignant lesion at anterior mediastinum.

Teaching Point Fifty to 70 % of all extragonadal germ cell tumors are located in the mediastinum. Yolk sac tumor is the most common mediastinal nonseminamotous germ cell tumor (60 %). ^{18}F-FDG PET/CT is rather effective and specific in detecting viable tumor in the residual mass after chemotherapy.

15.11 Case 11: Prostate Carcinoma Showing Invasion to Rectum

History A 64-year-old male underwent ^{18}F-FDG PET/CT for pretreatment evaluation of histopathologically proven prostate adenocarcinoma.

Findings

Interpretation Prostate carcinoma showing local invasion to rectum and adjacent tissues.

Teaching Point Prostate tumors are characterized by low metabolic activity and glycolytic rate, so the use of ^{18}F-FDG PET/CT in the diagnosis of localized prostate cancer has been frustrating. Possible indications of ^{18}F-FDG PET/CT might be staging of advanced prostate cancer with high Gleason score, detecting local recurrent or metastatic disease in some patients with biochemical failure, assessing treatment response, and providing prognostic information.

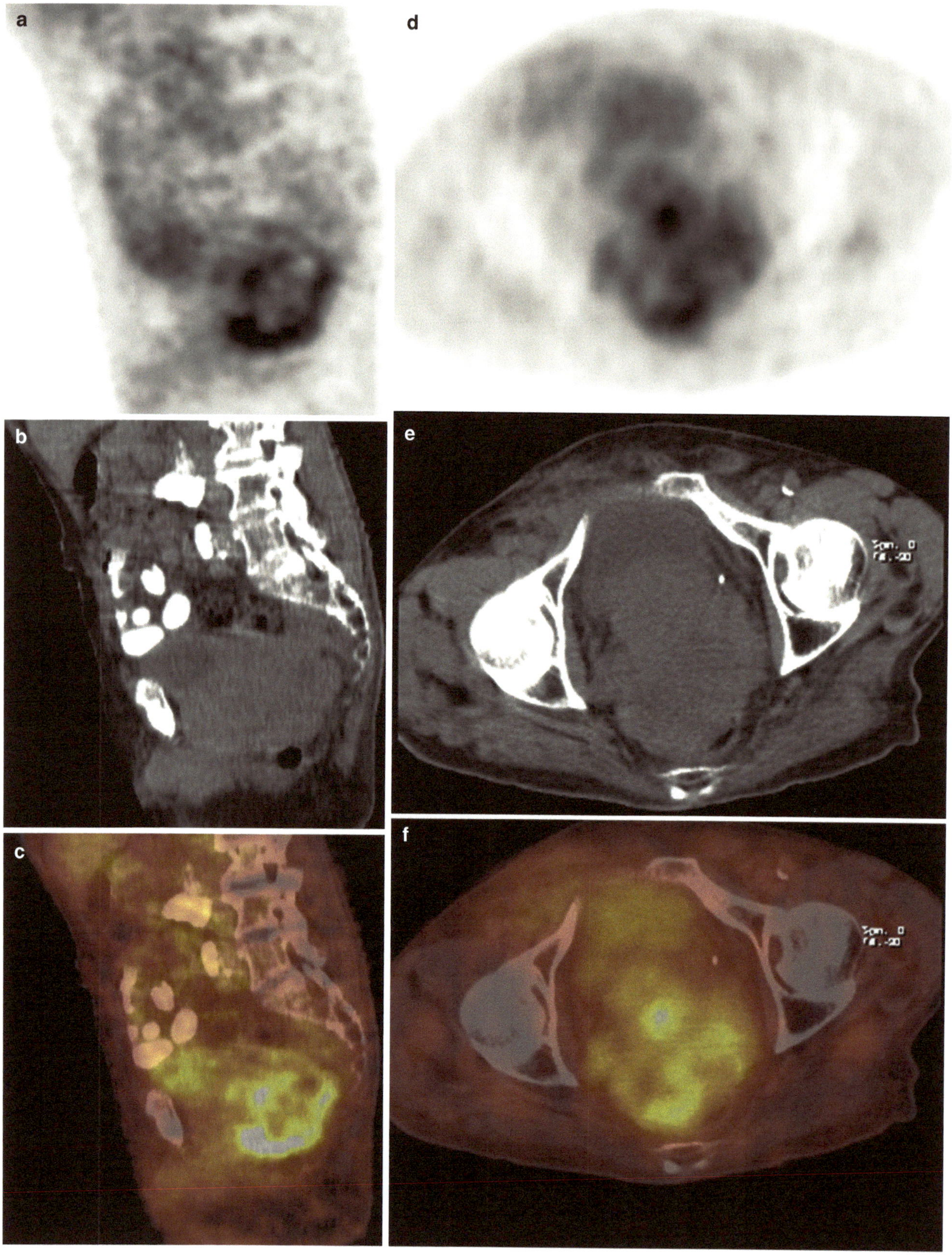

Fig. 15.19 Sagittal PET, CT, and fusion (**a**–**c**) and axial PET, CT, and fusion images (**d**–**f**) show moderately increased FDG uptake at the lesion in prostate gland which shows extension posteriorly to rectum

15.12 Case 12: Prostate Carcinoma Showing Metastases to Bone

History A 60-year-old male underwent ^{18}F-FDG PET/CT while he was being followed up for prostate carcinoma.

Findings

Interpretation Metastatic sclerotic bone lesions due to prostate carcinoma

Teaching Point Sensitivity of ^{18}F-FDG PET/CT in the detection of bone metastases is higher than bone scintigraphy (BS) when whole malignancies are concerned and it can be a substitute for BS in the assessment of bone metastases except prostate cancer. The most common organ for distant metastasis in prostate cancer is bone. ^{18}F-FDG PET/CT is variable in the detection of bone metastasis of prostate cancer and it was reported to be less sensitive than conventional bone scintigraphy. It is a well known fact that ^{18}F-FDG PET/CT is more sensitive in detecting lytic metastases than sclerotic metastases. In a group of patients with progressive bone metastases, in the subgroup of patients with blastic bone metastases, ^{18}F-FDG PET/CT detected fewer bone metastases than BS. In prostate carcinoma, ^{18}F-FDG PET/CT is superior to bone scintigraphy in discrimination of active osseous disease from lesions which are not detected on scintigraphy. It can be proposed that ^{18}F-FDG PET/CT is more specific than bone scintigraphy to detect active disease.

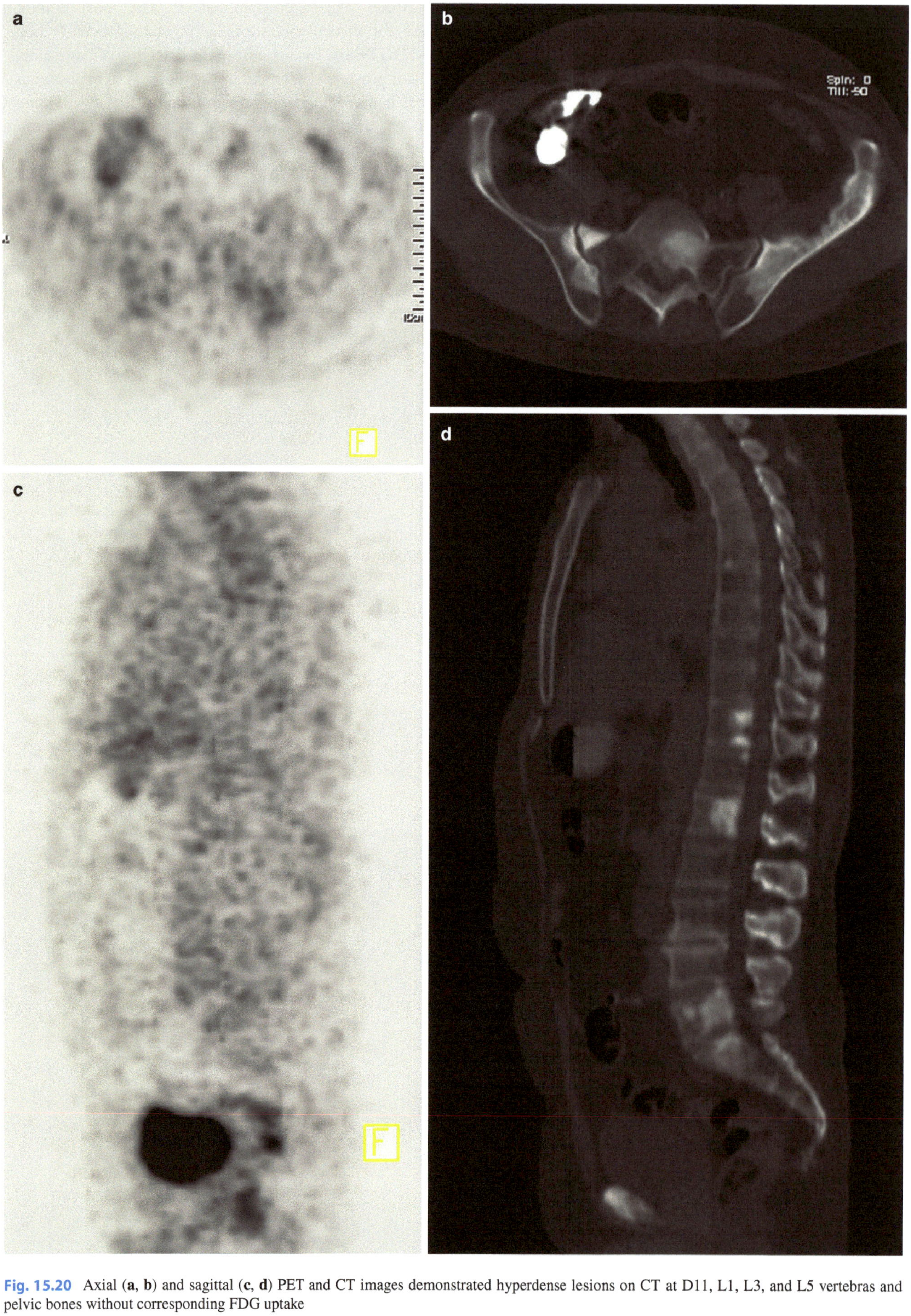

Fig. 15.20 Axial (**a**, **b**) and sagittal (**c**, **d**) PET and CT images demonstrated hyperdense lesions on CT at D11, L1, L3, and L5 vertebras and pelvic bones without corresponding FDG uptake

15.13 Case 13: Staging of Bladder Carcinoma

History A 73-year-old male with transitional cell carcinoma of bladder underwent transurethral resection 15 days ago and referred to ^{18}F-FDG PET/CT scan for initial staging.

Findings

Interpretation Intense FDG uptake at the lesion was suggestive of a malignant lesion.

Teaching Point Determination of depth of muscle invasion and degree of perivesical involvement is crucial in planning the treatment strategy of bladder carcinomas. PET has limited role in this aspect and it is not always possible to visualize primary bladder cancer on ^{18}F-FDG PET/CT because of physiological urinary FDG tracer activity.

- Possible uses of ^{18}F-FDG PET/CT can be preoperative staging, detection of pelvic recurrence, differentiation of fibrosis from tumor and identification of distant metastases.

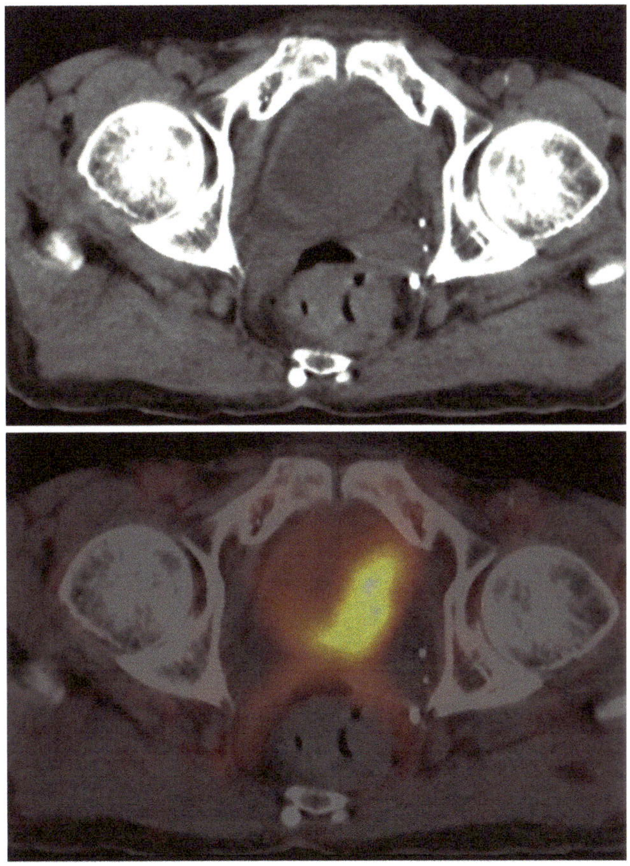

Fig. 15.21 Axial CT and fusion images showed FDG-avid left posterolateral bladder wall thickening corresponding to a primary urothelial neoplasm (SUVmax 13.9). There was not any other pathological activity in favor of local extension or lymph node involvement

15.14 Case 14: Staging of Bladder Carcinoma

History An 81-year-old male with underwent transurethral resection 6 weeks ago and having the diagnosis of bladder carcinoma referred to ^{18}F-FDG PET/CT scan for determination of initial treatment strategy.

Findings

Interpretation Malignant lesion at left posterior bladder wall and metastatic lymph nodes at left internal and external iliac regions.

Teaching Point Currently imaging of abdomen and pelvis with CT and MRI are standard tests for determination of lymph node metastases. ^{18}F-FDG PET/CT might have a role in the detection of lymph nodes with metastatic deposits which are not adjacent to bladder, and in one study 67 % sensitivity and 85 % specificity was reported.

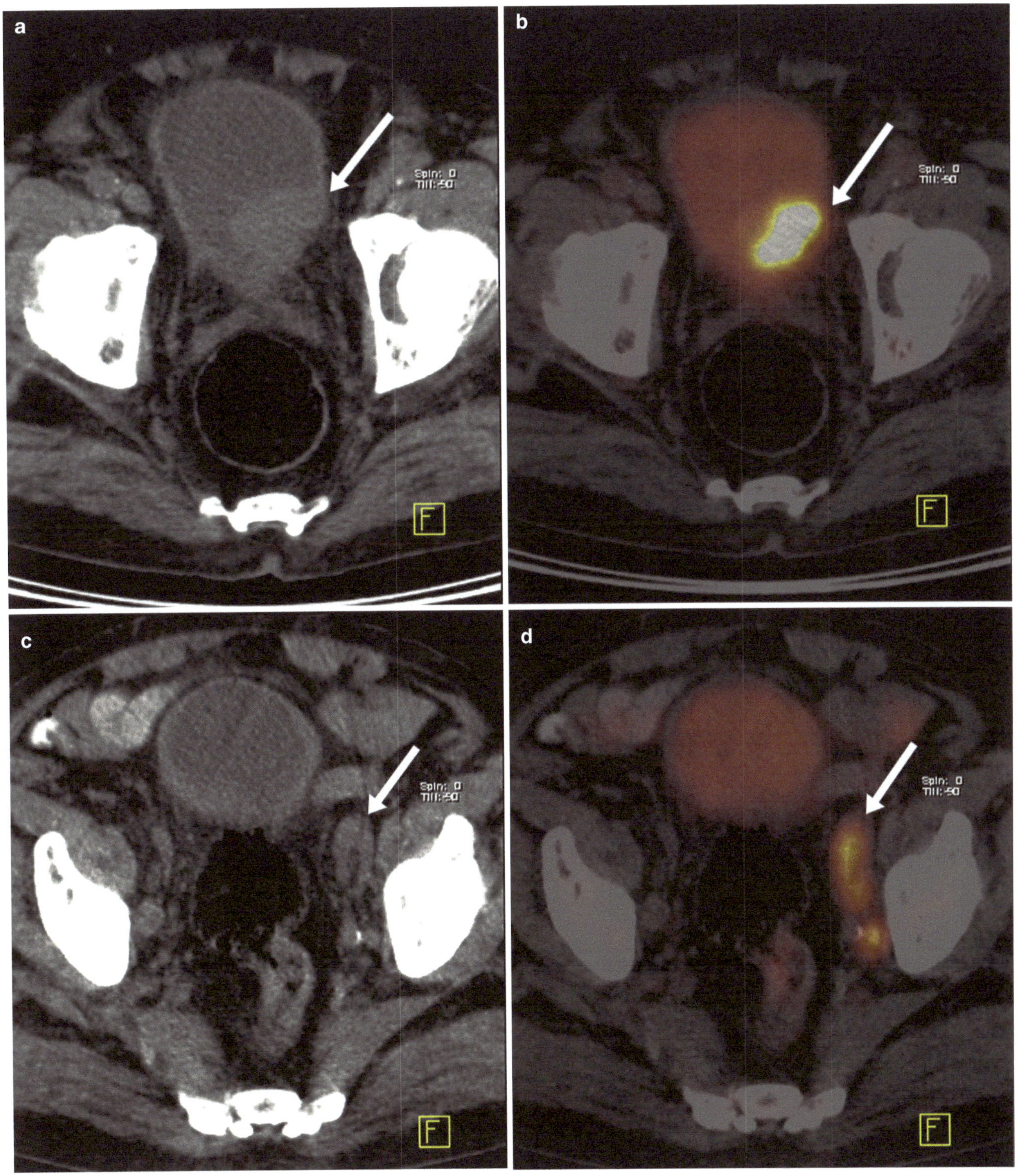

Fig. 15.22 Axial CT and fusion images showed intensely FDG-avid mass lesion originating from left posterior bladder wall (**a, b**) (SUVmax 45) (*arrows*). There were also hypermetabolic lymph nodes located at left internal and external iliac regions (**c, d**) (*arrows*)

Bibliography

1. Ak I, Can C. F-18 FDG PET in detecting renal cell carcinoma. Acta Radiol. 2005;46:895–9.
2. Bachor R, Kotzerke J, Gottfried HW, Brändle E, Reske SN, Hautmann R. Positron emission tomography in diagnosis of renal cell carcinoma. Urologe A. 1996;35:146–50.
3. Cook GJ, Houston S, Rubens R, Maisey MN, Fogelman I. Detection of bone metastases in breast cancer by 18FDG PET: differing metabolic activity in osteoblastic and osteolytic lesions. J Clin Oncol. 1998;16:3375–9.
4. Cremerius U, Effert PJ, Adam G, Sabri O, Zimmy M, Wagenknecht G, et al. FDG PET for detection and therapy control of metastatic germ cell tumor. J Nucl Med. 1998;39:815–22.
5. Dehner LP. Germ cell tumors of the mediastinum. Semin Diagn Pathol. 1990;7:266–84.
6. De Santis M, Becherer A, Bokemeyer C, Stoiber F, Oechsle K, Sellner F, et al. 2-18fluoro-deoxy-D-glucose positron emission tomography is a reliable predictor for viable tumor in postchemotherapy seminoma: an update of the prospective multicentric SEMPET trial. J Clin Oncol. 2004;22:1034–9.
7. Fogelman I, Cook G, Israel O, Van der Wall H. Positron emission tomography and bone metastases. Semin Nucl Med. 2005;35:135–42.
8. Hatcher PA, Anderson EE, Paulson DF, Carson CC, Robertson JE. Surgical management and prognosis of renal cell carcinoma invading the vena cava. J Urol. 1991;145:20–4.
9. Kang D, White Jr RL, Zuger J, Sasser HC, Teigland CM. Clinical use of fluorodeoxyglucose F-18 positron emission tomography for detection of renal cell carcinoma. J Urol. 2004;171:1806–9.
10. Karyagar S, Koc ZP, Karyagar SS, Ozulker T, Topal C, Karaguzel E, et al. Dual time F-18 FDG PET/CT imaging in the diagnosis of renal cell cancer. Curr Med Imaging Rev. 2014;10:134–9.
11. Liu Y. Diagnostic role of fluorodeoxyglucose positron emission tomography-computed tomography in prostate cancer. Oncol Lett. 2014;7:2013–8.
12. Majhail NS, Urbain JL, Albani JM, Kanvinde MH, Rice TW, Novick AC, et al. F-18 fluorodeoxyglucose positron emission tomography in the evaluation of distant metastases from renal cell carcinoma. J Clin Oncol. 2003;21:3995–4000. doi:10.1200/JCO.2003.04.073.
13. Mohapatra T, Arora A, Srikant K, Snehalata, Kumar N. A rare case of mature teratoma. Has FDG PET/CT a role to play?. Indian J Nucl Med. 2011;26:107–8. doi:10.4103/0972-3919.90265.
14. Montravers F, Grahek D, Kerrou K, Younsi N, Doublet JD, Gattegno B, et al. Evaluation of FDG uptake by renal malignancies (primary tumor or metastases) using a coincidence detection gamma camera. J Nucl Med. 2000;41:78–84.
15. Moran CA, Suster S, Koss MN. Primary germ cell tumors of the mediastinum. Part III. Yolk sac tumor, embryonal carcinoma, choriocarcinoma, and combined nonteratomatous germ cell tumors of the mediastinum—a clinicopathologic and immunohistochemical study of 64 cases. Cancer. 1997;80:699–707.
16. Morris MJ, Akhurst T, Osman I, Nunez R, Macapinlac H, Siedlecki K, et al. Fluorinated deoxyglucose positron emission tomography imaging in progressive metastatic prostate cancer. Urology. 2002;59:913–8.
17. Muros BT, Romero JRS, Rodriguez JGB, Parrilla RB. Maxillary sinus metastasis of renal cell carcinoma. ACTAS Urol Esp. 2006;30:954–7.
18. Nesbitt JC, Soltero ER, Dinney CP, Walsh GL, Schrump DS, Swanson DA, et al. Surgical management of renal cell carcinoma with inferior vena cava tumor thrombus. Ann Thorac Surg. 1997;63:1592–600.
19. Neves RJ, Zincke H. Surgical treatment of renal cancer with vena cava extension. Br J Urol. 1987;59:390–5.
20. Ozülker T, Küçüköz Uzun A, Ozülker F, Ozpaçac T. Comparison of (18)F-FDG-PET/CT with (99 m)Tc-MDP bone scintigraphy for the detection of bone metastases in cancer patients. Nucl Med Commun. 2010;31:597–603. doi:10.1097/MNM.0b013e328338e909.
21. Ozülker T, Ozülker F, Ozbek E, Ozpaçaci T. A prospective diagnostic accuracy study of F-18 fluorodeoxyglucose-positron emission tomography/computed tomography in the evaluation of indeterminate renal masses. Nucl Med Commun. 2011;32:265–72. doi:10.1097/MNM.0b013e3283442e3b.
22. Schöder H, Larson SM. Positron emission tomography for prostate, bladder, and renal cancer. Semin Nucl Med. 2004;34:274–92.
23. Seto E, Segall GM, Terris MK. Positron emission tomography detection of osseous metastases of renal cell carcinoma not identified on bone scan. Urology. 2000;55:286.
24. Shinagare AB, Jagannathan JP, Ramaiya NH, Hall MN, Van den Abbeele AD. Adult extragonadal germ cell tumors. AJR Am J Roentgenol. 2010;195:274–80. doi:10.2214/AJR.09.4103.
25. Skinner DG, Pritchett TR, Lieskovsky G, Boyd SD, Stiles QR. Vena caval involvement by renal cell carcinoma. Surgical resection provides meaningful long-term survival. Ann Surg. 1989;210: 387–94.
26. Sountoulides P, Metaxa L, Cindolo L. Atypical presentations and rare metastatic sites of renal cell carcinoma: a review of case reports. J Med Case Rep. 2011;5:429. doi:10.1186/1752-1947-5-429.
27. Wang HY, Ding HJ, Chen JH, Chao CH, Lu YY, Lin WY, et al. Meta-analysis of the diagnostic performance of [18F]FDG-PET and PET/CT in renal cell carcinoma. Cancer Imaging. 2012;12:464–74. doi:10.1102/1470-7330.2012.0042.
28. Wu HC, Yen RF, Shen YY, Kao CH, Lin CC, Lee CC. Comparing whole body 18-F-2-deoxyglucose positron emission tomography and technetium-99 m methylene diphosphate bone scan to detect bone metastases in patients with renal cell carcinomas: a preliminary report. J Cancer Res Clin Oncol. 2002;128:503.

16 Musculoskeletal Tumors

16.1 Case 1: Ewing Sarcoma

History A 26-year-old female underwent ^{18}F-FDG PET/CT after having diagnosed as Ewing sarcoma with a biopsy from a mass lesion located at left sacroiliac region.

Findings

Interpretation This finding is suggestive for malignant disease of bone invading surrounding structures.

Teaching Point ^{18}F-FDG PET CT demonstrated high sensitivity and specificity in pretreatment staging of Ewing sarcoma and may provide additional information that modify therapy planning. It is proposed that FDG PET could replace bone scan when the initial evaluation of the extent of disease is concerned.

T. Özülker, F. Özülker, *Atlas of PET-CT Imaging in Oncology: A Case-Based Guide to Image Interpretation*,
DOI 10.1007/978-3-319-18994-9_16

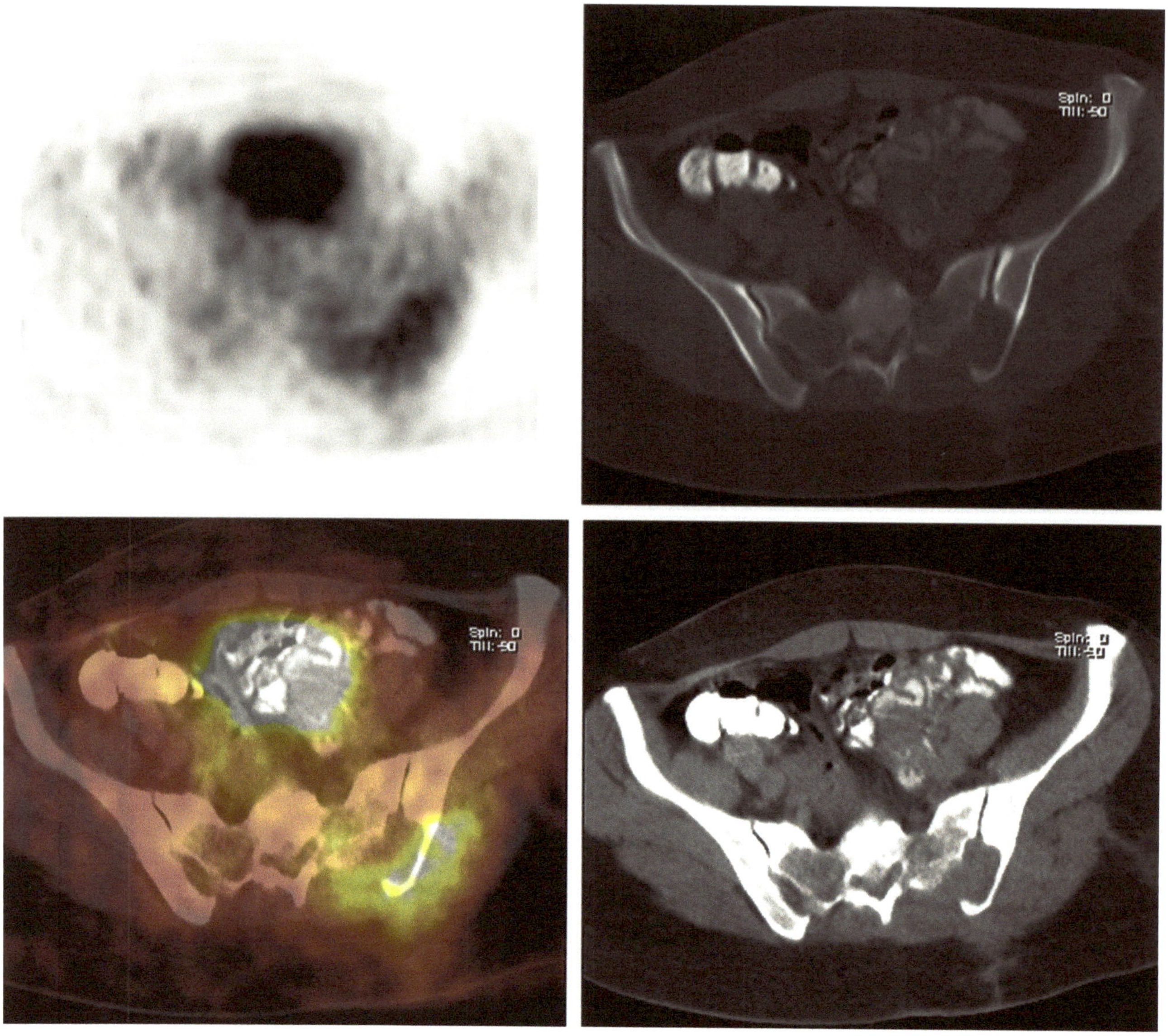

Fig. 16.1 Axial slices of CT, PET and fusion images show moderately hypermetabolic (SUVmax 5) mass lesion at left sacroiliac area invading gluteal muscles and obliterating sacral foramen

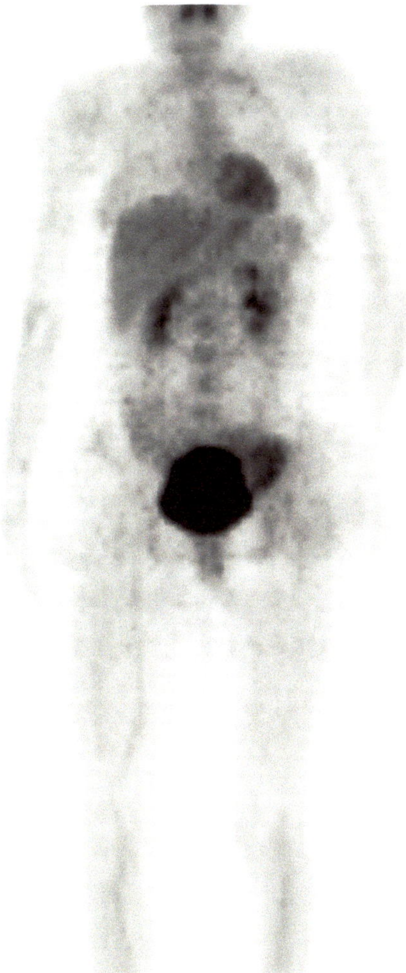

Fig. 16.2 MIP image

16.2 Case 2: Restaging of Ewing Sarcoma

History A 17-year-old female who was diagnosed to have Ewing sarcoma 1 year ago is now being evaluated with ^{18}F-FDG PET/CT for restaging, after having received chemotherapy and radiotherapy.

Findings

Interpretation Multiple hypermetabolic lesions consistent with widespread metastatic disease.

Teaching Point ^{18}F-FDG PET CT demonstrates high diagnostic accuracy for detecting recurrence in patients with primary skeletal Ewing sarcoma with a sensitivity of 95 % and a specificity of 87 %.

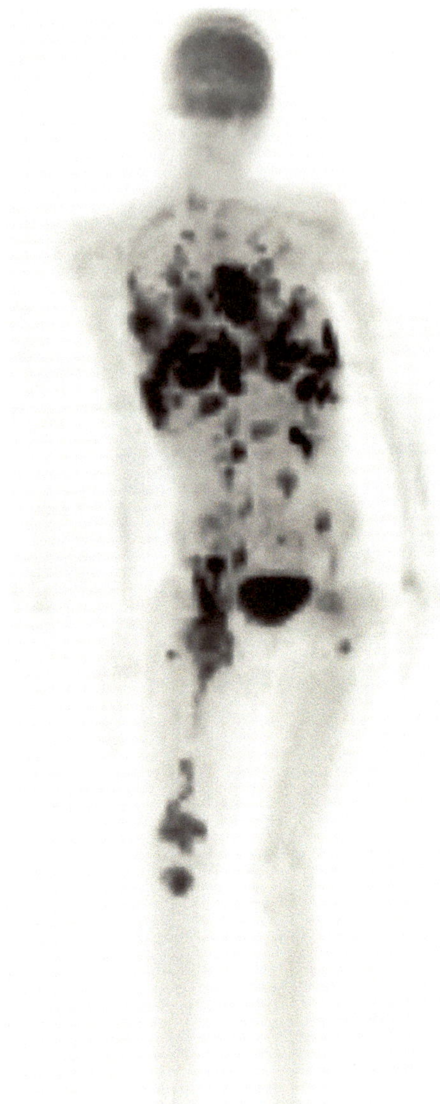

Fig. 16.3 MIP image shows multiple hypermetabolic lesions at pleural surfaces, lung parenchyma, mediastinal and intraabdominal lymph node stations, proximal and distal right femur, and proximal left femur (SUVmax 10)

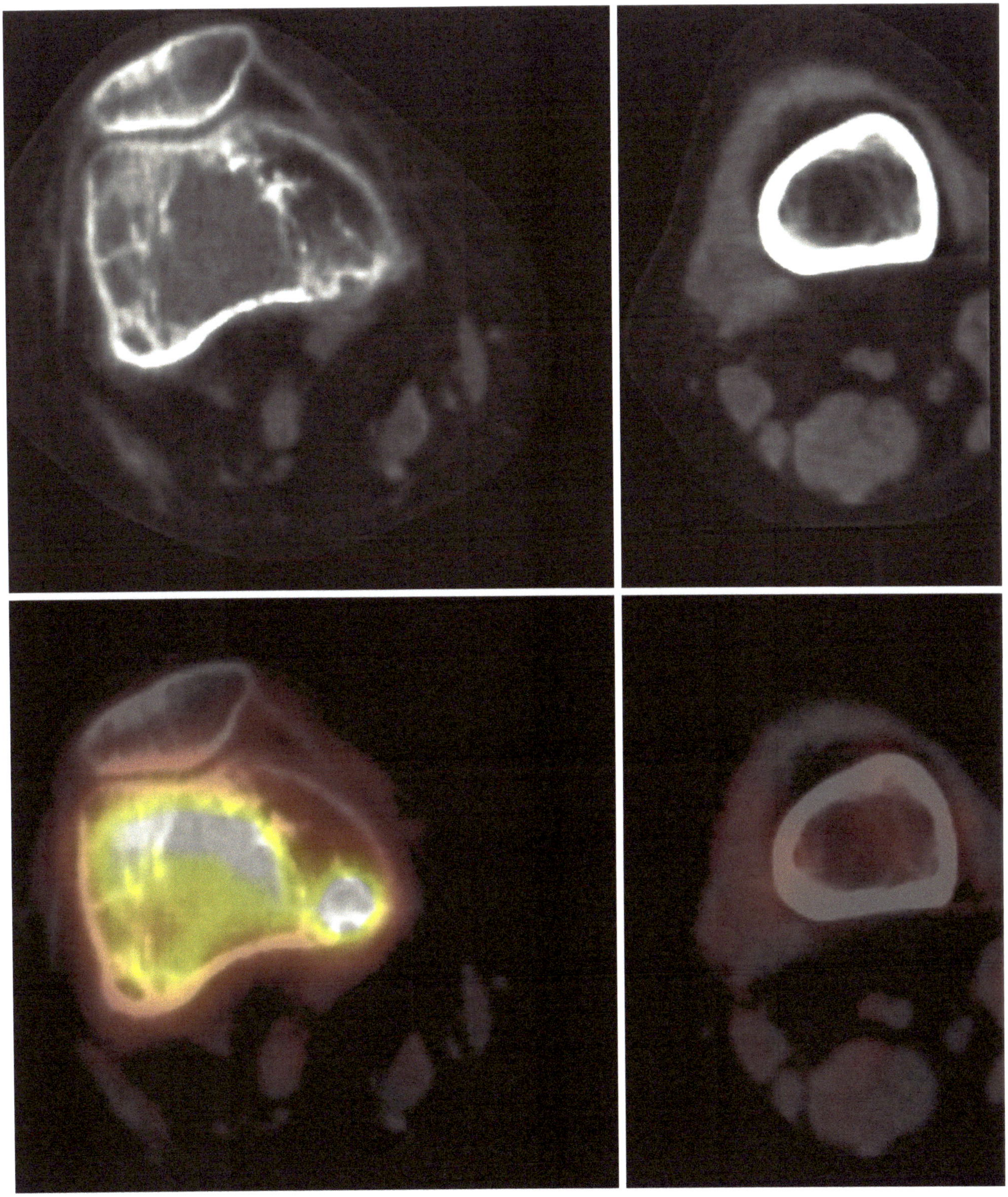

Fig. 16.4 Axial slices of CT and fusion images show increased FDG uptake corresponding to the lytic lesions at distal right femur

16.3 Case 3: Osteosarcoma

History A 29-year-old female who was diagnosed to have osteosarcoma at left femur underwent ^{18}F-FDG PET/CT.

Findings

Interpretation Hypermetabolic mass lesion at distal left thigh is compatible with primary malignant disease of bone. A focal increased FDG uptake located at intramedullary femur diaphysis above the primary lesion representing skip metastasis is seen. Right hilar lesion with FDG uptake is consistent with pulmonary metastasis.

Teaching Point Although, for osteosarcoma, FDG PET is less sensitive than bone scan for the detection of bone metastases and accuracy in detecting pulmonary metastases is lower than CT, bone and lung lesions in this case are correctly identified by PET.

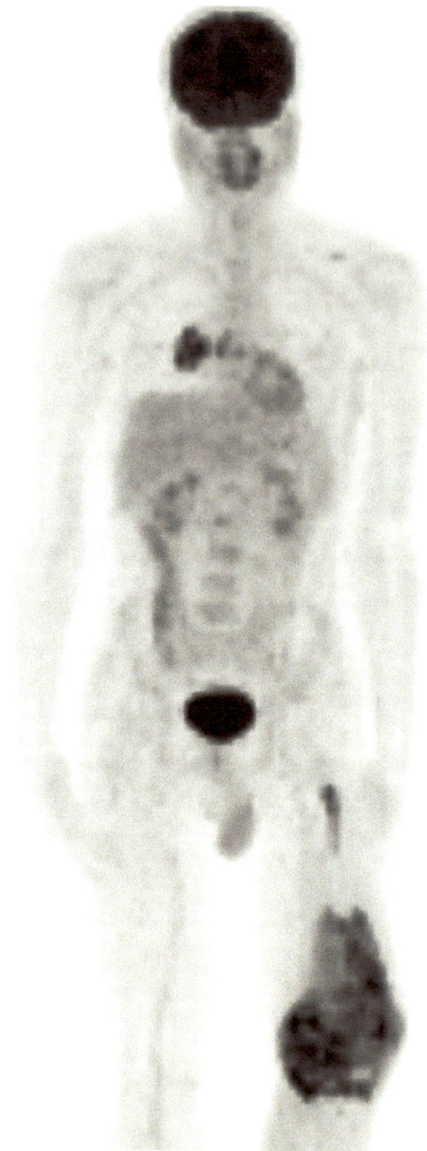

Fig. 16.5 MIP image shows intensely hypermetabolic expansile mass lesion at distal left thigh (SUVmax 10.7) and linear FDG uptake proximal to this mass (SUVmax 6.4). There is also hypermetabolic mass lesion at hilar region of right lung (SUVmax 10)

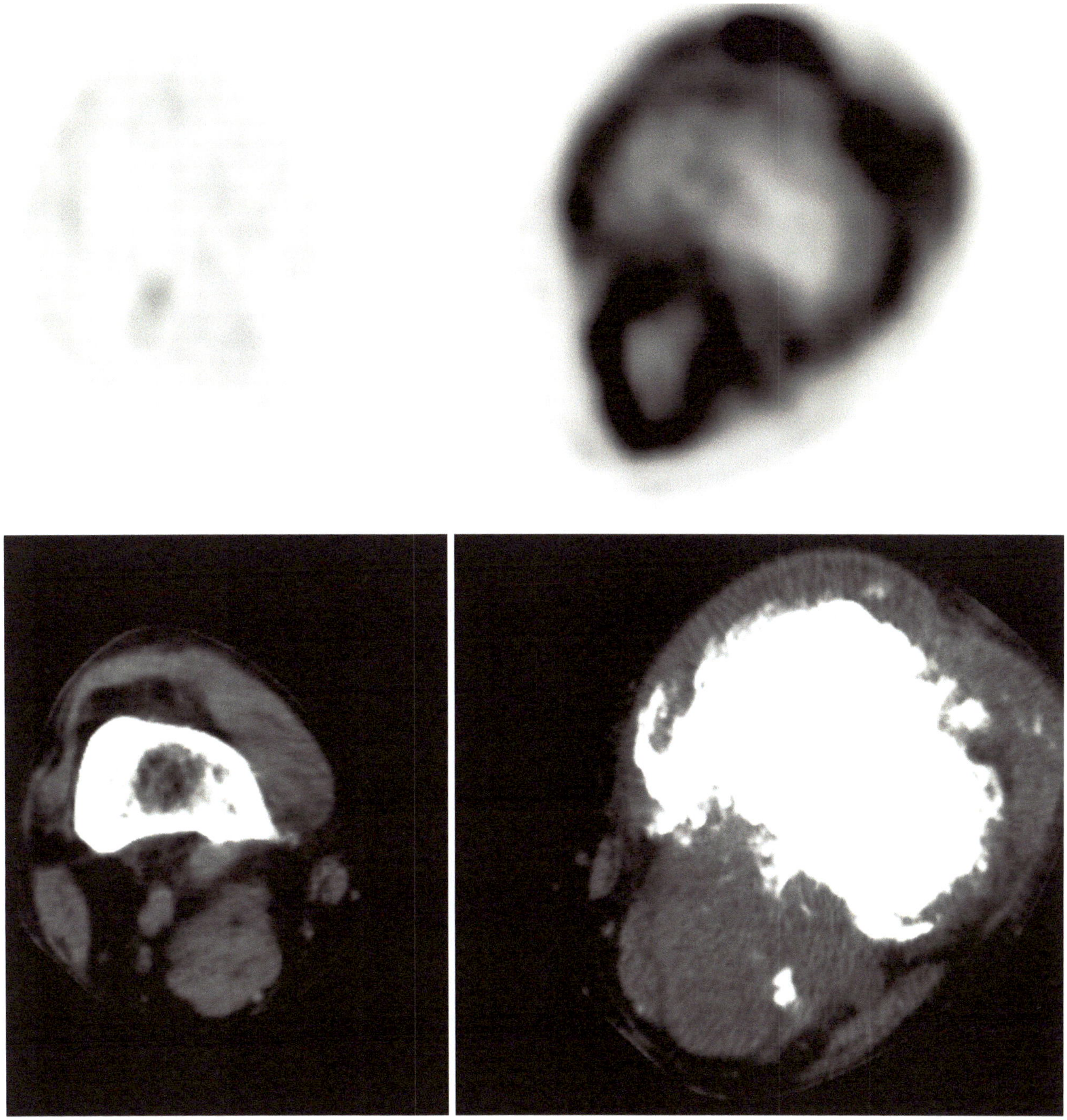

Fig. 16.6 Axial slices of PET and CT images show mass lesion at distal left thigh which shows bone destruction and involves calcified areas representing periosteal new bone formation. There is increased FDG uptake in circular fashion at mass lesion

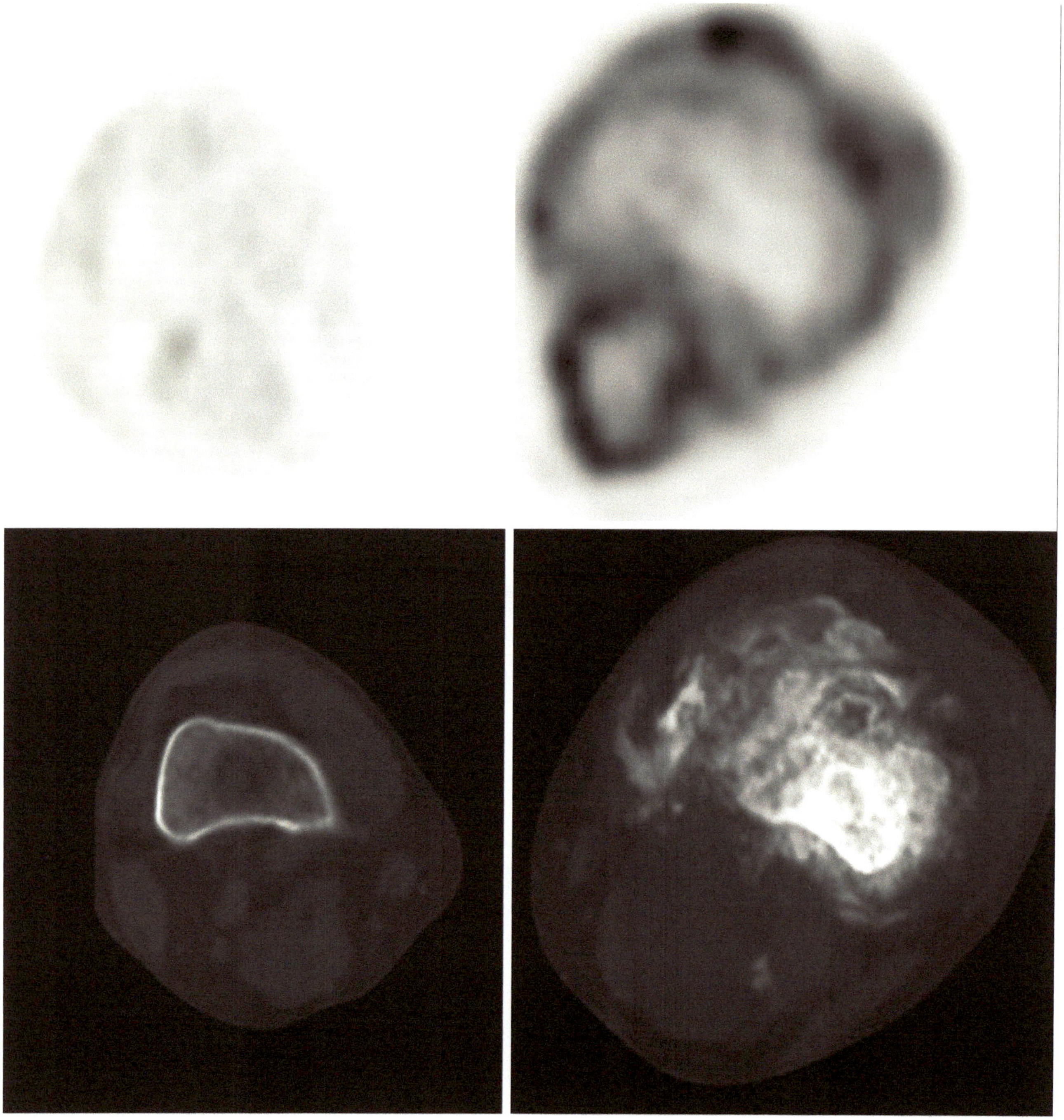

Fig. 16.7 Axial slices of PET and CT images show mass lesion at distal left thigh

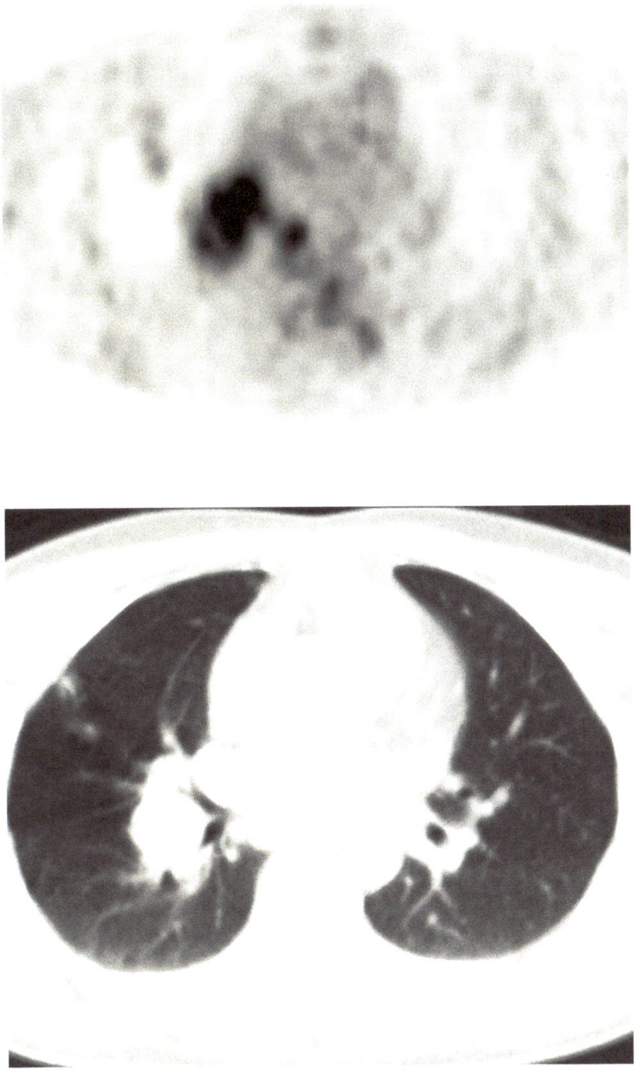

Fig. 16.8 Axial slices of PET and CT images show hypermetabolic mass lesion at right hilus

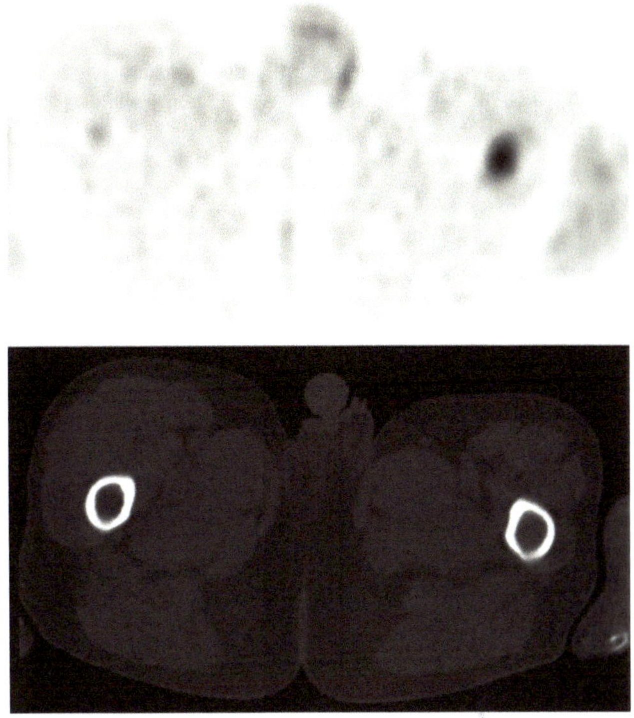

Fig. 16.9 Axial slices of PET and CT images display increased FDG uptake at diaphysis of left femur

16.4 Case 4: Solitary Plasmocytoma

History A 67-year-old male status post cervical vertebral body biopsy proven to be solitary plasmacytoma underwent ^{18}F-FDG PET/CT.

Findings

Interpretation Solitary plasmocytoma involving vertebral body. Moderate FDG uptake at lesion is an expected finding for plasmocytoma.

Teaching Point ^{18}F-FDG PET/ CT has a high performance for initial staging of plasmacytoma (98 % sensitivity, 99 % specificity). It has the advantages of performing whole-body examinations with the ability of detecting medullary and extramedullary lesions in one single examination.

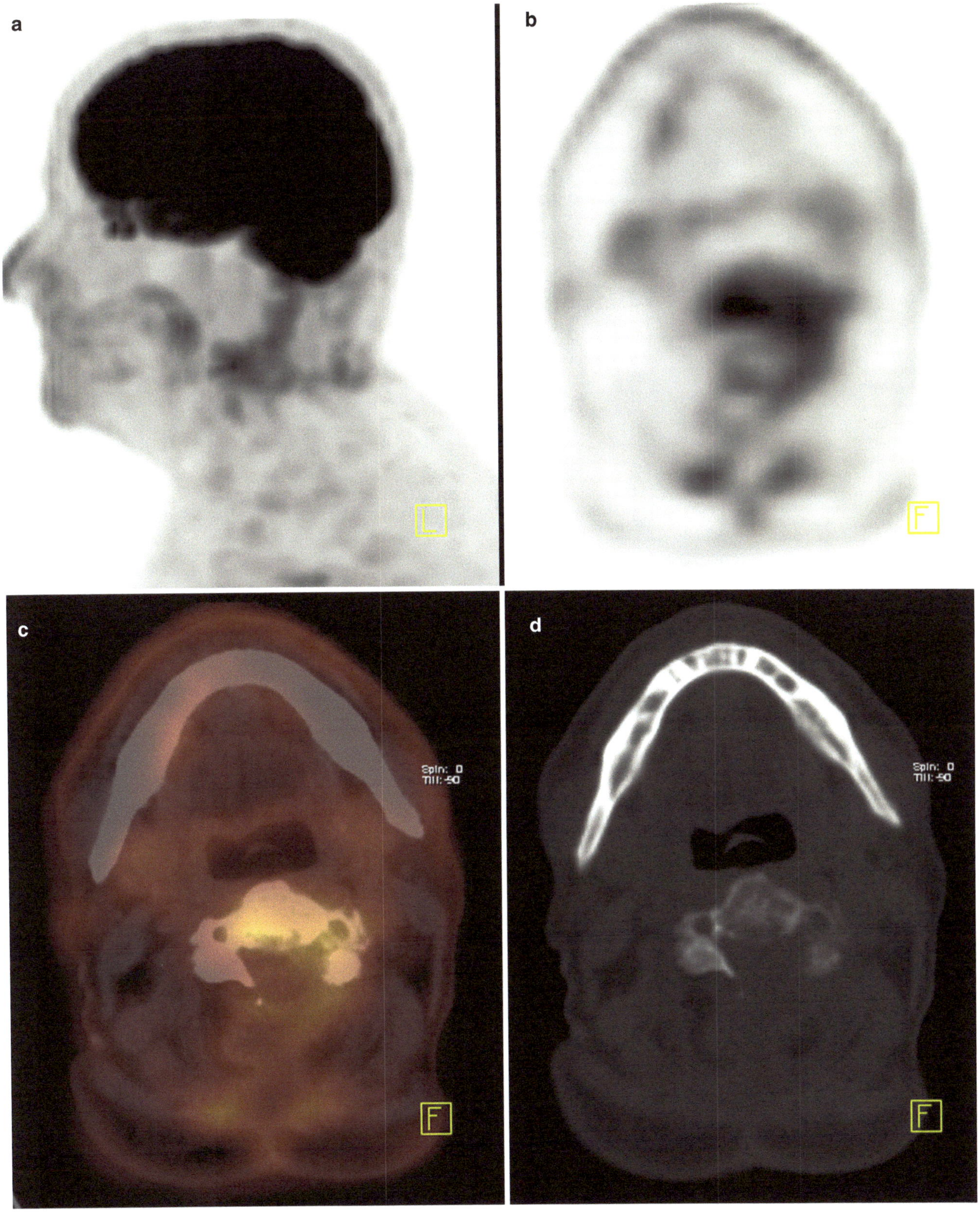

Fig. 16.10 Lateral MIP image (**a**), axial slices of PET, fusion, and CT images (**b–d**) shows moderately hypermetabolic lesion destructing vertebral body and invading posterior elements of vertebra. There is not any other pathological FDG uptake at whole body PET images

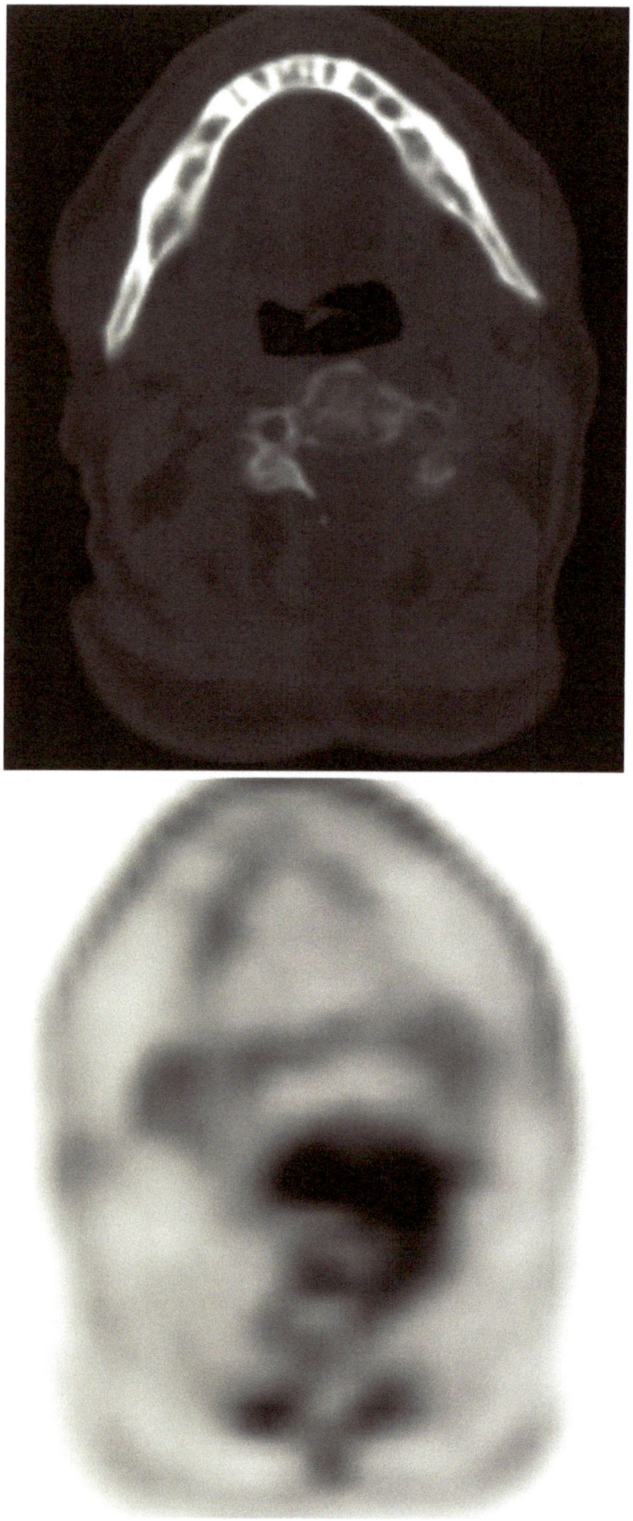

Fig. 16.11 Axial slices of CT and PET display hypermetabolic lesion destructing vertebral body

16.5 Case 5: Plasmocytoma

History A 57-year-old male who had the diagnosis of plasmocytoma underwent ^{18}F-FDG PET/CT for pretreatment staging.

Findings

Interpretation This is consistent with extensive active multiple myeloma.

Teaching Point Solitary plasmocytoma may be a local manifestation of multiple myeloma and ^{18}F-FDG PET CT may detect other unsuspected sites of bone involvement which are overlooked at other conventional imaging methods.

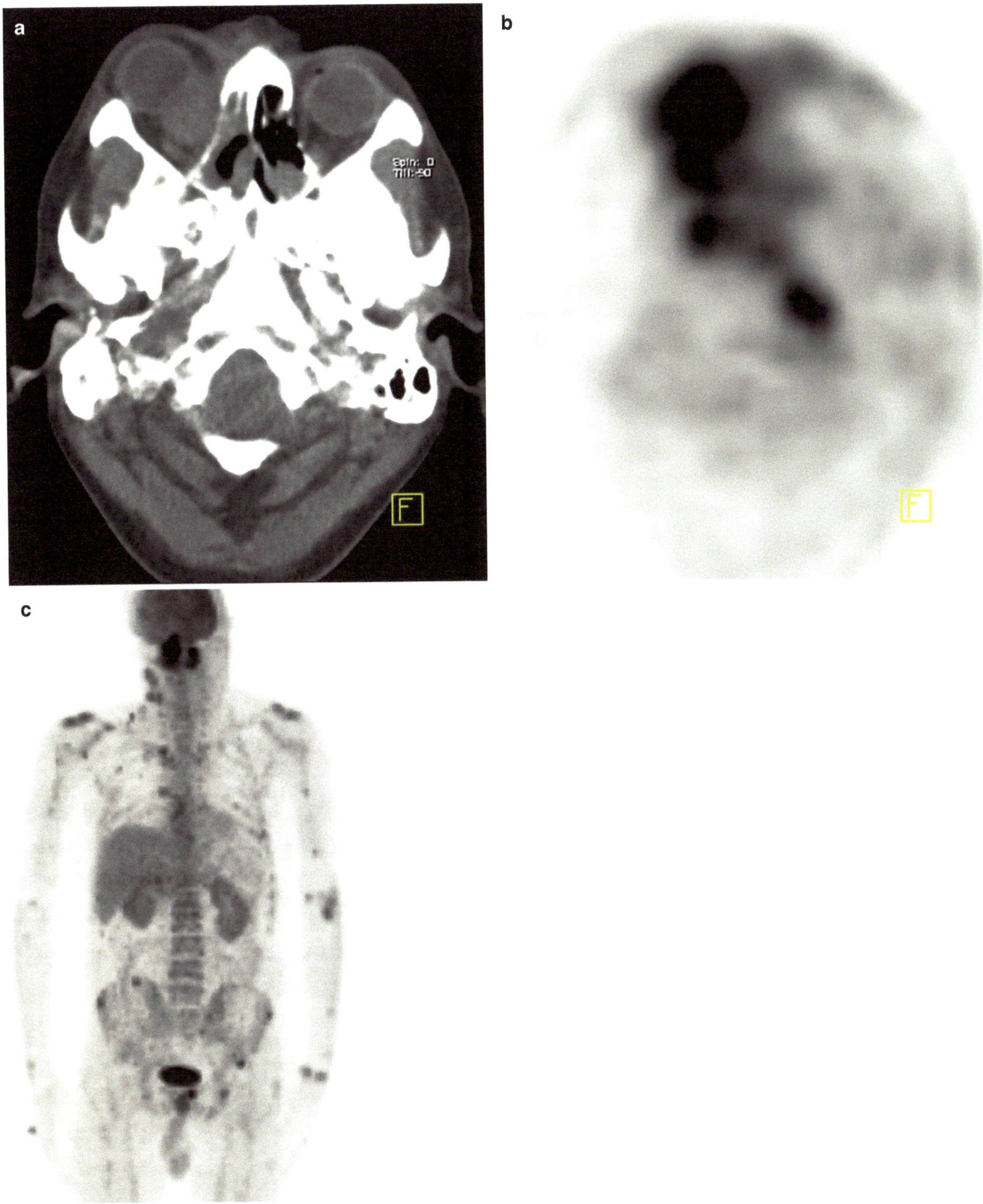

Fig. 16.12 Axial CT and PET images (**a**, **b**) show intensely hypermetabolic soft tissue lesion at right retroorbital area. MIP image (**c**) shows multiple moderately active randomly distributed pathologic hypermetabolic foci within the bony structures

16.6 Case 6: Multiple Myeloma

History: A 63-year-old male who was diagnosed to have multiple myeloma underwent ^{18}F-FDG PET/CT for pretreatment staging.

Findings

Interpretation This is consistent with extensive active multiple myeloma.

Teaching Point ^{18}F-FDG PET CT finds additional unanticipated bone lesions and upstage the patients in 33–43 % of multiple myeloma cases.

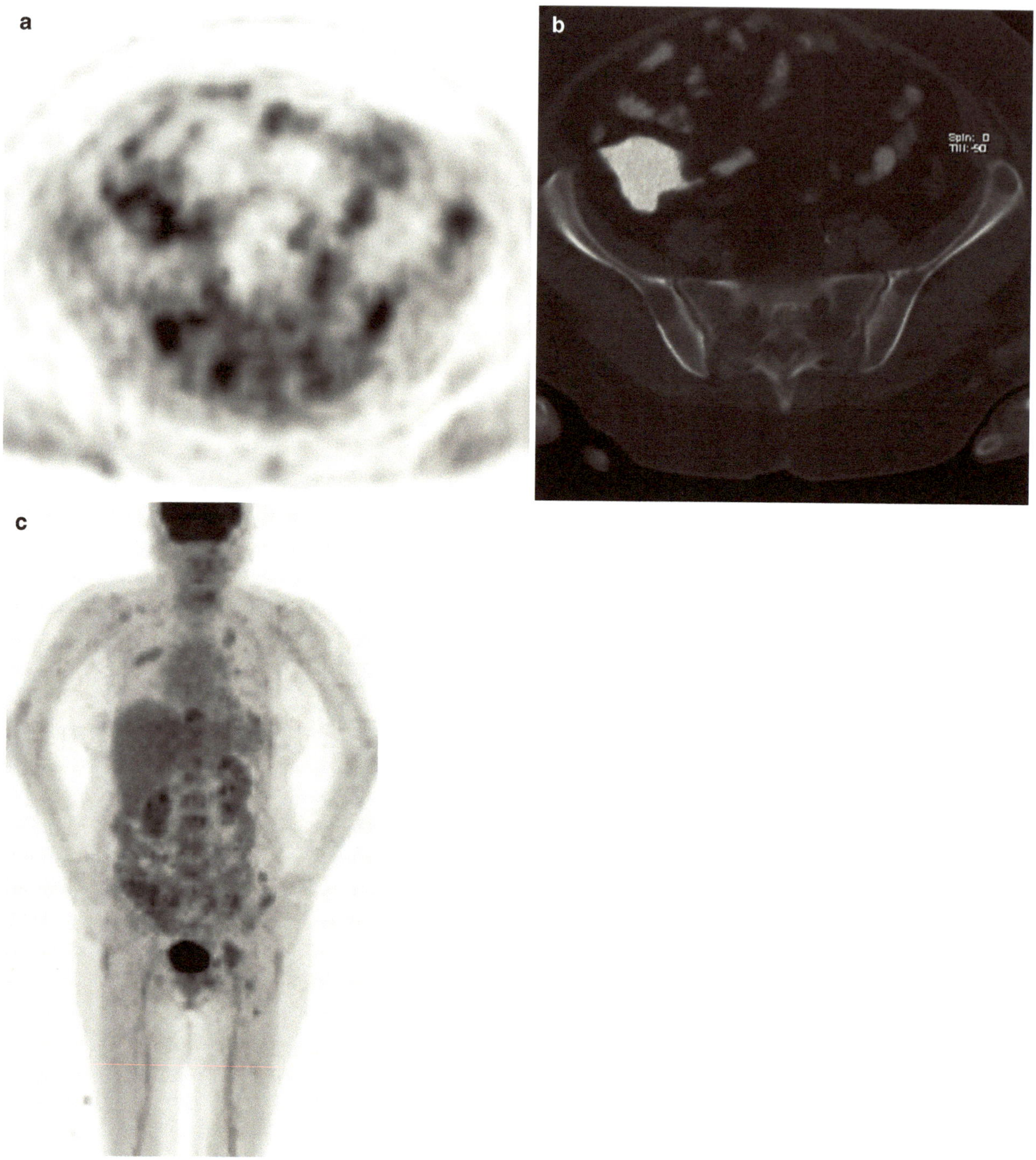

Fig. 16.13 Axial PET and CT images (**a, b**) show intensely hypermetabolic foci corresponding to lytic lesions at pelvic bones. MIP image (**c**) shows numerous foci of increased FDG uptake at bony structures

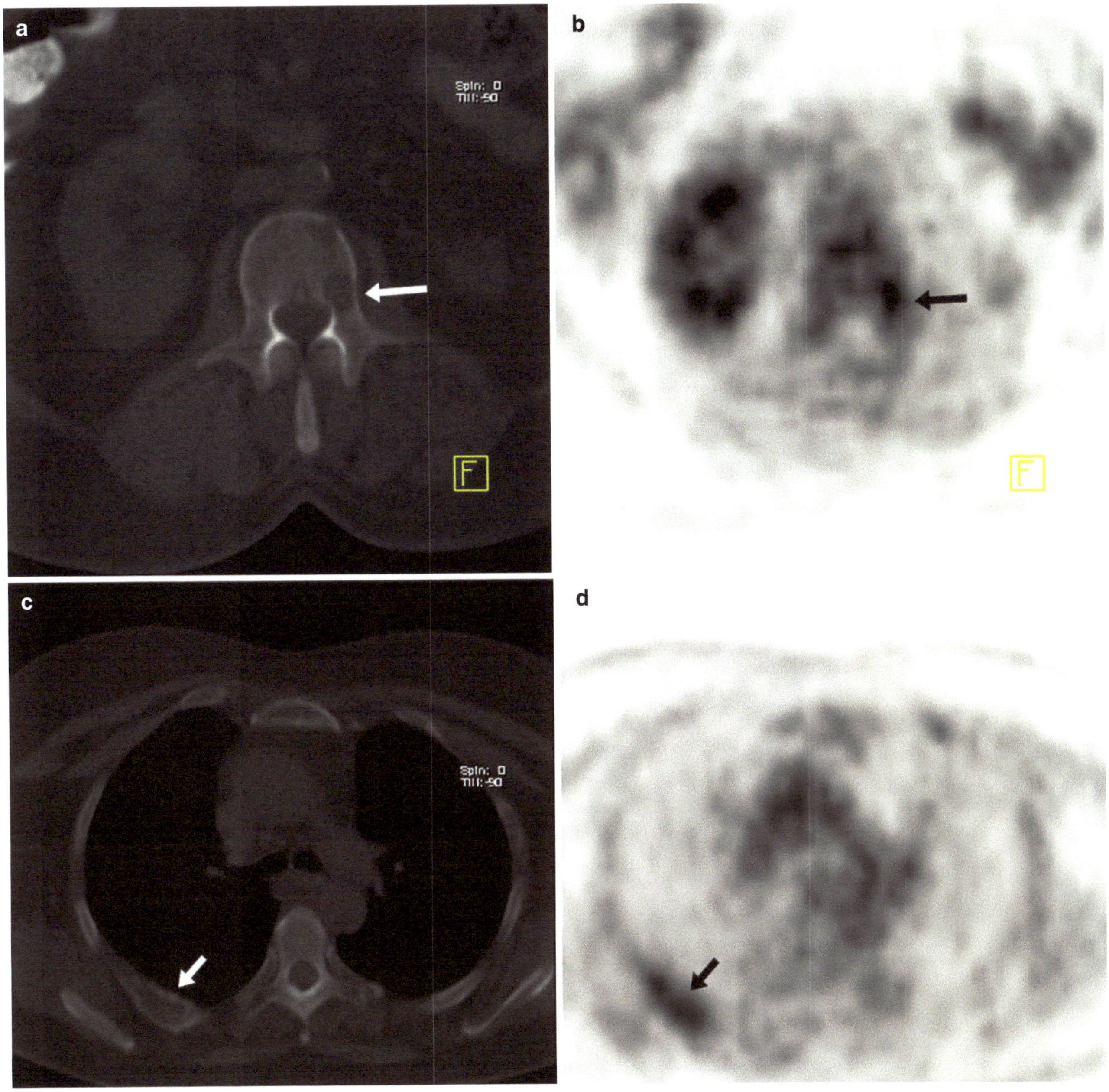

Fig. 16.14 Axial CT and PET images show increased FDG uptake at lytic lesions at vertebral body (**a**, **b**) and rib (**c**, **d**) (*arrows*)

16.7 Case 7: Sacrococcygeal Chordoma

History A 57-year-old female underwent ^{18}F-FDG PET/CT for characterization of sacrococcygeal mass detected on CT.

Findings

Interpretation Although the metabolic activity of the mass is subtle, the lesion is suspicious for malignancy when location and destructive nature is concerned.

Result The patient underwent surgery and histopathology revealed sacrococcygeal chordoma.

Teaching Point Chordoma is a rare malignant bone tumor derived from notochordal rests, and the most common site is the sacrococcygeal region. Chordomas are not FDG avid tumors, so chordoma should be considered when an osteolytic mass in the sacral region on FDG PET/CT is encountered, even if its metabolism is low.

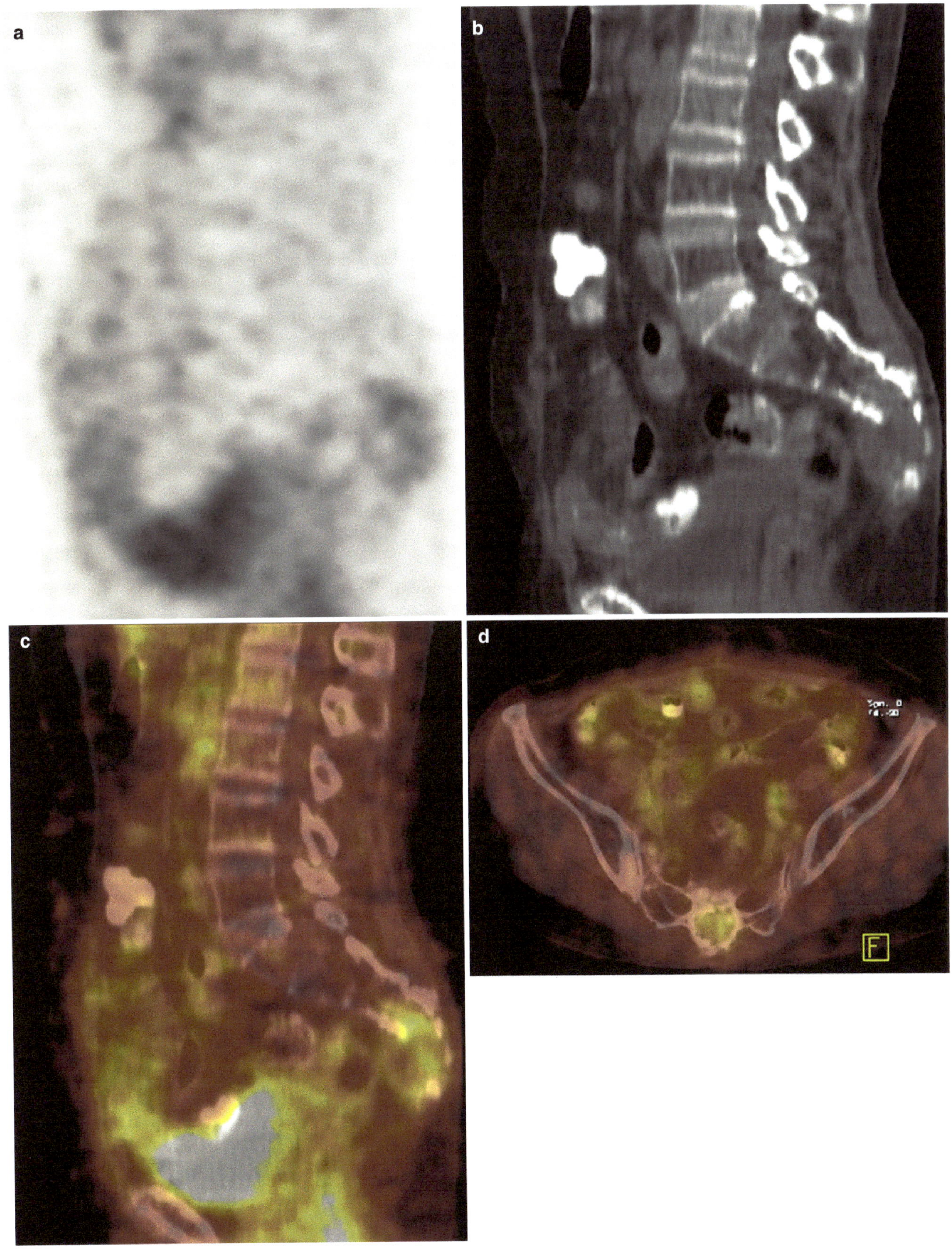

Fig. 16.15 Sagittal PET, CT, fusion (**a–c**) and axial fusion, PET, and CT (**d–f**) images show destructive mass at sacrococcygeal region and faint FDG uptake within the mass is observed

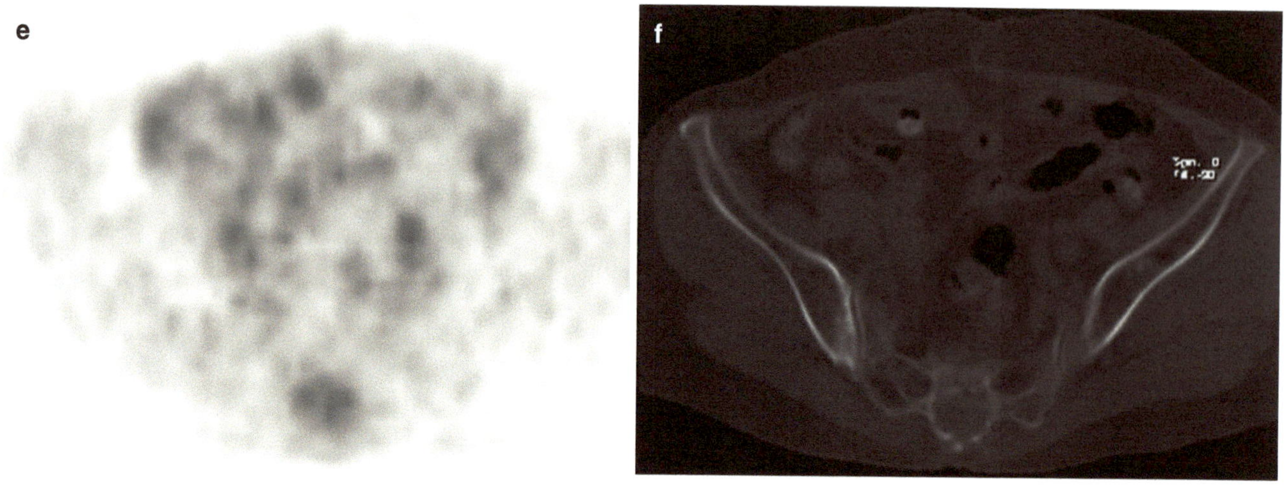

Fig. 16.15 (continued)

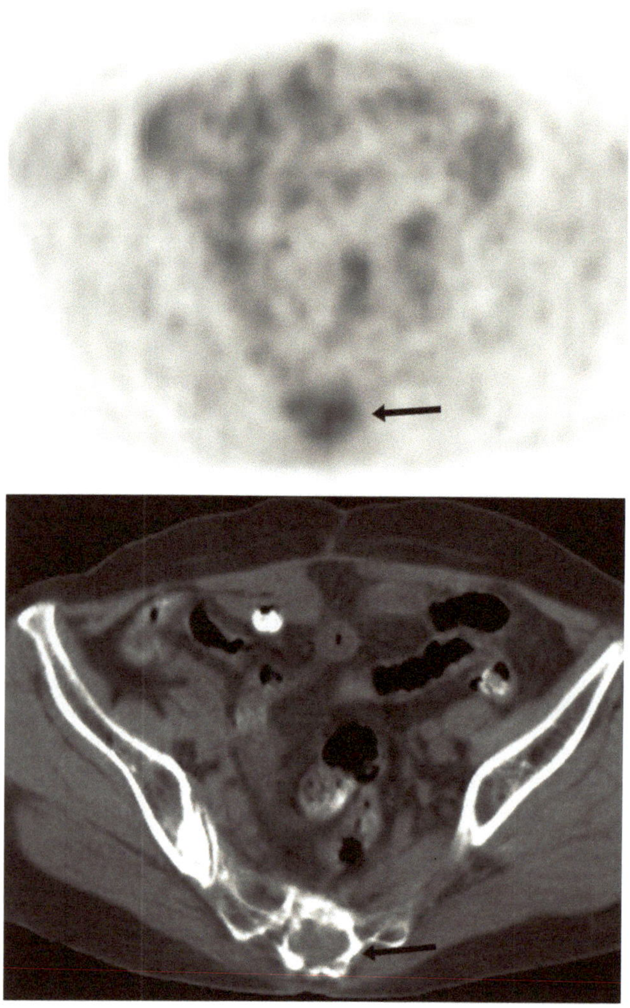

Fig. 16.16 Axial PET and CT images show subtle FDG uptake at sacrococcygeal region accompanying the destructive mass (*arrow*)

16.8 Case 8: Sacrococcygeal Chordoma

History A 65-year-old female who had been diagnosed to have sacrococcygeal chordoma and had received radiotherapy 7 years ago underwent ^{18}F-FDG PET CT for restaging.

Findings

Interpretation Hypermetabolic lesion at sacrum is compatible with recurrent disease and hypermetabolic foci at interaortocaval lymph node station are suggestive of metastatically involved lymph nodes.

Teaching Point Although radiotherapy is successful in terms of providing recurrence-free survival, these tumors are still associated with a high rate of recurrence, mostly being local. ^{18}F-FDG PET CT imaging has been proven successful in restaging of chordoma as well as monitoring the efficacy of radiotherapy.

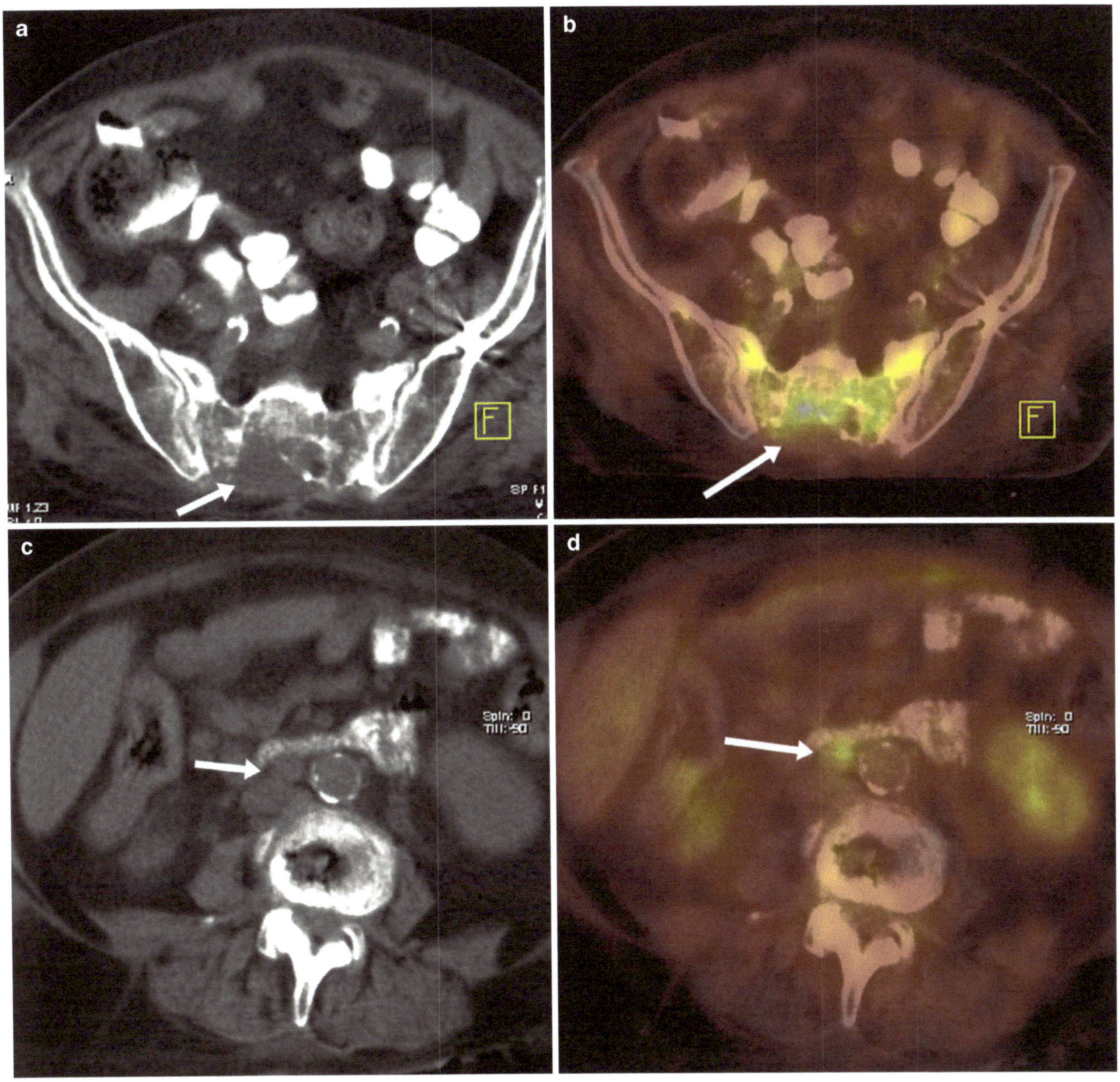

Fig. 16.17 Axial CT and fusion images (**a**, **b**) show destructive moderately hypermetabolic (SUVmax 6.5) mass lesion at sacrum (*arrow*), and hypermetabolic interaortocaval lymph nodes at the level of L3 vertebra (*arrow*) (**c**, **d**) (SUVmax 5.9)

16.9 Case 9: Therapy Response in Bone Metastases

History A 64-year-old male patient status post transbronchial biopsy diagnosed to have small cell lung cancer underwent ^{18}F-FDG PET/CT scan in order to identify any possible distant metastasis and complete the staging procedure. After the patient received six courses of chemotherapy a repeat ^{18}F-FDG PET/CT was performed for evaluation of therapy response.

Findings

Interpretation The FDG avid lesions in the skeletal system, which were not sclerotic initially, were transformed into FDG nonavid sclerotic lesions after chemotherapy. This was attributed to the direct effect of previous successful therapy for bone metastases, leading to the transformation of metabolically active disease, into blastic metabolically inactive metastases.

Teaching Point A ^{18}F-FDG negative bone lesion, which is sclerotic on CT, may represent posttreatment osteoblastic change rather than active tumor and BS might play a role in the discrimination of these two situations.

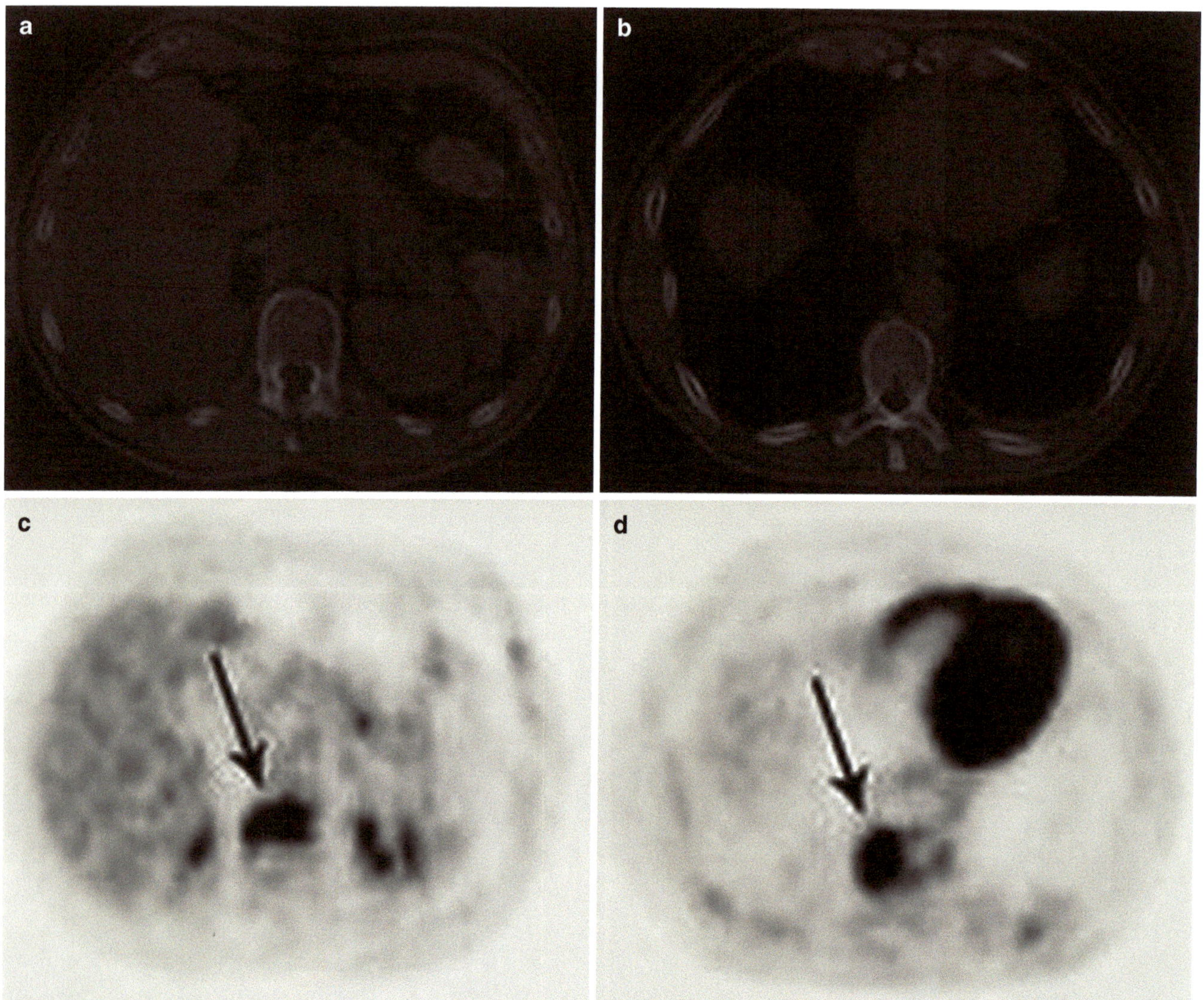

Fig. 16.18 Axial slices of PET and CT images from ^{18}F-FDG PET/CT scan show pathologically increased FDG uptake at dorsal vertebrae (*arrows*) (**a–d**) without any corresponding lytic or sclerotic lesion on CT images

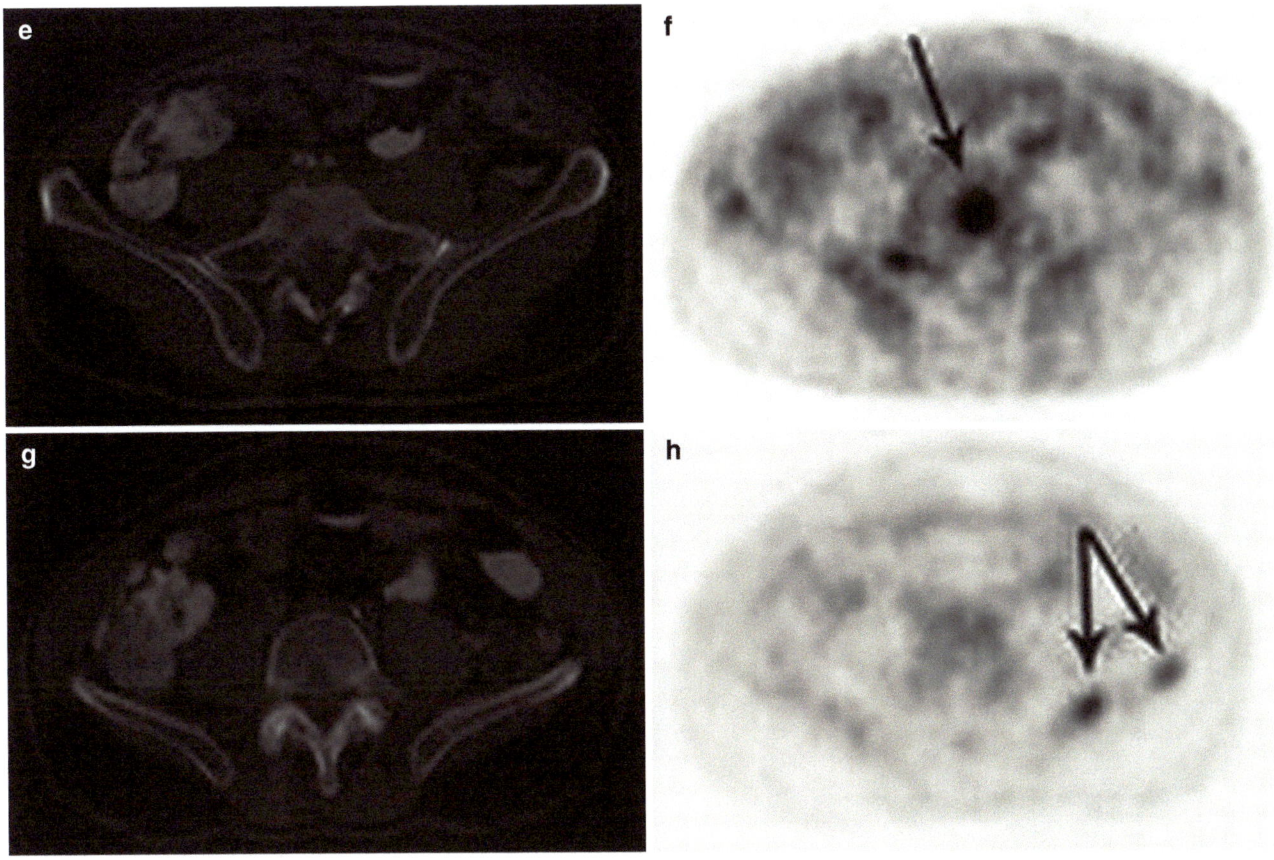

Fig. 16.19 Axial slices of PET and CT images from ^{18}F-FDG PET/CT scan show pathologically increased FDG uptake at L5 vertebra and left iliac wing (*arrows*) (**a–d**) without any corresponding lytic or sclerotic lesion on CT images

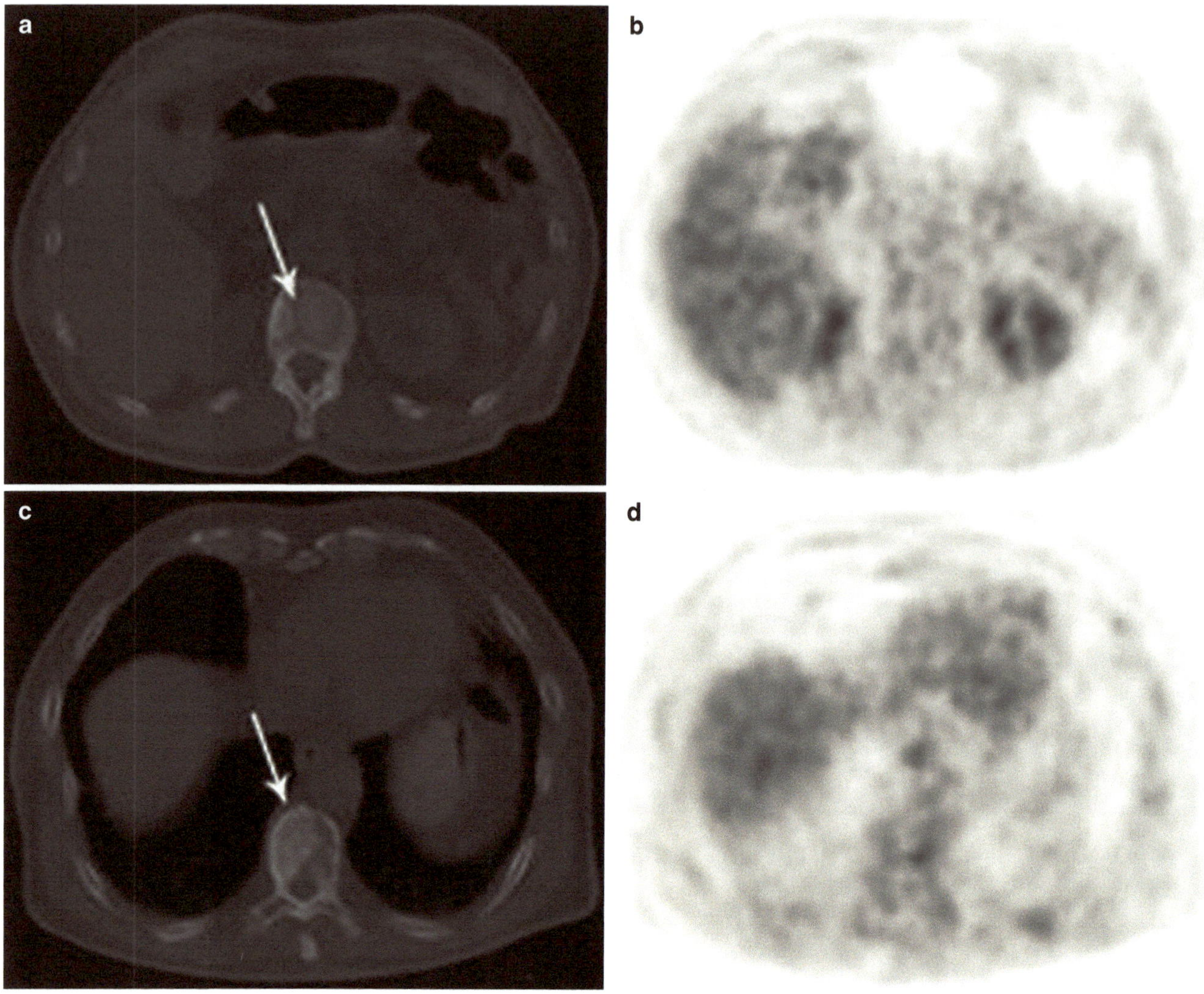

Fig. 16.20 ^{18}F-FDG PET CT scan after completion of therapy shows disappearance of FDG uptake at dorsal vertebrae but development of sclerotic lesions at the previous hypermetabolic sites (*arrows*) (**a**–**d**)

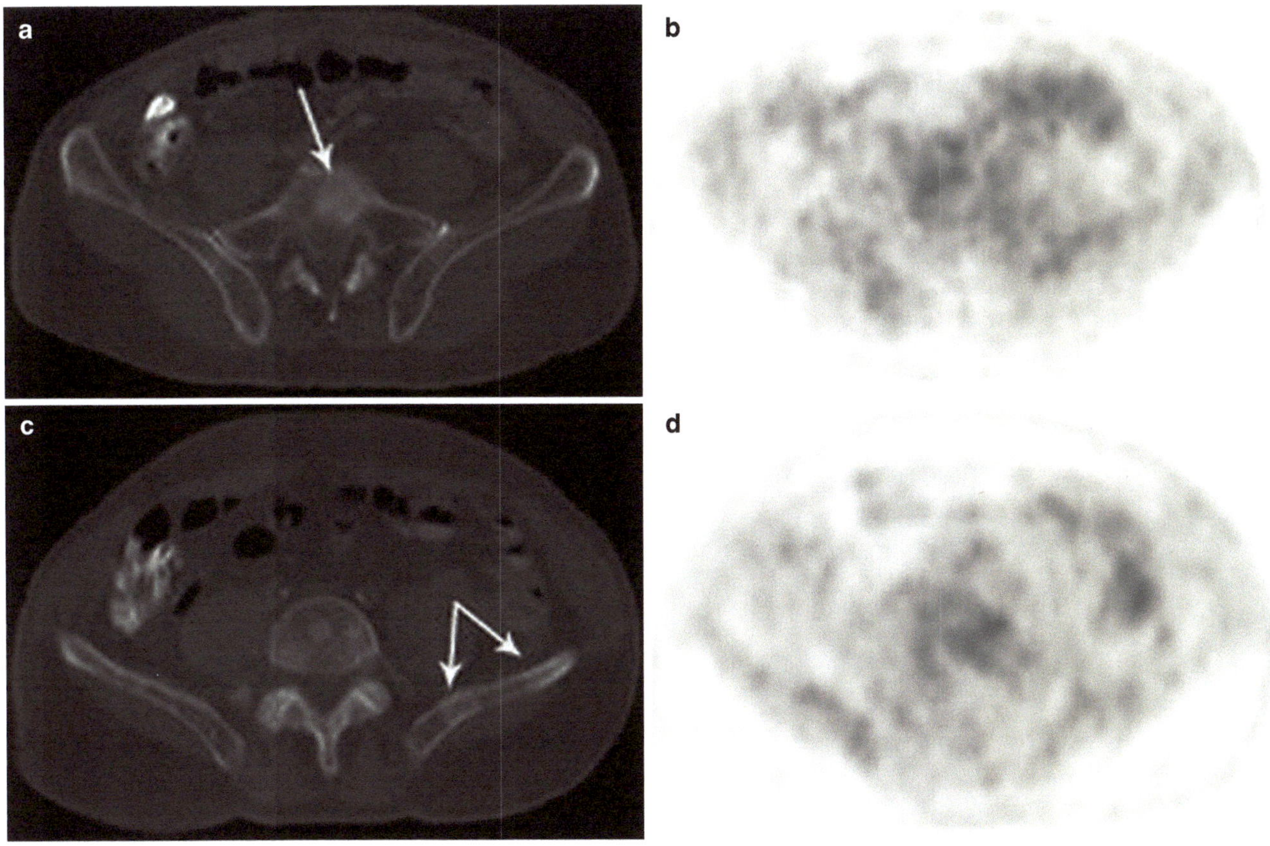

Fig. 16.21 ^{18}F-FDG PET CT scan after completion of therapy shows disappearance of FDG uptake at L5 vertebra and left iliac wing, but development of sclerotic lesions at the previous hypermetabolic sites (*arrows*) (**a**–**d**)

16.10 Case 10: Fibrosarcoma

History A 46-year-old female presented with a huge mass at right anterolateral abdominal region underwent ^{18}F-FDG PET/CT scan.

Findings

Interpretation The low FDG activity at lesion does not exclude malignancy because low grade sarcomas might not show significant FDG uptake.

Result Histopathology revealed fibrosarcoma.

Teaching Point ^{18}F-FDG PET/CT is a useful imaging modality in the evaluation of primary soft-tissue lesions. But it may not always distinguish low-grade tumors from benign lesions.

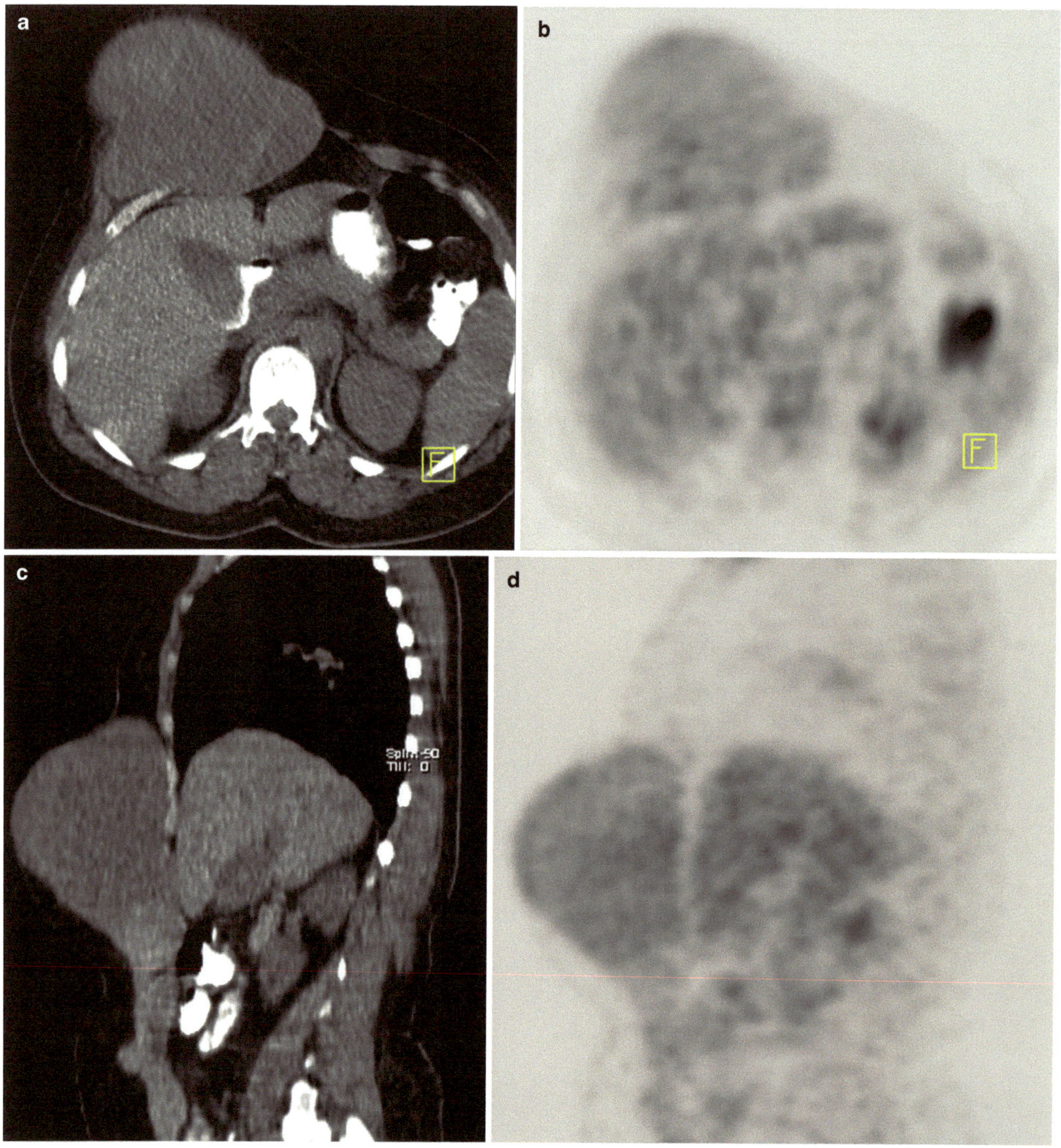

Fig. 16.22 Axial (**a**, **b**) and sagittal (**c**, **d**) slices of CT and PET images show faintly increased FDG uptake at mass lesion originating from right anterolateral abdominal wall. There is not any other pathological FDG uptake at rest of the body

16.11 Case 11: Staging of Synovial Sarcoma

History A 61-year-old male was diagnosed to have fusiform cell synovial sarcoma after a biopsy from mass lesion at left ankle. ^{18}F-FDG PET/CT is performed for the evaluation of the extent of the disease.

Findings

Interpretation This finding is consistent with primary malignancy.

Teaching Point There is a possible correlation between SUVmax values and patient survival in synovial sarcoma. In a study patients with synovial sarcoma presenting with a pre-therapy SUVmax greater than 4.35 were found to have an overall decreased survival.

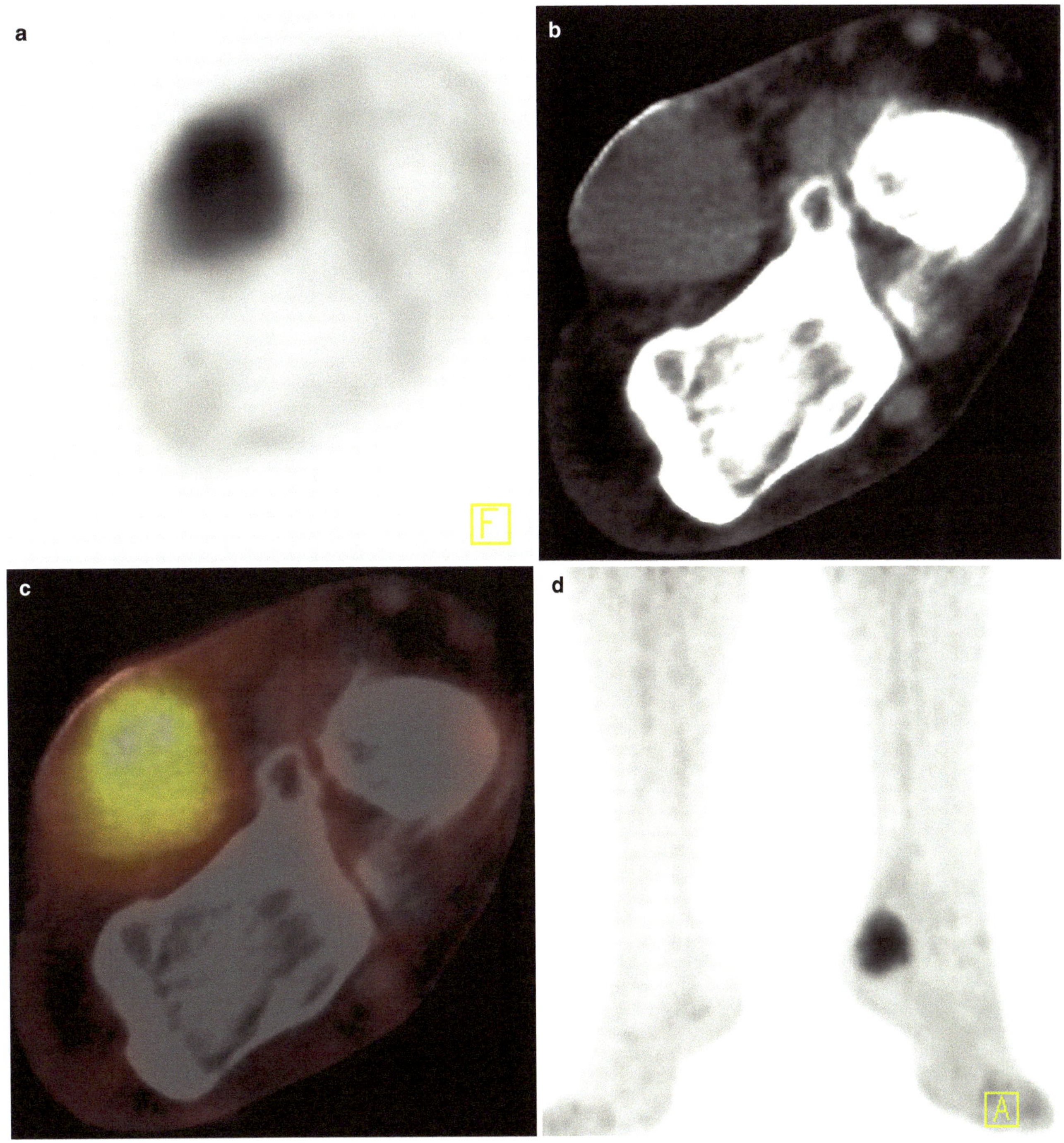

Fig. 16.23 Axial PET, CT, fusion (**a**, **b**, **c**) and MIP (**d**) images show a moderately hypermetabolic (SUVmax 4.7) mass lesion of soft tissue density measuring 40×37×32 mm at medial left ankle. There is no pathological FDG uptake other than this lesion

16.12 Case 12: Staging of Synovial Sarcoma

History A 67-year-old female was diagnosed to have synovial sarcoma after a biopsy from mass lesion at left distal thigh. ^{18}F-FDG PET/CT is performed for the evaluation of the extent of the disease.

Findings

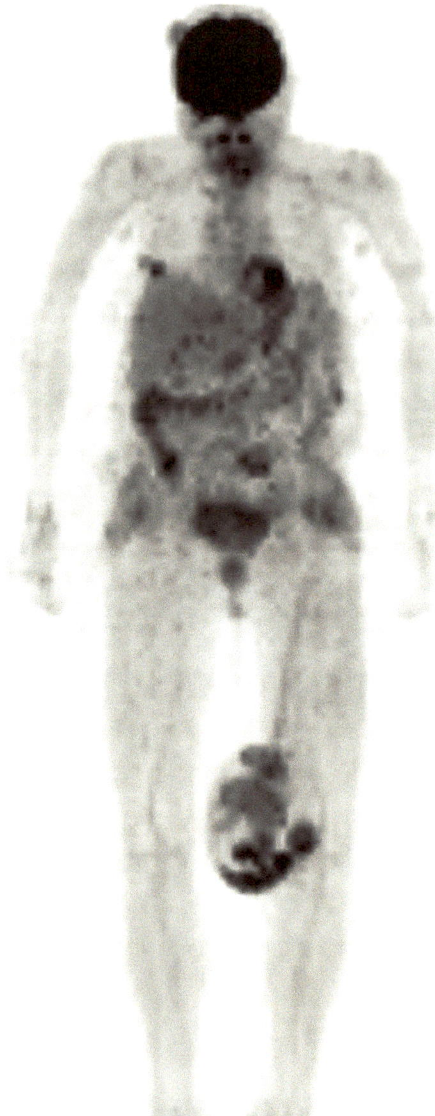

Fig. 16.24 MIP image shows mass lesion at left distal thigh with heterogenous FDG uptake. There are also hypermetabolic foci anteriorly at right hemithorax and right side of cranium

Interpretation Mass lesion at left distal thigh is consistent with primary malignancy. There is also local invasion to medial condyle of distal femur. The lesions at scalp, right thorax, and right lung represent metastasis.

Teaching Point Synovial sarcoma occurs most commonly in the lower extremities; presents as a large, well-circumscribed mass adjacent to joints, often with punctuate calcifications. It has a propensity for metastasis, most commonly to lung. These tumors are highly FDG-avid; locoregional and distant metastatic spread may be easily detected on whole body PET. FDG PET/CT is also effective in guiding biopsy by showing the most metabolically active part of the tumor.

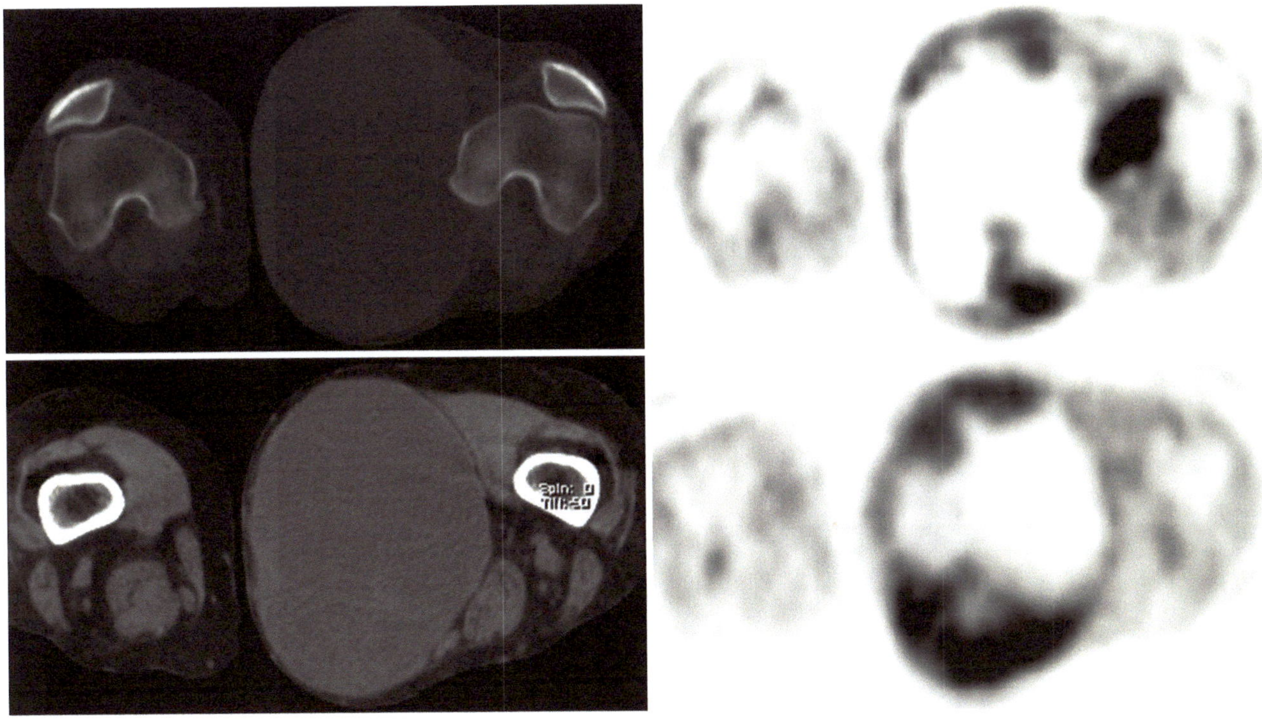

Fig. 16.25 Axial slices of CT and PET images show a mass lesion of soft tissue density at medial side of left distal thigh, with an hypometabolic center and moderately increased FDG uptake at periphery (SUVmax 3.4). Hypermetabolism at medial condyle of distal femur is also noted (SUVmax 3.4)

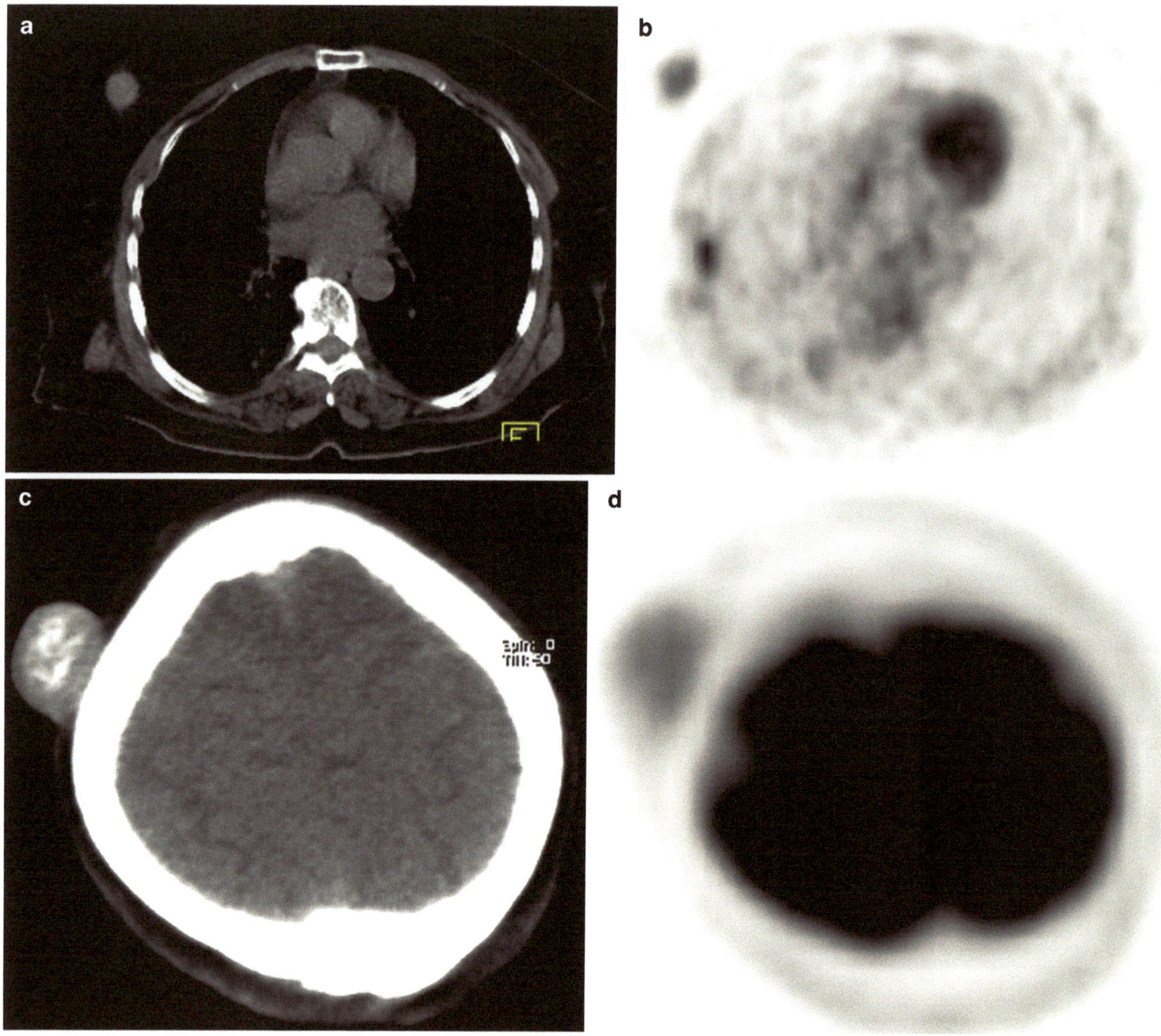

Fig. 16.26 Axial slices of CT and PET images from thorax (**a**, **b**) show hypermetabolic soft tissue lesion subcutaneously located at right anterior hemithorax. There is a mildly hypermetabolic soft tissue lesion with central calcifications in it, located at scalp of right anterior side of head (**c**, **d**)

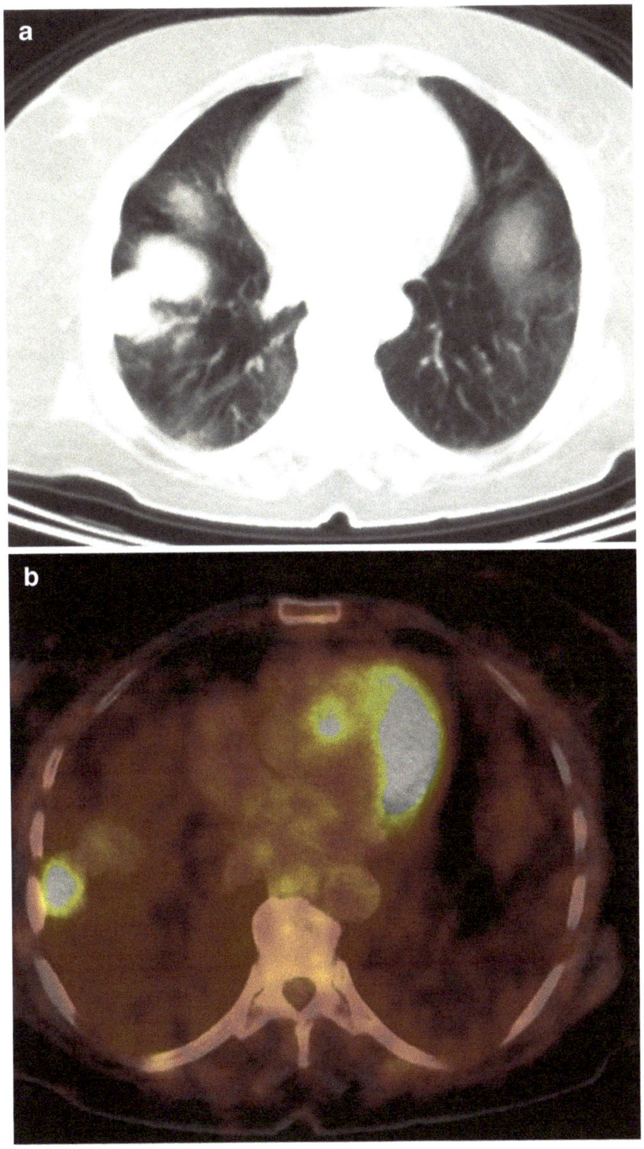

Fig. 16.27 Axial slices of CT and fusion images from thorax (**a**, **b**) show hypermetabolic pulmonary nodule at lower lobe of right lung (SUVmax 5.6)

16.13 Case 13: Staging of Liposarcoma

History A 56-year-old male presented with a retroperitoneal mass lesion was diagnosed to have liposarcoma after a tru-cut biopsy. The patient underwent ^{18}F-FDG PET/CT scan for staging.

Findings

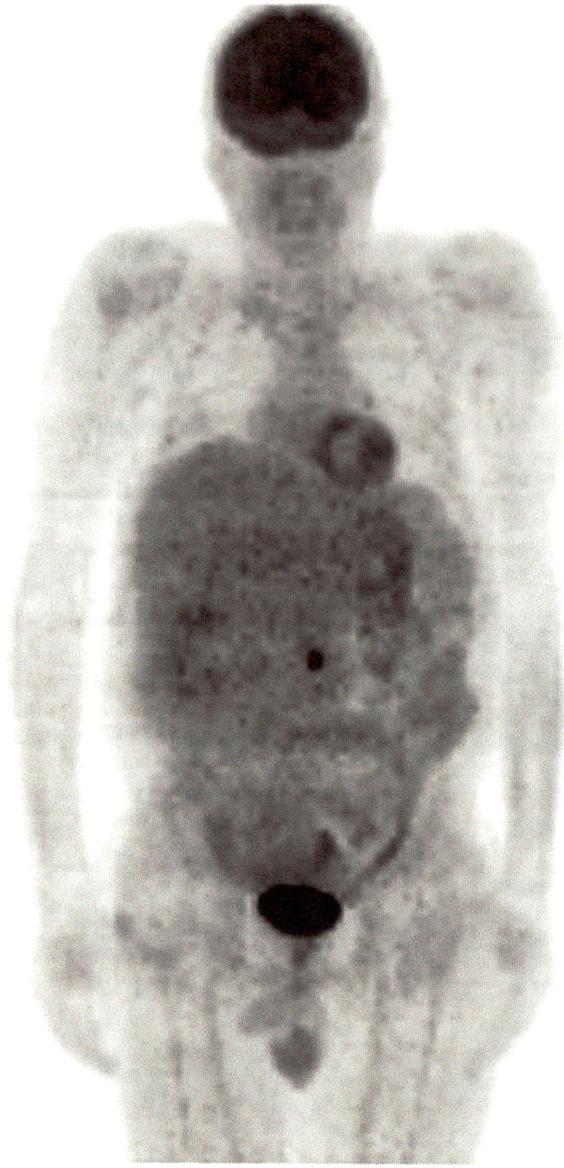

Fig. 16.28 MIP image shows faintly increased diffuse FDG uptake at right side of the abdomen, almost equal to liver uptake in intensity. A focal increased FDG uptake at midline of abdomen is also noted (SUVmax 6.8)

Interpretation Mass lesion at right side of the abdomen represents a low grade liposarcoma without FDG affinity. Hypermetabolic retroperitoneal lymph node is a suspicious finding, since it is not usual for a lymph node to show high FDG uptake when the primary lesion is not FDG avid.

Teaching Point ^{18}F-FDG PET/CT is not effective in well-differentiated liposarcoma which is not FDG avid, but may show relatively higher uptake at dedifferentiated liposarcoma.

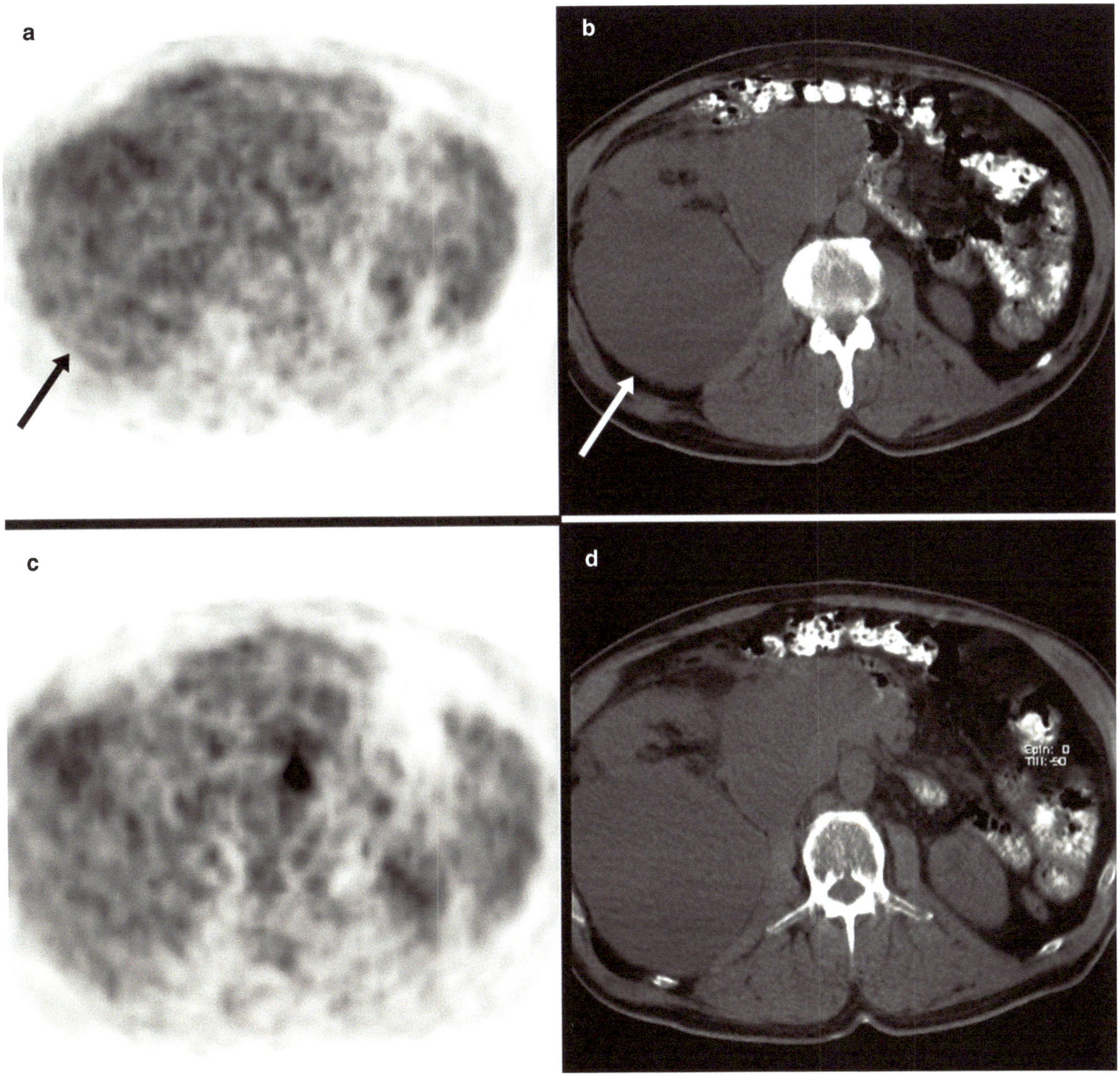

Fig. 16.29 Axial slices of PET and CT images (**a**, **b**) show a hypodense mass lesion measuring 22 × 11 × 10 cm at right side of abdomen (*arrow*). The mass lesion shows faint FDG uptake but there is a hypermetabolic focus corresponding a retroperitoneal lymph node (**c**, **d**)

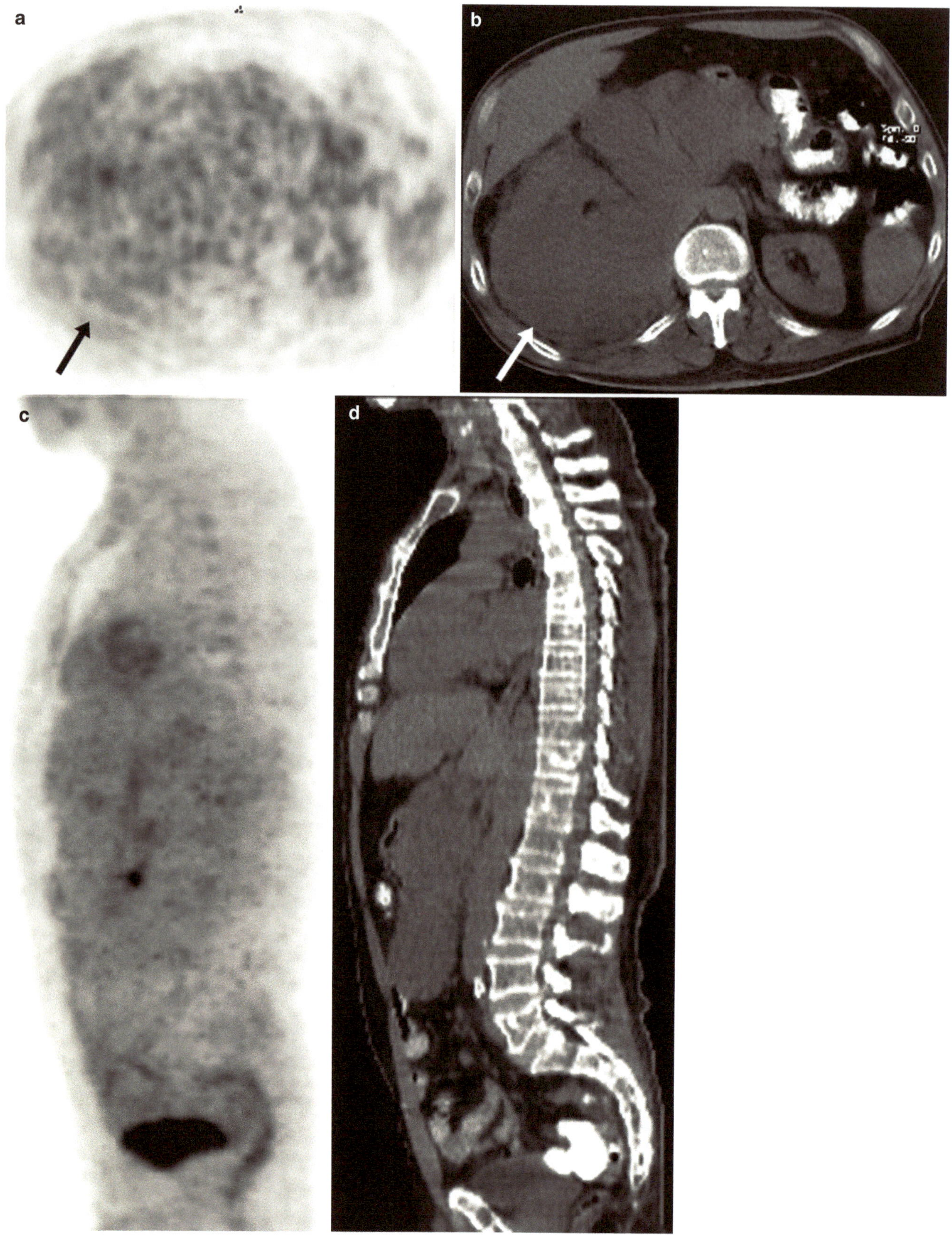

Fig. 16.30 Axial (**a**, **b**) and sagittal (**c**, **d**) images show mass lesion with low FDG uptake (*arrow*) and focal hypermetabolic retroperitoneal lymph node

16.14 Case 14: Lymphangiosarcoma

History A 60-year-old female who had lymphedema of right arm which is developed after right mastectomy performed for beast carcinoma underwent ^{18}F-FDG PET/CT scan for restaging.

Findings

Interpretation Multiple hypermetabolic foci that are detected at subcutaneous tissues of the right arm is not compatible with the usual metastatic spread pattern of breast carcinoma. These lesions deserve histopathological verification.

Result Biopsy from the lesion at right elbow revealed lymphangiosarcoma.

Teaching Point Lymphangiosarcoma is a rare vascular neoplasm which develops as a complication in patients suffering from chronic lymphedema of the upper limb following mastectomy and axillary lymph node dissection for breast cancer (Stewart-Treves syndrome). It may also arise in chronic congenital lymphedema.

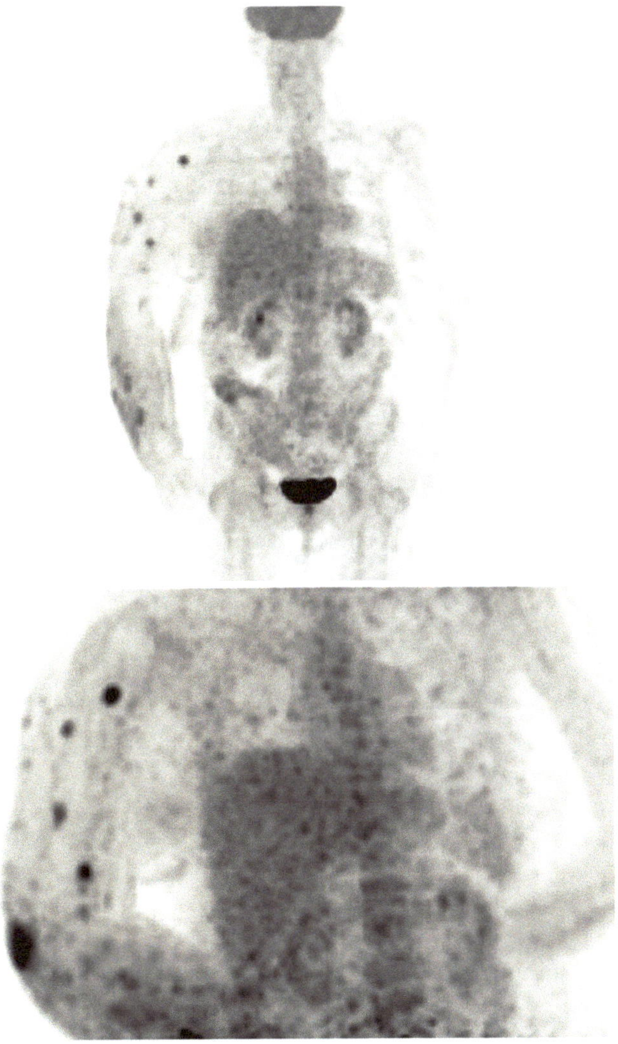

Fig. 16.31 MIP image shows several foci of FDG uptake at right arm. The swelling at right arm due to lymphedema is noted

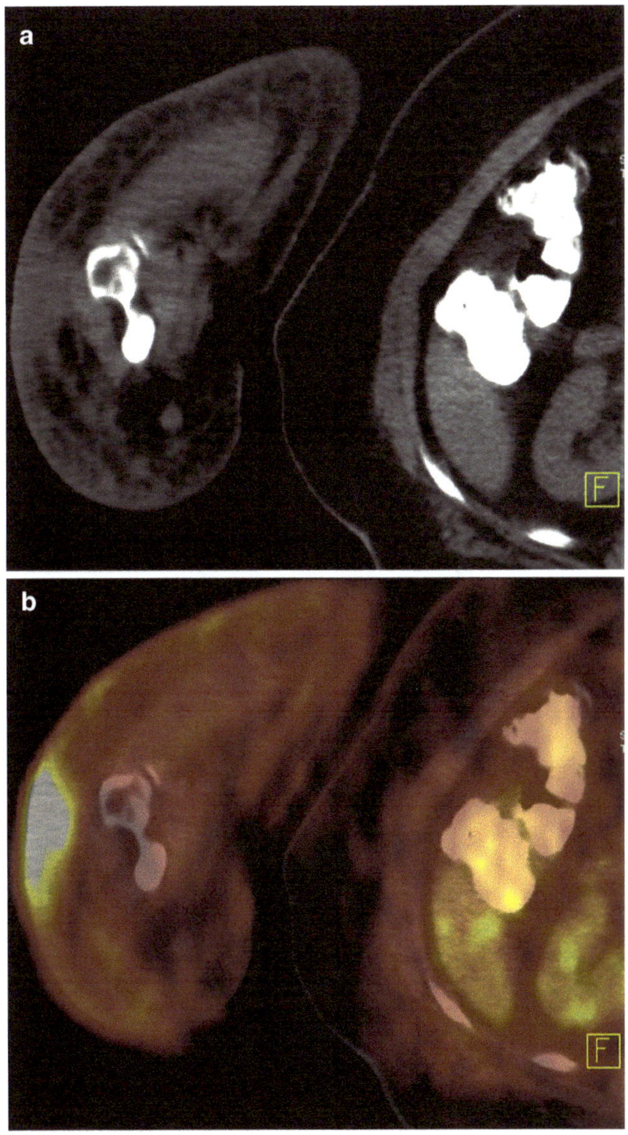

Fig. 16.32 Axial slices of CT and fusion images (**a**, **b**) show a hypermetabolic subcutaneous soft tissue density at right elbow

16.15 Case 15: Liposarcoma

History A 53-year-old female had the diagnosis of low grade myxoid liposarcoma after a biopsy from a retroperitoneal mass lesion. ^{18}F-FDG PET/CT was performed for staging and then the patient underwent surgical excision of the mass lesion followed by chemotherapy. Nine months after the completion of therapy a second ^{18}F-FDG PET/CT scan was performed.

Findings

Interpretation Mesenteric low grade myxoid liposarcoma which shows partial response to therapy.

Teaching Point According to NCCN 2014 guideline PET scan can be used in prognostication, grading, and determined histopathological response to chemotherapy for firm and deep lesions larger than 3 cm in patients with high grade extremity soft tissue sarcoma. There is only one case of mesenteric myxoid liposarcoma on ^{18}F-FDG PET/CT reported in the literature up to now. While evaluating patients with liposarcoma on ^{18}F-FDG PET/CT, the low FDG avidity of these lesions should be taken into account and the tissues which are rich in fat should be evaluated carefully for hypodense metastases.

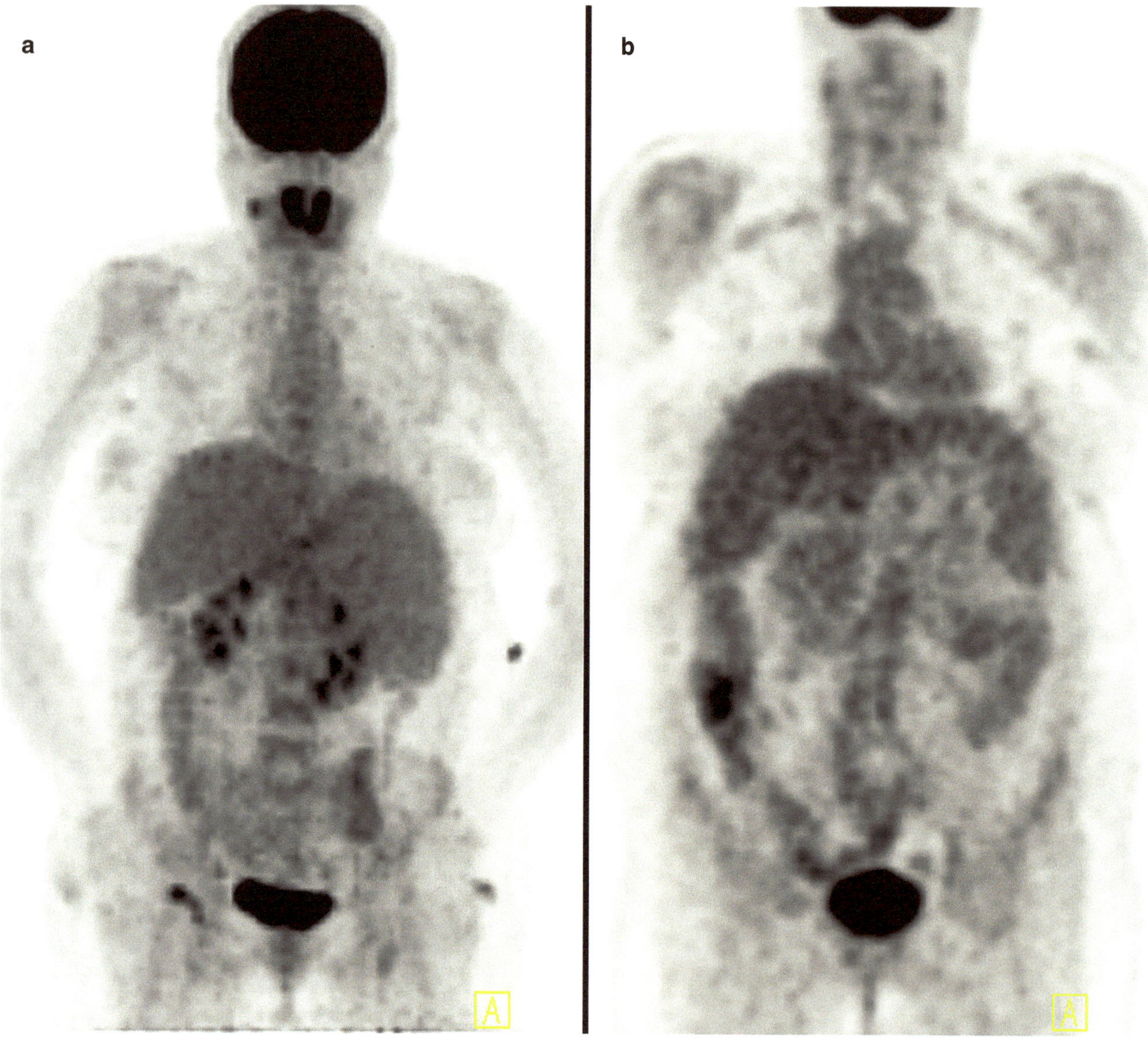

Fig. 16.33 MIP image before therapy (**a**) shows diffuse FDG uptake at the mass lesion located at left upper abdomen, with the intensity of the FDG uptake being almost equal to the liver (SUVmax 7.7). The lesion is smaller and shows less FDG uptake in the second MIP image (SUVmax 2.5) (**b**) that belongs to the study performed after therapy

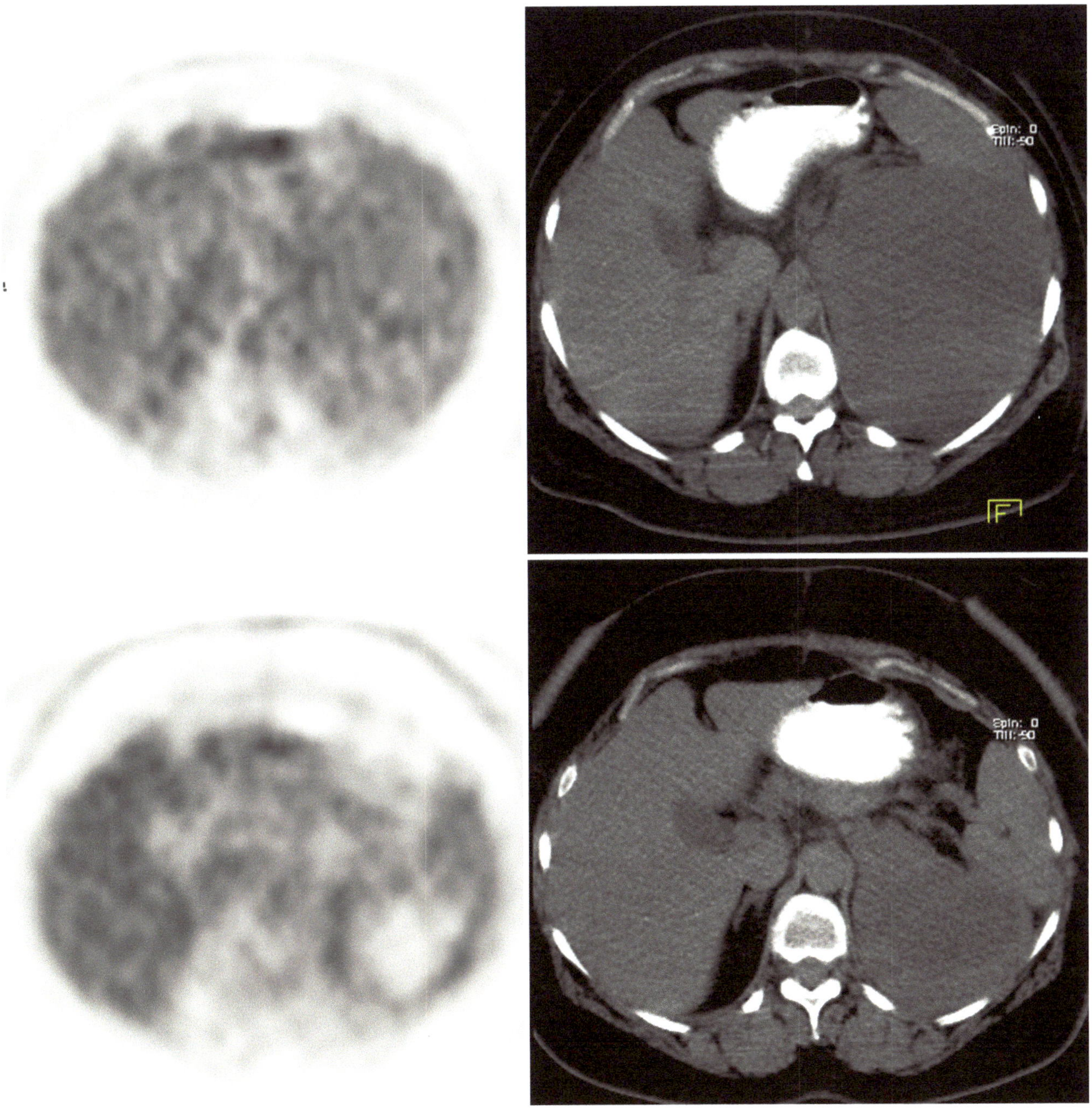

Fig. 16.34 Axial slices of PET and CT images before therapy shows the slightly hypermetabolic mass lesion at left side of abdomen which displaces the spleen anteriorly. The images after the therapy displays the decrease in size of the mass. The intensity of FDG uptake is also lesser and a hypometabolic necrotic center at mass is noted

Bibliography

1. Bakri A, Shinagare AB, Krajewski KM, Howard SA, Jagannathan JP, Hornick JL, et al. Synovial sarcoma: imaging features of common and uncommon primary sites, metastatic patterns, and treatment response. AJR Am J Roentgenol. 2012;199:208–15. doi:10.2214/AJR.11.8039.
2. Franzius C, Daldrup-Link HE, Sciuk J, Rummeny EJ, Bielack S, Jürgens H, et al. FDG-PET for detection of pulmonary metastases from malignant primary bone tumors: comparison with spiral CT. Ann Oncol. 2001;12:479–86.
3. Franzius C, Sciuk J, Daldrup-Link HE, Jürgens H, Schober O. FDG-PET for detection of osseous metastases from malignant primary bone tumours: comparison with bone scintigraphy. Eur J Nucl Med. 2000;27:1305–11.
4. Halaç M, Zincirkeser S, Sönmezoğlu K, Sağer S, Dervişoğlu S, Uslu İ. Diagnosis of a giant sacral chordoma by FDG-PET. Turk J Nucl Med. 2006;15:78–80.
5. Kara PO, Gedik GK, Sari O, Kara T, Yilmaz F. FDG-PET/CT imaging in a patient with lymphangiosarcoma. Clin Nucl Med. 2010;35:428–9. doi:10.1097/RLU.0b013e3181db4d0f.
6. Lisle JW, Eary JF, O'Sullivan J, Conrad EU. Risk assessment based on FDG-PET imaging in patients with synovial sarcoma. Clin Orthop Relat Res. 2009;467:1605–11. doi:10.1007/s11999-008-0647-z.
7. Nanni C, Rubello D, Zamagni E, Castellucci P, Ambrosini V, Montini G, et al. 18F-FDG PET/CT in myeloma with presumed solitary plasmocytoma of bone. In Vivo. 2008;22:513–7.
8. Newman EN, Jones RL, Hawkins DS. An evaluation of [F-18]-fluorodeoxy-D-glucose positron emission tomography, bone scan, and bone marrow aspiration/biopsy as staging investigations in Ewing sarcoma. Pediatr Blood Cancer. 2013;60:1113–7.
9. Ozguven S, Aras M, Inanir S. Mesenteric metastases of purely myxoid liposarcoma: an unusual behavior of primary tumor depicted on fludeoxyglucose positron emission tomography/computerized tomography. Indian J Nucl Med. 2015;30:82–3. doi:10.4103/0972-3919.147556.
10. Ozülker T, Ozülker F, Küçüköz Uzun A, Tatoğlu T, Ozpaçacı T. Evaluation of response to therapy in a patient with lung cancer: correlation of sclerotic bone lesions with F 18 FDG PET/CT and bone scintigraphy. Mol Imaging Radionucl Ther. 2011;20:29–33. doi:10.4274/MIRT.20.06.
11. Sabet A, Ahmadzadehfar H, Huertos Lopez FJ, Muckle M, Schmiedel A, Biersack HJ, et al. Detection of chordoma recurrence by F-18 FDG-PET/CT. Iran J Radiat Res. 2012;10:109–10.
12. Salaun PY, Gastinne T, Frampas E, Bodet-Milin C, Moreau P, Bodéré-Kraeber F. FDG-positron-emission tomography for staging and therapeutic assessment in patients with plasmacytoma. Haematologica. 2008;93:1269–71. doi:10.3324/haematol.12654.
13. Schirrmeister H, Buck AK, Bergmann L, Reske SN, Bommer M. Positron emission tomography (PET) for staging of solitary plasmacytoma. Cancer Biother Radiopharm. 2003;18:841–5.
14. Sharma P, Khangembam BC, Suman KC, Singh H, Rastogi S, Khan SA, et al. Diagnostic accuracy of 18 F-FDG PET/CT for detecting recurrence in patients with primary skeletal Ewing sarcoma. Eur J Nucl Med Mol Imaging. 2013;40:1036–43. doi:10.1007/s00259-013-2388-9.
15. von Mehren M, Randall RL, Benjamin RS, Boles S, Bui MM, Casper ES, et al. Soft tissue sarcoma, version 2.2014. J Natl Compr Canc Netw. 2014;12:473–83.
16. Yamamoto H, Sugimoto S, Miyoshi K, Yamamoto H, Soh J, Yamane M, et al. The role of 18F-fluorodeoxyglucose (FDG)-positron emission tomography/computed tomography (PET/CT) in liposarcoma of the chest wall. Kyobu Geka. 2014;67:4–8.

17 Skin Cancers

17.1 Case 1: Basal Cell Carcinoma

History A 84-year-old female status postsurgical excision of a lesion from skin of nose proven to be basal cell carcinoma underwent ^{18}F-FDG PET/CT scan.

Findings

Interpretation This finding is compatible with local recurrence of the disease.

Teaching Point Although there are limited data, ^{18}F-FDG PET/CT imaging might be able to image and identify basal cell carcinoma in the head and neck region. The histologic subtype of the basal cell carcinoma appears to affect the ability of detection with FDG PET, with the nodular histologic subtype being more FDG avid.

T. Özülker, F. Özülker, *Atlas of PET-CT Imaging in Oncology: A Case-Based Guide to Image Interpretation*,
DOI 10.1007/978-3-319-18994-9_17

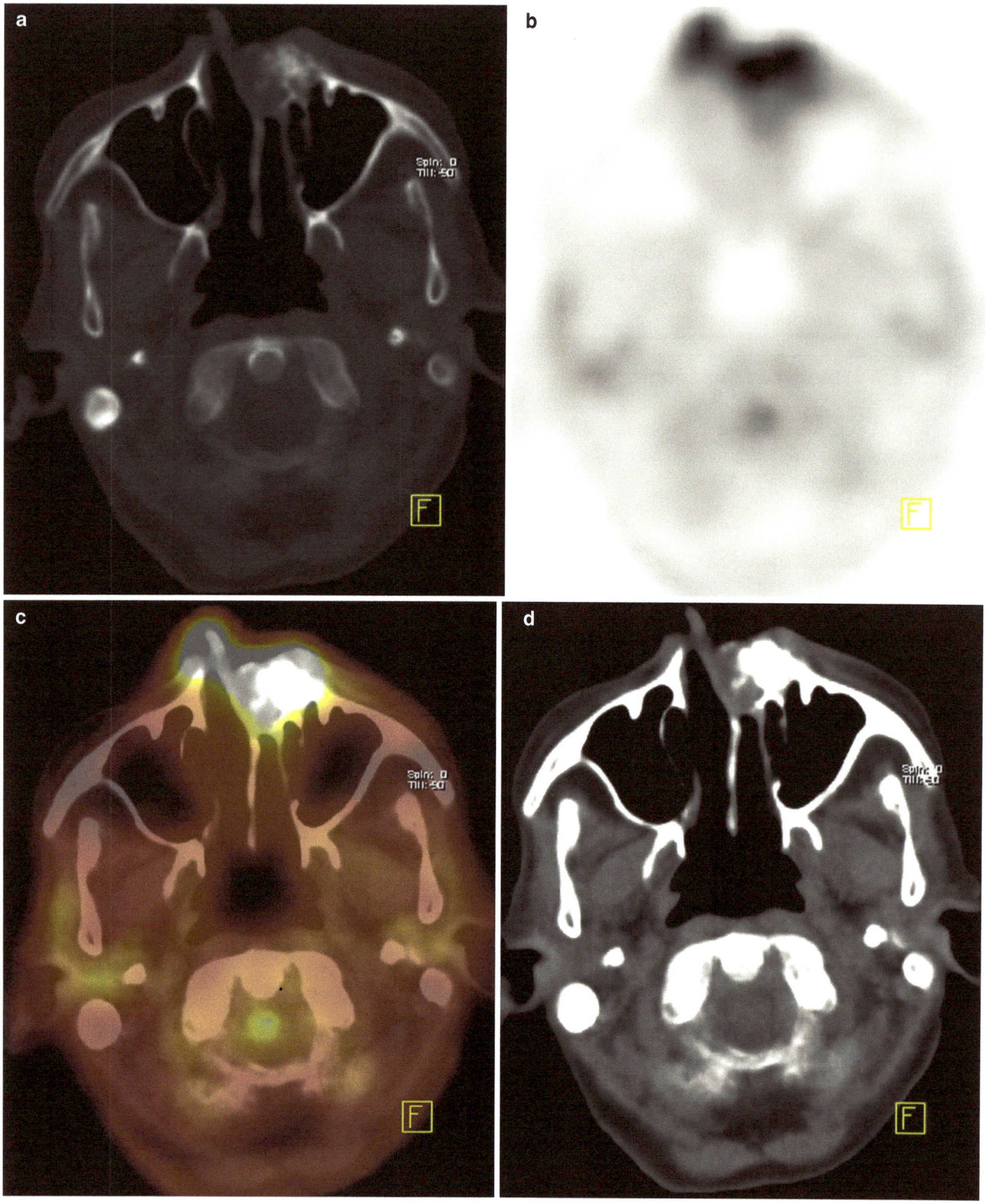

Fig. 17.1 Axial slices of CT, PET, and fusion (**a–d**) show significantly increased FDG uptake at left side of dorsum of nose (SUVmax 5.9)

17.2 Case 2: Squamous Cell Carcinoma of Skin

History A 77-year-old female who had been diagnosed to have squamous cell carcinoma of nasal skin following surgical excision, underwent ^{18}F-FDG PET/CT.

Findings

Interpretation Hypermetabolic lesion at left side of nose is compatible with local recurrence of the disease. Hypermetabolic lymph nodes are suspicious for lymphoproliferative malignant disease.

Result Biopsy from mediastinal lymph nodes revealed granulomatous disease.

Teaching Point ^{18}F-FDG PET CT might be a sensitive tool in detecting local recurrence in cutaneous squamous cell carcinoma but lack of specificity may cause false positive results in detection of lymph node metastases.

- Granulamatous diseases should always be kept in mind when multiple hypermetabolic lymph nodes are seen.

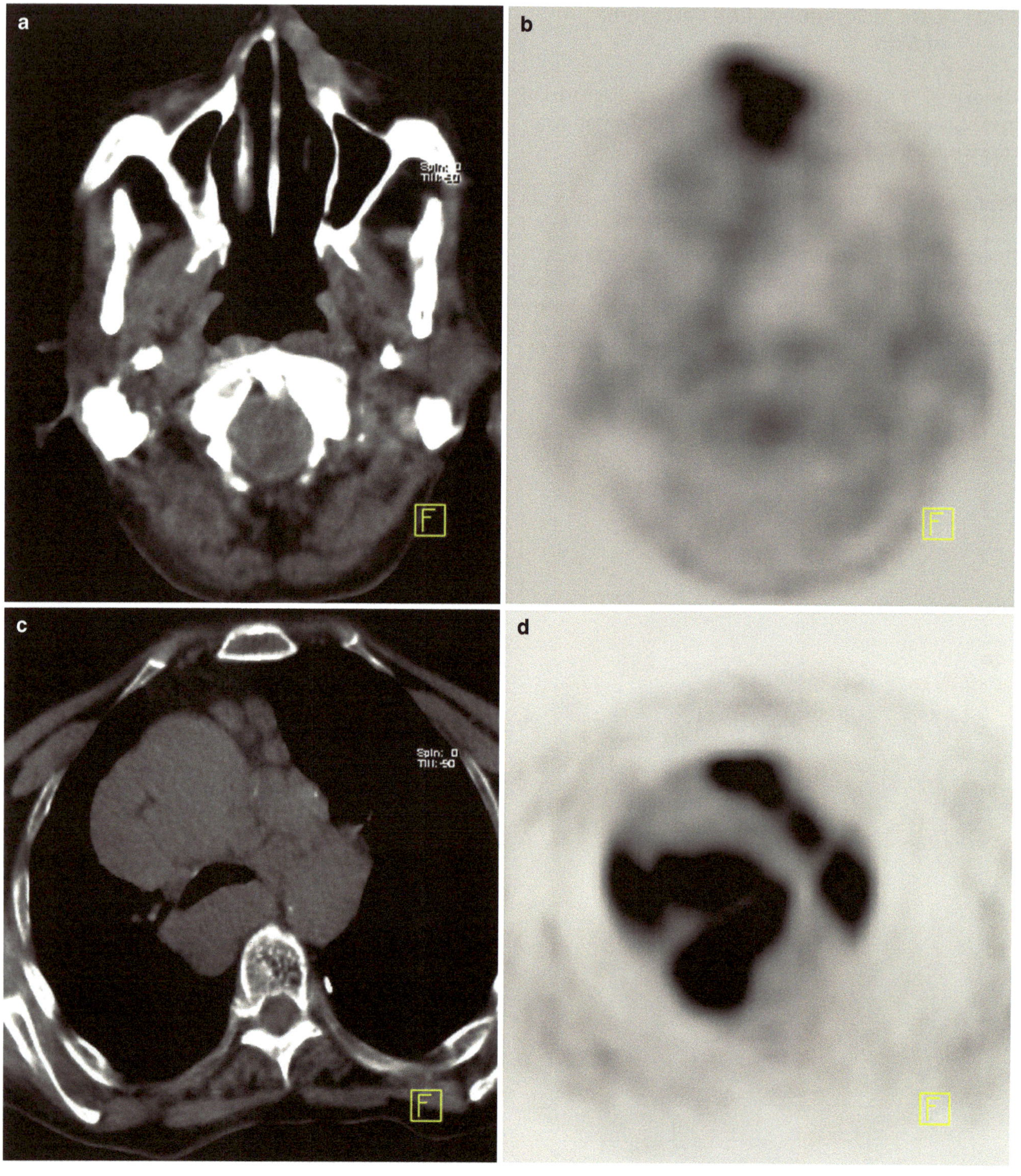

Fig. 17.2 Axial slices of CT and PET images of cranium (**a**, **b**) and thorax (**c**, **d**) show intensely increased FDG uptake at left side of dorsum of nose (SUVmax 8.7), multiple intensely hypermetabolic lymph nodes at mediastinum (SUVmax 16)

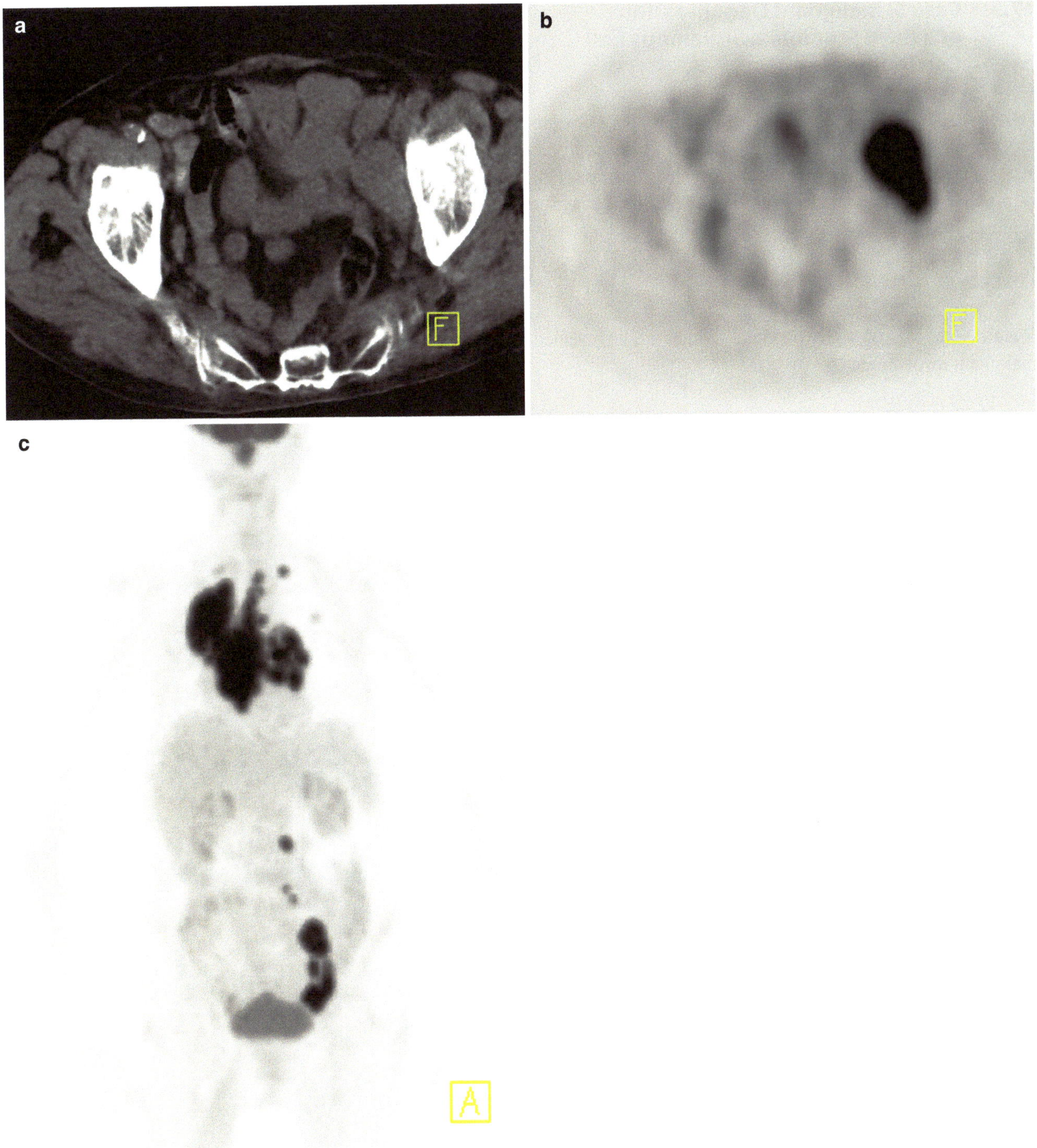

Fig. 17.3 Axial slices of CT and PET (**a**, **b**) and MIP (**c**) images show intensely hypermetabolic lymph nodes at left obturator area (*arrow*) and mediastinal and intraabdominal lymph node stations (SUVmax 16)

17.3 Case 3: Malignant Degeneration of a Burn Scar into a Squamous Cell Carcinoma

History A 36-year-old male had an electrical burn at right foot approximately 1 year ago. Biopsy from the exophytic lesion developed at chronic burn scar revealed squamous cell carcinoma. The patient underwent ^{18}F-FDG PET/CT scan for staging.

Findings

Result Excision of right popliteal lymph node revealed malignant involvement.

Interpretation Findings are consistent with malignant degeneration at burn scar and metastasis to popliteal lymph node.

Teaching Point Malignancy arising in a chronic burn scar, which is named as Marjolin's ulcer, develops in approximately 2 % of burn scars. ^{18}F-FDG PET/CT is useful in differentiating Marjolin ulcer from benign inflammatory conditions of chronic nonhealing ulcer in burn scars. It is also useful in the evaluation of the depth of invasion in Marjolin ulcer cases and detection of lymphatic invasion.

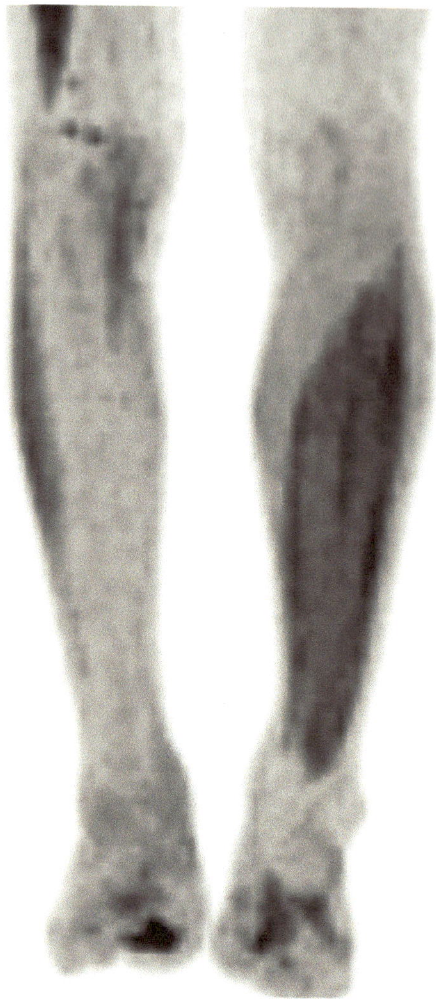

Fig. 17.4 MIP image show diffuse FDG uptake (SUVmax 11.8) at anteromedial aspect of left cruris. There is also focal increased FDG uptake at right foot

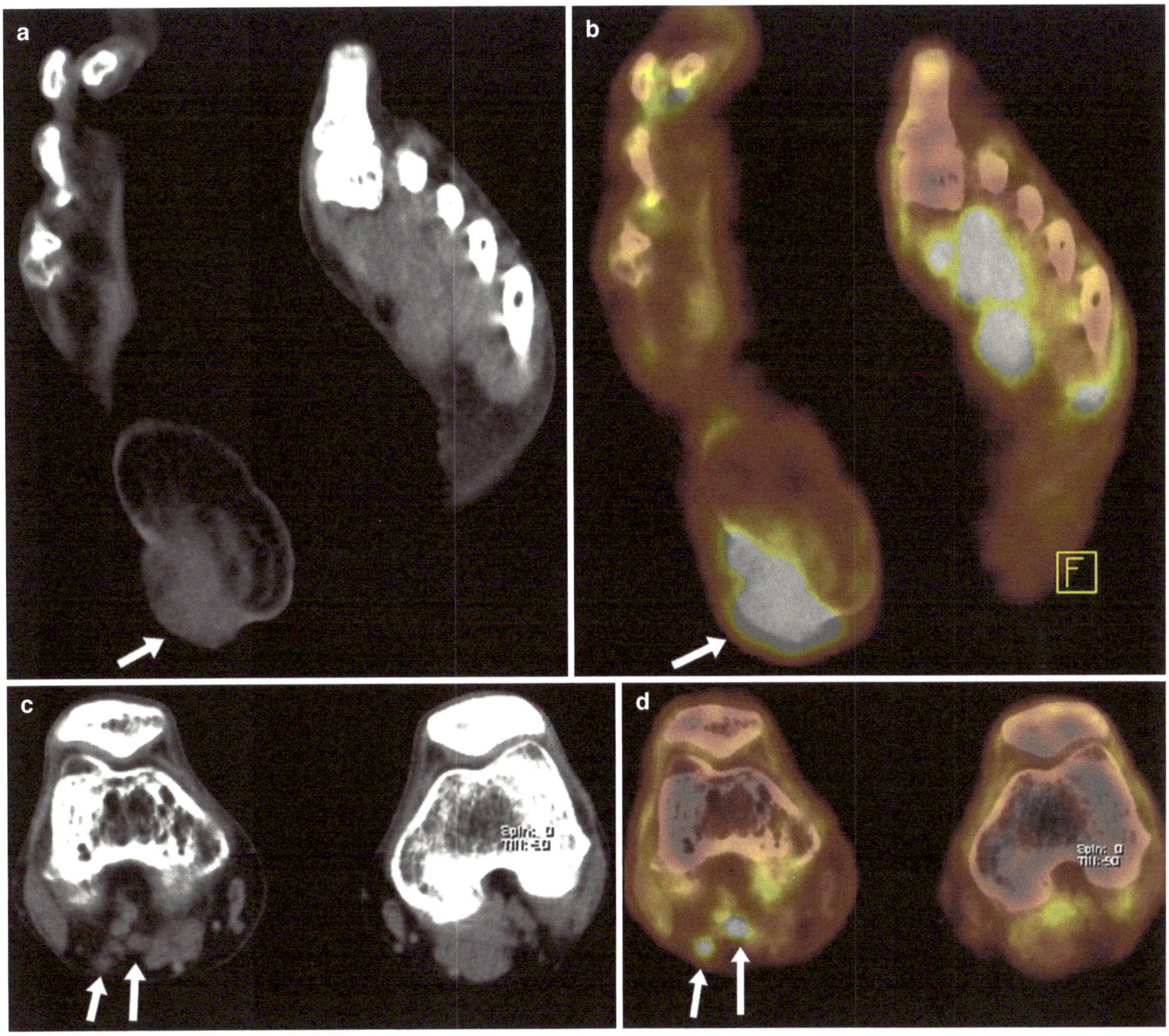

Fig. 17.5 Axial slices of CT and fusion images show intense FDG uptake at subcutaneous soft tissue lesion at right heel (**a**–**b**) and hypermetabolic right popliteal lymph node (**c**–**d**) (*arrows*)

17.4 Case 4: Restaging of Malignant Melanoma

History A 50-year-old female had the diagnosis of malignant melanoma after excision of a lesion from left arm 7 months ago. Left axillary dissection was also performed to the patient which revealed two metastatic lymph nodes. The patient received radiotherapy and interferon therapy 4 months ago and a ^{18}F-FDG PET CT is performed for restaging.

Findings

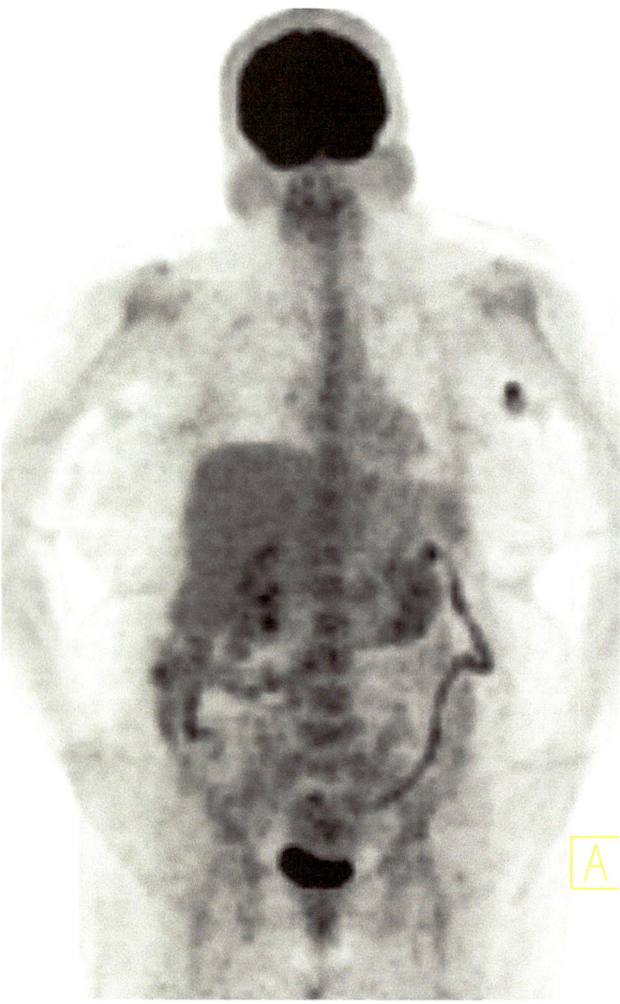

Fig. 17.6 MIP image shows hypermetabolic focus at left axillary region

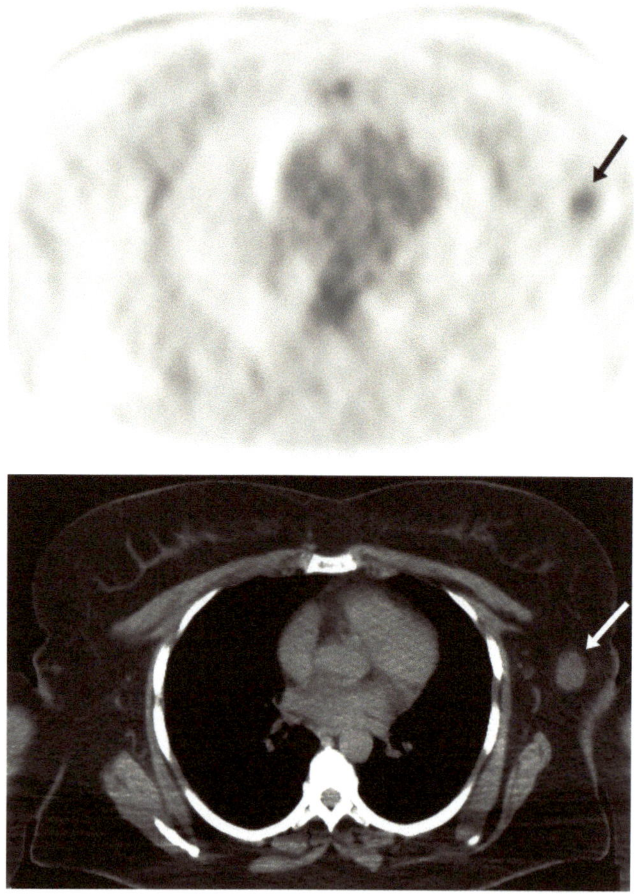

Fig. 17.7 Axial slices of PET and CT show moderately increased FDG uptake at left axillary fossa corresponding to an enlarged lymph node (*arrow*)

Interpretation This finding is compatible with recurrence of the disease with lymphatic invasion.

Teaching Point PET is useful in stage III disease with regional lymph node metastasis, has limited role in Stage I and II disease with low prevalence of lymph node metastasis. PET is a standard modality in evaluation of recurrent disease.

17.5 Case 5: Malignant Melanoma

History A 31-year-old male patient with a history of cutaneous malignant melanoma surgically removed from the skin of the left supraclavicular area 15 days ago underwent ^{18}F-FDG PET/CT study with the purpose of staging.

Findings

Interpretation These findings are compatible with metastatic disease at right atrium and gall bladder.

Result The patient underwent cholecystectomy and resection of the lesion at right atrium and histology turned out to be metastases of malignant melanoma in the right atrium and gallbladder.

Teaching Point The gallbladder is a rare site of metastasis for malignant melanoma (4–20 %) and primary malignant melanoma of gallbladder is also rare. Cardiac metastases are also rarely identified antemortem, despite the fact that malignant melanoma has a great propensity (38–50 %) for cardiac involvement, as indicated by autopsy findings.

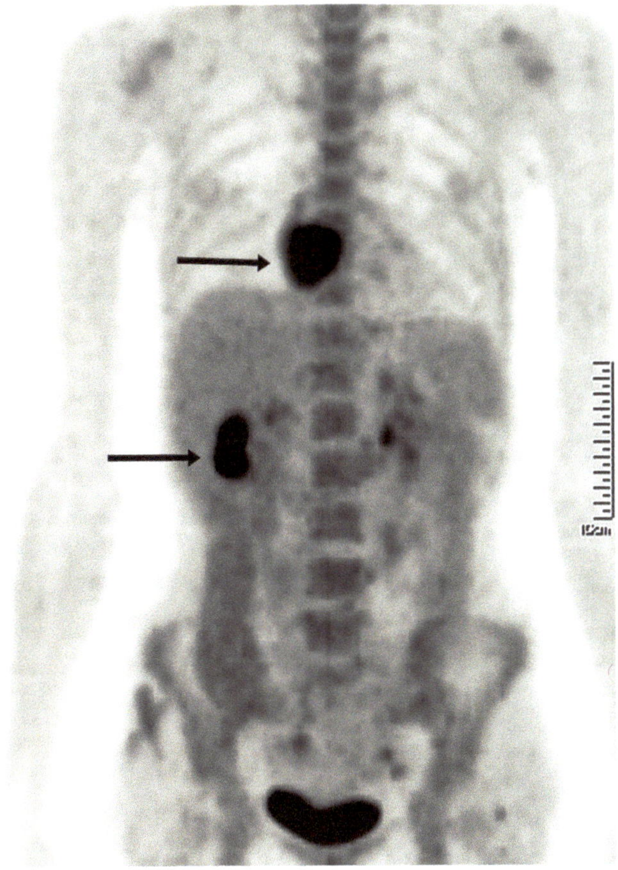

Fig. 17.8 MIP image shows mass lesions with increased FDG uptake in the right atrium (*arrow*), gallbladder (*arrow*), right adrenal gland, and subcutaneous tissue in the left side of the abdomen

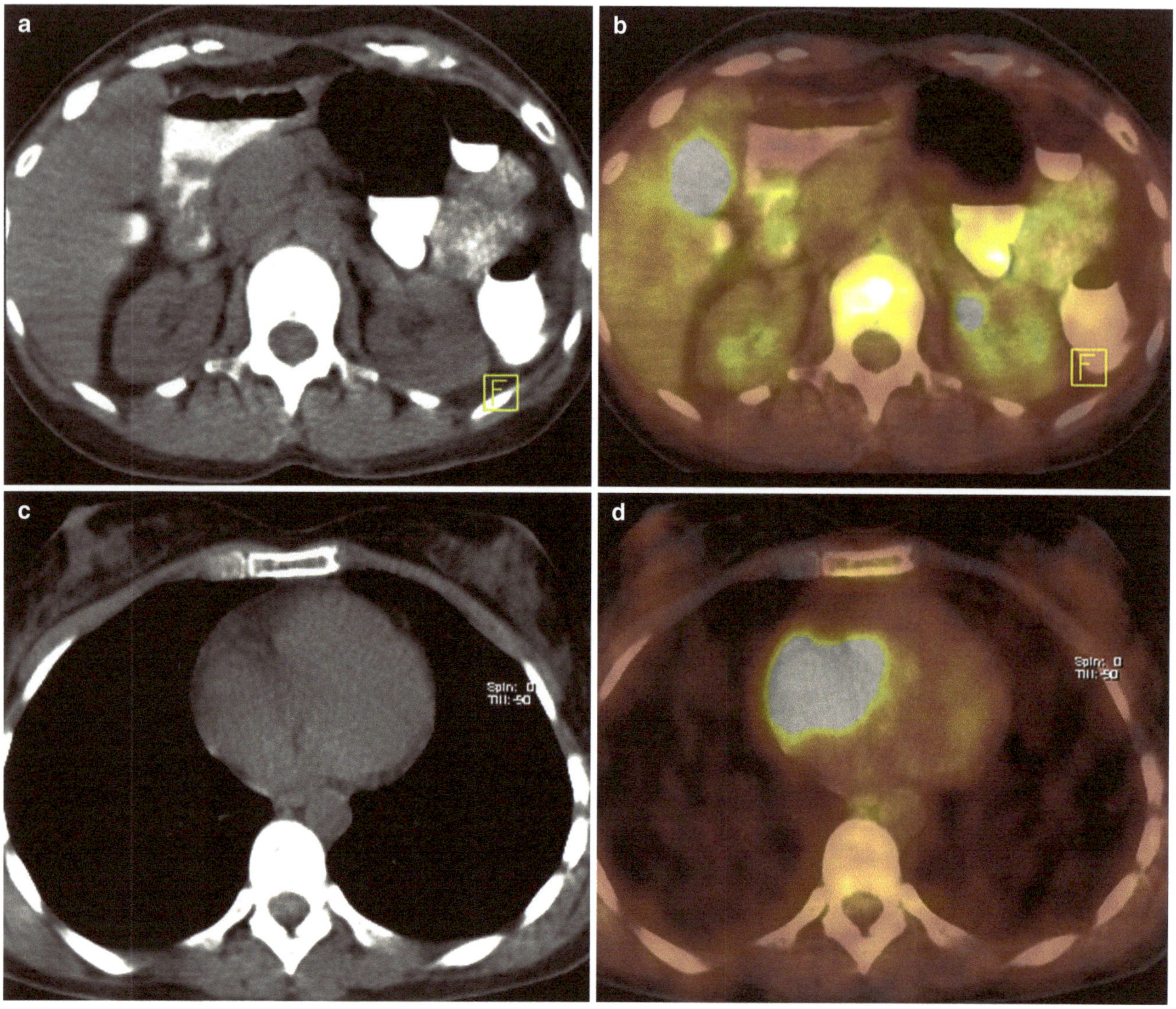

Fig. 17.9 Axial CT and fusion images show intense FDG uptake (SUVmax: 12.5) in the gallbladder in circular fashion (**a**, **b**) and intense pathological FDG uptake (SUVmax: 9.8) in the right atrium corresponding to a solid lesion (**c**, **d**)

Bibliography

1. Fosko SW, Hu W, Cook TF, Lowe VJ. Positron emission tomography for basal cell carcinoma of the head and neck. Arch Dermatol. 2003;139:1141–6.
2. Friedman KP, Wahl RL. Clinical use of positron emission tomography in the management of cutaneous melanoma. Semin Nucl Med. 2004;34:242–53.
3. Ko Y, Han YM, Hwang HS, Kang IW, Hwang DH, Lee ES, et al. Role of 18F-FDG PET/CT in the diagnosis of clinically suspected Marjolin ulcer. AJR Am J Roentgenol. 2012;199:1375–9. doi:10.2214/AJR.11.8398.
4. Kumar R, Alavi A. Clinical applications of fluorodeoxyglucose–positron emission tomography in the management of malignant melanoma. Curr Opin Oncol. 2005;17:154–9.
5. Ozülker T, Ozülker F, Cicin I, Ozpaçac T. A case of malignant melanoma with cardiac and gallbladder metastases detected by FDG PET-CT. Clin Nucl Med. 2009;34:948–9. doi:10.1097/RLU.0b013e3181bed02c.

18 Miscellaneous

18.1 Case 1: Carcinoma of Unknown Primary

History A 54-year-old female underwent tru-cut biopsy from mass lesions detected on USG at liver and histopathology revealed metastasis of adenocarcinoma. A ^{18}F-FDG PET/CT scan was performed to evaluate the extent of the disease and determine the primary site of malignancy.

Findings

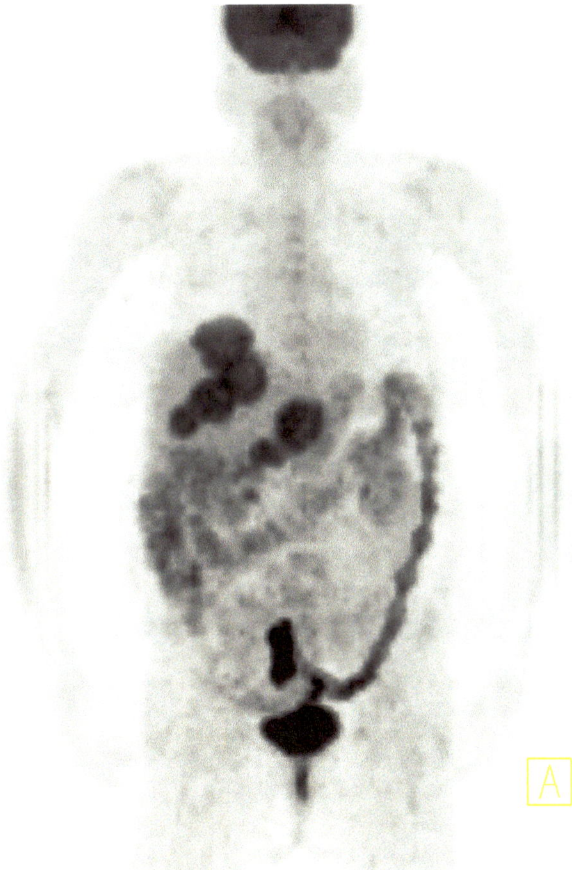

Fig. 18.1 MIP image shows intensely hypermetabolic mass lesions at both lobes of liver and a hypermetabolic lesion at sigmoid colon

Interpretation Hypermetabolic lesions at liver representing metastases from primary malignant lesion at sigmoid colon.

Teaching Point Adenocarcinoma is the most commonly encountered histology among patients with CUP. Most patients have a small primary tumor that can metastasize, and the metastases grow while the primary tumor usually remains small.

T. Özülker, F. Özülker, *Atlas of PET-CT Imaging in Oncology: A Case-Based Guide to Image Interpretation*,
DOI 10.1007/978-3-319-18994-9_18

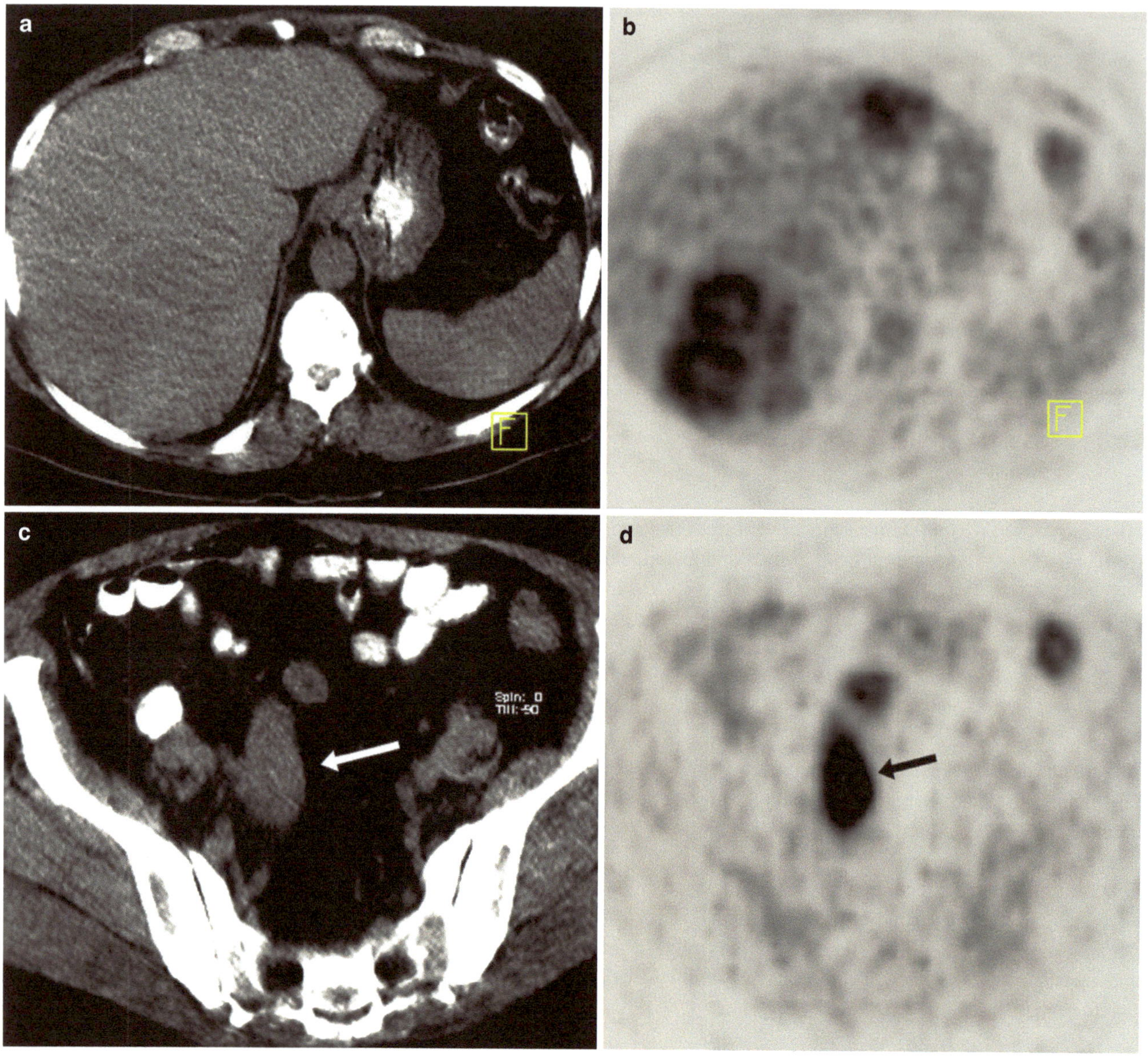

Fig. 18.2 Axial CT and PET images show multiple hypermetabolic mass lesions at both lobes of liver (**a**, **b**) and increased FDG uptake corresponding to the mass lesion at sigmoid colon (*arrow*) (**c**, **d**)

18.2 Case 2: Incidentally Found Prostate Adenocarcinoma

History A 71-year-old male who was being followed up with the diagnosis of lung cancer underwent ^{18}F-FDG PET/CT for restaging.

Findings

Interpretation Hypermetabolic lesions at right lung are compatible with primary lung cancer and there is also a metastatically involved right supraclavicular lymph node. Focal hypermetabolic lesion at prostate gland is suspicious for malignancy.

Result Biopsy from the lesion at prostate gland revealed adenocarcinoma.

Teaching Point Although prostate adenocarcinomas show generally no or mild FDG uptake, poorly differentiated cancers or those with a rapid cell turnover may exhibit increased FDG uptake and show FDG-avid areas within the prostate. Since the benign lesions can also show FDG uptake, it is not always easy to decide whether a hypermetabolic lesion at prostate gland is benign or not.

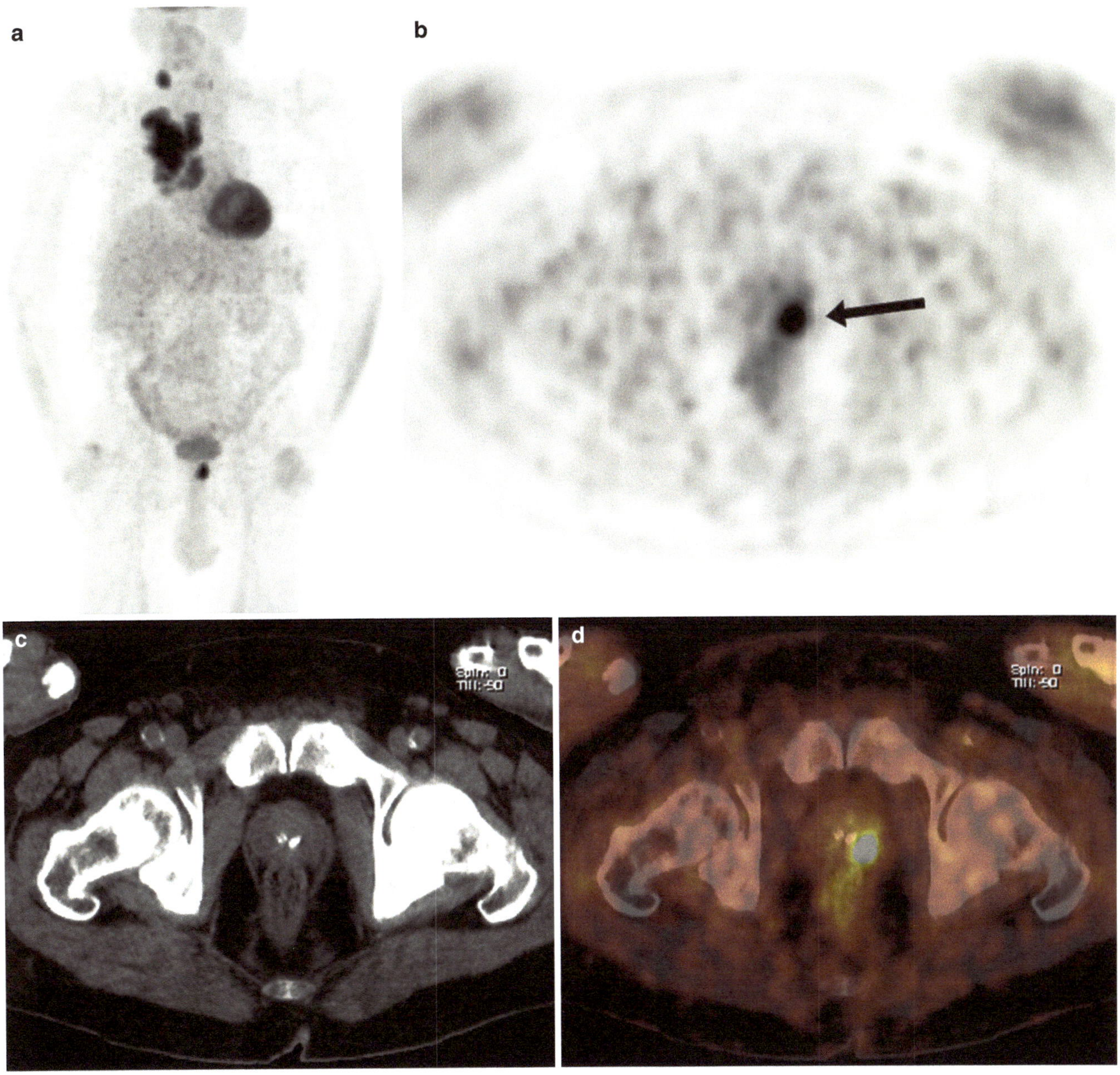

Fig. 18.3 MIP image shows intensely increased FDG uptake at right lung and a right supraclavicular lymph node (**a**). On axial PET, CT, and fusion images (**b**, **d**) there is incidentally found significantly hypermetabolic focus at prostate gland (*arrow*)

18.3 Case 3: Incidentally Found Sertoli Leydig Cell Tumor

History A 29-year-old female patient who was being followed up with the diagnosis of differentiated papillary thyroid carcinoma was referred to us for evaluation with ^{18}F-FDG PET/ CT.

Findings

Interpretation This is an unexpected finding and it is unlikely to be metastasis of thyroid carcinoma.

Result The patient underwent laparoscopic left pelvic mass resection, and the histopathology of the lesion revealed Sertoli–Leydig cell tumor. Together with a history of primary amenorrhea and MRI findings of absent uterus, short and blind end vagina, a diagnosis of androgen insensitivity syndrome (AIS) was made.

Teaching Point ^{18}F-FDG PET/CT can be used for the metabolic characterization of intraabdominal masses as well as staging of neoplasms in patients with AIS.

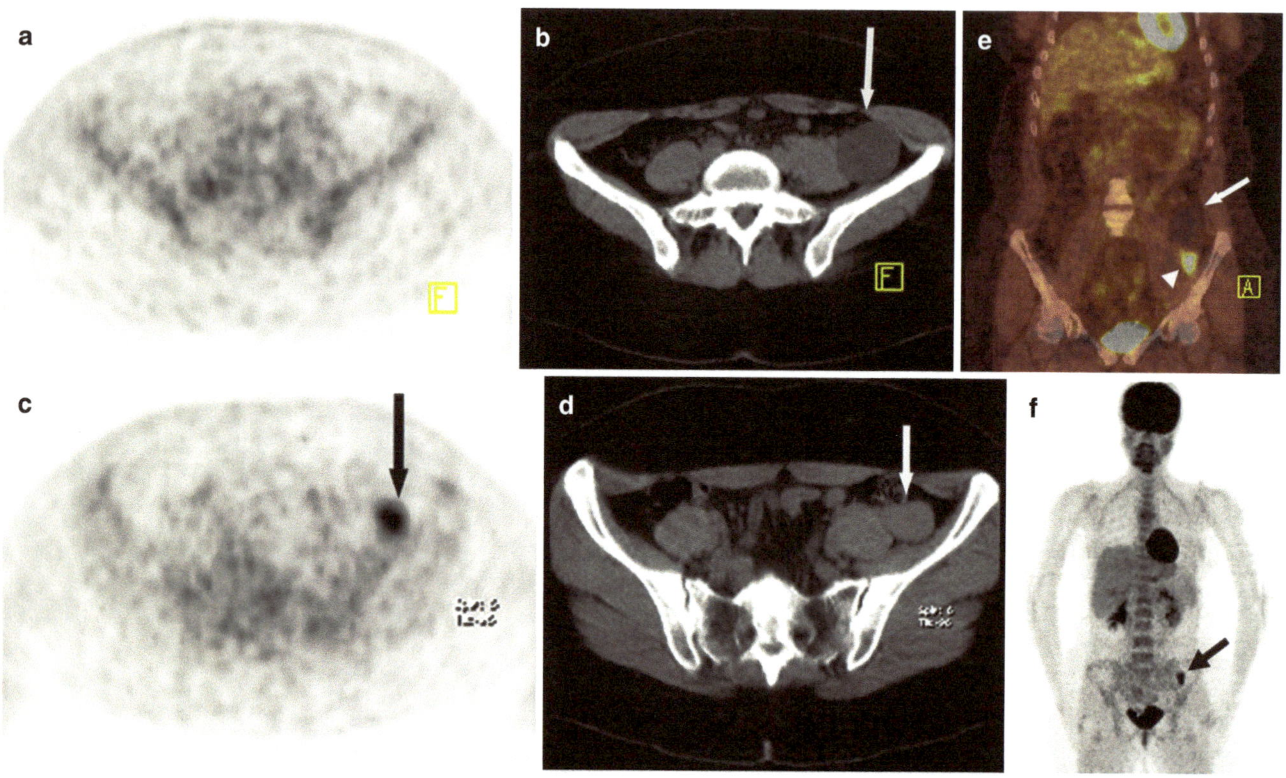

Fig. 18.4 Axial slices of PET and CT images showing a hypodense cystic lesion without FDG uptake (*arrow*) (**a**, **b**), an FDG avid solid lesion caudal to the cystic lesion (*arrows*) (**c**, **d**), coronal PET CT fusion image showing cystic lesion without FDG uptake (*arrow*) and solid lesion with moderate uptake located inferior to the cystic one (*arrowhead*) (**e**), MIP image showing pathologically increased FDG uptake at the left lower quadrant of the abdomen (*arrow*) (**f**)

18.4 Case 4: Paraneoplastic Syndrome Related to Small Cell Lung Carcinoma

History A 47-year-old male presented with neurological manifestations compatible with subacute sensory neuropathy. Since the patient also had paraneoplastic antibody anti-Hu, the case was found to be suspicious for paraneoplastic syndrome (PNS) and ^{18}F-FDG PET/CT scan was performed to explore the primary malignancy.

Findings

Interpretation Lung lesions are strongly suspicious for primary pulmonary malignancy. There are two foci of metastatic brain lesions.

Result Biopsy from mediastinal lymph nodes revealed small cell lung carcinoma (SCLC). The case is consistent with PNS related to SCLC.

Teaching Point FDG PET/CT is a highly sensitive (83–100 %) and specific imaging technique in the evaluation of PNS and it can be implemented at the initial evaluation or after failure of conventional imaging modalities.

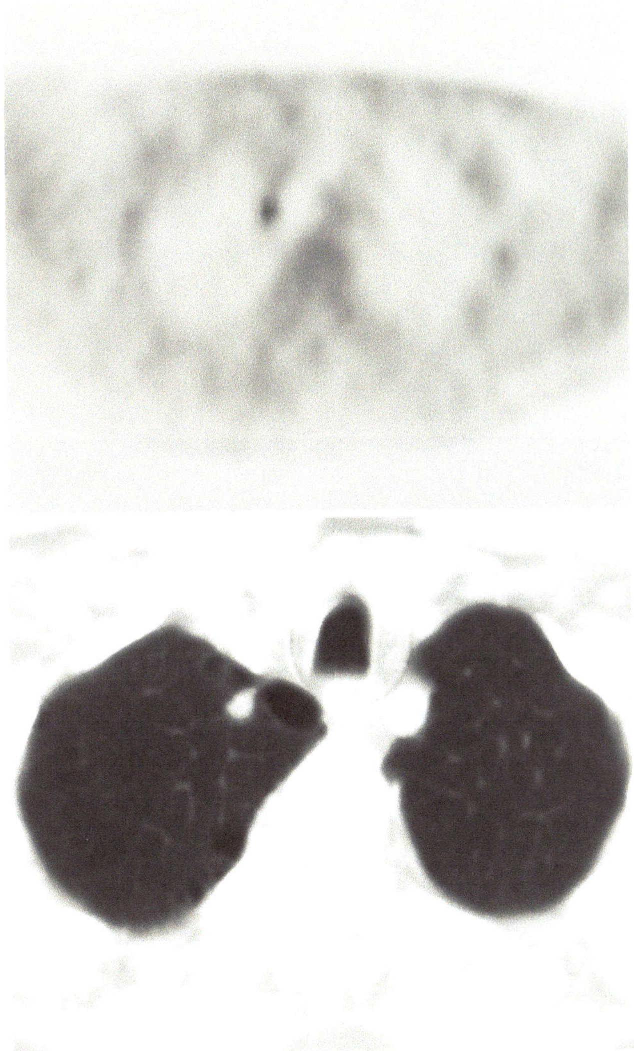

Fig. 18.5 Axial PET and CT images show slightly hypermetabolic lung nodule at apex of right lung

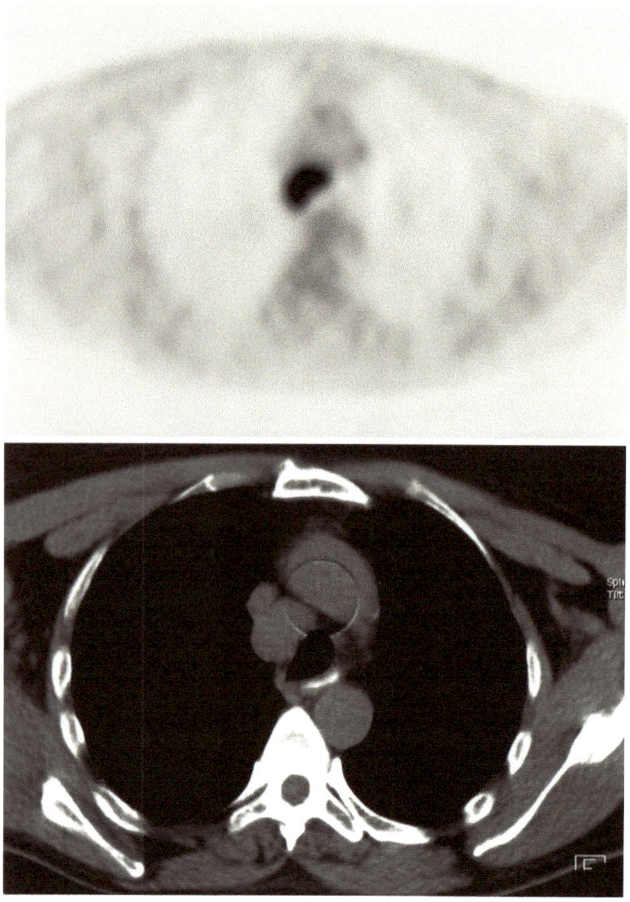

Fig. 18.6 Intensely hypermetabolic soft tissue lesion at right paratracheal region

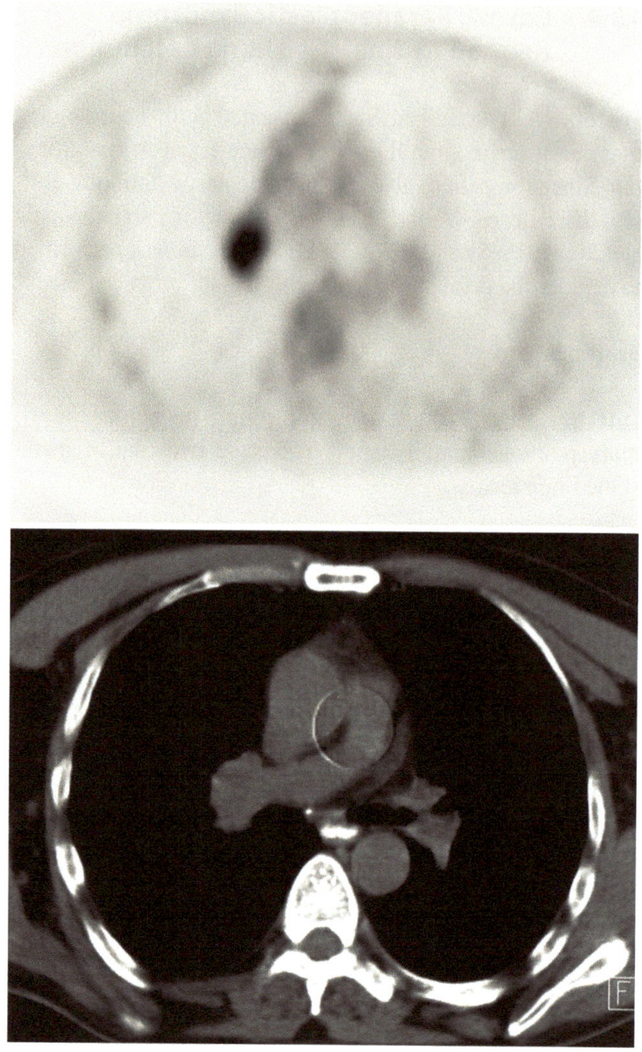

Fig. 18.7 Focal increased FDG uptake at right hilar region

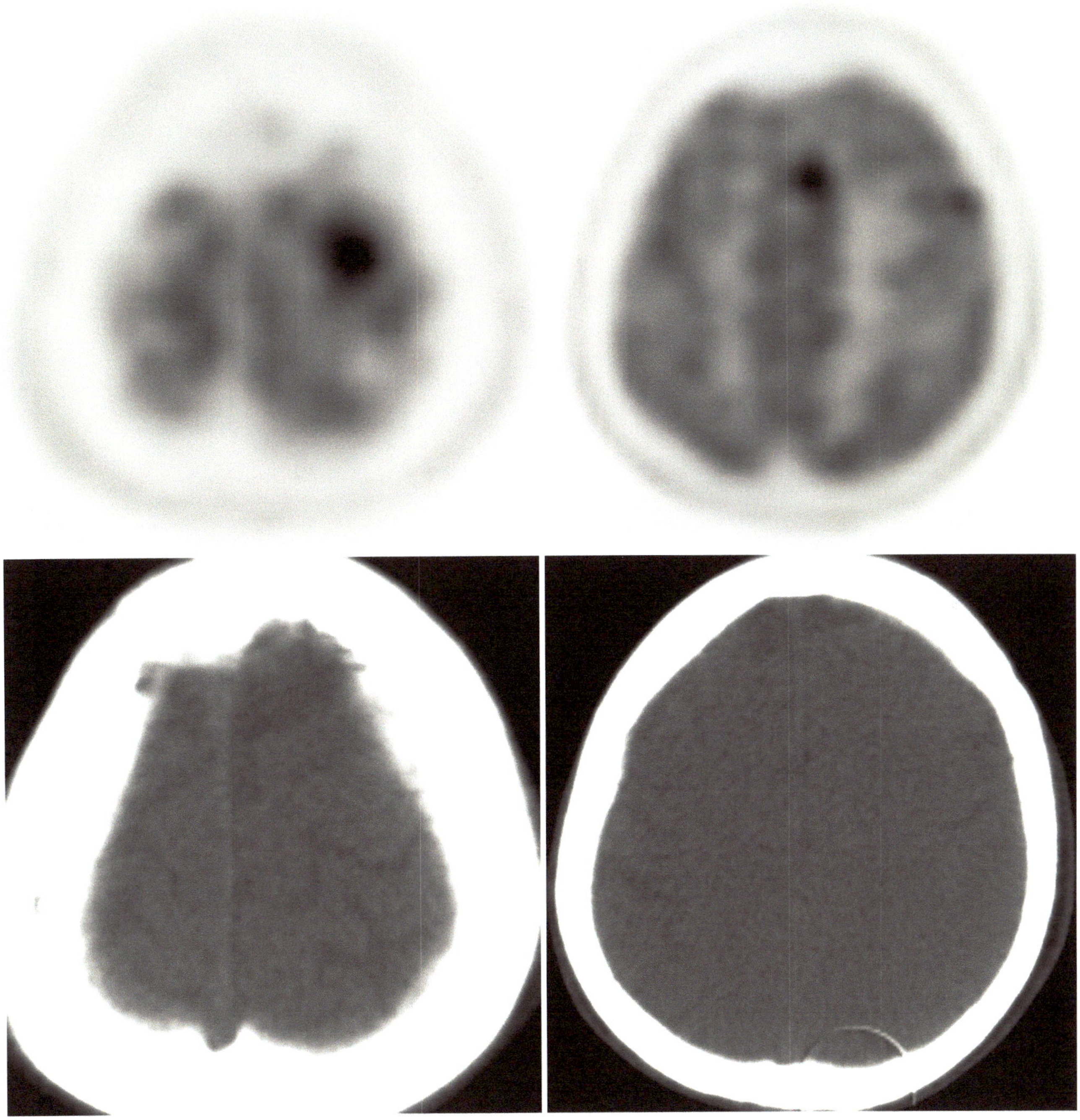

Fig. 18.8 Axial PET and CT images of brain show two hypermetabolic foci at frontal lobe of brain

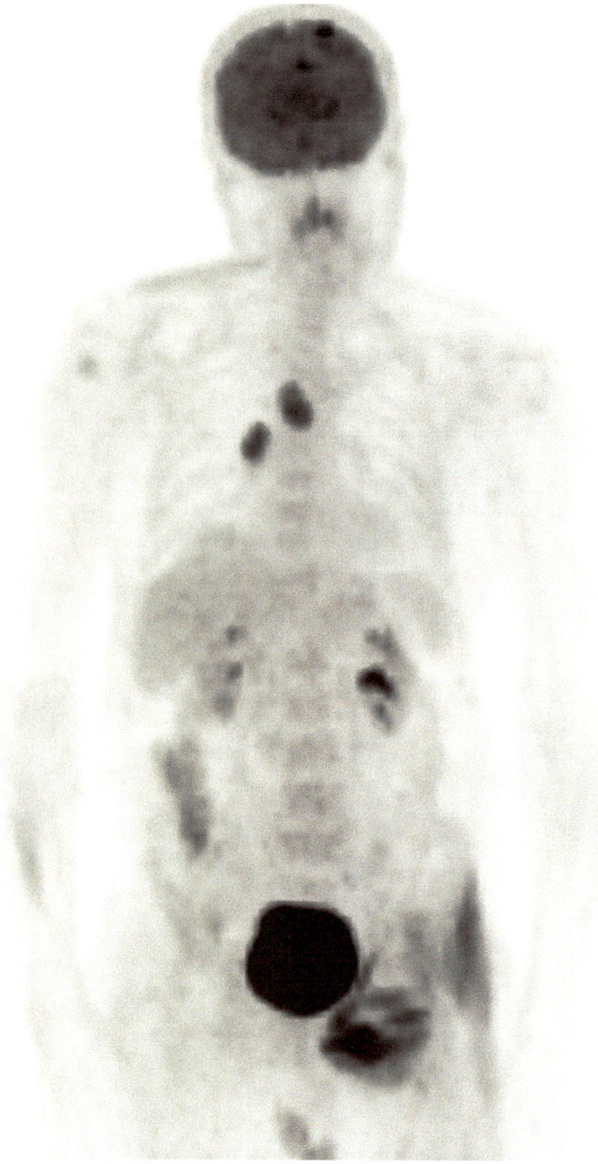

Fig. 18.9 MIP image

Bibliography

1. Greco FA. Cancer of unknown primary site: evolving understanding and management of patients. Clin Adv Hematol Oncol. 2012; 10:518–24.
2. Ozülker T, Ozpaçaci T, Ozülker F, Ozekici U, Bilgiç R, Mert M. Incidental detection of Sertoli-Leydig cell tumor by FDG PET/CT imaging in a patient with androgen insensitivity syndrome. Ann Nucl Med. 2010;24:35–9. doi:10.1007/s12149-009-0321-x.
3. Vaidyanathan S, Pennington C, Ng CY, Poon FW, Han S. 18F-FDG PET-CT in the evaluation of paraneoplastic syndromes: experience at a regional oncology centre. Nucl Med Commun. 2012;33: 872–80. doi:10.1097/MNM.0b013e3283550237.
4. Wong WL, Moule RN, Nunan T. Incidental fleurodeoxyglucose uptake in the prostate. Br J Radiol. 2010;83:902–3. doi:10.1259/bjr/28173921.
5. Younes-Mhenni S, Janier MF, Cinotti L, Antoine JC, Tronc F, Cottin V, et al. FDG-PET improves tumour detection in patients with paraneoplastic neurological syndromes. Brain. 2004;127:2331–8.

Index

T. Özülker, F. Özülker, *Atlas of PET-CT Imaging in Oncology: A Case-Based Guide to Image Interpretation*,
DOI 10.1007/978-3-319-18994-9

T

FSC
www.fsc.org
MIX
Papier | Fördert gute Waldnutzung
FSC® C083411

Kolibri 360 GmbH
Ferdinand-Jühlke-Straße 7
99095 Erfurt, Deutschland
produktsicherheit@kolibri360.de